Behavioural Sciences for Nurses:
Towards Project 2000

Behavioural Sciences for Nurses: Towards Project 2000

Evryl E. Fisher

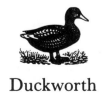

Duckworth

First published in UK in 1990 by
Gerald Duckworth & Co. Ltd.
The Old Piano Factory
43 Gloucester Crescent, London NW1 7DY

ISBN 0 7156 2336 2

British Library Cataloguing in Publication Data

Fisher, Evryl E.
  Behavioural sciences for nurses: towards project 2000
  1. Behavioural sciences
  I. Title
  300

ISBN 0–7156–2336–2

ACKNOWLEDGEMENTS FOR ILLUSTRATIONS

Page 40: H. F. Harlow, University of Wisconsin Primate Laboratory.
Page 105: Laddie Lucas, 38 Onslow Square, London.
Page 125 and 128: Hilgard, E. R., Atkinson, R. L. and Atkinson, R. C.
            Introduction to Psychology, 7th Ed. Harcourt Brace and
            Jovanovich.
Page 304: *Congress Report cover*, 1981. Edgar Wood Centre,
Manchester.
Opposite page 728: Photograph by Lord Snowdon—Camera Press,
Ltd. London.
Page 760: William Vandivert.
Page 179: 'Bringing Up Father'. King Features Syndicate.

Academic monitor: Colin Tredoux MA

Printed and bound in Great Britain by
Redwood Press Limited, Melksham, Wiltshire

To the thousands of lovable, white-uniformed women and men
who, in patience and tolerance, have
sat through my lectures; who have
stimulated, encouraged and taught
me so much,
And to my surgeon
whose skill and compassion
have enabled me to complete this work,
I dedicate this Book.

*In grateful acknowledgement of
the tolerance, kindness and erudition
of Richard Mein Ph.D., District Clinical
Psychologist, North West Hertforshire,
without whom this book would not have been possible;
and my colleagues at Leavesden,
Harperbury and Cell Barnes Hospitals
for their affection, support and
generous guidance.*

FOREWORD

by Phyllis Henderson

*Master of Nursing Science, Montreal University;
Lecturer in Behavioural Sciences, Nightingale School
of Nursing, St. Thomas' Hospital, London.*

The keynote to Project 2000

— is total care

based on sound knowledge of

BIOPHYSIOLOGY	PSYCHOLOGY	SOCIOLOGY	ECOLOGY
(the body)	(the mind)	(relationships with other people)	(relationship with the planet)

This book has been written for the Nurse 2000 who will require advanced skills in all these areas if she is to cope with her turbulent, changing world. Educational strategies are now being directed towards assisting nurses to be more analytic, flexible and better problem solvers.

Nursing no longer involves just the physical care of the sick and infirm. Today's nurse-practitioner, and even more so the nurse of the future, must have the skills to assess the total patient-client, his psychological and social behaviour, and how he interacts with the environment.

A major feature of this book is that it is specifically written for nurses entering into the new nursing programme. However, the author's special gift for explaining relatively complicated academic issues and technical information in simple, palatable, graphic, and often even humorous language, means that, without detracting from its scientific value, this book forms a most useful bridge between present qualifications for State Registration and the more formal, tertiary requirements laid down for Project 2000. While the spirit of Project 2000 encourages nursing students to select reading material from general academic sources, the Royal College of Nurses' programme does prescribe that books on nursing and behavioural sciences should, by virtue of the unique needs of the profession, be 'underpinned' to those needs. This is just such a book.

Formal sections on schools of psychology, learning, organic determinants of behaviour, behaviour-modification, scientific method and statistics; perception, memory and forgetting, are founded on sound scientific principles and are explained in clear, and even enjoyable terminology.

Selecting but a few salient topics, the section on the New Family introduces the student to sociological concepts such as monogamy and polygamy; the nuclear and consanguineous family; family structure — functions, pathology and rehabilitation. The New Family also highlights the important role of the midwife, specifically in relation to issues such as active labour, bonding, bereavement, contraception, the unmarried mother, and adoption — all within the nursing process. The scientific model of the nursing process prevails here, and in the rest of the book.

The nurse-practitioner in the community needs, in her training, to develop theoretical insight into sociological concepts such as norms, roles, folkways, social institutions, and role analysis. This need is ably provided for in this textbook.

Similarly, longitudinal community involvement requires insight into the life-long effects of Erikson's Maturation theory and Hirschowitz's crisis stages, which are discussed in Chapters 11 and 24.

Chapter 16 dealing with Sexually Transmitted Diseases extends from the physical and mental suffering of the 'old' diseases to the special problems encountered by patient, partner, family and those nursing AIDS victims.

The chapter 'Leadership — group morale and the role of the nurse-administrator' is deeply steeped in the nursing culture, and presents timely sections on conflict, prejudice and their resolution.

Of special significance is the graphic and vivid manner in which the author links scientific fact with everyday nursing situations — their problems, humour, achievements, sadnesses.

For the young nurse, who walks with patient-client (turned friend) and his loved ones, through the valley of the shadow of death, and performs last offices, the path is frightening and depressing — often the best nursing candidates seek escape in 'flight', torn by illogical guilt and anxiety, often converted to psychosomatic symptoms. They require interpretation, catharsis and support from colleagues, especially the ward-based psychiatric nurse, whose role is described in Chapter 26.

Traditionally the nurse is an expert in physical healing procedures. An innovation of this book is the extension of her role to encompass psycho-sociological diagnostic and therapeutic techniques, such as the professional interview, assertion training, stress management, and counselling (with special sections on groups, role playing, music and movement therapies).

This book was written to provide the student with comprehensive information required for that total patient/client care which is the basis of Project 2000. It is hoped that apart from its academic and practical value, it will provide the student with interesting and enjoyable reading. . . that it will accompany her on that great adventure from the hand-maiden role of Nurse 1900 into the academically enlightened, technically skilled, compassionate and insightful role of the Nurse-Practitioner 2000.

THE BEHAVIOURAL SCIENCES

Through the years there has developed a range of sciences attempting to understand the roots and nature of man's personal, inner and social behaviour. Anthropology, political science, economics, sociology, ecology, psychology are all relevant.

Because: (i) man cannot exist in a vacuum,
           (ii) individual and social behaviour cannot be separated,
the terms 'behavioural' and 'social sciences' have become interchangeable and complementary.

   This book attempts to overcome artificial barriers between these approaches to the understanding and enrichment of man in his personal and communal life.

   Surely we need the contribution and integration of all human sciences, and indeed all spiritual endeavour, if man is to live healthily, happily and in peace . . . even to survive . . . on this beautiful, but oh so demanding, planet with which he has been entrusted.

Does it really matter
If a nurse be he or she?
Do we care any less
What a patient's gender be?
To use both is oh so clumsy!

So reader, be not offended
No sexism is intended.
Please accept he or she
To be of equal noble calling.

Dear patient, be not pronoun-reliant,
For behold, you have become a client!

CONTENTS
LEARNING SUMMARY GUIDE
Page

xi

Psychological Preparation for Surgery: avoiding negative identification—tactile communication—anaesthetic trauma—role of the theatre sister—surgeon-patient relationship and general consent—nursing actions detrimental to patient confidence—the nurse's role in encouraging catharsis in patients and colleagues—guilt feelings and death. Special implications of cardiac surgery—Post-operative emotional trauma: Intensive Care Unit: Emotional trauma. Sensory disturbances. Post-anaesthetic confusion Intensive care psychosis. Staff stress—Mutilation of the body image due to surgery—Handling depression, anxiety and anger. Amputation and mastectomy: Post-operative mourning—effects on family—alternatives—Specific impact of cancer realization—The Emotional Support Sister in general wards.

tent levels of communication in professional/patient relationships. Conflict of communication needs, ward rounds—Imperviousness—Discrepancies of punctuation resulting in inappropriate patient expectation—Self-fulfilling prophecy, inappropriate introjection—Communicating Identification. Shyness and anxiety as communication blocks. Private Patients. *Techniques facilitating communication*—Communicating Respect, transcultural. *The Professional Interview:* Opening. Body. Closure. Impediments—The Trans-Cultural Interview. The interpreter in the communication triangle.

The nurse-patient/client relationship—(i) activity—passivity—(ii) guidance—co-operation—(iii) mutual participation—*Clients arousing Negative Feelings* in caregivers: Clingers. Demanders. Help rejectors. The Self-destructive Denier—Harrison: Balancing Humanism and Science—Empathy and its impediments. Buber's I—Thou relationship as key to the Nursing Process—Factors precipitating *Non-Compliance and Compliance*—Self-analysis in the Nursing Role viz-à-vis needs of patients, colleagues and personal satisfaction—*Unique nature of the nurse-patient relationship*, its impediments and satisfactions—Fulfilling conflicting needs within patient and nurse—Stress in the Healing Professions: features—contributors and etiology—the 'wounded healer'—depression—Neurotic Coping Mechanisms—Suicide—Alcohol—Help, and handling—Who is at risk? The role of professional. Fulfilling nursing's unique satisfactions.

procedures and genital surgery, sexual needs in convalescence—Negative effects of general ward placement—Advantages of group identification in visiting. (Teenage pregnancy: see the New Family Chapter 18.)

Breakdown: Prevention, Divorce, Custody, Rehabilitation

patient with unjustified hope?—Terminal paralysis—Trans-cultural communication: Muslim custom—Tactile communication—The dying child, his parents and his siblings—The adolescent—When
death is imminent who copes and how?—Reactions to switching off supportive machinery and donor
consent—Guilt feelings of staff, their flight reactions—Death-bed support of patient and family—
Differing levels of onset of death—Tactile comfort—Presence of loved ones—avoiding isolation—
Helping the bereaved family: depression and 'grief work'—Death of a child, the ultimate loss. Support
groups in the U.K. Griefwork. Bereavement in old age, middle age, teenagers, children. Funerals—
Alleviating staff distress—Emotional involvement in laying out the dead.

CHAPTER 1

APPROACHES TO MODERN PSYCHOLOGY

'An introductory course in psychology should give you a better understanding of why people behave as they do, and should provide insight into your attitudes and reactions.'

—Hilgard, Atkinson, Atkinson. *Introduction to Psychology* 7 ed.

So wide is the scope of psychology that it reaches almost every human thought and action. Because psychology attempts to solve why people act as they do, the scientific methods to which it aspires are being applied to an ever-increasing spectrum of problems ranged as widely as impediments to the nurse–patient relationship, the increasing divorce rate, international aggression, the measurement of intelligence and aptitudes, the relationship of pop music and discos to acquired deafness . . .

DEFINITION of this young and wide-ranging discipline is constantly being revised and modified.

Hilgard et al define psychology as *'the science that studies behaviour and mental processes'.*

The special value of this definition lies in its recognition of the two basic concepts of:

(i) an objective study of overt, observable activities or behaviour, such as involuntary withdrawal from pain;
(ii) the importance of understanding underlying mental processes that cannot be directly observed, but must be inferred from behavioural and physiological data such as emotions, thoughts and dreams.

Neurobiological approach:'Psychology is the science concerned with the mutual interrelation of organism and environment through the transmission of energy (ie stimulation–response).'*

The brain consists of twelve billion nerve cells enabling an infinite possibility of interconnections and pathways. To our knowledge, this organ, minute in relation to the Universe, may constitute its most complex structure. Clearly this most intricate of computers and accurate of filing systems was designed for the exertion of lifelong, reliable and intimate relationships between brain activity, experience and behaviour.

Disciples of this approach relate *an individual's reactions to physiological events within his brain and nervous systems.* These latter in turn are dependent on their unalterable, innate hereditary design.

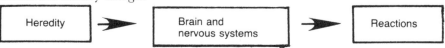

Heredity → Brain and nervous systems → Reactions

* Howard, Warren C. *Dictionary of Psychology.* Houghton Mifflin, Riverside Press

Neurological processes, they say, result in overt behaviour, eg

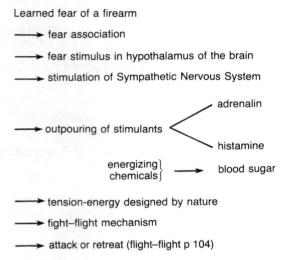

Learned fear of a firearm

⟶ fear association

⟶ fear stimulus in hypothalamus of the brain

⟶ stimulation of Sympathetic Nervous System

⟶ outpouring of stimulants ⟨ adrenalin / histamine

energizing⟩ chemicals⟨ ⟶ blood sugar

⟶ tension-energy designed by nature

⟶ fight–flight mechanism

⟶ attack or retreat (flight–flight p 104)

The intimacy of the relationship between brain activity, experience and behaviour has, in recent years, been highlighted by implantation of electrodes in varying cerebral areas, first in animals, and later in human beings. Electrical stimulation in the hypothalamus gives rise to overall fear and rage reactions; in the frontal lobe, to anxiety and vivid memories of the past—in other areas, to pleasure and pain. Surgical removal of these areas results in blunting of relevant reactions.

Electroconvulsive treatment relieves acute depression.

By means of surgically implanted electrodes, the brains of chimpanzees can be stimulated by remote radio control, the experimenter reversing dominant and submissive behaviour.

The electroencephalogram (EEG), picking up waves from the sleeping brain, has revealed that the individual shows 5 stages of sleep, each one producing characteristic brain-wave patterns.

From studying the subject's EEG pattern, the examiner is able to analyse sleep depth, dream stages, waking expectations, etc.

Evaluation

However, the complexity of the human organism defies accurate detailed analysis on the basis of neurological response alone.

Neurology alone cannot account for the values man places on his motivations.

Neurobiological investigation cannot answer

why a mother's love for her child is stronger than her own instinct for self-preservation?

why an adolescent is prepared to forgo food, sex, warmth, even life itself, for an ideal?

Clearly man does not live by bread (nor neurobiology) alone!

Other schools of psychology offer different approaches in investigating man's goals, loves, hates, fears, ideals and shortcomings.

Behavioural approach: 'Psychology is the systematic investigation of the behaviour of organisms.'*

The behavioural approach is based on observation of an individual's overt or external behaviour.

This school, founded by American psychologist John B Watson in the early 1900s, developed as a reaction against the concept of psychology as a form of inturned self-observation or 'introspection'.

Prior to Watson, psychologists hoped to reveal the mysteries of the *'psyche'* (Greek for mind) by minute analysis of their own reactions.

Basing his argument on great strides in the natural sciences, Watson maintained that psychology could not be considered a science until its data became *observable, measurable* and thus *objective.*

Self-observed perceptions and feelings are *subjective.* Watson based his school on the belief that *only study of what a person does, ie how he behaves,* can be sufficiently objective to constitute a science—hence his discipline is termed the Behavioural Approach.

During the first half of this century, Watson's Behaviourism played a dominant role in the development of psychological research.

His work was translated into concise and meaningful terminology by his Harvard disciple, B F Skinner. Skinner introduced:

1. The Stimulus → Response concept (S–R psychology)
2. A systematized classification of strength and frequency of reward and punishment. Rewards reinforce and thus maintain or strengthen man's responses: punishment modifies and changes behaviour patterns (see chapter 6), eg the idiom

    'The burnt child dreads the fire'

    may be translated thus in Behavioural terminology:

Stimulus + Punishment ⟶	Response
Fire + Pain ⟶	Avoidance behaviour
These come together until, through Association or Learning	
Fire alone ⟶	Avoidance
F + P ⟶	A
F ⟶	A
Generalized fear of fire ⟶	Generalized avoidance of fire

ie the child now avoids the fire even though specific punishment has not yet occurred.

If two exposures to this experience are necessary the formula becomes:

F2 + P2 ⟶	A
F ⟶	A

'Slow but sure wins the race' may be reduced to the following behavioural formula:

Stimulus + thoroughness ⟶	Response
Action + thoroughness ⟶	Prize
Conditioned by association	
Generalized thoroughness ⟶	Prize:
A + T ⟶	P
T1, T2, T3 ⟶	P

* Howard, Warren C. *Dictionary of Psychology.* Houghton Mifflin, Riverside Press

Evaluation

Behaviourism has been described as

Black Box Psychology

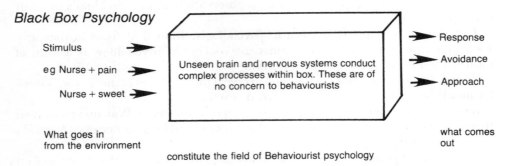

constitute the field of Behaviourist psychology

The Behaviourist Theory of Learning ('Conditioning' through Association—see chapter 6, pp 152) studies the effect of the environment on the establishment of learning by Association or Conditioning.

Shortcomings

Is environmental reward a more powerful welding force than punishment?

The scientific observer can *see* or *infer* when his subject is angry or happy—but *only the subject* may know how he *feels*.

These feelings, conscious or unconscious, are of no concern to the behaviourist.

He is concerned not with the intervening processes within the black box, but only with the ingoing stimulus and the outgoing response it arouses.

Contributions

Although limited, the Behaviouristic School did, by making psychologists aware of the need for measurement and objectivity, establish psychology as a science.

It also provided the theory upon which Behaviour Modification Therapy is based (see pp 152-165).

Modern therapy often seems to combine overt behaviourist learning with the insight operant in the cognitive approach.

Cognitive approach:'Psychology is the branch of science which investigates mental phenomena or mental operations.'*

This approach developed in response to the limitations imposed by the restrictive S → R concept. The restricted Behaviourist concept may suffice for simplest, most primitive biological organisms, but neglects many interesting, fruitful and important areas of human functioning.

What about people's thoughts, cumulative problem-solving; planning; remembering, decision-making—in fact what about the *important mental processing inside the box?*

If we consider the written word CAT we are looking at an arrangement of ink particles on white paper.

* Howard, Warren C. *Dictionary of Psychology*. Houghton Mifflin, Riverside Press

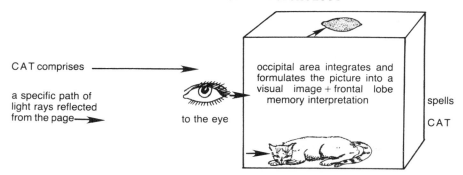

The Cognitive Approach is concerned with *internal functioning* within the 'black box'—with those processes which transform the sensory input into meaningful, usable information, thoughts and ideas. 'Cognition' therefore refers to perception, imagery, interpretation, problem-solving, remembering and thinking—to the drawing together, sifting out, generalization and reasoned utilization of perceptual input information.

Piaget, the giant of current developmental psychology, has stressed the cognitive approach in child development digging deep into learning processes; thinking, language ability, concept formation, techniques of problem solving and creativity (see pp 264-8).

Evaluation

The contribution of cognitive psychology lies in emphasis on *internal mental processing* which it has likened to electronic computer processing-selecting, comparing, combining and rearranging in the light of experience and memory.

The response output depends on the nature and quality of the processing machine, or cerebral structure, which we attempt to measure by IQ and other measurements of intelligence (see chapter 6, pp 144-7).

Psycho-analytic approach: 'Psychology is the science of the self or personal individual.'*

Concurrently with the growth in America of Behaviourism, in Europe Sigmund Freud was developing his psycho-analytic concept based on his *theory that much of man's behaviour is determined by innate (inborn) instincts or drives which are largely unconscious*. These unconscious instincts find expression in dreams, slips of speech, psychosomatic and neurotic, as well as socially approved behaviour such as artistic, literary and scientific activity.

In chapter 3 at page 60, there is a diagrammatic illustration of Freud's concept of mind-<u>function</u> (as opposed to anatomical structure):

Freud believed that all man's actions have a cause, but this cause is often founded on unconscious emotional motivation rather than on reason.

Through strict moralistic disapproval and punishment, the child is forced *unconsciously to 'repress'* or *consciously to 'suppress'* many childhood impulses or drives into the unconscious (Id).

* Howard, Warren C. *Dictionary of Psychology*. Houghton Mifflin, Riverside Press

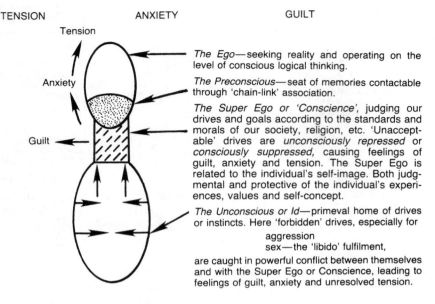

TENSION   ANXIETY   GUILT

Tension

The Ego—seeking reality and operating on the level of conscious logical thinking.

Anxiety

The Preconscious—seat of memories contactable through 'chain-link' association.

The Super Ego or 'Conscience', judging our drives and goals according to the standards and morals of our society, religion, etc. 'Unaccept-able' drives are *unconsciously repressed* or *consciously suppressed,* causing feelings of guilt, anxiety and tension. The Super Ego is related to the individual's self-image. Both judg-mental and protective of the individual's experi-ences, values and self-concept.

Guilt

The Unconscious or Id—primeval home of drives or instincts. Here 'forbidden' drives, especially for

aggression
sex—the 'libido' fulfilment,

are caught in powerful conflict between themselves and with the Super Ego or Conscience, leading to feelings of guilt, anxiety and unresolved tension.

Here they are in conflict among themselves, and against the Conscience (Super Ego), reinforcing distressing and debilitating tension, and hence neurotic and psychosomatic disorders. Man's strongest drives are

(i) The Life Instinct expressed in sexual fulfilment (The Libido).

(ii) The Death Instinct motivating aggression for survival, domination, killing and suicide.

Evaluation

Although Freud's theories are not based on scientific experimental assessment, they have exerted a profound influence on psychology. The do emphasize and attempt to explain the power and dynamics of strong emotions.

1.   While they would agree that the individual is not fully aware of some aspects of his personality and its manifestations, most psychologists are critical of Freud's geographical division of the mind into distinct functional areas.

2.   Freud's approach is somewhat negative in its emphasis on the inevitability in man of primitive animal instincts, such as aggression and the sex drive (libido), and their continuous struggle for expression against inhibitory social and religious restrictions.

    He saw no peaceful reconciliation of man's drives for aggression and primitive self-satisfaction.

Some of Freud's pupils and contemporaries, claiming his theories to be too orthodox and rigid, branched off to form their own schools. Most prominent among them were:

Carl Jung believed Freud's concept of the unconscious as the seat of man's basest, painful, even pathological mental functions to be too narrow and too rigid. In contrast Jung believed the unconscious to be the *creative companion* of the conscious Ego—the source of new energy and deeper meaning.

The health and vitality of the Ego depends on its communication and harmony, its compensatory relationship with the unconscious: eg the insignificant, isolated person may dream he is Zeus, the most powerful of mythical immortals.

It is not necessary always to interpret, dissect and understand the unconscious imagery which emerges in poetry, music, art and particularly in dreams: 'The peephole into the life of the soul'.

To attempt so to do causes anxiety, confusion and may freeze the ability to balance, to compensate for, the one-sided, anxiety-provoking intellectualization of the creative Ego. In order that they may fulfil their role, the inner harmony, creative imagery and emotions should be experienced, meditated upon, and accepted.

'What', one should ask, 'am I doing to make friends with my dream figures, to accept their feelings and the messages they bring from the seat of my inner needs?'

'If we accept with self-tolerance and understanding the hostility, anger, love, beauty of our inner images they will unconsciously change us and unify our personality.'

Jung divides unconscious imagery into:

1. 'Little Dreams'—ordinary imagery, resulting from the 'natural motions of daily living—dealing with daily events, personal life and hard, tangible facts'.
2. 'Big Dreams'—larger than life archetypes, immortal figures and myths drawn from the hereditary, collective Unconscious, that spiritual reality which transcends personal history, reaching far back into human beginnings, eg

> witches and fairy tales
> ancient heroes and gods of mythology
> the eternal wonders of nature—great mountains
> oceans, forests, deserts, even outer space visited by strange people
> animal figures, especially snakes and elephants

All these are endowed by the Jungian hierarchy with symbolism. Combined in various constellations, they form individual personality types, eg:

Uranus—the primordial father, caught in conflicting protection and violence towards his sons, wishing to devour them; in his realization of their desire to castrate the father figure he jealously denies them authority (the mythologically slanted Oedipus conflict).

Zeus—the thunderer, the strict dispenser of filial law and morality; his symbols were the eagle, the oak, the mountain tops.

Gaia—the primordial mother is constantly related to earth, seeds, water. She stands for fruitfulness, orderliness. She is the orderly, admonishing mother:
'You must pass your exams.'
'You must sit up straight.'

As opposed to Demeter, mother of the yielding earth, who loves her children so much, they must only be what they want to be.

Hera, who never punishes her husband Zeus, only women.

Aphrodite, the goddess of love and fertility, who demands the toll of her love—she is revengeful and punitive.

Personality classification ultimately depends upon the proportional dominance within the individual of his or her Archetypal constellation.

In Jungian terms, a mother's ability to nurture and to bond will depend upon her Archetypal dominance eg the Gaia mother is too strict, too obsessively orderly to achieve the warm spontaneity of the yielding Demeter mother.

Jung also described two fundamental personality types:

the outgoing, exuberant *Extrovert* who is able to socialize, express his needs and mourn his losses without inhibition

and the

withdrawn, 'private' *Introvert*, a more thoughtful personality, encountering difficulty in communicating, in forming intimate relationships and in expressing his feelings in such relationships.

Alfred Adler, who evolved the theory of the 'inferiority complex', associated with a self-concept (Super Ego) impaired through long-term criticism, failure and rejection.

Erik Erikson, who expanded Freud's developmental theories to encompass the entire life cycle. Erikson described an *inborn pattern of developmental stages,* each with its own growth tasks.

Mastery of life's growth tasks involves the resolution of a succession of eight *crisis watersheds.* In order that the individual may grow to his full 'Ego Identity' it is necessary that he overcomes *the maturational conflict* imposed by slipping away of the secure, comfortable familiarity of one stage and the fear, apprehension of failure and rejection created in him by the threat of the next. He proceeds to Ego Identity by *crisis resolution* through the interweaving of *introjection* and role model *identification* (see p 246).

The Humanistic approach

This approach developed from the existential philosophy of Kierkegaard, Nietzche and Sartre, all of whom emphasize those 'human' qualities which distinguish men from animals.

Foremost amongst these qualities are man's:

Freewill,
Drive towards Growth and Self-actualization.

In spite of familial, environmental and cultural obstacles, man's natural tendency is towards development of his fullest potential.

Evolved as a reaction against the genetic and physiological limitations imposed by the Neurobiological school; the impersonal, external control of the Behaviourist school; the primitive, inevitable struggle in which moral control loses to psycho-analytic concepts of aggression and irrepressible libido—in fact against all concepts of our technological society which tend to dehumanize man, *the Humanists believe every individual to be free to choose and determine his actions and hence his destiny.*

Owing to his freedom of choice, each person is responsible for his own actions. He cannot blame his heredity, his environment, his parents, or his 'bad luck' for what he is or does.

The Humanists reject the view that man is 'acted on' by forces outside his control. They do not agree with Shakespeare that 'all the world's a stage, and all the men and women merely players'.* They see man not only as an 'actor', but his own scriptwriter, director, and stage manager, governing his own destiny.

* *As You Like It* II. vii.

The Humanists emphasize experiences which make life meaningful and richer in 'the here and now', such as

sensory 'awareness'
interpersonal communication—verbal, visual, auditory, tactile
'encounter groups'
love
'consciousness'—expanding and mystical experiences through Eastern guru, extrasensory mediation, etc.

In antithesis to the Psycho-neurological and Behaviourist schools, the Humanists emphasize the individual's *subjective experiences*. How can man achieve self-actualization?

His self-concept and social constellation are considered more worthy of study and reconstruction than his overt actions.

Evaluation

1. In stressing the main goal of psychology to be human well-being rather than theoretical experimentation, the Humanistic school has made a valuable contribution.
2. However, to assume that current difficult problems can be solved by discarding the scientific approach, and all that has been learned from it, is to 'throw the baby out with the bath water'.
3. To pit resources unrealistically against limitations of innate ability, genetic predisposition to mental illness, gross physical mutilation, overwhelming environmental stresses, etc, is to condemn the individual to frustration, overwhelming guilt-feelings, and, at times, to deny him philosophical acceptance, support and relief.

Phenomenological Psychology
(by Christopher R Stones MSc PhD)

The derivation of Existential Phenomenology—from which has developed the field of Phenomenological Psychology—has been traced from two major nineteenth-century philosophers. The first, a Danish theologian and theoretician, is Soren Kierkegaard, who is generally held to be the father of contemporary Existentialism. The second is Edmund Husserl who is considered to be the founder of what was later to become known as the Phenomenological Movement. Although Existentialism and Phenomenology are different in that the former tends to be a doctrine of human existence while the latter has as its priority the study of human consciousness, they are nevertheless similar in that both reject the reductionistic predilections of the natural sciences (physiology, biology and so forth) with regard to describing and understanding human being.

Kierkegaard argued that we can best understand human nature by understanding that human existence is unique, unrepeatable and is thereby in principle always original and radically personal. However, this stance militates against any attempt to arrive at generalized laws and principles of knowledge. Consequently, Kierkegaard's school of existentialist thought cannot claim to be scientific, nor can it ever aspire to being scientific, since one of the hallmarks of a scientific discipline is that it endeavours to arrive at sets of generalized knowledge.

Husserl, on the other hand, strove to develop a philosophy which would be a rigorous science in that it would have as its base generalized laws and inter-subjectivity, but which would not attempt to emulate the reductionistic stance of the natural sciences. Husserl, proceeded by exploring the concept of *intentionality*. That is, that consciousness intends an object. Consciousness does not exist in and for itself but always intends an object beyond itself. For example, we do not just love, we love someone; we do not just blush, we blush for some interpersonal reason; we are not just aware, we are always aware of something.

And thus was born Phenomenology—an understanding of man through his phenomena. If consciousness intends an object, then the focus of the discipline should be on the object *revealed* and not on the person who is perceiving as if he were an encapsulated entity looking out onto the world. Being conscious implies being conscious of that which is revealed in one's dialogue with the world.

Under the influence of a more contemporary philosopher, Martin Heidegger, these two streams of philosophy, Existentialism and Phenomenology, were brought together in his work *Being and Time* (1962) to develop a philosophy of *being*. As such, Heidegger's Existential Phenomenology reverses the dualistic emphasis of Descartes's classic dictum 'I think, therefore I am'. Instead, the emphasis is placed on the question of being: 'I am, therefore I think.' That is, our being in the world precedes any thinking that we might do about the world.

Such a departure from tradition has great implications for the type of psychology that we might develop. The focus is neither one of idealism (with its emphasis on the encapsulated mental event) nor one of positivism (with the emphasis on observable and measurable behaviour), but rather on the issue of being-in-the-world. (*Note:* not a-being-in-the-world.)

Implications for Psychology

Once we are able to appreciate man as being-in-the-world—that is, man as and in relatedness—it then becomes possible to see why man cannot adequately be understood along intra-psychic lines nor as mere organism responding to stimuli (the fundamental tenet of Behaviourism). Rather, Phenomenology sees man as being in dialogue with a system of meanings. He does not respond to stimuli, but to the meaning that those stimuli hold for him. A red light, for example, is more than just a stimulus. It holds a multitude of meanings which emerge as a consequence of dialogue: stop! danger, the promise of illicit sexual delights and so forth. It is to these emergent meanings that man responds, not *bare* factual stimuli.

Given that man responds to meanings, the enterprise of hoping to further understand man by extrapolating from the results of animal studies is rejected by Phenomenology. By virtue of not being human, the animal is denied access to those meanings which are uniquely human, and it is these uniquely human phenomena that should be the epicentre of contemporary psychology. This is not to deny the substantiality of the human body and the commonalities that exist between man and sub-human species. But, it is argued, psychology must not be allowed to be the dumping ground for material not attractive or scientifically lucrative to other scientific disciplines. Such material is best left to those disciplines for which it is most suited: neurology, physiology, biology and the other natural sciences.

Evaluation

Phenomenological Psychology:

1. hopes to have overcome Cartesian dualism, that is, the theoretically hypothesized split between subject and object, inner and outer;
2. understands man as-relatedness rather than as-neurology, as-organism, as-mental-processor, as-driven-by-instincts;
3. argues against the endeavour to understand human psychology via animal experimentation. It argues for a truly human psychology;
4. shows that man responds to meanings not stimuli.

Eclectic approach: *'Psychology is the branch of science which investigates mental phenomena or mental operations.'* *

The Eclectic approach aims to evaluate the contributions of all schools—'to sort the wheat from the chaff'—welding that which is endorsed by scientific experiment or profitable usage, into a truly viable psychology.

This is the approach to which the writer adheres.

THE AIM OF PSYCHOLOGY is to collect data by:

1. Experimental methods designed to test theories

These methods involve submission of a *hypothesis* or assumption to be tested, in the hope of discovering a 'cause—effect relationship', eg that continuous exposure to loud pop music in discos impairs auditory discrimination.

AIM: To test the truth of this hypothesis by measuring the effect on the auditory discrimination of human subjects of repetitive loud sounds as measured in decibels on an audiometer.

METHOD: Within the *constant* disco environment, for a *measured* period of time, the subjects remain *constant*.

Their gyrating movements remain *constant*. The flashing lights remain *constant*. The *variables* to be studied are: repetitive *loud sounds* in relation to *efficiency* within a given sound range.

A variable is thus a condition 'injected into' an experiment so that its effect may be measured. The term 'variable' is used because the 'condition' may have different values—ie unlike the constants *it is free to vary*. The variable is usually a stimulus, the responses to which are under investigation. The auditory discrimination of subjects is measured in decibels on the audiometer to give the average *pre-experimental* auditory range—Finding A.

After exposure of one hour to experimental constants and the variable (repetitive loud sounds), the audiometric test of discrimination is readministered to give the average *post-experimental* auditory range—Finding B.

* Howard, Warren,C. ed. *Dictionary of Psychology*. Hougton Mifflin.

The *criterion* of measurement is thus the fineness or range of decibel discrimination on the audiometer.

The difference between the pre-experiment discrimination range (Finding A), compared with the post-experiment discrimination range, (Finding B), represents an objective measurement of the effect of repetitive loud sounds on auditory discrimination (Finding E):

$A - B = E$

CONCLUSION: If the difference (E) is positive in favour of larger Finding A, (ie a greater discrimination range pre-experiment) then it may be concluded that exposure to the variable, ie repetitive loud sounds impairs auditory discrimination.

EVALUATION: Assuming the finding to be positive, and thus indicative of impaired auditory discrimination, as a result of loud discos, this finding must now be assessed with reference to:

1. *Its significance*

Is the difference between scores A and B on sound discrimination large enough to be *meaningful*, or could it have occurred simply by chance?

By means of a statistical procedure it is possible to conclude that, due to the experimental variable (ie repetitive loud sounds) pre- and post-test scores deviate enough to be 'statistically significant', and not just coincidental.

Finding the 'statistical significance' of an experimental result is the process of determining whether the result could have been obtained simply by the operation of chance factors.

2. *Its reliability*

The reliability of experimental findings indicates the extent to which they are:

(i) reproduceable, established by administering the test to the same subjects on two different occasions;
(ii) consistent.

The closer the agreement between two scores, the closer their relationship and the higher their mutual reliability.

Statistical reliability is thus *the self-consistency of a test or other measuring device.**

If an experiment yields different results:

(i) on different occasions,
(ii) in the hands of different administrators, then its findings are said, in the statistical sense, to be unreliable.

eg the particular audiometer used to measure decibel discrimination pre- and post-experiment may be unstandardized, ie not sufficiently rigid in its measurements, giving different readings on different occasions.

Hence results are too variable for reliable discrimination. Unless a stringent and standardized criterion yielding comparable results is applied, retest results may be too different for reliability.

Certainly some variability is unavoidable.

---

* Howard, Warren C. *Dictionary of Psychology*. After the work of Aristotle and his followers

In order to *evaluate the degree of relationship* (and thus the reliability) between two scores or sets of scores, an index of this relationship is provided by the statistical device termed the *'coefficient of correlation'*.

The *coefficient of correlation is a numerical index indicating the degree of correspondence between two sets of paired measurements,* and usually designated by r.

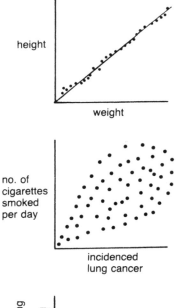

Correlation (r) = + 1 means a perfect positive relationship between pre- and post-test scores, indicating complete agreement.

r = − 1 means a perfect negative correlation, or complete disagreement between experimental scores.

r = 0,5–0,7 does reflect a positive relationship and a degree of reliability which may be acceptable in certain more flexible experimental situations.

eg as between university attainment and vocational success.

(r = 0,70 reflects nearly double the degree of relationship of r = 0,50. This is because r values express a relationship—not a percentage.)

r = 0,8–0,9 or above, represents an excellent level of reliability and is an appropriate criterion for eminently reliable experimental results.

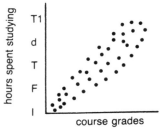

Returning to our example, r = 0,85 between test and retest scores would certainly indicate a strong positive relationship between repetitive loud sounds and decreased auditory discrimination in the sound range investigated.

Experimental devices increasing reliability include:
repeating the experiment as performed originally.
repeating the experiment using different sources of noise, eg a drum or bugle.

For example, the following diagram might represent the relationship (r) between two sets of experimental scores obtained using different sources of sound—the high correlation shows that the relationship between auditory discrimination and loud noise is constant across different sources of sound.

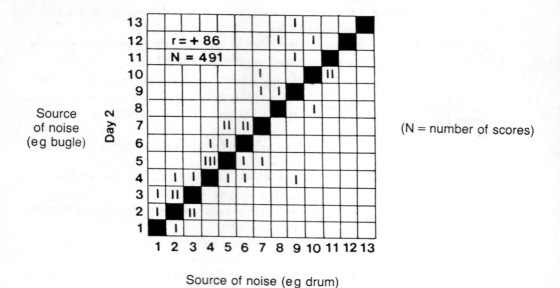

Source of noise (eg drum)

3. *Its validity*

Is the assumption that reduced auditory discrimination is the *result specifically of exposure to the variable, ie repetitive loud sounds, justified?*

In fact, is the experiment *testing what it is designed to test?*

Experimental results are valid only if they measure what they are intended to measure.

Could the difference in measurement be, in fact, due to factors other than loud noises such as the effects of bright lights or constant gyrating movement?

To be predictive, the structure of an experiment must ensure that *the variable is responsible* for changed measurements. *Validity is thus 'the predictive significance of a test for its intended purpose.'**

A widely used method for testing the validity of experimental data is the *'control' device* where a group, eg of teenagers matched for age, sex, etc, is subjected to the same experimental constants, with the exception of the variable, namely repetitive loud noise.

If one group (control group) is not exposed to the loud noise (experimental variable) but also shows reduction in auditory discrimination, then we cannot conclude that the loud noises were responsible for the reduction in auditory discrimination in the other group (experimental). However, if only the exposed group shows a difference in sound discrimination we *can* conclude that the experimental variable (loud noise) is responsible for the difference.

(If we take away the loud noises will we obtain the same reduction in discrimination?)

* Hilgard E R, Atkinson R C, Atkinson R C. *Introduction to Psychology* 7 ed. Harcourt Brace Jovanovich

If the criterion of sound discrimination is not affected by the constants of flashing lights and gyrating movement, then one is justified in assuming that it is the variable, namely repetitive loud sounds, which is responsible for the measured reduction in auditory discrimination. Indeed, experiments are designed so that *control* and *experimental* groups are *equivalent* except with respect to the critical experimental manipulation. Therefore, if differences are observed between the groups they are thought to be due *only* to the manipulation.

Establishment of the validity of assuming 'carry over' of findings on animal experiments to humans is a major concern in experimental psychology.

Are we justified in assuming the carry over of learnt behaviour in animals to occur in humans?

Hopefully, scrutiny of the validity of an experimental, or test, result will help solve this problem.

2. Experience: direct observation, subjects' reports, introspection, psychosomatic reactions, etc

(a) The Observational Method

Careful observation of human and animal behaviour, and conscious thought processes, was often the precursor of more exact experimental procedures, as well as for its own intrinsic value. An example is observation of dolphins in their natural environment.

Because this method is vulnerable to the observer's preconceived beliefs and wished outcomes, training involves methods of accurate observation, description and interpretation.

Check-lists, continuum criteria, tables and questionnaires all assist standardization of observation and thus investigation reliability and validity.

(b) The Survey Method

Some topics have long been considered unsuitable for laboratory experimentation.

An example is that of human sexual motivation and activity. Until Masters and Johnson (1966)* devised techniques enabling direct laboratory observation of human sexual activity, Kinsey's surveys, 'Sexual Behaviour in the Human Male' (1948) and 'Sexual Behaviour in the Human Female' (1953), were the standard works on this subject.

Kinsey and his co-workers analysed information obtained from thousands of individual interviews.

Their respected surveys involved:

(i) The application of carefully compiled, pretested and standardized questionnaires by interviewers especially trained in their use.
(ii) Statistical analysis to ensure that the sample surveyed really did *constitute a representative sample of the population as a whole* (inappropriately but technically termed a *'random sample'*).

* Masters W H, Johnson V E. *Human Sexual Response*. Little Brown

(iii) Sophisticated analysis of survey data.

(iv) Expert interpretation of findings.

What Kinsey achieved from the survey method in the field of sexual behaviour, Gallup had pioneered in his poll of political opinion . . . a prediction of political opinion which has almost taken over from the ballot box!

The national census, market research and surveys of community health needs are examples of the survey method.

3. Test Methods

Standardized tests of intelligence, aptitudes, interests, and scholastic achievement are usually based on comparison of the subject's own scores relative to those obtained by the population as a whole.

Complicated statistical analysis ensures that the sample upon which scores are standardized really is random, representing the population as a whole, and that the test material really does measure what it is supposed to measure, rendering the test 'valid'. Retest and split-group techniques must ensure that the test is 'reliable'.

4. Case Histories

The case history (usually applied in Data Collection and Assessment stages of the Nursing Process, Chapter 9) aspires to be a scientific biography of the subject.

Although they may be augmented by official records, such biographies are (and for therapeutic purposes should be) based on the individual's own memories of his life events. Because a personal biography usually only becomes of scientific import in response to some life-crisis or other unforeseen event, it may be dependent on distortions and oversights.

Where, by virtue of predicted scientific study, eminence or other selective factor, the desirability of personal biography is foreseen, a case history usually becomes a *longitudinal study* over a period of time. This procedure,

(i) enabling periodic observation, interpretation and, hopefully measurement.

(ii) being relatively independent of the errors of retrospective memory,

is usually more scientifically meaningful than the personal case history.

The disadvantage of longitudinal studies lies in accumulated wastage of material which may be irrelevant when the particular life-crises or other precipitatory event arises.

Confirming and illustrating the very wide scope of psychology are its widely *variant fields of practice*, namely:

EXPERIMENTAL AND PHYSIOLOGICAL PSYCHOLOGY

Although psychologists in other fields also use experimental methods, those who specialize in experiment and research are primarily concerned with developing and applying precise methods of measurement and control in such areas as perception of, and reaction to, the environment, how human beings learn, remember, respond emotionally; recogniton and importance of primary drives and motivations.

Concerned with the relationship between biological processes and behaviour, they have developed sophisticated methods of experimentation in fields such as:

the interaction between anxiety and physiological change;
sexual stimulation and the Autonomic Nervous System;
the effect of drugs upon perception and motor control.

Two new and intensely active areas of experimental psychology are:

(a) the neurosciences, concerned with such problems as

anatomy and cellular structure of the brain, intake, processing and output functions of specific brain areas, the effects of cerebral impairment;

(b) psychopharmocology, which is concerned with the study of effects of drugs, both destructive and therapeutic, upon perception, motor co-ordination and emotional experience.

Methods of experimentation and statistical evaluation which experimental psychologists utilize have been outlined above.

DEVELOPMENTAL PSYCHOLOGY

Developmental psychology is concerned with the changes that occur as a function of *growth* and *development* in relation to:

inborn maturation potential,
environmental stimulation and growth opportunity,
the relationship between early and later behaviour.

Developmental psychology is the field of child guidance, education; counselling and psychotherapy: reactions to health, sickness, ageing and bereavement.

Life itself, for better or for worse, is a growth experience!

SOCIAL PSYCHOLOGY

'No man is an island, entire of itself; every man is a piece of the continent, a part of the main. Ask not for whom the bell tolls. It tolls for thee.' JOHN DONNE (1573-1631)

Because human development takes place in relation to others, social psychologists are concerned with *the manner in which interaction with other people influences attitudes* (p 110) and behaviour.

Communication (inter alia chap 7)
Patterns of individual conformity to group requirements (inter alia p 49)
Group behaviour, especially group development (p 170); introjection, identification and conflict (pp 106-110); therapeutic dynamics (chap 26)
Propaganda, prejudice and aggression
Market consumption patterns
Community living and organization (chap 10)
are all areas of social psychology.

CLINICAL PSYCHOLOGY

This branch of practice consists of the application of psychological knowledge to the *diagnosis and treatment* of emotional and behavioural problems such as anxiety and neuroses, juvenile delinquency, marital problems, drug abuse, mental retardation, etc.

Psychotherapy, the therapeutic tool of clinical psychologists, takes many forms and usually involves delving into early and unconscious experiences; reliving traumatic experiences within a deep, long-term relationship (inter alia pp 65, 609-613).

Counselling, operating in the 'here and now' of the problem presented, is a more surface-level interpretative, supportive, guidance technique.

In most countries, clinical psychologists require two university degrees, a specialist diploma and a term of internship at a teaching hospital before registration with their professional body. Formal training is of approximately six years' duration.

Application of certain individual tests, such as diagnostic intelligence tests, tests of organic brain impairment and projective techniques (inter alia pp 65, 609-613) is confined to psychologists thus registered.

Clinical psychologists work as part of a mental health team, in psychiatric and general hospitals, child guidance clinics, prisons, marriage guidance services, university student guidance facilities, private practice, etc.

(For differentiation between the roles of clinical psychologist and psychiatrist see The Psychiatric Team, p 605.)

SCHOOL AND EDUCATIONAL PSYCHOLOGY

This is the field of *'guidance teachers'* in possession of a university degree majoring in both teaching subjects and psychology, followed by a specialized teaching diploma recognized by the state department of education. Training is of four years' duration.

These specialized teachers conduct:

group intelligence, personality and interest tests
group and individual scholastic attainment tests
group and individual guidance in fields of:

> academic difficulties and subject choice,
> emotional and behavioural problems

They also act as a link between the school system and parents, and as a resource service to teachers.

They are not usually permitted to conduct diagnostic tests of individual intellectual ability, organic cerebral impairment, or deeper emotional or patho-logical functioning, which problems should be referred to registered clinical psychologists and sometimes psychiatrists and neurologists.

Guidance teachers who are in possession of a specialized university diploma in *Remedial Education* may apply some tests of motor, language, spatial, visual and auditory functioning and conduct individual remedial programmes for children with specific learning problems.

Remedial teachers are usually members of a team, including a neurologist, a registered clinical psychologist and a social worker.

Educational Psychologists have specialized in child development, learning techniques (Chapter 6), learning problems, research on teaching methods, curriculum development and teacher training.

Industrial Psychologists should hold a university degree in psychology, preferably with sociology, statistics and personnel management, plus a university diploma in industrial psychology.

Important skills in this profession include industrial research aimed at *job analysis* detailing all procedures, visual-motor and personality traits, intellectual requirements, in any given job.

This information is compiled into a *job description*, and a set of tests and questionnaires constructed and validated to measure applicants against standardized job requirements or norms. It is now the function of the industrial psychologist, to *'match the man to the job'* and to compile appropriate job-training programmes.

This approach differs from that of the *Vocational Counsellor* whose function it is to *'match the job to the man'* in aptitude, interest and personality.

The industrial psychologists is involved not only in personnel selection and training in order to achieve maximum productivity but also in maintaining optimum

work conditions
motivation
goal achievement (wage increases, promotion, etc)
job satisfaction

THE NURSE-COUNSELLOR

Recognition of the:

particularly wide range of intellectual, visual-motor, social and other skills required in various fields of modern nursing,

unique and intense stress areas encountered by both the student and professional nurse, and thus the importance of opportunity for catharsis and counselling,

has led to this new concept of an especially trained professional outside the nursing hierarchy.

Appropriate training will probably include:

a university degree in nursing,
followed by a specialist diploma in personnel management,
educational or industrial counselling, social work or an allied discipline.
(See inter alia p 193, chaps 7, 9, 10, 26.)

The *Pastoral Counsellor* is a clergyman possessing a qualification in psychology and/or social work. He uses his understanding of psychological diagnostic and therapeutic techniques within a religious background.

His long-term association with omnipotent love and forgiveness, and a better life hereafter, may enhance his role, in relief of guilt, isolation, suffering, disaster and death (see pp 577, 537).

CHAPTER 2

PERSONALITY DEVELOPMENT AND FUNCTION

'The integrated organization of all the cognitive, affective, conative and physical characterization of an individual as it manifests itself in focal distinctness to others.' —Warren C Howard *Dictionary of Psychology.*

To psychologists, who like to think of themselves as 'experts in human behaviour and mental processes', the word 'personality' has a special technical meaning. In psychological language, *personality* refers to the *total person*. It is the summation of his individual.

> Anatomy and biochemistry,
> Heredity,
> Life story (including sociological processes).

It includes a person's body and mind, loves and hates, abilities and interests, speed of reaction and length of memory.

Personality is all that a person has been, is, and hopes to be.

Body and mind cannot be separated; neither can function without affecting the other. By virtue of the Autonomic Nervous System, mental processes are closely related to a person's physical condition and vice versa.

The Type Theory

Kretschmer attempted to classify personality on the *basis of body build:*

The endomorph, short and plump, was said to be relaxed, a good mixer, even tempered and jolly.

The ectomorph, tall, thin, spare, was classified as restrained, self-conscious, somewhat austere, withdrawn, of studious bent and prone to solitude.

The mesomorph, heavy-set, muscular, was classified as noisy, insensitive, tough and somewhat 'thick', preferring physical activity to more intellectual pursuits.

However, scientific efforts to link (or correlate) personality characteristics with physique have been fruitless, except in a direct cause → effect role.

> eg A fat stocky girl feeling inferior to languid, long-legged beauties, may become shy and isolated, or seek compensation in intellectual achievements or a 'clown' role.

Swiss psychiatrist **Carl Jung** attempted to classify personality by *psychological criteria* impelling from within, rather than by physical features.

He divided all personalities into two types, viz:

1. *Introverts* whose behaviour pattern, especially in times of emotional conflict, illness or environmental crisis, is one of withdrawal.

   Introverts find socialization somewhat difficult turning in on their own company, sometimes to the point of isolation. They prefer working on their own, often in thoughtful or creative activities, and find active participation in team projects stressful.

2.   *Extroverts* who, turning to others in times of stress, grief or need, usually find emotional outlet and support. They are good mixers and flourish in group projects. They usually choose, and enjoy outgoing, people-orientated activities and careers such as the theatre, advertising and public relations.

The main disadvantage in trying to classify people by 'type' is the multiplicity, rather than simplicity, of human nature. The *endless variations in personality combinations* result in most people falling outside the confines of personality classification.

Somewhat simplistic but often workable is the **A and B personality** theory.

A-type personalities

are self-assertive, aggressive, impatient: more prone to stress-related disorders such as anxiety and neurotic symptoms, especially perfectionism and psychosomatic disorders. They present with above-average risk for coronary thrombosis.

A-type personalities are driven to do more than one thing at a time.

They are compulsively competitive and distressed when unable to win. They tend to rush things and take on the burdens of others—they find it difficult to delegate responsibility.

They need to:

(i)   plan carefully in order to reduce their task burden;
(ii) programme for mental and physical relaxation;
(iii) discuss with others more streamlined task processing and allotment.

B-type personalities

(i)   less inclined to aggressiveness;
(ii) present with overtly calmer behaviour; are more 'laid back';
(iii) plan well to reduce task pressure and share burdens.

Although these individuals may not achieve as much as their A-type counterparts, statistics show they can expect increased life expectancy of approximately 14 years. Exponents of this type of A–B classification insist that neither type is 'better' nor 'smarter', but merely constitutionally different.

Thorsen of Stanford University has structured a model for:

identifying Type A and Type B individuals;
conditioning Type A, by a behaviour modification process, to adopt more 'laid back', Type B behaviour patterns, e g when stressed by driving in the fast lane purposefully to move over into the less pressurized inner lane.

By repetitive rewarding of Type B behaviour Thorsen claims to have cut the group death rate from stress-related illness by one-third to one-half.

The Trait Theory

A more meaningful concept is the trait theory which sees personality as an *individual cluster* of relatively permanent and consistent characteristics such as intelligence, aggression, friendliness, excitability, independence, integrity. Within a cluster, each individual characteristic or trait can be represented by continuous dimensions or scales.

A trait is thus a relatively permanent, measurable characteristic or dimension of personality.
Personality definition involves:

1. a meaningful description of the individual's trait cluster;
2. measurement of relative trait importance.

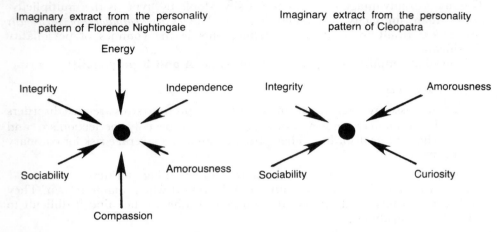

Important pioneer work in this field is that of **Raymond Cattell** who, on the basis of direct observation, standardized questionnaires and personality tests, identified 16 factors which he believes to be the basic ingredients of personality.

Labelled according to traits at both extremes of their continuum, Cattell's 16 components of personality are as follows:

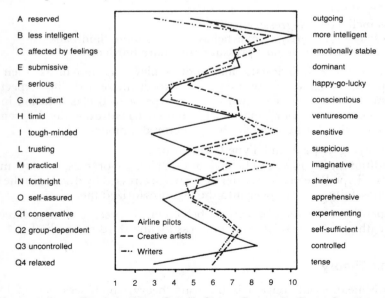

A reserved	outgoing
B less intelligent	more intelligent
C affected by feelings	emotionally stable
E submissive	dominant
F serious	happy-go-lucky
G expedient	conscientious
H timid	venturesome
I tough-minded	sensitive
L trusting	suspicious
M practical	imaginative
N forthright	shrewd
O self-assured	apprehensive
Q1 conservative	experimenting
Q2 group-dependent	self-sufficient
Q3 uncontrolled	controlled
Q4 relaxed	tense

— Airline pilots
-- Creative artists
-·· Writers

Vocational personality profiles derived from Cattell's Sixteen Personality Factor Questionnaire (1973)*

* From Hilgard E R, Atkinson R L, Atkinson R C. *Introduction to Psychology.* 7ed. Harcourt Brace Jovanovich.

In order to endow his Sixteen Personality Factor Questionnaire with practical purpose, Cattell has calculated the average score clusters for vocationally adjusted members of professional groups such as airline pilots, artists, writers, teachers, etc. Youngsters meeting these average or 'norm' score combinations should function well, personality-wise, in the appropriate career indicated.

Cattell's reason for selecting the term 'factor' derives from his use of the statistical technique of *factor analysis* which enables the investigator to analyse out or 'extract' from a given whole or *general factor*, such as intelligence or personality, the largest number of component 'special factors'. Very low intercorrelation scores (r) indicate the uniqueness of each separate factor extracted.

Sophisticated use of factor analysis enabled **Hans Eysenck**, Hungarian-born research psychologist at London's Maudsley Hospital to construct his *dimensions* of personality traits.

Like most investigators of personality, he extracted the two basic factors of introversion and extroversion, which he characterized as:

Introversion	**Extroversion**
stability	instability
calm, well adjusted	moody, anxious temperament
reliable	unreliable

Further factors analysed out resulted in the following dimensional diagram:

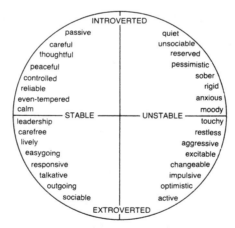

Eysenck's dimensions related to personality traits

A major limitation upon the usefulness of the trait approach is the possibility that an individual may react differently in response to widely variant environmental circumstances. A patient who presents as controlled and calm in the face of physical pain may prove frightened, moody and aggressive when faced with death.

Conclusion

Personality analysis is *not* a trustworthy predictor of human behaviour.

What is more important and significant is the *interaction between individual differences and changing enviromental situations.*

In order to understand more fully the complexity and countless variations of personality combinations, let us turn our attention to a more detailed study of the basic ingredients of personality, namely:

1. ORGANIC STRUCTURE.
2. HEREDITY.
3. THE LIFE STORY.

> culture
> geography
> social milieu

1. THE ORGANIC STRUCTURE IN RELATION TO EMOTION

Clearly one's metabolic rate, whether it be accelerated or sluggish, will affect one's personality pattern, resulting in an energetic, active, enthusiastic person or a stodgy, lazy, slow-reacting one.

Glandular Secretions (eg thyroxin, estrogen and testosterone output) tend to influence personality traits such as energy, determination, amorousness, etc.

Whether one has usually experienced a feeling of *physical strength* and well-being; whether one has had to adjust to pain and dependence, will affect the whole individual as described in the personality pattern.

Clearly the individual whose *appearance* resembles that of Apollo will have a very different perspective on life from one who looks like Frankenstein's monster.

The brain communicates

1. with the outside world via the **Central Nervous System** comprising afferent sensory fibres bringing messages into the brain for interpretation,
    efferent motor fibres taking instructions out to the musculature for execution.
2. The **Peripheral Nervous System** with nerve tracts stretching out from the brain and spinal cord to all parts of the body.

    The Peripheral Nervous System is divided into

    (a) The *Somatic Nervous System* transmitting information including pain, temperature-change, pressure outwards to initiate organ activity. Such activity includes voluntary movements as well as adjustments in balance and posture.

    (b) The *Autonomic Nervous System* consists of:

    > (i) The Thoracic–Lumbar or Sympathetic Nervous System (stimu-lating). (See opposite page.)
    > (ii) The Cranial–Sacral or Parasympathetic Nervous System (soothing).

The Sympathetic Nervous System is intimately connected by nerve fibres with

(i) the hypothalamus, main cerebral seat of emotion (whence its name) and
(ii) the pituitary 'master gland' which, by producing the largest number of different hormones, 'orchestrates' hormonal, and thus psycho-physiological reactions.

The *hypothalamus* and certain parts of the limbic system are linked via the Papez circuit to the neo-cortex.

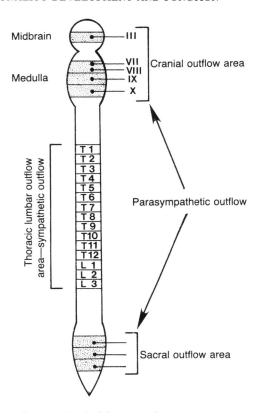

Midbrain — III

Medulla

VII — Cranial outflow area
VIII
IX
X

Thoracic lumbar outflow area—sympathetic outflow

T 1
T 2
T 3
T 4
T 5
T 6
T 7
T 8
T 9
T10
T11
T12
L 1
L 2
L 3

Parasympathetic outflow

Sacral outflow area

The Hypothalamus and Sympathetic Nervous System are concerned with

(i) the satisfaction of biological and emotional needs and drives, such as the need to relieve hunger or thirst; the need for love fulfilment, for the expression of hate and anger; for relief from fear and pain (homeostasis, pp 89-93);

(ii) the stress which results when insurmountable environmental obstacles frustrate the fulfilment of emotional drives (inequilibrium).

Drives to fulfil biological and emotional needs (especially those concerned with man's primeval needs of survival and reproduction) stimulate an increase in the brain's gross electrical responses measurable on the electroencephalogram. Appropriate arousal signals are conveyed by nerve fibres from cerebral seats of emotion, hunger, respiration, etc, via the *Sympathetic Nervous System* to the involuntary internal organs, stimulating them to mobilize that *biochemical tension-energy* which is designed by nature to satisfy these needs. The individual is then said to be in a state of tension.

TENSION is thus a state of mobilized biochemical energy, the purpose of which is to fulfil the needs of the organism.

STRESS is a state of prolonged tension-energy.

ANXIETY is a strong precipitator of tension and stress.

May defines *anxiety* as '*diffuse apprehension that is vague in nature, and associated with feelings of uncertainty and helplessness*'.

When the individual perceives his *very being to be threatened*, feelings of isolation, alienation and insecurity invade his personality.

Experiences provoking <u>anxiety</u> invade the child, spread and grow throughout life, to conclude with the fear of helplessness and rejection in old age, and culminating with the greatest fear of all, the great, unknown threat of death.

'It is all-pervasive, and every corner of human endeavour is affected by anxiety. It is closely related to the terms "<u>anger</u>" when defined as "grief or trouble", and "<u>anguish</u>" which is described as "acute pain suffering or distress". *Anxiety is a multi-dimensional concept and it is manifested as a somatic, experiential and inter-personal phenomenon.* It therefore involves one's body, perceptions of self, and relationships with others.'*

Signals of danger, sexual desire and those physical and emotional needs concerned with man's survival and basic satisfactions, are conveyed via the hypothalamus to the Sympathetic Nervous System. Appropriate signals are conveyed from the middle brain to the suprarenal gland, resulting in the *outpouring of adrenalin and noradrenalin, histamine and blood sugar* into the bloodstream.

Blood enriched by stimulants and energizing chemicals enables automatic, split-second muscle activity. This peak-level energy is termed *Tension-energy*.

Tension-energy is designed

(i) to mobilize the organism for the expression of the *Fight* ←→ *Flight* reaction necessary for man's primeval functions of survival by *Fighting* off the enemy or, where the latter is too strong, by *Flight* from the enemy;

(ii) for *reproduction*.

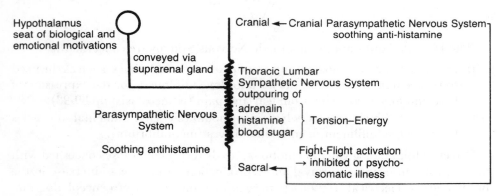

Heartbeat accelerates, blood pressure rises, sugar and fat reserves are tapped and moved into the muscles; hydrocortisone is activated. Red blood cells are pumped into arteries to give the body more energy. The blood-clotting factor is raised so that wounds may close more easily—a dramatic vestige of man's primeval mobilization of tension-energy for survival.

Tension energy is characterized by *overactivity* in all body processes, except that involved in bowel elimination—for primitive man did not have time to defecate while fighting off enemies or running in the opposite direction!

---

* Stuart G W , Sundeen S J. *Principles and Practice of Psychiatric Nursing.* St Louis, Toronto, London: C V Mosby Company, 1979.

Being part of the *Autonomic Nervous System*, the *Sympathetic Nervous System* is autonomous or self-governing. Because it is involuntary, the individual's 'will-power' can do little to arrest its train of action, once begun.

The following table summarizes areas of overactivity resultant upon stimulation of the Sympathetic Nervous System by *danger, basic bodily needs* such as the relief of hunger, thirst, escape from pain; *emotional needs* such as relief from anxiety, expression of anger, hate and the satisfaction of love, honour status fulfilment, etc.

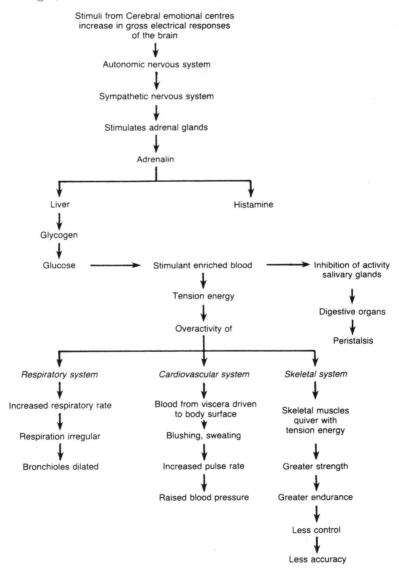

The manner in which stimuli from cerebral emotional centres are conveyed via the suprarenal gland and Sympathetic Nervous System to various internal and external bodily functions is the basis of *psychosomatic involvement, by which emotional*

stimuli are converted into physical or organic change. (See also Cannon–Bard and James–Lange theories of emotion, pp 89-93.) However, the interflow between mind and body still holds many mysteries.

The specific psycho- (from the Greek word *Psyche* pertaining to the mind) somatic (organic or pertaining to the body) involvements of tension and stress have only recently begun to emerge, based on the pioneering investigations of **Selye**, an Austrian, appropriately possessing doctorates in both philosophy and medicine. Working in Montreal, Selye sought a new hormone in the ovaries of cows. He became side-tracked when, in his experiments on animals, he observed that *all reacted the same way to every kind of injection*, whether from the ovaries, spleen, kidneys or even poison. He discovered that hunger, noise, fear, light blows on the back of the head, electric shocks, or even fights, produced the same chain of reaction.

He concluded that there exists a kind of '*general alarm* for all imaginable contingencies. A blow on the neck, an extra-marital adventure accompanied by guilt feelings, a busted straight in poker, a jump into a safety net, the award of a medal, an attack of flu, a shot in the leg, a missed putt, all produced the same stress count-down, the identical reaction from nerves that mobilize hormones to enable the body to survive'.

Selye points out that the *comprehensive reaction* to fear and other emotional upheavals in primitive man 'takes place in us today just as it did in our Stone Age ancestors. And for us, just as for them, it can be the means of saving our lives by jumping away from a fast-moving motor car, or, in contrast, taking our lives in a serious pathological psychosomatic illness'.

All too often these days, *the alarm reaction is an empty exercise.* Whatever the stressors may be, in our highly technical modern society, they all prepare our organisms for Fight or Flight, ie for strong physical activity. 'But what do we *do*? Nothing! What man, having just been reprimanded by his boss, utters a loud yell and lifts his office desk over his head? On the contrary, *in spite of the preparation for high performance activity, our bodies remain completely motionless.*'

Whereas primitive man could reduce his psychosomatic tension reactions by appropriate physical outlet of his tension energy, modern man, in his complicated social set-up requiring *constant inhibition of his natural reactions*, is frequently (often unconsciously) *forced to 'push' his tension energy 'underground'.* Here it causes areas of festering overactivity, experienced at first as general restlessness and lack of well-being, eventually turning into long-term biochemical change and eventual somatic or physical pathology.

Whereas primitive man was able to externalize his psychosomatic tension in purposeful, outgoing physical activity, modern man is forced to contain long-term psychosomatic tension to the point of extended internal stress erosion.

Primitive child could go out and kill the snake he feared, but modern child does not solve his problems by direct physical tension release in killing a feared schoolteacher. Primitive man could throw a constantly irritating mother-in-law over a cliff; modern man must bear his tension internally, with resultant gastric ulcer. Primitive man reduced his tension energy by physically attacking his aggressive neighbour, but modern man cannot find similar stress release in killing the stockmarket which is holding him in long-term suspense.

Classically his *tension goes underground*, to result in the following classification of typical psychosomatic stress results:

I. Cardiovascular System:
—tachycardia
—hypertension
—raised blood glucose level

II. Gastro-intestinal System:
—nervous dyspepsia
—peptic ulceration
—chronic constipation
—ulcerative colitis

III. Excretory System:
—increased urinary output
—skin eruptions, eg: eczema

IV. Respiratory System:
—hyperventilation
—possible bronchospasm
(leading to asthma)

V. Muscle System:
—increased tone
—'fibrositis'

VI. Nervous System
—headache (tension type)
—irritability
—insomnia

Selye emphasizes that stress situations in a large, modern city are very different from those encountered by our primitive ancestors. While they experienced only brief terms of exceptional stress situations, followed by pauses in which to regain balance between the Sympathetic and Parasympathetic Nervous Systems, (see Homeostasis, p 103), to recover and relax, modern man is subjected to a barrage of permanent, long-term environmental irritants.

Experimentation with rats has shown that persistence of the cause of stress without periods of 'easing off' and recovery (homeostasis), results in a state of physical exhaustion which may lead even to death.

Death from exhaustion is not in such cases due to failure of energy reserve. Rather does it occur because the organism has passed the limit of its capacity to adjust.

No one would argue with the necessity for allaying the painful effects of stress. Some researchers believe the biochemical sequelae of stress to be immuno-suppressive, exposing the body to infection and other invasions.

Among others, Myrin Borysenko of Harvard Medical School, has demonstrated that excess adrenalin can significantly depress the body's immune system. His colleague David McClelland, has presented complementary research endorsing that love and joy, in stimulating the parasympathetic nervous system to secrete soothing antihistamine, help boost the immune system. Thus it would seem that the happy and relaxed patient (and nurse) stand a better chance of resisting invasion, from the common cold to cancer.

But that cannot be the whole story. Sickness is not reserved for the sad and the stressed, and the cheerful do not always recover.

Research workers in the field of psychosomatic medicine believe that certain psychosomatic illnesses are commonly encountered in persons of particular personality 'types', eg

1. *Exact and exacting persons,* who are over-meticulous in their work, tend to develop tension headaches.
2. *Worriers:* tense, anxious people who cannot tolerate insecurity, tend to develop duodenal ulcers.

3.	*Over-tidy, compulsively clean people* tend to develop ulcerative colitis.
4.	*Over-dependent people*, fearing separation from mother or mother-figure, tend to develop asthma.
5.	*Persons with a deep-seated emotional conflict* (usually between dependence and aggression) tend to develop hypertension.
6.	*Persons needing love and protection* tend to develop peptic ulers.

For many years Wolff & Wolff studied, through an open fistula, the gastric juices of their laboratory attendant, Tom. Very distinctly, his stomach content and its colour changed with his mood variations.

It is only when tension-energy is expended (by direct or underground expression) and the opposing *Parasympathetic Nervous System* (cranial and sacral Autonomic Nervous System), *stimulating secretion of soothing anti-histamine*, restores balance that an individual's distressing psychosomatic symptoms are relieved. The Sympathetic and Parasympathetic Nervous Systems act in 'seesaw'-like opposition to each other.

Inequilibrium is the state pertaining when:

the Sympathetic Nervous System is dominant, the organism being disturbed by biochemical over-activity designed to change behaviour so as to restore equilibrium, ie to achieve homeostasis (see pp 89–93).

Equilibrium is the state pertaining when:

the Parasympathetic Nervous System is dominant. The organism, soothed by anti-histamine, is lulled to a feeling of restful well-being. By the process of homeostasis nature tries to restore equilibrium.

The Parasympathetic Nervous System can be stimulated by patting, stroking, fondling, rocking movements in the sacral and cranial areas of the Autonomic Nervous System. This reaction is initiated by the mother when she fondles, nurses and soothes her baby, and in adulthood is brought to fruition by the sex partner.

Implications of the psychosomatic link between cerebral seats of emotion, and biological needs, are examined in later sections dealing with the mother–child relationship, feeding, midwifery and, later, with motivation.

Clearly then, *an individual's personality is much affected by the 'trigger-like' excitability or, alternatively, by the placidity of the Sympathetic Nervous System* he inherits.

People whose tension-energy and drive 'get things done', or who are easily 'worked up', have highly reactive Sympathetic Nervous Systems. Stodgy, placid people, who are seldom aroused, exhibit slow-reacting or sluggish Sympathetic Nervous Systems. Neither group is to be praised or blamed for its own individual pattern.

Anxiety is differentiated from fear, which reaction has a specific source or object which the person can identify and describe. Anxiety is a more diffuse overall reaction.

Anxiety is communicated interpersonally, eg if a nurse is talking with a patient who is anxious, she will need to guard against herself becoming anxious. Factors predisposing the extent of anxiety lie in the individual's inherent frontal lobe and Sympathetic Nervous System reaction patterns and his previous life experience.

Erikson (see chapter 11) and others have shown that physical and emotional disorders tend to cluster around periods of major life-change crisis.

Life-change Scales were developed to measure stress in terms of these changes. Holmes & Rahe, having interviewed 400 men and women of varying ages, backgrounds and marital status, constructed a classic Life Change Scale. In that minority groups in the United States, and people in both underdeveloped and highly industrialized countries, give much the same ratings to stressful events, this scale is considered to be fairly universally applicable. Events are ranked in order from the most stressful (death of a spouse: 100 points) to the least (minor violations of the law: 11 points). When their life-change units amounted to between 200 and 300 points over a period of one year, more than half the subjects encountered health problems during that period. When scores rose above 300 points, 79% of the subjects became ill the following year.*

Life-change Scale†

Life event	Life-change value	Life event	Life-change value
Death of spouse	100	Change in responsibilities at work	29
Divorce	73	Son or daughter leaving home	29
Marital separation	65	Trouble with in-laws	29
Jail term	63	Outstanding personal achievement	28
Death of close family member	63	Wife begins or stops work	26
Personal injury or illness	53	Begin or end school	26
Marriage	50	Change in living conditions	25
Fired from job	47	Revision of personal habits	24
Marital reconciliation	45	Trouble with boss	23
Retirement	45	Change in work hours or conditions	20
Change in health of family member	44	Change in residence	20
Pregnancy	40	Change in schools	20
Sex difficulties	39	Change in recreation	19
Gain of new family member	39	Change in Church activities	19
Business readjustment	39	Change in social activities	18
Change in financial state	38	Mortgage or Loan less than $10 000	17
Death of close friend	37	Change in sleeping habits	16
Change to different line of work	36	Change in number of family get-togethers	15
Change in number of arguments with spouse	35	Change in eating habits	15
Mortgage over $10 000	31	Vacation	13
Foreclosure of mortgage or loan	30	Christmas	12
		Minor violations of the law	11

† This scale is also known as the Holmes and Rahe Social Readjustment Rating Scale.

* Holmes, T H & R H Rahe 'The Social Readjustment Rating Scale.' *Journal of Psychosomatic Research* **11:** 213–18, 437. 1967.

STRESS MANAGEMENT: common stress precipitants include

<u>Change of:</u>
place (especially in migration, job transfer, hospitalization)
tasks
physical condition
alert the organism to anxiety:

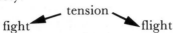

How can we render change less threatening?
Sue Breton* recommends the following tension/stress reducing techniques

1.   Establishment of, and adherence to, <u>routines</u> which
      provide   (i)   reassuring familiarity (see also nursing process pp 224-230)
                        (ii) safer structure to reduce feelings of frightening rootlessness,
                        (iii) break threatening tasks and exposures into smaller, more tolerable and thus manageable units

    Familiar religious services and prayers may soothe and convey feelings of superhuman protection. Regular exercise, meals and good sleep provide temporary escape, a "breathing" space between waves of internalized anxiety and panic, and thus constitute demonstrations of mastery, comfort and well-being.

2.   Spatial imagery to break down the frightening, or depressing, whole into more containable and manageable parts.

    "Imagine you are sweeping your fears away from the whole big field of your life into a small box. There they are closed in, ready for resolving in special "worry" and "problem solving" time. For the rest keep your mind on the clear, manageable field of every day life."

3.   *Relaxation* slipping into self hypnosis adapted to the client's own personality and life story.

    "You are lying under the warm sun beside the gentle, rhythmic waves of a never ending sea. The sunset rays are a golden path to eternity.
    Clench and tighten all your muscles . . . hands, feet, neck. Let go slowly.
    Now the muscles of your face are loose and heavy and relaxed.
    Your back is sinking through the sand.
    Your arms—your hands, your fingers are heavy and loose.
    Your legs, your thigh, your knees your feet are heavy and loose.
    The light of the sun is gentle, warm—
    It is carrying you away to peace and emptiness.
    When you awaken
       your fears of e.g. punishment
                    cancer
       will be smaller
       you will overcome them
       they will recede

* Breton, Sue (Cardiff); From Panic Attacks to Stress Management. The Evolution and Generalization of Treatment Technology Techniques. An address delivered to the General Meeting of the Association of Clinical Psychologists in Private Practice. London, Sunday September 18th 1988.

Individually designed self-hypnotic tapes

  (i) provide the client with repetitive, self-administered stress and panic relief for individually spaced self training routines.

 (ii) preserve the client's
                self esteem
                self generated power.

4.   Biofeedback is a scientific approach to anxiety management. A biofeedback machine measures physical response to stress, and flashes a signal to the person using it when his or her anxiety level starts to rise. Over a period of time the person can learn to lower the signal by consciously relaxing until able to control feelings of anxiety without needing to use the machine. A newer development is chemically dyed adhesive paper spots recording tension levels.

5.   **Assertion training**
    Many people who are insecure and lack confidence in their dealings with others suffer from anxiety. Assertion training gives people greater confidence and a more positive outlook on life. It helps them *express their feelings, needs and opinions so they stand the best chance of being understood and getting what they want from a relationship or situation.* It is especially useful for women who are by tradition conditioned to behave passively in some situations. Assertion training especially role play teaches identification of needs and rights. It expresses *assertiveness* without being *aggressive.* Some local authorities now offer day and evening classes in assertion*

Peplau[†] identified anxiety as:

  (i) <u>mild anxiety</u>—that tension of everyday living which, by mobilizing bio-chemical energy
      alerts the organism for action;
      increases the perceptual field and attention span;
      motivates:
          problem-solving
          creativity
          overcoming of obstacles
          learning
          growth

 (ii) <u>moderate anxiety</u>—which concentrates on immediate problems and fear imprints moderate anxiety:
      focuses on trouble area,
      narrows perceptual area,
      blocks out periphery.
    The subject sees, hears and grasps less of his general environment; selective attention may be extended back to the task in hand by environmental prodding.

---

* MIND Publications National Association for Mental Health 22 Harley Street, London WIN 2 ED: Anxiety—Fact Sheet Nog.

† Peplau, H. Interpersonal Techniques: The Crux of Psychiatric Nursing. *Am J Nurse.* 62.53.54 June 1962.

(iii) <u>severe anxiety</u>—the subject loses his mental shift, and perseverates or focuses his attention and activities intensely on his problems, fears and conflicts
If he fears his indigestion is due to cancer *he may think of nothing else*. All his behaviour is aimed at getting relief from his fears, problems and conflicting needs. He may need respite from his predicament in order to overcome his fears, work out his problems and resolve his priorities—to clear his mind.

(iv) <u>panic</u>, is the fourth level of anxiety. It is associated with awe, terror and dread. Terrifying details are blown out of proportion and take over the subject's thought processes
Involuntarily Exaggerated biochemical tension-energy
overcomes controlled activity → loss of voluntary, directed control
'Panic involves the disorganization of the personality. It is a state in which a person can no longer function as an organized human being . . . . It is a frightening and paralyzing experience for the individual in which he is unable to communicate or function effectively. It is incompatible with life and if it continued over a long period exhaustion and death would result.'*

Panic attacks

The sufferer will experience some, or all, of these symptoms:

1. <u>Recognition of panic 'imprints'</u>
  (i) reality danger and its terror reaction, eg the impact of cancer diagnosis
 (ii) obsessional images

An obsessional image is that *mental picture* of the past, or distressing threatening present (visual, auditory, sensory), which will not go away. It may consist, for example, of compulsively reliving a traumatic experience, or fear, of being trapped in a burning building. Any related stimulus, such as the glow of a red light under a door, *may trigger a panic response*. The more the sufferer tries *not* to think about it, the more terror will pervade—even to the exclusion of all else. The accuracy and persistence of fear imprints illustrate the manner in which they may become as powerful as delusions of 'the real thing'.

Fear feeds upon itself. Other obsessional thoughts may complicate the web of terror: some illogical dreaded 'sacrifice' may 'save' others by stalling the fire.

'If I jump off the balcony the others will be saved.'

Thus guilt-fixated, 'forbidden', often destructive thoughts reinforce panic stimuli and the *dread they precipitate:*

'Oh no—here it comes again!'

(See Obsessive compulsion pp 62-63,119.)

2. Mobilization of biochemical tension-energy as for 'Fight or Flight' acutely disturbing psychosomatic changes (pp 32 et seq) to reinforce the terror cycle:
accelerated breathing → hyperventilation
                        carbon dioxide insufficiency
panting, breathlessness

* Stuart, G W and Sundeen, S J. *The Principles and Practice of Psychiatric Nursing.* Mosby. St Louis, Toronto, London 1979.

racing heart
dizziness
chest pain
shaking and trembling
cold shivers, 'right down to my bones'
hot flushes and sweating
nausea and vomiting
tension across the shoulders
'a tight band around my head', tension headaches or migraine.

3. 'Flight' via the adjustment mechanism of *dissociation* (p 130), ie distancing; the feeling of being outside looking in.

4. Feelings of inescapable helplessness: 'I'm trapped—there's no way out for me!'

5. Inability to concentrate on anything other than the dreaded fear stimulus and its offshoot ramifications:
   inability to manage the task in hand
   reinforced panic: 'I can't break out—I'm going to fail my exam!'
   inability to concentrate, blocking vocational goals and ability to give of oneself in intimate relationships.

6. 'Flight' escape into drugs or alchohol; withdrawal into fantasy compensation, obsessive eating or anorexia. Actual physical escape.

7. Feelings of hopelessness, worthlessness, depression.

8. Depression.

9. Suicide.

Handling the attack

1. Have ready a strong, demanding 'Intrusive', ie a *'safe' substitute thought sequence*, such as a multiplication table, a clothes list for a holiday, a grocery shopping list. Draw the panic-blocking thought out and *concentrate hard* on it until the 'danger' stimulus has receded.
   "Body searching" compulsions, followed by fear slanted perceptions of imagined lumps or swellings are common in persons who have suffered actual cancer or a frightening scare. Fear and obsessions feed on themselves. The more intense the search the greater the terror. Sometimes it is possible to break into the terror or cycle by
   (i) concentration on a substitute invasive thought (see above) or soothing scene
   (ii) purposefully resisting "examining" until the danger of escalating symptoms abates.

2. To counteract hyperventilation it is necessary to *restore carbon dioxide balance*. Avoid breathing quickly. It is important to breathe smoothly and slowly. Where possible, breathe into a paper bag. Breathe out in small steps:
   breathe in
   hold it
   exhale slowly—one step every 3 seconds
   repeat.
   Relaxation Technique see p. 499
   Do not gulp—rather swallow a few times.

3.   If the attack is aggravated by environmental pressures, try to *escape for a few minutes* to resolve anxieties and conflicts and restore proportions. The sluice room is often a convenient haven!

The Behaviourist approach

Some panic states are 'eliminated' by *repeated confrontation and intellectualization of comforting evidence of solution*. For example:

to overcome anxiety about accuracy of blood grouping it is usually helpful to recheck your records, reassured by the confirmatory witness of a colleague-with repetition of successful experiences panic should recede.

Increased exposure to the feared stimulus within a 'safe' supportive relationship may show that nothing terrible happens.

blood group test **+** fear of mistake → panic attack
blood group test **+** fear **+** check and comforting support → success
repetition of association with success experience → new 'conditioned' response
blood group test → success expectation → confidence
                                        → panic reaction elimination
(Learning by conditioning pp 152 et seq; Systematic desensitization p 161; see also application in the paediatric ward p 165.)

Reinforced generalized self-confidence usually diminishes panic. But remember:
Careful efficiency is excellent.
Compulsive rechecking is sick!
So let go! Move on!

Psychotherapy

Tracing back the image or life imprint to its source—the original, repressed or suppressed, fearful, painful guilt-laden, humiliating experience from which its disorganizing associations emanate.
Insight. Catharsis. Re-education (The Psycho-analytic Approach chapter 3, pp 60 et seq).

Usually varying combinations of 'on-the-spot' insight (cognition), behaviourist and in-depth psycho-analytic methods, ie the *Eclectic approach*, are the most fruitful. Probably no one can ever completely overcome ingrained fear. One aims to *teach ways of coping with fear*, which should minimize pain and interference with everyday living.

2. HEREDITY AND PERSONALITY

There is increasing evidence of the importance of *heredity* in the formation of individual personality. There has long been genetic evidence to prove that external physical attributes (such as height, complexion, hair texture, nose shape), as well as glandular and other internal structures, are inherited. These physical attributes interacting with the enviroment, affect personality structure.

The *innate*, probably genetically determined capacity to learn, to solve problems, to adapt to and overcome the enviroment, is currently termed *'Fluid Intelligence'*.

The amount of *knowledge acquired* or achieved is termed *'Crystallized Intelligence'*.

Identical twins, who, because they have developed from the same original germ cell, are endowed with the same set of genes, tend to possess similar intelligence patterns. Non-identical twins, on the other hand, who do not share the same set of genes, present intelligence only as similar as that found in ordinary siblings. (Opposing evidence is presented in the work of Kamin (1974): *The Science and Politics of IQ.*) For the nature and measurement of intelligence see p 144.

Persons with endogenous mental handicap certainly tend to produce mentally handicapped offspring.

The manner in which special talents in sport, the arts, mathematics, etc 'run in families' is borne out by statistics, and by the observation that no amount of practice and stimulation will turn the average club member into a Wimbledon champion, nor an adequate newspaper reporter into a Shakespeare. Such abilities are either familial, or depend on some chance combination of genes unlikely to reproduce itself exactly in successive generations. Many aptitudes may rest on an inborn structural superiority of the muscular system or special neural integration.

Certainly the potentiality for certain types of physical and mental illness appears to be inborn. Diabetes mellitus, for instance, 'runs in families'. Schizophrenia (the most common psychosis) is now thought to result from faulty metabolism in which there is an hereditary component, probably in the form of an enzyme block. Metabolism being incomplete, unmetabolized food becomes toxic, clouding brain function.

Just as the myriads of Nature's gene combinations have designed each individual to be of different external appearance, so is he unique in his psychological design. No two patients, or nurses, react exactly the same way in similar sets of circumstances.

The environment and the life story consititute the mould in which the individual's hereditary potential is confined or brought to fruition.

Heredity may be compared to a liquid contained in the bottle of enviroment. We shall see that heredity and environment—like two blades of a pair of scissors, or the two sides of a coin—are both equally important and cannot, in reality, be considered independently.

3. THE LIFE STORY: THE MOTHER–CHILD RELATIONSHIP

Little Frederik, 9, died of homesickness . . . in the hardest possible way. His starved, dehydrated, exposed body was found under a thorn tree, 45 km from Aroab, where he had been sent to stay with his aunt by his mother and stepfather.

His home was in Koes, a tiny hamlet 100 miles away, and ten days ago, after weeks of crying for his mother, he set out to return to her. Barefoot, wearing only a shirt and shorts, Freddie walked along the dusty road dividing the hostile Namib and Kalahari deserts.

His shrivelled little body was found under a thorn tree. He had given up the fight and died of exhaustion, hunger and thirst.

This section should be read in conjunction with 'Bonding—The Mother–Child Relationship' in the chapter on the Psychology of Midwifery, pp 390-412.

The human infant comes into the world in a state of extreme helplessness, much more so than most animals. He would quickly perish except for the loving care of his parents, especially his mother. For nine months he has been living a happy, comfortable, parasitic existence, eating, sleeping, eliminating all day, being rocked and kept pleasantly warm in his dark, cosy, watery intra-uterine environment. Within a few moments of birth he must learn to breathe for himself, to switch over to his own circulatory system, to adjust to temperature changes and to his first primitive fears—loud noises, loss of balance, and sudden bright light. Within a few hours he must switch over to his own digestive system. At no time of life, except in death, does physiology undergo such change.

Our experiences—events, triumphs, sorrows, the contacts we have with others—all help to mould us as we grow. One reason each of us reacts so differently lies in the widely variant sequence of events to which life exposes us. Even siblings do not share the same environment; whether a child be first or last born; whether he be handsome or ugly; healthy or sickly; clever or simple, will all affect the way in which he is treated by his family.

Some developmental stages appear to be more receptive to outside influences than others. Our relationships and experiences with people surrounding us in *early life*—parents, brothers, sisters, teachers, friends, grandparents—appear to be particularly (and permanently) influential, establishing the pattern of our adult fears, dislikes, loves and hates, pessimism or optimism.

Experiences during the first six years of life, which few people can remember, are extremely important in moulding personality, for they are 'stored' in various levels of unconscious functioning (see chapter 3). The baby's first intense contact outside of himself comes through *the nursing relationship and feeding*.

When feeding goes well the mother figure is associated with prompt relief from hunger pain, gentle touch and a feeling of warm physiological well-being; when feeding goes badly (usually through rigid, arbitrary four-hourly feeding, under-feeding, digestive upsets, etc) mother is associated with deprivation and frustration—emotions which spread out to attach themselves to other human beings, setting the stage for social complications, emotional isolation and other maladjustments.

Tactile comfort Relief from hunger pain ↓ Physiologically satisfying, happy, feeding associations ↓ Good mother–child relationship ↓ Other happy, well-adjusted social relationships	Prolonged hunger pain Long crying, deprivation of tactile comfort Unsatisfying feeding associations ↓ Deprivation, frustration, aggression spread out ↓ Other unfulfilled, unhappy, aggressive relationships

Crying is not simply a distress signal, but Nature's powerful communicator. Studies have shown that infants as young as eight weeks appreciate their ability to make things happen through crying. The functions of crying include:

attempts to cope with environmental limitations and restrictions,
relief from helplessness resultant upon his immature visual–motor skills,
the child's attempt to console himself in the face of hunger, pain, loneliness.

Crying, by giving him some control over his environment, *should teach a child optimism*—that he is competent, loved and cared for. If his cries go unanswered he feels distresed, confused and powerless. So nurses and mothers should learn to understand and answer children's cry-messages: The story of an experienced paediatrician who, in the middle of the night, asked a distraught mother to put her child on the phone in order to 'speak for himself' and from the nature of his cry successfully diagnosed earache, is not unfounded.

The pitch and rhythm of a baby's cry hold promise as a diagnostic indicator of

neurological disorders,   anger,
stomach ache,   trauma etc.

Her response to her baby's cry tells much of a mother's relationship with him. Having empathy with his distress is very different from the anger, impatience and general stress-reaction exhibited by a mother in danger of becoming a baby batterer.

Dr Susan Crockenberg, Associate Professor of Human Development at the University of California, summarizes the work of several researchers thus:

'The more responsive a mother is to her baby, the less it cries, the more securely attached it gets to its environment, and the more readily it develops trust.'

That a self-regulated, fully fed, warmly dressed baby, experiencing an abundance of physical contact, and a warm satisfying relationship with one special figure, has a good chance of becoming a contented and well-adjusted adult, and that with opposite conditions the reverse also applies, has been illustrated by much careful research, among the most interesting being that conducted on other species of animals.

A pioneer in the field of animal studies was <u>DAVID LEVY</u>, whose experiments on litters of puppies demonstrated the close relationship between bodily needs and emotional satisfaction. In his famous *Six Puppy Experiment* Levy divided the litter thus: (See opposite page.)

This was a pioneer among experiments showing that *early maternal deprivation and the denial of spontaneous access to sucking situations, caused permanent personality changes.*

<u>WILLIAM C MENNINGER</u> of the Menninger Foundation, the world's largest training centre for psychiatrists, says 'Satisfaction not only comes from the taste of food itself and the relief of hunger, but from the process of eating, or, more specifically, sucking. Even more satisfaction comes from the cuddling that goes with the nursing period, and from the adult attention necessary for the feeding process. The presence or absence of these satisfactions leaves a deep imprint on the baby's personality.'

There are many people who are *never able to satiate their need for mouth activity* as a chief source of satisfaction, indulging in compulsive gossiping and eating, in gum-chewing, chain-smoking or excessive drinking—often these are people who have been deprived of satisfying mouth activity at the appropriate babyhood period. While breast-feeding does provide special tactile satisfaction and warm interflow emphasis is *not* on the indispensability of breast-feeding but rather on the indispensability of sucking, nursing, fondling, physical closeness and 'adult attention', which *stimulate the Parasympathetic Nervous System to secrete anti-histamine*.

SIX PUPPIES

CONTROL GROUP	EXPERIMENTAL GROUP	
2 puppies breast-fed	4 puppies bottle-fed (no access to mother)	
	Artificial Feeding	
2 puppies were permitted *to suckle on mother's breast* whenever they so desired.	2 from teats with moderately large holes.	2 from teats with very large holes.

RESULTS

Thrived well. Little sucking activity except from mother's nipples.	5 minutes per feed. Frequently engaged in vigorous, destructive sucking and chewing on various objects; more restless than breast-fed puppies.	2 minutes per feed. Engaged in continuous vigorous, destructive sucking and chewing activities, even on each other's bodies.
Played in a lively manner, rested contentedly and showed normal tolerance of frustrated desires.	Could not bear frustration, in the face of which they became angry and aggressive: (i) Inability to bear frustration, (ii) sudden displacement of anger and aggression on objects and people persisted throughout life.	Restless, fought, snarled, irritable, combative, lost weight; finally in their unsuccessful efforts to find satisfying substitute mouth activity and physical warmth, they bit each other to death.
Were able to postpone a desired satisfaction, such as the relief of thirst.		
Proved amiable pets for children, being free of sudden outbursts of aggressive behaviour.		

Outpouring of anti-histamine counteracts the disturbing effects of Sympathetic Nervous System arousal, resulting in feelings of soothed well-being.

Artificial Feeding, provided that

(i) it conforms to the baby's own individual requirements rather than to a rigid, often irrelevant four-hour schedule,

(ii) it is conducted in leisurely manner, by the mother herself, to the accompaniment of cuddling, nursing, etc,

(iii) the teat hole allows for sufficient sucking activity (it should not permit more than 20 drops per minute when the bottle is inverted),

need not impede healthy personality development. It is certainly preferable to pressure exerted on the mother to breast-feed if, through a lifetime of 'shame' associations, she has come to look upon breast-feeding with distaste and disgust; or when, through jealousy of her own mother's breast-feeding of a sibling rival, she has developed feelings of resentment and hostility towards breast-feeding.

Fortunately, young mothers today are less vulnerable to false prudery and more receptive to joyful participation in natural functions. Opportunity to talk out emotional problems; explanation, reassurance and support usually smooth the way to the special close bond inherent in successful breast-feeding. (See Breast Feeding, p 405.)

The baby feels hunger as generalized pain.

The emotional satisfaction and feeling of physical well-being which come with eating remain, in most people, an integral part of their personality. At birth, his mouth is the infant's most highly developed voluntary organ. He gets his earliest pain-relief, pleasure and satisfaction from mouth activity—and from the maternal fondling, and feeling of warm love and security which come with sucking. When Princess Diana slipped her finger into William's mouth she performed a happy service to babies around the world!

From his earliest days the baby learns to associate

(1) relief from hunger pain,
(2) fondling stimulation of the Parasympathetic Nervous System → soothing anti-histamine → physiological well-being,
(3) mouth activity, and mouth satisfaction,

   with mother love, safety and security.

Hence, all his life, especially when he is under stress, he will seek mouth satisfaction, both for its own sake and for its association with mother love, safety and security.

When an obese person is put on diet we are denying him not only food but, more important, the adult equivalent of that mother love, security and well-being which have always accompanied mouth activity. It is no wonder he becomes resentful, depressed and tense, often 'taking out' or displacing (p 121) his frustrated tension-energy on the nurse who brings him that despised lettuce leaf and slice of tomato!

In times of stress a person may become a chain-smoker (to die of lung cancer), or a 'compulsive eater' (to die of coronary thrombosis)!

Besides healing, modern medical knowledge has, alas, taken from living many of its spontaneous, natural joys and comforts.

The close connection between eating and emotional satisfaction has, of late, been emphasized by neurological research indicating *anatomical proximity between seats of emotional satisfaction, and the sense of physical well-being which accompanies a full stomach.* Both centres are situated in the hypothalamus.

When we deny a patient mouth satisfaction such as a bedtime feeding bottle, smoking or eating, we may remove his main source of satisfaction and comfort at just that time when, being in pain, fear and tension, this symbol of mother love, safety and security is most needed. The data collection stage of the Nursing Process should avoid such errors.

It is reasonable to believe that the long, foodless period from 6 pm to 7 am which characterizes the hospital night adds to the night-time burden of pain, noise and anxiety, rendering hospital nights so restless, so long, so demoralizing. Here again one would submit a plea for emphasis on 'patient needs' rather than on rigidity of ward procedure. In fact, adapting to patient needs, several overseas hospitals are serving later main-meal dinners and night-time snacks from the disposable thermostatic containers developed for air-travel.

We are familiar with the comfort afforded the stressed patient by a 'nice warm cuppa'. In understanding the real significance of mouth activity, the desirability of giving the patient a cup of tea, a piece of cake, a cigarette(for a child a sweet or a cool drink) on admission, or in other stressful circumstances, is self-evident. For, *in offering mouth satisfaction we are also giving a deeply ingrained symbol of affection, acceptance, safety and security.*

Knowledge of the manner in which, under natural circumstances, eating and sleeping go together is a powerful support for the time-proven principle of self-regulated or 'self-demand' baby feeding. This method also provides more mouth activity, frequent fondling and mammary stimulation.

It is sometimes necessary for his health that the mother deny her child favourite sources of eating satisfaction (as, for instance, in the case of a *diabetic child*). Mouth satisfaction being so deeply associated with the mother figure, in withholding the preferred food she is, at a symbolic level, denying him that maternal love, warmth and comfort upon which he has come to rely. At an *intellectual level* he may accept the medical explanation for this denial, but *intellectual acceptance* is far removed from *emotional acceptance.*

In order to preserve her relationship with her child, a mother will need to spend considerable thought and time on other compensation activities which will reassure him of the warmth of her love. Permissible substitute mouth activity, such as sugarless chewing-gum or biltong, is often comforting and reassuring.

To a lesser, but still significant degree, necessary *withholding of mouth satisfaction* in dieting, presurgical preparation, etc, *imposes a strain on nurse/patient relationships*, to counteract which the astute nurse will seek opportunities for substitute assurances of her goodwill and affection. She will also request that the anaesthetist instruct to *minimum individual denial requirements*, rather than submit patients to the strain of unnecessary group restrictions.

Research workers, while admitting that opportunity for spontaneous suckling (either on the breast or on an appropriate artificial teat) is of importance, have isolated other important aspects of the young animal's need for maternal closeness. Harlow, for instance, experimenting on monkeys, divided his subjects into:

1. The control group—comprising monkeys with free access to their natural mothers.
2. An experimental group deprived of mother and mother substitute.
3. An experimental group deprived of the natural mother, but provided with:

    (a) a wire mother subsitute, to which food was attached,
    (b) a wire mother substitute, covered with cotton wool and soft towelling (providing substitute 'cuddly' tactile satisfaction).

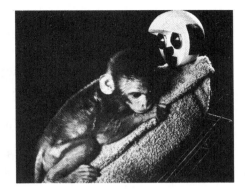

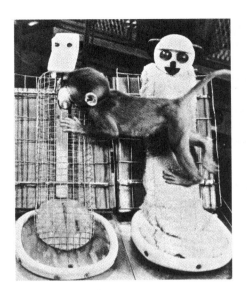

'Although fed via the wire mother, the infant spends more time with the terry cloth mother. The terry cloth mother provides security and a safe base from which to explore strange objects.'

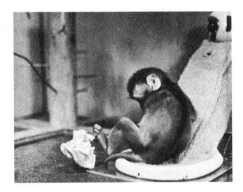

Result of Harlow's experiments

1. All experimental monkeys showed a preference for the substitute figures rather than no mother at all.

2. Monkeys comprising group 3 showed a marked and 'statistically significant' preference for the towel-covered 'cuddly' artificial mothers, despite the fact that the wire mother became associated with feeding satisfaction. Some died of starvation rather than give up their places on the cuddly subsitute mother.

This experiment demonstrates the primary importance of *tactile experience* with the mother substitute. On the introduction of a grotesque, fear-stimulating toy, the monkeys fled to their cuddly substitute mothers, clinging frantically for reassurance, although they had never known a real mother figure.

In forms of surgery and burn treatment, where handling of the patient is reduced to a minimum, he may suffer from *tactile deprivation*. Even though he may *understand* the reason for withdrawal of physical contact, he may *feel* rejected, anxious and guilty lest he has become 'untouchable'.

Visiting parents and friends should be encouraged to make tactile contact with the patient. A patient is quick to respond with pleasure and reassurance to the nurse who holds his hand or puts an arm around his shoulder.

Old people, now deprived of physical expressions of warmth and love, find some substitute comfort in physiotherapy.

Long-term results of maternal deprivation

The 'experimental', 'maternally deprived' monkeys demonstrated:

(1) *lack of adjustment* in adult life;

(2) severe sexual and parental maladjustments, including

   (a) *impotence:* lacking exposure to sexual activity, there was inability to participate therein;

   (b) *infertility*—both physiological and through disinterest in sexual relationships;

   (c) the fact that those who did evetually, through various interventions, reproduce, showed *deficient maternal reaction* towards their own offspring. Having no experience of warm physical stimulation and response, they were unable to tolerate the needs of their offspring for loving attention. Having developed no patterns of self-control they reacted with aggressive frustration to their offsprings' persistent demands for physical attention, even trying to kill them. In fact several did batter their babies to death. *In order to give love, one has first to know love;*

(3) that emotional maladjustments can be pin-pointed in actual psychosomatic conversion changes; endocrine functioning of maternally deprived animals was adversely affected to the extent of *permanent ill-health* and *premature death.*

Post-mortem examination of these animals showed that, lacking fondling and warm physical contact which in mothering or sexual activity stimulates the Parasympathetic Nervous System to secrete soothing anti-histamine, the Parasympathetic Nervous System itself was physiologically underdeveloped. Absence of Parasympathetic and anti-histaminic dominance, deprived the monkeys of respite periods of quiet, soothing calm. In contrast the stress-associated Sympathetic Nervous System was overdeveloped. Impaired endocrinological balance, resulted in the animal literally burning itself out with tension-energy.

A recent confirmatory study of rats demonstrated that maternally deprived rats showed a stronger anxiety-reaction on exposure to a frightening situation than normally reared rats. This anxiety reaction, accompanied as it was by psychosomatic changes, produced increased stimulatory Sympathetic Nervous System endocrine secretion. The experimentally deprived rats manifested a markedly shorter life-span than did the control group, in whom the stimulatory Sympathetic Nervous System and soothing Parasympathetic Nervous System were more normally balanced.

Research into the effects on human beings of *maternal deprivation* is consistent with that conducted on lower animals.

Examples of events which may have a traumatic effect on the all-important mother-child relationship are:

(a) apparent transfer of love to a new sibling (which, in the elder child, causes jealousy, guilt feelings, anxiety, and general insecurity);

(b) placement in an orphanage, boarding-school, etc;

(c) abandonment (for this is how the child sees it) to strangers in hospital in time of pain and crisis, especially where parents are denied the opportunity of frequently visiting, loving and comforting their children.

In 1956 <u>H Rheingold</u> conducted an experiment to demonstrate the generalization of social responses from the mother figure to other persons. His subjects were 16 six-month-old institutionalized infants.

The experimental group

(i) was tended by only one investigator (*the substitute mother figure*) for eight hours of five days for eight consecutive weeks,
(ii) received more frequent feeding.

The control group was cared for in typical institutional routine, without an individual substitute for mother figure.

Progress tests were applied to all infants at each week of the experiment, plus four additional weeks thereafter. The tests assessed:

(i) auditory responsiveness to three kinds of people, viz the mother substitute, the tester, a stranger;
(ii) visual-motor development on the basis of postural development;
(iii) intellectual development as indicated by cube manipulation.

Results

The experimental group showed much more auditory and social responsiveness to the original stimulus, viz mother figure. Increased responsiveness spread also to extended stimulus—viz the tester and the stranger. The experimental group also presented more smiling, facial reaction.

In contrast with the dramatic effect on social and auditory behaviour, the experimental group manifested *no significant difference on tests of motor development*.

The experimenter believed that the frequency of *individualized contact*, and *reciprocal* and playful social *stimulation*, were of primary importance in stimulating social responsiveness.

Child development experts believe the infant to be attached to the mother figure not only as the result of satisfying *tactile* perceptual experiences and afferent sensation of *hunger-relief* but also by satisfying association with the 'visual schema' or mental image created by her face.

He acquires a *well-organized mental picture* of, and close association with, the whole mother schema, with consequent tendency to:

1. *React with fear to people who differ from his mother schema*, eg strangers and even father. This fear reaction to people other than mother is termed 'stranger anxiety'.

In the context of considerable *experience* and *time* for positive conditioning, anxiety tends to be eliminated, and a more positive 'stranger approach' response built up.

2. *To react with anxiety if the familiar mother schema is absent*. This is termed 'anxiety as a reaction to discrepancy', the discrepancy being resultant upon removal of the familiar mother figure.

The opportunity of making a *'doing something' response, which will again make the mother figure available* to the baby, appears to allay his anxiety.

To illustrate his relief-reaction Rheingold placed a group of 10-month-old children in a strange room under four sets of circumstances:

Result

1. With mother   The infants did not cry.
2. With a stranger   The infants cried within one minute
   (no mother)   of being placed in the room.
3. With toys   The presence of the stranger and
4. Completely alone   toys did not help to alleviate fear.

The strangeness of the room, being inconsistent with the child's 'schemata' or mental image, produced fear, but mother's presence protected the child from anxiety.

To demonstrate the importance of a response which will bring the child into visual or physical contact with mother, Group 1 was connected by an open interleading door to the same room which caused Groups 2, 3 and 4 to cry. Children in Group 1 often crawled into the same strange empty room but did not cry on arriving there. They just investigated and returned to their mothers.

Unlike Groups 2, 3 and 4, children in Group 1 were able to alleviate their fear by 'doing something', namely by returning to mother.

Separation anxiety thus appears to have three components, viz:

 (i)   the discrepancy or schema lack, which results from separation from mother,
 (ii) disruption of habitual response to mother,
(iii) the inability to make a response which will make mother again available.

With time, maturity and favourable experiences teach him that the *can do* something to restore mother's presence, and thus overcome his separation anxiety.

The *mal-effects of long-term hospitalization* have been very closely studied. Results have shown a well-defined clinical entity known as *hospitalism* and defined by Spitz as 'the evil effect of institutional care of infants, placed in institutional care from an early age, particularly from a psychiatric point of view'.

The main features of this condition are:

(a) a failure to gain weight properly, or to grow well in stature, despite the ingestion of a scientifically well-balanced diet;
(b) such infants sleep less and more fitfully than do children even in over-crowded homes;
(c) they pass stools more frequently and appear more prone to infection than do children in the community;
(d) their intellectual development is slower than that of 'control' non-hospitalized children with similar IQ scores.

This latter observation is, no doubt, due to:

(a) lack of opportunity for self-care and observational experienes pertaining in the outside world;
(b) lack of exposure to the example and standards set by more mature family members—the institutional child, largely confined to the company of his own age group, does not have opportunities to copy the more mature behaviour of older children and closely associated adults;
(c) lack of that stimulation to further effort provided by the doting interest and warm praise of family members.

This depression of intellectual growth applies also, as we shall see, to institutionalized mentally defective children.

In the course of two studies Spitz concealed small movie cameras in the cots of his hospital subjects—from these 'candid camera' strips he compiled 'Grief', a film which has become a classic in child development libraries throughout the world.

Following on the work of Spitz, Goldfarb, one of the world's most eminent social psychologists, conducted a now famous *study of the lasting effects of long-term institutionalization*. He compared the fate of children institutionalized for long periods in the first three years of life, and then transferred to foster homes, with those who had been in foster homes from birth. From these studies he observed the following long-term results of early deprivation of the mother, or constant mother substitute:

(a) retardation of intellectual processes—'deprived' children had difficulty in grasping songs, rhymes, stories, number concepts, and in sizing up social situations;

  Psychometrically the institutionalized children presented with mean IQ 68 as compared with mean IQ 96 in the foster-raised controls.

(b) absence of normal patterns of self-control. The children were over-active, unmanageable and given to persistent temper tantrums;

(c) the children were always demanding affection and attention from staff, visitors, etc. They were insatiable in these demands, but were unable to employ the self-control essential to the maintenance of long-term relationships. Their social lives were filled with shallow, fleeting relationships never reaching fulfilment;

(d) there was about them an emotional 'flattening'. They had little reaction to failure, appeals for conformity, or disapproval. They manifested little 'drive', sustained ambition and initiative.

When he followed these children into adolescence and adult live, Goldfarb found that within this group there was an abnormally high rate of habitual crime. They did, indeed tend to become psychopathic, lacking normal social values, social conscience, self-control and responsibility.

Authorities now maintain that this chronic and serious lack of social conformity is often due to the absence of a strong mother–child relationship.

The mother–child relationship as the nucleus of socialization processes

Resulting from the baby's early hunger-relief, pleasure-attachment to the mother-stimulus:

1. Through association, positive outgoing pleasure responses will spread to other people (Similarly, negative hostile responses, such as those resulting from unhappy withholding feeding situations will also spread out to others.)
2. The infant develops very organized schemata (Piaget's term for mental image) for mother, combining her voice, shape, face, form etc.

However, these association responses will not 'spread out' to stimuli very different in origin.

To illustrate these hypotheses, Sackett, Porter & Holmes in 1965 divided monkeys into three groups:

Experimental Division

Year I	Year II	Year III
Group 1. Those reared by human beings for first *three weeks* of life and then isolated in wire cages. This group had no contact with monkeys until CA 1 year.	All monkeys lived in wire cages with regular opportunity to play with other monkeys.	Each monkey placed in circular chamber—human on one side, monkey on other. Monkey could choose to— (i) join the human (ii) join other monkey (iii) stay in centre
Group 2. Reared by natural mothers until CA 1 year.		
Group 3. Those isolated at birth, neither seeing nor touching humans nor monkeys until CA 6 months; then placed in wire cages until CA 1 year.		

Overall Results

Group No. 1. The early association with the human being had apparently resulted in persistent human attachment, even though it had occurred only in the first three weeks of life.	Group No. 2. Most often found in association with another monkey.	Group No. 3. The isolated monkey remained virtually isolated, approaching neither monkey nor man.

It is accepted that generalization of responses from earliest objects to later similar objects pertains also in the human infant.

We have noted that in 1956 H Rheingold conducted an experiment demonstrating the generalization of social responses from the mother figure to other persons.

Goldfarb emphasized that within the first six years of life the child is expected to take upon himself the fundamentals of that code of socially-accepted behaviour which we term 'civilization'. He is expected to have moved from his self-indulgent, intra-uterine parasitic life to a life governed by communal responsibility and a high degree of personal subjugation and self-control. By the time he turns 6, he is expected to have taken unto himself the *sacrifices involved* in keeping clean, eating at certain times, taking his turn, telling the truth—all of which are difficult.

The first voluntary sacrifice usually demanded of an infant occurs when, at about 18 months, the sympathetic mother puts him on a 'potty' and indicates that she would like him to defecate therein.

To the infant the *special person of greatest emotional importance is the mother*, who since birth has relieved his hunger pangs, nursed, comforted and protected him, and *to whom he has attached feelings of love*. When she asks him thus to inhibit his natural impulse for self-relief, to voluntarily bear discomfort, even though this be temporary, she is asking no small sacrifice. But he learns that *if he conforms he will be rewarded by demonstration of that love* upon which, if his relationship with her is good, he sets great store. From this successful infantile experience he soon learns the satisfaction to be gained by conformity. *He learns that small sacrifices now bring the long-term reward of love and acceptance.*

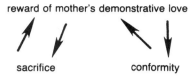

reward of mother's demonstrative love

sacrifice   conformity

So kids, like grown-ups, need plently of kisses and cuddles.

Developing patterns of conformity spread out from his relationship with his mother to the family, the school, social groups and society as a whole. For the human personality may be likened unto a quiet, calm pond into which one casts a stone. From the central core there will spread out concentric circles, each ripple reproducing the pattern of the original impact.

Thus behaviour which has fulfilled its purpose, and succeeded in the early, impressionable years in obtaining the highly prized reward of mother's special love and praise, and later of popularity and social achievement is reinforced, to emerge in fixed behaviour patterns.

DEVELOPING PATTERNS OF CONFORMITY

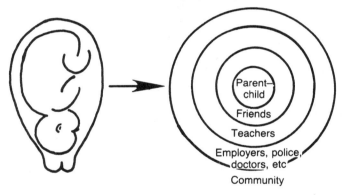

Continuing into childhood this association of mother with her love-rewarding relationship and reliable protection, he turns to her for the refuge, solace and security she spells for him whenever life becomes too hard or frightening. Where punishment has associated mother with pain, the relationship is imperilled and no longer serves its important function as motivator for conformity.

In the world of the *institutional child*, on the other hand, there is *no special person of his own whom he loves enough or who is sufficiently important to him to warrant sacrifice.* Lacking an all-absorbing relationship through which to work, he lacks that special love-object whose love-reward is sufficiently important to provide incentive for establishing patterns of conformity.

The duty nurse who places him on a potty means little to him. *She* has not removed his hunger pains, loved and comforted him from his earliest hours. He feels no desire to please her. Why should he make himself uncomfortable for her? So he balks at toilet training and other conformity sacrifices.

He goes into the world with *no particular love-object* and, in fact, often with resentment towards the community as a whole. Lacking incentive to please those around him, he goes through life with no motivation to please anyone, or any social institution. Soon his lack of conformity brings him against the law, reinforcing his hate of society as a whole. He is now well on the way to a psychopathic record.

Of course, psychopathology is not always due to maternal deprivation. Subnormal intelligence and hormones are possible etiological factors. Marginal brain damage associated with an abnormal EEG and reduced frontal lobe control is classically associated with psychopathic behaviour and subclinical epilepsy.

In 1965, motivated by a similar study in English State hospitals, Dr Patricia Jacobs conducted a chromosome survey at the Scottish maximum security hospital at Carstairs. Pertaining to XYY patterns, among 315 male inmates, 10 had an extra Y chromosome relative to XYY occurrence 1 in 1 000 male births in the general population.*

Such hospitals house a large proportion of patients committed for criminal offences involving violence. In fact, histories reveal that fluctuation between passive inadequacy and impulsive behaviour which characterizes the psychopathic personality. The theory that the Y chromosome is a developmental decelerator would also account for the pathological immaturity of persons carrying the chromosomal pattern XYY (see p 335).†

An excess of aggressive male inheritance may be associated with disproportion-ate violence. Nevertheless follow-up studies fail to replicate chromosomal etiology of psychopathology.

While the hospital population studied was admittedly highly selective, geneticists do consider these findings a significant lead.

During the 1939–45 war, Dr John Bowlby showed that many children were emotionally more *adversely affected by 'evacuation'* to the country, and thus by *separation from their mothers,* than by exposure at their mothers' sides, to the grimmest *air-raids.*

'Evacuated' children were characterized by psychosomatic tension symptoms such as excessive sexual self-arousal (masturbation), thumb sucking, nail-biting, head-banging, urticaria, asthma, etc. They also showed a marked tendency to *distrust, inability, to make lasting friendships, compensatory stealing, lying* and *aggressive behaviour,* which behaviour patterns persisted into adulthood.

Summarizing: if the mother–child relationship is weak, distorted; demanding or rejecting or disrupted, by, for exmaple, hospitalization, the 'maternally deprived' child may tend to:

(a) become anxious and insecure

(b) become over-demanding and ungiving in his relationships within the family, within his environment, and within society as a whole, for our responses and attitudes to the world spread out in fixed behaviour patterns emanating from the all-important early mother–child relationship.

   If he has not learned to give and receive love in the mother–child

---

* *Sex Determination, Mental Subnormality, Crime & Delinquency in Males*—W H Price Medical Research Council Clinical and Population Cytogenics Research Unit and University Dept of Medicine, Western General Hospital, Edinburgh 4.

† Professor Christopher Ounsted, Director, Child Develpment Centre, Oxford.

relationship, he may always encounter difficulty in forming lasting friendships and in achieving outgoing loving sexual fulfilment of marriage;

(c) show socially irresponsible behaviour. When early positive patterns of conformity have not been formed in the mother–child relationship, the adult may lack self-control and social responsibility. His inability to postpone immediate personal satisfaction, for the reward of ultimate approval, eventually culminates in psychopathic behaviour. He goes through life 'grabbing' whatever he desires as long as he possibly can, irrespective of distressing consequences or punishment, for negative as well as positive behaviour patterns become firmly entrenched (undersocialized aggressive;

(d) become so unhappy in his real environment that he may form patterns of frequent escape into a compensatory, unreal dream world, until fantasy overcomes reality. When this fantasy world predominates he is headed for mental illness. This quiet, withdrawn behaviour may well be misinterpreted by hospital staff as 'settling down'. Withdrawn behaviour is convenient to the staff, but may well deny the child that emotional outlet, love and reassurance which he needs, and without which his anxieties, depression and resentment may well fester within him;

(e) become so deprived of his mother's love and support when he most needs them that, at an emotional level, he may come to distrust and even to hate her. These feelings of resentment may spread out to other members of the family (especially younger siblings of whom he may already be jealous), and thence to society as a whole. Sometimes a child manifests this resentment by appearing to reject his mother when she comes to visit. In actual fact he is 'punishing' her for 'abandoning' him;

(f) lack normal sources of interest, warmth and comfort. He thus establishes patterns of turning to his own body for comfort in excessive sexual self-arousal, thumb-sucking, head-banging, nail-biting, etc;

(g) artificial intellectual retardation; his intellectual growth may be inhibited by lack of normal opportunities for:

   (i)   mimicking the more mature behaviour of older family members;
  (ii)   stimulation through the doting appreciation of his own family;
 (iii)   automatic learning within the community.

For futher discussion of the detrimental effects of hospitalization and the alleviation thereof, refer to chapter 13, 'The Emotional Effects of Illness upon Children'.

The kibbutz experiment

Addressing the symposium 'Children of the Dream Revisited' at the 94th American Psychological Association Convention, Wahington DC, August 1986 two Israeli psychiatrists, Meshulam Piaves of the Ann Martin Childrens Centre, Piedmont, California and Moshe Yotvat Talmon of the Kaiser Permanente Medical Group, Hayward Ca, author of the book *Growing Up on a Kibbutz: The*

Family System Perspective, discussed the merits and disadvantages of separation in the 'childrens' house'.

Piaves:

> 'We had a *secure, familiar and safe* childhood. I knew everyone around me. I was never alone. We grew up confident and aggressive. We were productive and decisive. Through the years we managed to *stick together through "thick and thin"*. I never knew a key—I never learnt to hide anything.'

But on the negative side:

> 'I never had anything to hide. It was very hard to share every sweet—every toy. We became very *object-orientated*.
>
> We knew who our parents were and what they did, but not about their feelings—their relationships. The emphasis was on what you did, not who you were—"My father is the bookkeeper." The first question was not "Who are you?" but "To what kibbutz do you belong?" *Personal identities were underdeveloped.*
>
> *Lack of close personal relationships made it difficult to form, and keep, our own intimate relationships as we grew up.*
>
> The fact that we bathed, ate and slept with the girls made it difficult to form romantic attachment. Even our dreams were not our own. We were expected to have *group goals,* so that *personal creativity and academic ambitions remained underdeveloped.'*

Talman:

> *'We did not have strong enough emotional tools to develop a sense of "self".*
>
> The *emotional restraint* of the kibbutz environment, the *social pressure on the kids, was enormous.* It was hard to individuate and scary to have a strong group identity, but not enough self-esteem to build one's own personal emotional life nor to make one's own decisions.
>
> We *lost* the principle of each according to his own, and the *ability to fulfil our own psychological needs.'*
>
> What has happened to Bettelheim's 'Children of the Dream'?
>
> About 50% have left their kibbutzim (plural), 5–6% have left Israel.
>
> Their record as army leaders rises far above their record of academic, creative and spiritual achievement.

Current reforms to promote healthier development are the result of pressure from the girls who grew up on the kibbutz, and 'could not bear to separate—to sneak a glance of their children round windows and doors. Now 75% of kibbutz children live overnight with their parents. Parents are becoming more involved in their children's lives, and individual identity is coming into its own.'

The working mother (The latch-key generation)

The necessity for mother to work outside the home may cause separation anxiety and maternal deprivation, not only at pre-school level, but during primary school years. The child comes home agog with the news of the day, or tired and eager for the loving comfort of mother's arms.

In his article 'Working Mother and Problem Childhood' (1970) Dr I Mirvish pens a poignant picture of the homecoming schoolboy.

'As he approaches home, he makes a sudden charge, opens the front door wide, flings down his satchel, calls out "Ma, I'm home", and waits for the answering voice . . . lunch is not the same if there is no response to his "Ma, I'm home" signal. He feels rejected, a lost child, deprived of the warm comradeship he so ardently expects. He wants to tell his mother . . . of the marbles he has won, or of his friend's tortoise, of the beautiful new model jet in the shop window. . . . How is he to occupy himself in the next few hours? He is lonely, he is bored, he roams about. Who knows what company he keeps or how he is taken advantage of? He may take to pilfering or stealing, either for adventure (for kicks) or to "buy love" with stolen money.'

No mother likes to picture her child as a lonely 'drifter'. The decision to forgo the maternal role of homemaker is a serious one, not to be lightly undertaken. Some mothers work for 'excitement', 'stimulation' and extra luxuries. They seek to rationalize their guilt feelings rather than face squarely their avoidance of those responsibilities which should make these the most fulfilling years of their lives. To many, morning work is the ideal solution.

The mother who, by virtue of financial pressure, is *'forced'* to work full time in order to support her family, is quite another matter, and deserves the support and help of her family and community.

What compromises can she make?

Perhaps there is a nearby granny, a motherly neighbour who may like to supplement her income by caring for the youngster. Many private schools provide 'day boarder' facilities. There is evidence that working mothers need not, in ordinary circumstances, fear alienation of the mother–child relationship by carers.

Concerned with assuring a warm relationship with a mother-substitute, as well as efficient intellectual stimulation, kibbutz child-care centres provided facilities for studies by Rabkin and Rabkin 1969; Nahir and Yussen 1977. Research showed that being separated from the mother for *most of the day does not appear to weaken the mother–child attachment.* When kibbutz children (who spent nights at home) were observed in a strange situation at age two and a half, they were just as concerned about separation from the mother as were United States children raised at home (Maccoby and Feldman, 1972).

When kibbutz children were left with mother and a stranger they appeared more secure than when left with the carer and a stranger. Similar results have been found when day-care children in the United States are compared with home-reared children.

There appears to be little difference between the two groups, either in the amount of protest shown when left by the mother in an unfamiliar room, or in the tendency to seek closeness to the mother when tired or upset (Kagen et al 1978).

The attachment to the mother appears to be a special bond that is unrelated to the number of hours per day the child spends with the mother.[*]

* Reported Hilgard E R, Atikinson R L, Atkinson C A. *Introduction to Psychology* 7 ed. Harcourt Brace Jovanovich.

The experimenters may well, however, have added 'within limitations', in that *long periods of separation may result in maternal deprivation* and the conflicting, anxiety-ridden and emotional maladjustments therewith associated.

Clearly, in any case, the environmental situation should cater for the *primary importance of the mother-figure in times of intensive intimacy* such as morning waking, evening feeding, bathing, settling for the night, etc. The provision of after-school facilities should be a primary aim of Community Nurse and social worker. To resort to boarding-schools is indeed very sad, for, from the child's point of view, they differ little from other institutions, the detrimental, psychological and psychosomatic results of which have been discussed in detail.

Certainly the working mother herself is often under considerable stress from 'introjected' (p 106) social disapproval and resultant guilt feelings.

In their study 'Social Support and Resentment in Employed Parents', Nora W Wong and Marybeth Shinn, New York University* attempt to answer two qustions, namely:

1.   What is the relationship between

    (a)   positive social interactions   vs   *(b)*   negative social reactions
       (social support)   (resentment: criticism),

    in a sample of employed parents combining a job with parenting?

2.   Which type of social interaction

has the stronger relationship with well-being?

Method

The study was based on data collected in 1984 as part of a larger investigation of employed parents (M Shinn, New York University). Questionnaires were completed by 495 married men and women who had at least one child aged 16 or younger living at home. Respondents were employed at one of eight New York City organizations representing three industries: retail sales, insurance and government agencies.

Respondents were asked to report (i) levels of social support and resentment from the spouse and supervisor, (ii) levels of stress and well-being. Social support was defined as the frequency with which the spouse or supervisor provided emotional or problem-focused support. Resentment was defined as the frequency the spouse or supervisor was critical or resentful about efforts of combining job and parenting.

1.   *Results* reveal considerable ambivalence and sensitive reaction.

2.   Across the board *resentment was the most powerful variable:*
    'For both married men and married women, the average amount of variance accounted for in well-being by resentment was much higher than for social support.'

3.   *Married men* were most acutely affected by spouse resentment. Supervisor resentment was largely irrelevant.

4.   *Married women* showed a wider range of social interactions:
    spousal support
    spousal resentment   were all important in determining either well-being
    supervisor resentment   or stress.

---

* Presented at the 94th convention of the American Psychological Association, Washington DC, August 1986.

The investigation emphasizes

(a) the negative value of social resentment in provoking parental stress
(b) the positive value of social support in avoiding parental stress.

In her study 'Shift Work, The Family and Child Maladjustment' Sara Deutsch of Abbott House, Irvington, New York* investigated 84 families, each family consisting of a male postal worker (employed on either a 'day' or 'non-day' ie 'shift work' schedule), his wife, and their target child, aged between 4 and 16, in the New York City metropolitan area. Workers and their spouses participated in a brief interview and completed a series of self-report questionnaires.

Results

1. Considerable variation in 'non-day' families' responses indicated that shift work was *not* objectively stressful to all families.

2. The relationship 'r' (see p 13) between:
   (i) shift work per se and individual worker strain was not 'statistically significant' (p 12)
   (ii) shift work and worker *choice of schedule* was 'statistically significant'.
   Thus *whether or not work is seen as stressful is an important variant in job stress.*

3. 'While workers themselves may be able to cope with the demands of shift work, *spouses may be more stressed* because they are the primary ones who must deal with the demands of shift work upon the family, as well as maintain the family while the worker is on the job.
   These findings suggest that the link between the negative effects of shift work upon the family and child may be through the spouse, rather than the shift worker.'

4. *Benefits:*
   While there certainly were costs associated with non-day hours for those families who do not like such hours, shift work did afford the following benefits for many participants:
   (a) Because one parent could always be with their children, better child management was possible. Almost one-third of the non-day families mentioned this benefit.
   (b) Increased family income.
   (c) More time was available for workers to spend on housework and errands, having weekends off from work.

5. For both day and non-day workers, decreased time spent in childcare activities with the target child was 'significantly related to child maladjustment'.

Thus increased hours of parent contact afforded by shift work may well prove advantageous to mental health.

Psycho-analytical concepts of personality development emphasize the long-standing effects, at varying levels of consciousness, and intensity, of:

(i) *'the birth trauma'* consequent upon expulsion from the warm, comforting and secure womb, into the harsh outside world. Feelings of rejection, hostility,

* Presented at the 94th convention of the American Psychological Association, Washington DC August 1986.

guilt and anxiety attach to and spread from, the all-important mother figure. 'Gentler methods' of childbirth (see p 393), 'rooming-in', breastfeeding, self-regulated 'demand' feeding, sucking, holding, and general warm close- ness help counteract the mal-effects of the birth trauma. (See also pp 38.)

(ii) From birth to approximately 18 months: the *'oral or mouth-centred stage,* in which feelings of gratification and security or, conversely, rejection and deprivation are centred on sucking and eating. (See 'mouth activity' and 'the role of the feeding relationship' in personal and social adjustment, p 404.) Failure to satisfy oral needs may lead to stressful inhibition or obsessive indulgence in mouth activity such as drinking or smoking.

(iii) Approximately 18 months to 2 years: *'the anal stage'* in which pleasure and satisfaction or, conversely, guilt and anxiety are centred on sensual experiences associated with excreta. Toilet training is associated with rewarded 'giving' or punished 'withholding'. Orthodox Freudians would maintain that a child who has been introduced to bowel control around 18 months, and urinary control around 2 years, in a relaxed and non-demanding way, will grow up confident, loving and giving.

'Mummy loves me and everything I do. So other people will too'. In contrast, one who has been subjected to a rigid, punitive toilet regime will carry over a pattern of:

anger displaced (p 121) from parental pressure
'compulsive' fear of soiling and offending (p 121) spread to withholding in other areas such as refusal to share sexual and other pleasures
fear of relaxed giving, to the point of social withdrawal
and withholding meanness
'Mummy thinks my motion and I both bad and dirty. I won't give out anything.'

(iv) Approximately $2\frac{1}{2}$ to $4\frac{1}{2}$ years: The sex drive or Libido becomes more clearly defined. This is the *'erotic'* or *'phallic' stage* in which pleasure or (when shamed) guilt feelings and anxiety, are centred on sex organs and their activities (including curiosity and sexual *self-arousal or 'masturbation'*). Disapproval or punishment lays the foundation for persistent feelings of deprivation and resentment in the girl, and castration-fear in the boy (see p 283). Disapproval imperils that self-esteem basic to mental health.

Thumbsucking is an appropriate source of comfort and pleasure in the 'oral' or mouth-centred stage. Similarly exploration and pleasure in *handling the genitals* (masturbation) is appropriate to the 'erotic' or 'phallic' stage. 'Masturbation' may, in fact, constitute an important 'learning experience' in the achievement of ultimate sexual fulfilment.

Naturally these pleasures or deprivations persist, and overflow into other developmental stages. Throughout life there is, in stress or deprivation, a tendency to regress to immature satisfactions such as thumbsucking or sexual self-arousal. Should such behaviour assume problem proportions, direct attack such as provoking, shaming or inflicting punishment will only serve to increase the underlying stress responsible in the first instance for the tension rather than relieving it. One should instead *seek underlying causes* such as maternal deprivation, sibling rivalry and feelings or rejection, school anxiety, night fears, etc, seeking to remove the cause rather than the symptom. The imposition of guilt feelings may result in repression, persistent anxiety and the development of neurotic symptoms. Distraction by other activities may break the cycle temporarily.

(v) Approximately 3 to 6 years: the *'Oedipus'* stage in the boy, and the *'Electra' stage in the girl*, in which the child experiences feelings of passionate love and sexual desire towards the parent of the opposite sex. Punishment or shame by the same sex "rival" parent may entrench or 'fixate' feelings of rejection, hostility, guilt and anxiety. These feelings spread out from the 'rival' to disturb positive identification with same-sex role models, eg to the girl, mothers are cruel and selfish to the boy, men are bullying and brutish.

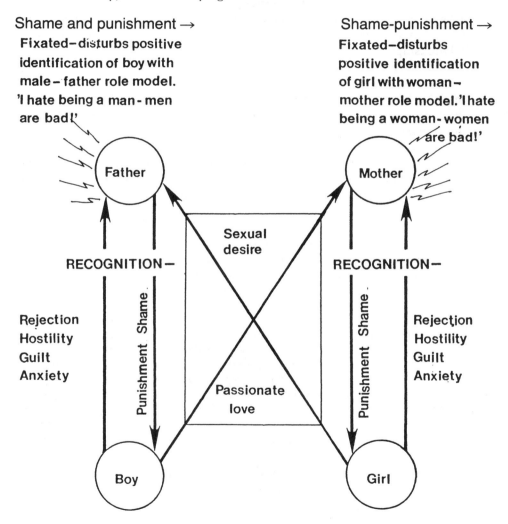

Shame and punishment →
Fixated–disturbs positive identification of boy with male – father role model. 'I hate being a man - men are bad!'

Shame-punishment →
Fixated–disturbs positive identification of girl with woman – mother role model.'I hate being a woman- women are bad!'

Father   Mother

Sexual desire

RECOGNITION–   RECOGNITION–

Rejection   Punishment Shame   Punishment Shame   Rejection
Hostility   Hostility
Guilt   Guilt
Anxiety   Anxiety

Passionate love

Boy   Girl

* In mythology Oedipus unwittingly married his mother, who, on discovering this, hanged herself. Oedipus blinded himself and went into exile from his Kingdom of Thebes. Electra was in love with her father Agamemnon who was murdered by her mother Clytemnestra.

Hamlet's double-pronged agony lay not only in his beloved mother's insensitivity, and his hate and jealousy towards his stepfather, but also in his own frustrated search for a successful and admired male figure with whom to 'identify' and upon whom to model himself. Some men, at a conscious or unconscious level, compare their wives unfavourably with their mothers. "Mother cooks better—she's more feminine. . . ." They fantasize that their mothers are better in bed and they are guilt-stricken.

In the context of developmentally appropriate *fulfilment* of 'oral', 'anal', and 'erotic' satisfactions; *acceptance, support* and *reassurance* in 'Oedipus' and 'Electra' attachments, the child passes through each stage, establishing patterns of healthy fulfilment, enjoyment or compromise, and the ability 'to give' and 'to take' in love relationships.

Conversely, punishment and threats of rejection, will result in tantalizing taboo. Feelings of conflict, guilt and anxiety, especially when reinforced by 'abandonment' to hospital, illness or surgery, may result in *fixation upon*, or *regression to*, an inappropriate, immature developmental stage, and the possibility of permanent inhibition of healthy personality development. (See Psychotherapy, p 609 et seq.)

All the while there should be developing that increasing sense of *self-worth, personality integration and self-governing power* which Freud terms the *'Ego'*. A self-respecting, healthy Ego or self-concept, is basic equipment in that battle and *reconciliation between personal and social demands* which ensues throughout life.

A sound, secure, loving and accepting parent-child relationship probably constitutes the best insurance policy against failure to develop patterns of social conformity, and thus exposure to social rejection, frustration, guilt anxiety and sorrow. The child who grows up knowing that he is loved, that he can rely on his parents to accept him for what he is; whose parents are able to demonstrate their affection; who is not crushed by early and excessive disciplinary demands; a childhood in which the developing youngster feels safe to experience and express strong emotions, to express his ambivalence without fear of guilt-laden disapproval; parents whose loving relationship motivates the wish to identify strongly and constructively—the girl with her mother in preparation for womanhood, the boy withhis father in preparation for manhood; the youngster whose most important lessons in self-discipline are to be found in the constant example of his loved and admired parents—all these contribute to the formation of that important *self-concept* or *self-respect* which is the basis of mental health.

If we are to understand a person's reactions to the favours and blows of life, in health and in illness, we must remember that Man is, throughout his life, the product of his existence in many spheres.

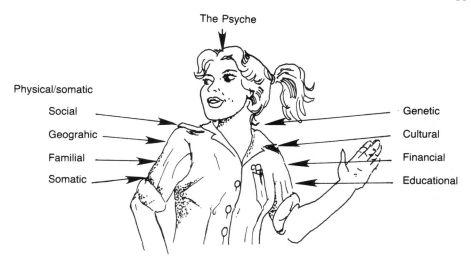

Various theories, structures or models are interpreted within these frames of reference.

CHAPTER 3

DEEPER LEVELS OF EMOTIONAL FUNCTIONING

(especially in illness and hospitalization)

How, one may ask, can events such as premature or stressful toilet training, or an unfortunate hospital experience, at say 2 years old, cause permanent personality changes, affecting our adult reactions long after the so-called 'traumatic' event is consciously forgotten?

We know that people do things, and experience emotions, for which they have no logical explanation. We know also that no one fully understands oneself and that a large part of one's personality cannot be voluntarily controlled. Often without reason we love one person and hate another.

Psychoanalysts believe that the human personality seldom recovers completely from the 'birth trauma' accompanying expulsion or 'rejection' from the maternal womb. We continually seek reassurance of loving acceptance and protection, first from our mother, then from our family and society. In times of crisis and sadness we seek to return to the womb. The patient in pain and distress regresses to a curled up foetal position: in grief people seek comfort in rocking their bodies to and fro.

Freud's psychoanalytical explanation of these phenomena is the most feasible so far submitted, and constitutes the psycho-analytical school's most valuable contribution. It is the one tenet of that school which has stood the test of time, to become fundamentally acceptable to most schools of psychological thought.

LEVELS OF EMOTIONAL REACTION—PSYCHO-ANALYTIC THEORY

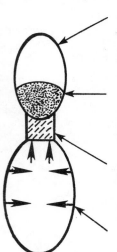

The Conscious:
Freud's reality-seeking Ego
The seat of that mental activity of which we are *aware* and can, to some extent, control. This is the controlled behaviour level presented to the outside world. Associated with self-esteem.

The Preconscious or Subconscious:
The seat of *Memory* from which we can usually draw material at will, through *Association* into consciousness.
Material here contained is usually of a fairly innocuous nature.

The 'Super Ego', Conscience or Censor strives for perfection. It guards and cuts off the 'unconscious' from the 'preconscious'. The 'conscience' suppresses 'forbidden' material into the 'unconscious' in accordance with society's morals and values.

The Unconscious or Id seeks pleasure-satisfaction:
That part of the mind with which, under ordinary circumstances, we have no direct communication. Contains basic drives, eg aggression and sexual energy.

This tenet should be seen as explanatory of function rather than anatomical location.

The human mind may be compared to an iceberg, only the uppermost tip of which protrudes into the outside world.

The true man, his life story, fears, loves, hates, dreams and conflicts lie below the surface usually presented to the undiscriminating onlooker.

Leaning heavily upon and, one certainly hopes, exaggerating the aggressive swing of ambivalence, is current American work on 'narcissism'.

In their book *Narcissism and the Text: Studies in Literature and the Psychology of Self* (New York University Press 1988) Lynne Layton and Barbara Ann Shapiro claim that men and women are not gentle creatures whose only wish is to be loved. Rather are they capable of defending themselves very strongly if attacked.

> 'They are, on the contrary, creatures among whose instinctual endowments is to be reckoned a powerful share of aggressiveness. As a result, their neighbour is for them not only a potential helper or sexual object, but also someone who tempts them to satisfy their aggressiveness on him, to exploit his capacity for work without compensation, to use him sexually without his consent, to seize his possessions, to humiliate him, to cause him pain, to torture and to kill him.'

While this scientifically unproven theory must surely lack proportion, it does bring to the fore many basic, primitive and potentially destructive universal needs.

Where, as in

(i) fear, anger, pride, humiliation, pain, bereavement within the patient,
(ii) frustration, anxiety, exhaustion, helplessness, sadness, and, it must be admitted, sometimes the professional power-needs of the nurse,

behaviour controls are reduced, the negative and very human needs of 'narcissism' may be laid bare, certainly imperilling the nurse–patient relationship.

Into the *Unconscious* part of the mind (Id) *the Conscience* (Super Ego) suppresses all those primitive, aggressive, 'shameful' and frightening thoughts which, being unacceptable to his self-image (Ego), the individual cannot face or acknowledge.

The *unconscious* is, however, far from dormant, as within its sphere, unacceptable 'bad' drives battle with 'good' drives and with the 'conscience'. This is what we term *conflict*.

The 'bad' unacceptable drives are in a state of constant struggle to escape or 'get by' 'the censor' or 'Conscience' (Super Ego) which guards the entrance of the preconscious (memory). The psycho-analytical school distinguishes between

Suppression

> as a *conscious* activity of inhibition by the conscious or the Conscience, while still remaining dynamic.
> in contrast with,

Repression

> as an *unconscious* inhibitory process by which perceptions and ideas which would be too painful to consciousness (The Ego) are pushed into the unconscious (The Id).

Freud's repression hypothesis proposes that some emotional experiences in childhood are so traumatic that to allow them to enter the conscious, even many years later, would cause one to be totally overwhelmed by anxiety.

But forbidden or untenable drives and experiences are far from dormant.

This suppressive or repressive power of the conscience or censor has a direct relationship with feelings of *guilt, anxiety* and *tension*, both psychosomatic and psychoneurotic.

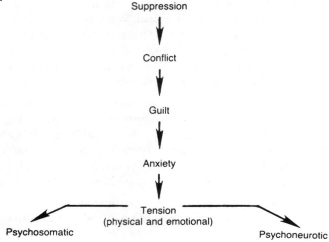

Obsessive compulsions: The Oxford Dictionary reaches the core of the matter when it defines the verb 'to obsess' as 'to haunt, preoccupy, fill the mind of'. DSMIII classification defines obsession as 'recurrent thoughts that enter into the patient's mind against his will'.

While a certain degree of social conscience is necessary if one is to live happily with one's fellows, overdemanding parents, some religious misinterpretations, and other environmental pressures tend to reinforce the inhibitory Conscience (super ego), until it 'works overtime', causing the individual to be crippled by his suppressed feelings of festering guilt, shame, anxiety and tension—both psycho-somatic and psychoneurotic. The range of psychoneurotic symptoms, all of them painful and persistent, is wide, including anxiety neuroses, crippling feelings of inferiority and depression, obsessive thoughts, cleanliness compulsions, etc. A person possessing an 'over-worked conscience' may grow up fearful to perform (or even think about) the simplest and most innocent actions, for fear of punishment and rejection. Sometimes the individual forces himself to perform actions (such as continual hand-washing) which are displeasing, or even hateful to himself, in order to guard himself from partaking of, or even thinking about, those primitive satisfactions about which he feels consciously or unconsciously guilty.

He feels that as long as he performs this burdensome task he will be protected and 'cleansed' from his own suppressed desires. At the same time, through the suffering and sacrifice entailed in the 'task', he will guard himself against divine punishment. These 'safeguarding', 'cleansing', appeasing or self-punishing acts are termed Obsessive Compulsions. Although they might relieve temporarily, obsessional compulsions feed upon themselves, and the underlying fear grows and spreads. Stress management (p. 32) seeks to break into, and eliminate the stress→compulsion→stress chain.

COMPARISON OF NEUROTIC PRESENTATIONS

Diffuse fears	Developed anxiety states	Obsessive compulsive	Hypochondriasis	Post traumatic stress	Phobia
eg fear of dying fear of rejection fear of the future feelings of inferiority	Highly developed, ingrained anxiety states resultant upon vulnerability plus the individual's own life-situation eg school phobia claustrophobia	External } + Vulnerable stimulus } personality feelings of *guilt* and *anxiety* original, and transferred. Repetitive 'dread ideas' and attempts to assuage by ritual performance	Exaggerated reaction to real or imagined internal somatic symptoms eg tension headaches + imagined symptoms → terror of cerebral haemorrhages	Outside range of normal human experience, eg disaster crisis	Excessive fear originally attached to specific object or situation A may be displaced, transferred or extended to object or situation B. The patient tries to escape by the avoidance mechanism of 'Flight', eg Fear for father as a mountaineer (complicated by the hate swing of ambivalence) experienced as phobia for lifts. Irrational fear of a specific object, activity or situation → persistent avoidance behaviour.
				Psychologically traumatic experience, e g divorce	

To quote a case which illustrates the impact of inhibited drives on personality structure and personality functioning:

Mary T was a good, quiet little girl, of the type praised by parents, teachers and nurses (but viewed with some misgivings by psychologists). Mary never 'answered back', never fought and gave no one any trouble at all. She was, in fact, so good that one was often scarcely aware of her presence. This behaviour pattern was naturally most acceptable when the new baby began to demand much of her mother's time. No one noticed Mary becoming increasingly quiet and withdrawn.

One day when her mother was cleaning out the attic, she found a large trunk crammed to overflowing with small pieces of paper torn exactly 2,5 cm × 2,5 cm. Eventually this handiwork was traced to Mary, who admitted that she *hated* tearing the paper into these precise little squares. Her parents realized there was something amiss in a little girl who, for no apparent reason, subjected herself to the onerous task of tearing all those thousands of small pieces according to rigid self-imposed requirements. In interviews with a child-psychologist, Mary was eventually able to verbalize that *suppressed* hatred and aggression, guilt and anxiety which she had managed to conceal from her parents. As in all close relationships, Mary was *ambivalent* towards her baby brother, her feelings for him swinging, pendulum-like, between love and hate.

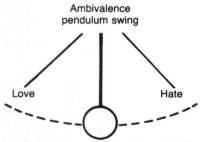

But, like many people who easily develop an 'overworked conscience' in their 'love periods', Mary came to feel acutely guilty and anxious about the aggressive feelings dominating her 'hate periods'.

The realization that she sometimes hated her baby brother for 'stealing' the all-important parental love and attention; that, in fact, she often wished he were dead, *had so frightened her that she pushed it into the unconscious part of her mind.* But here the death-wish was far from dormant, constantly conflicting with the censor or conscience and causing guilt-feelings and anxiety lest she should be punished for her 'evil' thoughts.

To assuage this anxiety, she did something that she hated as a 'sacrifice'. Being the type of person who cannot easily express her hate, love and anxiety at a direct or conscious level, she set about placing the anger of 'The Powers that Be' by the painful and distasteful task of precise paper tearing.

Mary embarked upon psychoanalytically orientated psychotherapy involving the following basic processes:

1. She was encouraged through projective techniques (miniature toys and story-telling designed to *trick* the Conscience) to 'associate' or 'chain-link' back to her earliest feelings about the new baby, being supported and reassured, as she finally brought them and their associated emotions through the preconscious into consciousness. (ASSOCIATION)
2. The significance and meaning of the paper tearing as a safeguarding ritual were interpreted to Mary (in simple terms) as a compulsion designed to stave off punishment by the 'powers that be'. 'She feels that if she tears the paper God will forgive her for hating her brother'. (INTERPRETATION)

3. Her play and the feelings it revealed were carefully repeated to Mary until she accepted them as her own, saying 'that little girl is me'. She was in fact encouraged to *'relive'* her feelings and, in so doing, was *emotionally* reassured as she *re-experienced* her painful emotions. This re-experiencing of emotionally traumatic events is necessary if *emotional level acceptance* (as opposed to merely *intellectual acceptance*) is to be achieved. (IDENTIFICATION) 'If you want to, you can tread on the boy doll'. Nothing bad will happen. God understands.

4. Mary was encouraged to talk about (Ventilate) her formerly 'forbidden' feelings of hate and hostility. *The relief that comes of talking out* one's fears, guilt feelings, anxieties, is termed 'Catharsis'. (or ABREACTION) The aim is to exhaust or 'burn out' the painful emotions.

5. Mary was reassured that the 'hate' swings of her natural love—hate ambivalence were universal and perfectly normal. She need have no guilt feelings about her hatred of her brother. (REASSURANCE)

6. The therapeutic contract: Mary was confronted with her old emotional reactions and asked to live through different ways of facing her hostilities and fears. 'You could tell your brother you're cross with him'. When you try different ways of handling your fears and anger, we will discuss them together to see which are best for you.

7. Attempts were made to teach Mary less guilt-laden, more self-accepting and constructive emotional reactions to perfectly normal motivations and feelings. (RE-EDUCATION)

The psychotherapeutic technique entailed in taking the patient back to the original emotional suppression or repression causing her symptoms; of dragging the 'ghost' out of the cupboard into the light of day; showing fears to be groundless and bad feelings to be common to most human beings, illustrates the operation of the various layers of emotional functioning.

It is often helpful to centre therapeutic focus upon the client by asking him to draw himself at the centre of a spider's web surrounded by his own internalized map of significant relationships, traumatic experiences, guilt stimuli, fears, obsessions, sorrows and satisfactions. This is amended as therapy proceeds.

We are all familiar with the picture of the earnest analyst busily scribbling notes beside his patient, prone on 'the couch'.

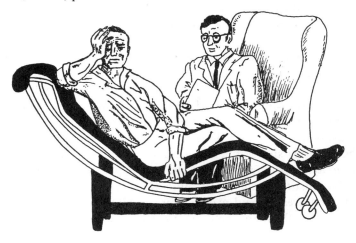

The analyst uses his own preferences of a classic approach:

'1.   Please relax completely. (It is helpful to tense and relax each muscle group from feet to neck and head. Relaxation tapes or focus on a fixed object (perhaps a weak light) may promote relaxation of physical and mental barriers.)

2.   Close your eyes. Bring to the forefront of your mind that image, or experience, which most frightens or distresses you.

3.   Hold the image (usually from the past) as long as you are able, feeling again the fear, guilt, hurt, pain, rejection attached. (For example, to an imprint of child abuse.) Within the safe confines of this room, and our confidential relationship, everything you do or say is acceptable and justified—you are free to talk, or cry out, all your grief, terror, remorse, pain and anger.

4.   All these *images are figments of your imagination*. They can no longer harm you. Continue bringing back your image again and again.

Confront it; learn that its power to hurt you is diminishing until it disappears of its own accord or entirely loses its power over you.

Grade the diminishing power of the image on a scale of 1 to 10.

You will find the stress level decreases the more you allow yourself to live through your trauma, anxieties and attempted solutions, eventually fading out altogether. Then you will face your previously distressing image stimuli with minimal stress'.

After each session the client may feel drained. But with the pain of discovery usually comes a healing peace, a feeling of completeness. If the image or imprint returns it must be confronted and tackled until it is finally eliminated.

Distressing images passed are, of course, easier to deal with than those long-term traumatic and heartbreaking realities with which we must live painfully, and with compromise, as we pass through life. Here there is no elimination—only an ability to tolerate.

Sometimes the inhibitory or suppressive action of the conscience is so strong that hypnosis, or drugs such as dilute sodium pentothal, are necessary to encourage that state of half-sleep in which the power of the Conscience is reduced, enabling 'forbidden' material to be brought through the vigilance of the censor or Conscience.

Sometimes the 'forbidden material' can only 'get through' disguised, or symbolically clothed, as in <u>dreams</u>, when the power of the conscience is reduced by sleep. In fact, the very nature of dreams—in which we allow ourselves to indulge in behaviour to which we would never admit in our waking hours, or in which we see clearly faces and places of long-forgotten—illustrates the persistent power of material stored away in the Unconscious.

For psychotherapy to be successful, intellectual insight is not alone sufficient. *The patient must learn to feel differently*. Bridging the gap between *intellectual insight* and *emotional acceptance* constitutes the main difficulty in psychotherapy, and is the reason for many failures. Freud called this crucial part of the process of psychotherapy 'working through' the patient's defences, namely:

Resistance

An impediment to successful analytical therapy lies in 'resistance' which constitutes the client's attempt to remain unaware of his anxiety-producing defences.

The term 'resistance' was originally used by Freud to describe unconscious opposition to exploring, or recognizing, suppressed, or repressed, material which is either *too painful to face* or which still serves a *defensive purpose*.

Resistance results from *ambivalence* and thus reluctance, or learned avoidance, in verbalizing, or even experiencing *conflicting aspects of the 'self'*.

Sometimes it constitutes an angry or fearful *defence against the therapist* who 'presumes' to probe prematurely or too deeply into the client's inner life.

Resistance may take the form of:

   (i) feelings of self-devaluation, depression and hopelessness—'What's the use? I'm not strong enough to change'.
  (ii) pretended recovery
 (iii) intellectual inhibition:
       'There is nothing worrying me'.
       'I don't want to think about my problems—it upsets me'.
       'I couldn't keep my appointment—I was too tired'.
  (iv) irrelevant, 'side-tracking' small talk: 'stalling'
   (v) intellectual understanding, even glib psychoanalytical 'interpretation', in the face of unabated symptomatology—'OK—so I've got an unresolved Oedipus complex—but I still can't communicate with my father'.
  (vi) long, awkward silences
 (vii) contempt for normality 'OK, so I'm a nut—who wants to be normal anyway?

Transference

During interflow between therapist and client, the latter re-experiencing her traumatic emotions may seek to spread and share her burden of guilt and anxiety by transfering or displacing (p 112) them upon her therapist. If this process is recognised, mirrored, resolved and integrated into her mental functioning transference may prove a helpful mechanism.

Counter Transference

Refers to the manner in which the therapist experiences and reacts to her client's problems and behaviour. If they arouse emotional upheavals in her own past, she may ask to consult with a colleague to assure her own objectivity and professional skills.

Shame and embarrassment in procedures (Diagram P 343)

An important example of the distressing potency of suppressed guilt feelings lies in the patient's acute emotional reaction to the use of bed-pan and bottle, and to procedures involving the handling of sex organs or organs of elimination. In spite of the nurse's logical explanations as to the necessity for such procedures, the patient involuntarily resists, becomes angry, resentful, tearful, or is unable to relax. His personal space is being invaded.

The roots of his strong attitudes of shame and embarrassment lie in the early and rigid demand for cleanliness and sexual disinterest to which most infants in our society are subjected. Very early the infant is given the impression that his faeces are unclean, unacceptable and even revolting to the all-important mother figure. He soon develops the impression that the organs of elimination which produce this unacceptable product are dirty, bad and shameful. Because the sex organs are so closely situated on his body, these feelings of shame and guilt implanted in the unconscious mind by early, often forgotten incidents, spread, persist and grow, producing feelings of acute, traumatic embarrassment, resentment and shame, when the patient is stripped of his defences. Forced public exposure of those organs of elimination and sex around which, through the years, he has built a strong protective wall of defensive privacy constitutes a distressing and invasive experience. (See also Sexually Transmitted Diseases p 340.)

Many patients report that the emotional ordeal, the humiliation, the feeling of mental assault entailed in such common procedures as enemata, catheterization, preparation for surgery, PV examinations, etc far outweigh the physical sufferings in their illness.

Understanding the illogical, but long-standing, deep-seated nature of her patient's feelings of embarrassment, shame and humiliation, the nurse will not persist in reasoning, nor indulge in rebuke. Rather will she do all in her power to reduce onslaught on her patient's deepest emotions. She will use screens carefully and supply dressing towels to cover genitalia. Verbalized reassurance to the effect that the patient is free to 'finish off' a full-wash for him or herself should come early in the procedure. This will avoid mounting stress as the wash proceeds.

The trauma of public defacation is indeed very distressing. Although it may be easier to offer a bedpan, many patients prefer, as soon as possible, to be helped to the toilet. The provision of aerosol deodorants facilitates important tension relief.

Some hospitals, realizing the acute psychological trauma entailed in preparation for abdominal or genital surgery, prepare the patient, already unconscious, in a special anteroom to the theatre—a merciful and enlightened example of how knowledge, compassion and ingenuity can eliminate an illogical but nevertheless potent horror of hospitalization. One-way vision rooms and closed-circuit TV would spare the patient the ordeal of exposure to a student audience while undergoing PV examination.

'The child is father to the man': the structure of personality reaches far back into earliest experiences.

The human personality has been compared to an iceberg, only the tip of which sticks out into consciousness. Some understanding of the mountainous bulk lying below the surface should increase our compassion, and our tolerance, for the fellow-traveller we encounter in the often painful and perverse sea of life.

Overcoming anxiety(see also Managing Anxiety, pp 33-35)

Psychological preparation for surgery. To a patient there is no such thing as a 'routine' consent form

'Are patients really informed before signing operation consent forms? How many are properly prepared for the hospital experience or presented with the choice of alternative treatments? Medicine has become so slick and impersonal that people feel like helpless cogs in implacable machinery. Good communications is a finely tuned balance of silence and sound, an *ability to listen and to talk*.'*

How many receive this interflow in the patient—professional relationship? (Chapter 7.)

It is important to <u>encourage 'feedback'</u> by requesting comment upon, or repetition of, information as to the nature of proposed treatment or surgery, and how the patient conceives its aftermath. Some patients are reassured by taking written notes or requesting these of professionals.

Often real anxieties are revealed in the last moments of the interview when departure is imminent: 'You don't think it's cancer, do you Sister?'

Some professionals suggest that the patient be asked to *draw his concept* of surgical procedures and their outcome as a means of assessing 'real informed' consent. They insist on the necessity for *'worry work'* to include anxiety ventilation and catharsis and, in the case of children, tangible experience in a simulated hospital setting (pp 269 et seq).

In spite of *intellectual-level reassurance* the difficulty encountered in changing people's *feelings* about their fears is a major 'stumbling block' in reassuring anxious patients.

Intellectual ———— **?** ———— Emotional acceptance
insight

In many cases, our reassurances are nullified by early fearsome experiences which, 'festering' in the unconscious part of the patient's mind, are shooting forth illogical, but nevertheless potent, terror associations. The anxious patient who is continually compelled to demand our attention and reassurances deserves our sympathy and support rather than impatient censure.

Logical, patient reasoning and reassurance may not remove fear of surgery from the mind of the patient who, as a child, was subjected to the terror of insensitive, emotionally traumatic handling in ward or theatre, screaming separation from mother . . . the black anaesthetic mask . . . awakening in pain.

Although at a conscious level he may have 'forgotten' the original frightening incident, the experience is permanently stored away, 'festering' in the unconscious part of his mind, plaguing him with the terror associations pertaining thereto. Hospital arouses many stimuli to repressed terror associations.

When intellectual explanations and reassurances fail to relieve the anxiety in a patient (or relative) it becomes necessary to <u>attempt deeper-level emotional reassurance</u>. The nurse should take time to 'chat' with her patient, turning conversation to past hospital experiences, his attitude towards his house doctor, his parents' feelings about matters medical, frightening books he has read or films he has seen, etc, thus attempting to *reach, talk out* and *relieve,* the real underlying origins

* Donna Wurzel, radio commentator, on Communication in a Medical Setting. July 1983. Further details available from the author.

of his fear-associations. Some patients are helped towards *positive identification*, and thus emotional-level reassurance, by introduction to a cheerful, convalescent patient who has recently undergone similar surgery. 'If it has gone well for him', he may feel, 'it will go well for me too'. The advisability of this technique will depend on the sensitivity and sophistication of the patient.

'Negative identification' should be avoided. Certainly patients going to theatre should not see others emerge unconscious or attached to drips, drains and other frightening apparatus.

The comfort of *tactile communication* derives from deep and primitive love and reassurance associations in the mother–child relationship. The caress of a loved one, the warm, friendly hand-grasp of an involved nurse, may well impart deeper-level reassurance than intellectual information, important though the latter may be.

The need for touch as a caring and reassuring expression is never outgrown. One should not forget that men too need tactile reassurance.

Illness is an estranging process. Dr Carol Englander, medical director of World Health Associates in Massachusetts, writes:

> 'When people don't get touched they feel there's really something wrong with them. A touch can transform a fearful patient. A person suddenly feels "I'm not isolated. Somebody's willing to reach out to me", and for someone who is sick or frightened, that's very important.'

Often the *reassuring presence of a trusted friend or relative* in whom the patient has, through a long-term relationship, developed *feelings* of confidence, can impart deeper-level emotional reassurance than the impersonal, intellectual reassurances of the greatest surgeon. The psychological approach does not, of course, preclude *appropriate tranquillization*.

In assigning 'routine' (if such a term can be applied to the highly charged pre-operative nurse-patient relationship) *preparation procedures* to the less qualified, professional, staff 'miss out' on a valuable opportunity for establishing meaningful communication. The anxious patient 'hangs on' to every remark and gesture, placing heavy responsibility on the intelligence and experience of the nursing staff.

A patient commenting on the behaviour of a pleasant, cheerful and kind assistant-nurse deprecated the responsibility with which she was burdened. The nurse explained the procedure of covering her wedding ring with plaster, as a precaution 'in case you are "confused" and hit out at things while you are coming round'—hardly a reassuring picture.

'At least,' she said, 'if indeed I *was* ever to awaken, I had hoped to emerge from the anaesthetic with reasonable dignity and peace.'

Death and anaesthesia are indivisible in the patient's mind. No one really believes he will wake up from an anaesthetic. In his mind he must face giving himself over to death. Even if he does not die, he is losing control over his body and his future, if he has one. Alleged fear of post-operative pain may mask deeper *fears of mutilation*. The innovation of a pre-operative visit by the theatre sister is no doubt helpful in establishing human contact, but in the final analysis *real assurance lies in the patient's relationship with his surgeon—the man who holds the knife!* Only he may counteract the deeper fears—fears of the unknown escalated by insistence on 'routine' 'general consent'. Meaningful and direct patient–surgeon communication is vital to effective pre-operative reassurance (see also p 68).

Professor Ephrahim Siker (May 1983), President of the American Board of Anaesthesiology, speaks strongly against the paucity of communication, which is often limited to a perfunctory 'You are going to feel a little prick in your skin'.

Although the patient is mildly sedated, he is certainly alert enough to be concerned about what is being done to him, but usually too intimidated to ask: 'Do you know that I'm still awake? Do you understand that I'm frightened? Why is nobody talking to me?'

Even Dr Jean Horton, honorary secretary of the Association of Anaesthetists, admits fear, although, at an intellectual level, she knows that

> 'anaesthesia is far, far safer than crossing a road . . . Some patients worry about an impending general anaesthetic for months in advance, starting from the day notice of admission to hospital drops through the letter box. It isn't just the *fear that they may never wake* . . . they often fear they're going to *talk in their sleep and reveal their life's secrets* . . . If they're really worried there's no need for them to suffer in silence . . . they won't be considered daffy. We recognise that patients are scared and we're here to offer all the comfort and reassurance that's needed.'

Very clearly for such reassurance to be effective there must be a team effort, including the effort of the man who 'holds the knife' and who alone can give effective reassurance with regard to the possibility and extent of post-surgical mutilation.

Patients and relatives are quick to sense the *nurse's competency and attitude to her professional responsibilities*. If she is slow, sloppy and disinterested she will not convey feelings of confidence.

Conversely, if she is skilled, conscientious, efficient, caring and optimistic she will spread feelings of safety.

Nursing actions detrimental to patient confidence

1. A *judgmental attitude, verbal disapproval* of the patient's behaviour and *rough tactile handling* sets him on the defensive, increasing his isolation and anxiety.
2. Mocking, *criticizing*, or in any way focusing upon his anxiety in the presence of others.
3. *Taking offence*, or for any other reason withdrawing from the patient.
4. A nurse who *lacks insight* into her own behaviour and feelings, *'displacing'* (p 121) anger or anxiety upon her patient or *'over-idealizing'* (p 117) his ability to cope with his fears.
5. Exposure to the *fear-provoking situation* of other patients leading to *negative identification* (p 108). A patient who lies between moaning, pain-ridden people tied to fearful contraptions, is hardly likely to face surgery with anything other than depressed terror.
6. Adoption of an authoritarian attitude.

The nurse's role in encouraging catharsis in patients and colleagues.

No one expects the nurse to be a professional psychotherapist. But within the relatively long-term contact involved in nursing procedures, in the context of respect, sympathy, friendliness and, above all, *absence of moral judgment*, she has special opportunities for establishing the kind of friendly relationship which encourages CATHARSIS, *the relief that comes from talking out one's anxieties, resentments, etc.*

It is often in her relationship with a junior nurse that a patient will obtain the relief that comes with verbalizing her anxieties, depressions and hostilities following, for example, the emotionally traumatic experience of a hysterectomy.

Often, too, in the course of nursing procedures, the patient will speak of basic, stress-producing circumstances such as an unsympathetic, anxiety-laden work situation, or a nagging, tormenting, interfering mother-in-law!

These may well constitute circumstances reinforcing those biochemical changes which, via the Autonomic Nervous System, constitute a fundamental cause of his gastric ulcer or coronorary thrombosis.

Through her more prolonged contact with the patient, the tactful, friendly and compassionate nurse, who is a *good listener*, may obtain valuable *insight* into her patient's *real problems* and stresses, which, conveyed to other members of the hospital team, such as the physician, psychiatrist or social worker, may help bring long-term improvement in the patient's personal and social adjustment, and thus in his physical health.

It is certainly beholden upon senior staff to encourage juniors to afford catharsis, and to take seriously their contributions to the hospital team.

Acceptance of the normal *swing between love and hate* which constitutes *ambivalence* (and consequent tendency to suppress hate) helps in achieving understanding and relief of those acute *guilt feelings* and thus anxiety-tension, which accompany death. A nurse may sometimes feel involuntary hostility towards a particular patient. Should this patient die, she is liable to expiate her illogical, but nevertheless powerful, guilt feelings in anxiety lest, through some omission or mistake, she is herself responsible for his death.

The opportunity for catharsis and simple reassurance as regards the universality of guilt-feelings in the death situation, often does much to reassure colleagues and relatives, thus easing at least one tension-laden aspect of death.

(See Care of the Dying, p 534; Conversion, p 126.)

Special implications of cardiac surgery

Owing partly to the side-effects of imunosuppressant drugs, gross psychological disturbances may characterize post-operative presentation from even the first or second day.

Etiology is apparently related to blood lactose metabolism. Patients become euphoric and even present characteristics of manic psychosis, including delusions and hallucinations. Confused thought processes and disorientation in time and space are typical.

Overt over-reactions include distress and even attempts to remove and destroy equipment such as drips, monitors and catheters.

African patients in particular tend to be confused and frightened, perhaps due to their unfamiliarity with powerful and overwhelming medical machinery. Language and cultural differences render communication difficult.

The strength of emotional reaction to heart surgery is, no doubt, aggravated by the manner in which literature, religious writings and folklore have, through the ages, focused upon this organ, man's emotions, his vulnerability, the very fountainhead of his life. It is this central core of his being that is being invaded by the surgeon's knife.

Professor Christiaan Barnard* comments graphically on the emotional effects of heart surgery:

> 'Your heart *is you*, in the most personal sense. There is a shocking feeling of dismay at the thought . . .
> The surgery itself, apart from the physical trauma, represents a *massive invasion of privacy* in entering the chest's cavity, removing body organs and replacing them with others . . .
> Who is stable in the face of major surgery? The psychological damage alone makes the surgery pale into insignificance.'

POST-OPERATIVE EMOTIONAL TRAUMA

Intensive care unit

No matter how well the patient is *prepared at an intellectual level, the emotional trauma of waking to find oneself pinioned* by immobilizing wires and tubes, and bombarded by a barrage of frightening instruments, weird noises and muffled voices, certainly *cannot be over-emphasized*. Nursing procedures constantly interrupt rest and diminish privacy and dignity. The patient's predicament is intensified by his inability to ascertain the extent of his mutilation.

He is trapped between the terror of dying, pain, anger at personal diminishment, and a regression to childhood helplessness. Helpless dependence is encouraged by the strong, mother-role of the intensive care nurse:

> 'Patients in the intensive care unit are submitted to both sensory over-stimulation and sensory deprivation—over-stimulation by noise, light and new things, but deprivation through the lack of touch, spoken word and reassurance.'
> Many are in terror of what has been done to their bodies.

Fifty per cent of patients become disoriented about time—most prefer a calendar they can read rather than a clock (Hackett 1968).† While it is important that staff mention time, dates, etc the patient's most meaningful and intimate link with the reality (and hope) of the familiar, sunny outside, world lies in the visits of his loved ones. They prove he is not forgotten, that they still love him.

They punctuate his stressful, isolated days and give him hope of ultimate escape from this weird, tense, pain- and death-laden 'vault'. (They should, of course, be guided with the request that they avoid tiring him with home troubles, financial problems, etc.)

---

* Professor Christiaan Barnard 1982.

† Hackett, T *et al*. 'The coronary care unit—an appraisal of psychological hazards.' *New Eng J med* **279** (25). 1968

'Recently I saw an example of family dedication that certainly saved the life of the patient . . . She was the wife of a middle-aged car accident victim . . . Before we could even think of his basic problems, we had a half-dozen other ills to combat, not the least being the problem of avoiding lung complications from broken ribs . . . She rarely left his side, and probably broke every rule in the nursing handbook. But it was she who gave the alarm when a breathing tube blocked. And she was the one who noticed when a drip pulled out. She fought with him through all the crises, talked to him when consciousness flickered back . . . Her example gives me cause to wonder. Is our fascination with well-run institutions and an expert for every problem not perhaps leading us astray? Costs of staffing such giant gadget boxes have overrun the budget. Perhaps it's time to bring the family back into the hospital, and throw out part of our clean, clinical approach.'

During ward rounds he is discussed as if he were a feelingless, endangered laboratory specimen. Within the relatively cramped conditions of the ICU he may easily overhear a frightening prognosis for a fellow-patient and introject it to himself.

Intimate functions become common property, and in some insensitive situations he is stripped of the last shreds of his personal dignity, being forced to lie naked in the unisex environment. Little wonder that, thus traumatized, deprived of normal sensory information, pain-ridden, depressed, confused and disoriented, he may verge on the psychotic. (See p 585.) In fact, Hackett *et al* (1968) claim that 30–70% of patients in intensive care units do develop ICU psychosis.

Although he is constantly measured, prodded, turned and invaded, all too often the patient enjoys but little meaningful communication. In a study of ICU communication patterns Nobel breaks down the pattern of ICU communication as follows.*

65% of all communication is related to the patient's treatment and care. This usually occurs in medical jargon, short unconnected sentences or commands. 18% of the total communication concerns the personal affairs of the staff. Only 14% of the communication is directed at the patient, consisting mainly in short verbal exchanges (frequently directional in nature) or non-verbal communication.

This type of sparse and impersonal communication certainly reduces the patient's status to that of a half-witted outsider, relative to professional identification of the staff.

Dr A E Gasperi of Matteo, Italy, currently practising in Maputo, reports thus on the 'outcome of Intensive Care—Psychological and Physical Sequelae of Resuscitation.' A survey of 201 patients presented the following two most important patient-complaints:

'Lack of involvement by nursing staff, especially on Monday after the weekend football game'—no doubt an observation adaptable to other cultural situations;
Humiliation due to enforced nudity, claimed to facilitate mechanical devices.

---

* 'Communication in the ICU—Therapeutic or Disturbing.' *Nursing Outlook* **27** (3). March 1979.

One certainly hopes that most patients are provided with the dignity of at least a sheet, which surely cannot make that much difference to nursing procedures.

Loss of privacy is aggravated by *negative identification* with the traumatically ill and dying. This poses the no doubt surmountable architectural problem of placing staff in a strategic position for seeing patients (while the latter are), as far as possible, screened from each other) perhaps in a raised centrifugal position. (See also Avoiding Regression, p 123.)

In spite of painful, confusing and diminishing experiences within the ICU, many patients present with considerable ambivalence when informed of their transfer to the general ward. Encouraged by the strong maternal role of the nurse to regress, they have learnt to feel safe and well cared for within the highly technical and impressive safeguards prevailing in the unit. They fear that, on transfer, they will not be so well cared for—an anxiety easily *introjected by loved ones* and requiring much reassurance, including actual physical transferral and introduction by the ICU staff to the general ward.

Post-anaesthetic confusion or 'delirium' is largely resultant upon the temporary toxic effect of anaesthetic agents especially upon a brain rendered vulnerable by old age, alcoholism, drug addiction; underlying predisposition to schizophrenia or depression, and organic pathology such as cardiovascular abnormalities, and infections especially where operations are of longer than four hours' duration.

Women appear to be more vulnerable than men. Because she returns (sometimes precipitously) *to her pre-operative state*, a terrified patient may well return to consciousness in panic, aggravated by her physiological ordeal and possibly mutilated body-image.

This observation, consistent with higher incidence of post-operative 'delirium' in emergency surgery, emphasizes necessity for *effective pre-operative emotional-level reassurance* (unlikely when 'prepping' is allotted to untrained personnel) *and a positive supportive relationship not only as between patient and nurse but very emphatically as between the patient and her surgeon who holds the knife*. Specific agreement on the extent of surgery, and appropriate definition on the 'consent form', are basic to pre-operative confidence. Imagine the trauma of expecting a Caesarian delivery and awakening to a dead child and a hysterectomy!

'What have they done to me?' is the panic query with which, even in the context of a sound surgeon–patient relationship, the frightened patient frequently returns to consciousness.

Many patients would prefer the inconvenience (and slight risk) of a second anaesthetic, to unexpected mutilation and permanent impairment of quality of life. Some may wish to obtain a second opinion.

Gillis points out that 'amputations, hysterectomies and mastectomies . . . cause disturbance of the body-image which requires considerable psychological adaptation.* And that's 'putting it mildly'!

'Intensive care psychosis' (see also Post-operative trauma)

According to Hacket *et al* (1968), 30 to 70 per cent of patients in Intensive Care Units develop ICU psychosis.[†]

---

* Gillis, L. *Guidelines in Psychiatry*. David Philip (1978).

† Hackett, T *et al*. 'The coronorary care unit—an appraisal of psychological hazards.' *New Eng J med* **279** (25). 1968.

Predisposing factors consist in
the *patient's pre-existent personality* and psychological make-up, eg a patient who, pre-operatively, suffers from endogenous depression certainly stands a high chance of suffering post-operative reactive depression;
length of time under anaesthetic;
length of time on the cardio-pulmonary bypass machine also appears to predispose to ICU psychosis;
the *extent of pre-operative anxiety* and *post-operative mutilation.*

Presentation

Signs and symptoms of the ICU syndrome are at first mild, consisting in sleeplessness and hyperactivity.

The patient then becomes disoriented and frightened and often attempts to interfere with treatment apparatus. Physical restraints aggravate his panic and anger.

There are frequently perceptual distortions and illusions when the patient sees and hears things that are not there. His remarks and behaviour become inappropriate and he may well resist co-operation strongly.

Etiology

Patients are afraid—afraid of the new, weird, noisy and light-shot environment; strange people, *pain* and *physical restraints.*

The highly sterile and mechanically technical atmosphere commonly pervading intensive care units has brought with it *psychological disorientation,* stress and even paranoic symptoms which cannot be attributed to anaesthesia or drug therapy. Man is at the mercy of machines! A special transcultural trauma!

Disorientation may be due to *sensory deprivation* such as lost hearing aid or bandaged eyes, predisposing strongly towards post-operative panic and confusion. *The patient's body is 'invaded'* and immobilized by wires and tubes, and he is subjected to a barrage of frightening instruments, *weird noises* of monitors, muffled voices frequently discussing his condition in technical terms he does not understand. During *ward rounds* he is discussed, often in frightening terms, as if he were a feelingless laboratory specimen. *Nursing procedures constantly* interrupt his rest and diminish his privacy and dignity. He is subjected to *negative identification* with the traumatically ill and dying. It is not surprising that acute tension and distress, even paranoia, commonly occur in the ICU.

Treatment

This takes the form of

Phenothiazine medication;
emotional support, reassurance and active steps to counteract perceptual disorientation and emotional isolation;
allaying fears—either by intellectually oriented preparation or counteraction of the traumatic surgical and recovery trauma;
reassuring presence of long-term 'significant' family and friends.

Prognosis

If all goes well, symptoms tend to recede four or five days after admission to the ICU or after discharge from it.

According to Nobel, there is a 'statistically significant' correlation between patients who develop ICU psychosis and mortality rates.

Prevention

Ward administrators and architects are increasingly urged to provide windows for day-night time orientation, taped music, pleasant décor and familiar, reassuring environmental stimuli. Visits by reassuring family and friends are encouraged.

Emphasis is on the necessity for *shortening intensive care stay* and, for psychological reasons as well as to avoid infection, attempts are made to remove extraneous equipment from the patient's body within 72 hours.

Surveys of *patient opinion* show reassurance that the individual can be seen by the staff at all times to be his predominant requirement when dangerously ill.

At the same time, he is much distressed by loss of privacy, and negative identification with the traumatically ill and dying. This poses the no doubt surmountable architectural problem of placing staff in a strategic position for seeing patients (while the latter are, as far as possible, screened from each other) perhaps in a raised centrifugal position. (See also Avoiding Regression, pp 123-124.)

Staff stress

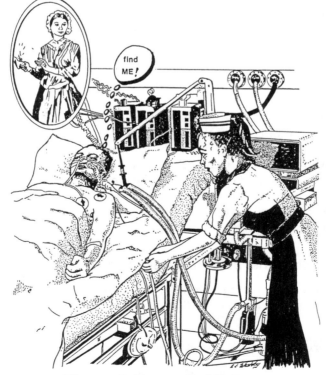

"You never had to cope with all this!"

There are always new sisters and nurses who are frightened . . .

> 'Not only must the nurse be alert, she must be one step ahead. The staff are continuously doing potential lifesaving tasks. One mistake could thus be fatal. Furthermore there is a constant threat of a crisis which can happen at any time.'

Added to the stress born of long-standing crises and the guilt and anxiety arising when death is pronounced inevitable, the ICU staff are burdened by the acute and persistent stress of *unresolved conflict*:

> 'What does the nurse do if she has made a mistake? Does she admit ignorance or incompetence, reducing her professional status and, more important, her own self-concept?
> If she does not admit her mistake, she will not lose face, but she will feel guilty lest the mistake could have been rectified. Either way she faces crippling anxiety and guilt.'

What can be done to help her in this tension-fraught 'cleft stick' situation? The answer lies in communication and mutual support.

> 'The ideal situation would be regular *group meetings* with the same leader, so that *direct communication* can take place. The staff should be able to tell each other of their faults and help each other to correct them. This is unfortunately very difficult as misunderstanding and victimisation may develop in such groups.'

Such caution is certainly justified—especially within the context of self blame and anxiety, and thus *temptation to project guilt feelings* one upon another.

> 'Nurses must reassure each other and therefore allow colleagues to express their fears and emotions. Time must be taken to listen without being judgemental. Words of encouragement and positive reinforcement must be given.*

What has been said of the intense *need for communication and mutual support* within the ICU certainly applies to the *long-term stress and split-second efficiency pertaining in the theatre*. Of very special importance is the theatre *staff's warmth of communication with the patient*, who will certainly enter this terrifying situation *in crisis*, overt or covert.

Although his *memories* of the theatre will be short and condensed, they *will certainly always feature among the most critical in his life*. The theatre nurse who can convey to him, in his extremity, involvement, confidence, reassurance and warmth will certainly be long remembered.

Depression and other psychological effects of major surgery

The finding of Moffic and Paykel (1975),[†] to the effect that 24% of hospital in-patients are at least mildly depressed, impresses as an underestimation.

---

* Gudrun Dannenfeldt 'The Psychological Aspects of Intensive Care Units.' *Curationis* 5 (3). September 1982.

† Moffic H S, Paykel E S. 'Depression in Medical In-patients.' *British Journal of Psychiatry* 1975; **126**: 346—53.

Depression may be reactive as a result of physical and emotional trauma, or it may be endogenous (constitutional) perhaps 'triggered' by the trauma of illness and hospitalization (pp 591-2).

Bedside handling includes:

(i) opportunity for catharsis, empathic listening, tactile support by both staff and loved ones. Sometimes it is necessary to guide the patient towards his trauma and provide him with tools of emotive expression (words, toys, paints). The reader is referred to chapter 7, especially pages 188-190: Techniques facilitating communication.

(ii) acceptance of slow emergence from withdrawal, anger, feelings of hopelessness and reassurance that depression, however deep, will pass. *This is no time to react personally to, or team up against, the patient's anger and aggression.*

(iii) bolstering of self-worth and building of ego-strengths by extracting and encouraging environmental supports, interests, creativity. (See Nursing Process, chapter 9 especially pp 228-232, 514-516.)

(iv) suggestion of 'booster' anti-depressant medication such as Tofranol.

Body image is the sum of the conscious and unconscious attitudes the individual has towards his/her body. It includes present and past perceptions, as well as feelings about size, function, appearance and potential. (See p 501.)

While it is true that patients need privacy in which to come to terms with themselves, especially in the case of mutilating surgery, they certainly also need the nurse's understanding, support, cheerfulness and affection. Not all enjoy the support of a loving, caring family or community situation; not all share a happy prognosis. *Sometimes, in fact, the nurse, who spends so much time with her patient, who shares the 'night watch', wonders whether the prognosis warrants the suffering, mutilation and pain to which he is subjected.* She finds it difficult to support and encourage her patient in an optimistic and constructive attitude to such surgery. Her lot may be eased by readiness of surgeons to include her in discussions of the necessity, and prognosis, of her patient's surgery.

Research conducted at Oxford showed that, even without surgery, an anaesthetic produces protein disbalance for up to fourteen days thereafter. Consequent physical debility results in further reduction in post-operative resilience to physical pain and emotional trauma.

Euphemisms used by some surgeons may cause the patient to underrate the effect and implications of surgery. Terms such as 'bypass' and 'investigation under anaesthesia' do little to prepare the patient for the reality of post-operative loss. On the other hand, many patients might shrink from consent were they to be made fully aware of the physical and emotional trauma that lies ahead. Is this not their prerogative? Will the nurse who conscientiously interprets the implications of specific surgery be held culpable if legal consent is refused or withdrawn? A nurse of the author's acquaintance who explained the true implications of 'commodore' surgery to a cancer patient was dismissed when he withdrew consent. What is the true professional role (and protection) in these circumstances? What does the patient's disillusionment with the nurse's information do to her relationship with her client? These questions lie at the heart of a professional–client relationship.

The body image is so deeply ingrained that the personality, in order to defend itself against a threat so overwhelming as body loss, must 'deny' (see p 115) or 'dissociate' itself from (see p 130) anticipating this reality. *Finding it impossible to conceive of personal mutilation, true emotional-level preparation is virtually impossible.* After surgery the patient sees himself as broken, incomplete, inferior.

According to Jung (p 7), a pupil of Freud, the 'group unconscious contains universal prototypes such as the beautiful Fairy Queen, symbol of Good—the ugly, deformed witch, symbol of Evil. Through negative identification the crippled patient may see himself as ugly, evil and untouchable.

The following five factors influence amputees and their actions:

1.   loss of ability to work;
2.   loss of self-confidence;
3.   the state of dependence which is caused by an amputation;
4.   effect on sexual life;
5.   loss of confidence in ability to defend oneself and to resist others.

Normally, people need around ten days in which to prepare themselves for an amputation.

Loss of self-confidence is aggravated where capacity to work is affected. A labourer does not have the education to do office work. It is very difficult to rehabilitate a person to do something which he does not have the training (nor sometimes the intelligence) to do. (See also ch 22, Rehabilitation after Major Body Loss p 501.)

The phenomenum of phantom limbs is not due only to persistent CNS afferent receptor images, but also to *the unconscious need of the patient to cling to his own body image.* This is especially true following amputations and similar traumatic losses after the age of five years.

The patient's anxiety is heightened by the emotion of loss. *He sometimes mourns a lost limb as if it had been a beloved relation.* He will need to be reassured that the limb was not wantonly discarded. Patients are even comforted by the knowledge that the limb had decent burial. Loss and mourning must be accepted by the patient and taken into account by the hospital team and relations before a rehabilitation programme is undertaken to facilitate other intact functions. (See p 502.)

The emotional, social and sexual mal-effects of colostomy and iliestomy are certainly also destructive to body ego. According to Katherine Jetter, rehabilitation counsellor, 'It is beyond description what incontinence does to any man's ego and dignity' (see The Nursing Process, pp 224 and 520).

While the patient may show her anxiety and anger to the rest of the hospital team, she may irritate staff by her contrasting attitude to her surgeon. While some patients do feel genuine respect and gratitude for their surgeon, others may, at a conscious or unconscious level, fear or hate him. In his presence they seek to 'deny' their anxiety by false bravado or hide their anger and aggression lest (in their imagination) they displease him, incur his wrath and hence be subjected to further painful and mutilating surgery (see also The Wounded Healer p 200). This phenomenon of *reaction formation* towards the surgeon, bending backwards to please him lest he counterreact, is quite well known.

Others are bitterly angry with their surgeon and, by association, with his team.

Loss of body image—with special reference to mastectomy

The trauma, or even threat, of mastectomy, involving loss of a woman's main external evidence of femininity, is perhaps as threatening, or as intensely distressing, as the comparable castration fears or loss felt in men. The woman knows that her breasts constitute an essential of successful love-making.

Breast reconstruction does not restore tactile sensitivity. Also it often involves surgery (and scarring) in the remaining breast to reduce and equalize. It may fail due to silicone rejection and ulceration.

Irrespective of attempts at explanation and reassurance through the intellectual approach, the devastating effect of entering the operating theatre a whole woman, to emerge as a permanently mutilated one, cannot be over-estimated, varying only in the manner, either overt or covert, of its presentation according to personality differences and the real life situation. To the happily married woman, the trauma of mastectomy may be rendered less devastating—though she too may fear that henceforth kindness rather than passion, will motivate her husband's sexual approaches. Perhaps with justification, she may doubt her husband's ability to continue the former intensity of his sexual involvement.

'Following breast amputation, Barbara went through a month of radiation and a year of chemotherapy sessions—one week on, five weeks off. And Patrick received a crash course in the sexual problems that beset a mastectomy couple in a society that places a lot of emphasis on breasts.

The operation was just the beginning of a complex web of continuing problems. Even though Barbara has been free of cancer since 1981, some wounds still haven't been healed; the scars reach far deeper than those on her chest. They reach to the center of a male–female relationship.

Patrick, a writer from Arizona, agrees to talk openly about the sexual problems that can plague the partners of women who have undergone mastectomies. But he insists on retaining anonymity to save his wife from embarrassment and to allow himself to be completely candid.

When he's telling it honestly and openly, Patrick will say that in a way, his wife wasn't the only one who lost a breast. He lost one, too.

"I've always absolutely adored womens' breasts. It's been a great part of my sexuality. I love to feel them, and I love to kiss them, and I love to see them.

"What does a mastectomy mean for a male? It means that you're cut off for the rest of your married life as long as your mate lives. Yes, you continue to love her as a person, as a spirit, as an individual. Yet in your own sexuality there is a love—and a need—for breasts."

Patrick emphasizes that he's not talking about intercourse, but about the erotic (and often nurturing) pleasure of touching and holding a woman's breast.

And what does it mean for a female? Patrick sits silently for a moment. Then, just above a whisper, he tries to explain: "My wife is very self-conscious about the way she looks. She'll wear a high-necked nightgown, dress in another room, take baths or showers by herself. She feels that she's been mutilated and doesn't want me turned off by seeing a chest that doesn't have a breast on one side.

This doesn't mean I haven't seen her scar. I've seen her scar but not since she first came home. One of the great joys of my life had always been watching my wife dressing. I always enjoyed that. But I haven't seen a naked woman now for six-and-a-half years . . .

Another problem, certainly an unspoken one, is do you want to kiss that breast? You know in your mind that you can't catch cancer, but the thought goes through your mind.

And then, of course, you're beset by feelings of guilt for even thinking about that. But I'm sure it all goes through the mind of every man who's married to a mastectomee''.'*

The single woman is alone and uncomforted in her distress. The mutilation of her body may well herald the end of whatever hope she may have entertained of establishing a loving and intimate relationship. For her there is no sharing, no comfort to rebuild the self-image of her womanhood.

Some women seek catharsis in talking about their reactions to mutilating surgery, a mechanism used in an attempt to motivate others to some form of overt, constructive adjustment by group identification.

Others are less apt in covering their real emotional reactions, withdrawing permanently, physically and mentally, from social, familial and sexual relationships. Differences in overt manifestation depend on individual personality, and should not arouse the nurse's moral judgement.

It is true that artificial appliances may enable the mastectomy patient to create a reasonable external image. Facing the mutilated image is another story. Years after amputation many bath in the dark, shrink from facing their wounds, and from any sort of intimate physical contact.

The patient may weep overtly, or inside of her. She may withdraw, or become hostile and aggressive in her resentment towards the healthy people who surround her—a reaction for which she may despise herself, but which is involuntary. Frequently a mastectomy occurs simultaneously with the depressing and debilitating symptoms of the menopause, with a consequent overlay of menopausal anxiety and depression.

Post-operative mourning in the older person is very apt to include a general mourning for loss of youth, of loved ones, opportunity and health. The patient is confronted by distressing 'moments of truth'; she may well encounter her first brush with death and mortality. Henceforth every bump or lump may press the panic button, body searching becomes a burden to the patient and her family (see AIDS).

Frequently the patient's reactions 'split off' into ambivalent, contrasting channels. One part of the personality may try 'bravely' to go on living; the other wants to die, with the flesh and lost body-image she mourns. Yet another is filled with anger which she takes out on hospital staff and other healthy people surrounding her (see Displacement, p 121).

Thus she may refuse the help of the hospital team; she may also consistently refuse food. In a public ward, she may yearn for the privacy afforded by closed curtains. Attempts should be made to meet her needs by placing her bed in a corner, thus keeping clear the nurse's view of the ward.

Rose Kushner, a medical writer for more than twenty years and a former research assistant at the John Hopkins School of Medicine, had a mastectomy in

* Mastecomee Mates—When a partner needs a shoulder to lean on. *Cope Magazine for Cancer Patients, their Families and Physicians*. September 1986, Vol No 2. PO Box 51722, Boulder, CO 80322–1722, USA.

1974. Her anger at the lack of information available to women prompted her to write *Breast Cancer: A Personal History & An Investigative Report*, published by Harcourt Brace and Jovanovich, and, in September 1985, *Alternatives—New Developments in the War on Breast Cancer*. She emphasizes two-step and local surgery.

Mrs Kushner also set up the Breast Cancer Advisory Center and Breast Cancer Hotline in Kensington, Maryland, USA. (Phone 0911-301-949-2530)

An article entitled 'Breast Cancer: Surgery & Survival,' published in *Harper's Bazaar Magazine*, October 1976, reads:

'After breast surgery of any kind, women of every age suffer various kinds of psychological trauma. These depend on a woman's age, marital status and the extent of her disease . . . Those women who, as far as anyone knows, are 'cured' have varying psychological problems. Young, unmarried women worry about getting and keeping boy friends or husbands. Older widows or divorcees have the same worries, intensified by the loss of youth, and attractiveness. Removal of a breast is another sign to them that they are nearing the end of their appealing years. Married women with young children—that is, married women whose husbands stand by them—seem to be more concerned with avoiding a recurrence and with "who will look after my children?" Of course, there must certainly be hidden fears that the loss of a breast will drive their husbands away, but—according to interviews—these are hidden and not uppermost in their minds. However, older married women whose husbands may already have begun to stray to younger girl friends, or who have become totally preoccupied by their jobs or businesses, do suffer sexual anxiety. Their children are usually grown and gone from the house, their husbands' attentions have drifted elsewhere, and they consider having a breast amputated one more thing that will drive their husbands away.'

In 1981, in an article on the family relationships of mastectomy patients (*Israeli Journal of Medical Science* 17-993-996), Dr Wellisch suggested that one aspect of a mother's distress may stem from envy of her daughter's intact body, causing rivalry, guilt and anxiety.

At a conference on 'Early Breast Cancer: The Psychological Perspective,' co-sponsored by Long Island Jewish Medical Centre, SUNY at Stony Brook, New York, and Memorial Sloan Kettering Cancer Centre, Wendy Schain PhD, consultant with the National Institute of Health, stated:

'There was a time (before lesser surgery such as lumpectomy and wedge resection) when most of what we saw clinically or heard anecdotally was a daughter whose mother died of breast cancer and the horror of the image of the mutilating procedure and the way that mama died.'

Dr Schain quoted the declaration of a teenaged daughter from California: 'I am very uninterested in sexuality. Why should I get involved when I am almost certainly going to lose my breasts as time goes on?'

'Are they avoiding the self exam? Are they fearful about being sexually excited about their breasts because they fear they may lose them? Are they hyper vigilant and need constant reassuring?' asked Dr Schain.

Shelley E Taylor PhD, professor of psychology at the University of California, maintained that daughters most 'at risk' for poor psychological adjustment, and, indeed, intensive emotional suffering and threatened body-image, are those whose mothers had had extensive surgery, including mastectomy and, to a lesser extent, more difficulty with radiation or chemotherapy.

Sometimes the mother–daughter relationship is imperilled, and even broken.

Of 78 mothers interviewed by Dr Taylor's researchers no son left home, but daughters did, temporarily or permanently. 'They cited the fear of inheritance as the cause. As one of these mothers said: "I feel she is rebelling, and doesn't really want to have anything to do with me, because she feels that perhaps she herself will become a cancer victim."' (See Flight adjustive mechanism pp 26, 104.)

Younger girls generally feel the same way as sons—extremely fearful that their mother would die. Reaction to stress takes several forms—anger, defensiveness, aloofness, denial (chapter 5).

Anxiety and distress for their daughters is also a major cause of concern for husbands of breast cancer patients. Dr Wellisch maintained:

> 'The number one, very fist thing the husband wanted to talk about was . . . their worries about their daughters getting breast cancer.'

Dr Wellisch now routinely schedules a two-hour consultation session, spending the first hour with the daughter alone, and the second hour with both mother and daughter.*

Perhaps because most doctors are men, some experience difficulty in identifying with the extent and intensity of a woman's reactions to mastectomy, with consequent tardiness of research into this area of enormous import. However, research of the past thirty years has shown that, in many spheres of breast cancer, the statistical chance of developing secondaries is no greater in a well-conducted lumpectomy than in amputation.† Many eminent authorities believe that preservation of the regional glands provides indispensable lymphatic drainage and antibody protection.‡ Chemotherapy and other complementary therapy have extended confidence in lumpectomy and partial mastectomy. Mercifully a growing number of highly skilled and sensitive surgeons are using the lumpectomy technique in cancer therapy. Were more women aware thereof, they would, no doubt, be less reluctant to seek treatment. Two-stage surgery enables consideration of options.

An important milestone in favour of lesser surgery is the publication in the *New England Journal of Medicine* Vol 312 No 111 14 March 1985, of Bernard Fisher MD and associates' 'Five Year results of a Randomized Clinical Trial Comparing Total

---

* From a leader article, *Psychiatry Clinical Psychology Practice.* Vol 1 No 2 April 1986

† NIH Consensus Development Conference. 'The Treatment of Primary Breast Cancer: Management of Local Disease.' Sponsored by National Cancer Institute and Office for Medical Applications of Research, NIH, 5 June 1979. Conference Summary vol 2 No 5.

‡ Peters, Vera M. 'Wedge Resection with our without Radiation in Early Breast Cancer.' *International Journal Radiation Oncology Biol Phys.* **2**: 1151–6. 1977. United States: Pergamon Press. Princess Margaret Hospital, Toronto, Canada.

References:

Kushner, Rose. Breast Cancer Advisory Center, 9607 Kingston Road, Kensington, Maryland 20795, USA, provides a wide range of literature and a 24-hour telephone service: 0911–301–949–2530.

Crile, George. *What Every Woman Should Know About the Breast Cancer Controversy.* New York: Macmillan. 1973.

Mastectomy and Segmental Mastectomy With or Without Radiation in the Treatment of Breast Cancer':

> 'Life-table estimated based on data from 1 843 women, indicated that treatment by segmental mastectomy, with or without breast irradiation, resulted in disease-free, distant-disease-free, and overall survival at five years that was no worse than that after total breast removal. In fact, disease-free survival after segmental mastectomy plus radiation was better than disease-free survival after total mastectomy, and overall survival after segmental mastectomy, with or without radiation, was better than overall survival after total mastectomy.'

Says Dr Samuel Hellman, the physician in chief at New York City's Memorial Sloan-Kettering Cancer Center: 'In my judgment, the most important fact about breast-saving surgery is that it has resulted in women being less fearful and, therefore, more willing to consult physicians when they feel a lump. They no longer assume they will automatically lose their breast. I believe that this gives us a chance to see patients earlier, when the disease is more curable.'

Specific emotional impact of cancer realization

The cancer patient's reactions to diagnosis will probably place him in crisis and thus expose him to the classic stages of

1. Impact phase
2. Turmoil—recoil phase
3. Emotionally wounded phase
4. hopefully, and where applicable, Adjustment and Reconstitution phase. (Chapter 24 p 563.)

Reacting to the death encounter, he will be exposed to the agonies of

Awareness
Denial
Bargaining
Anxiety, sometimes amounting to terror
Depression and Grieving
hopefully, Acceptance (Chapter 23 pp 534 et seq.)

Frequently surgery brings the *realization of serious or fatal illness*. Life will never be the same again. Patients are becoming more sophisticated; they know, or at least they *feel*, themselves to walk in the shadow of death. <u>Henceforth every physical irregularity could herald a recurrence or escalation.</u> Long-term plans and hopes melt away. One is jolted out of one's dreams of marriage, child-bearing, seeing a son graduate or a grandchild's face. Even one's financial plans flounder on the implications of the expenses incurred by long-term illness. (See Cancer Rehabilitation—the Damocles Syndrome p 520)

One is cut off from the rest of humanity.

Because of the connotations of cancer in our society, there may well be an emotional reaction of inturned repugnance. <u>One feels unclean.</u> One fears that others even one's loved ones will find one untouchable. Patients have been known to further mutilate their bodies—tearing out stitches, sticking cigarette butts into wounds . . . perhaps to purge their feelings of uncleanliness . . . perhaps to punish a body that has turned rotten.

The sensitive patient senses the fear her condition arouses in others, who would wish to run away and dissociate themselves from the distasteful, frightening involvements of cancer. One senses this even amongst some of the staff, who perform their duties diligently, efficiently and skilfully, but with the least possible personal contact.

One lies and wonders what one has done to be thus singled out and isolated, in a cell of soul-searching, guilt, anxiety and depression. Resentment towards the healthy, integrated, optimistic, whole people around one mounts. Their remarks such as 'Pull yourself together,' 'Think of others worse off than yourself,' 'It's a matter of mind over body,' anger or embitter.

Hildegard Knef,* the Austrian cabaret star, describes poignantly the patient's post-operative reaction to the realization of cancer:

> 'I see myself falling, blindly running into fear, intractable raw fear; fear of being excluded, of being incapable of rehabilitating into a world of fearless diffidents; fear of the drawbridge that's up, separating me from those who know nothing of pain. Its fear's poison, fear's pride. I go to a party and look around, thinking is there anyone else there with a *verdict*. There's a new symptom. I'm to be X-rayed the day after tomorrow . . .'

One knows there is no real help in anyone. Only God lives in X-ray rooms.

In the context of the reality horror, or depression, demands for co-operation from physiotherapist, nurse, radiotherapist may well appear paltry, annoying and pointless.

Individual consideration by the team, support system and patient himself of his ego-strengths, life situation and resources, burdens and goals is certainly of import before embarking on a long, frightening, pain-ridden programme of chemo- or radiation therapy. Isolation from loved ones, mutilation, sensory bombardment and encasement in frightening apparatus, nausea, pain and negative identification (pp 108-111) with the terminally ill constitute serious, sometimes overwhelming suffering. Justification can only be attempted in the light of team consideration of the patient's prognosis, life history, personality and life circumstances.

The role of the emotional support sister in the general wards

From a presentation by psychiatric nursing sister Debbie Tyrrel-Glynn (March 1981).

Ranking the demand for her services, she presented the following 'need scale':

(1) *Orthopaedic wards*—the 'Why me?' syndrome.
    After lying many weeks in restricted, painful and uncomfortable positions, patients are not infrequently informed of treatment failure and poor prognosis, plunging them into despair.

* Hildegard Knef 'The Final Role.' *Fair Lady Magazine, 15 September 1976.*

(2) *Haemotology*—young people struck down without hope, face long periods of 'heavy' and traumatic treatment. Heartbroken, guilt-laden parents dread the final parting.

(3) *Cancer wards*—'Where I have learnt to respect the supportive strength of *denial*. While we are taught to work for acceptance, often I feel I have done my best if I can leave the patient and his family with some little hope of something good . . . Patients cannot be left alone in terminal wards. Sometimes, two days before a patient unknown to me dies, I am called in to hold his hand and see him through this all-engulfing experience. I must save him from dying with no relationship . . . You must have the courage not to leave the patient and his family. Often I must attempt to support and comfort patients facing the many horrors of mastectomy.' (*Author*: This role will require increasing soul-searching, tact, and strong personal integrity, as women begin to learn about treatment controversies, and their right to information about their options, including 'lesser surgery' (see p 81ff).)

(4) *Transplant wards* where the patient may be 'cut-off' from meaningful human contact for six weeks on end, suffering the mental disintegration that accompanies sensory deprivation.

Among the special qualities required of the 'emotional support sister' are an ability to:

(i) accept patient's needs of *repetitive* catharsis and verbalized reassurance,

(ii) accept flexibility,

(iii) adapt to, and make herself belong in, a wide range of difficult and stressful situations, frequently involving patient-loss in death,

(iv) accept personal isolation and frustration of her 'belonging' needs,

(v) constantly accept the 'on site', 'lifebuoy' psychotherapeutic role,

(vi) accept adjustment/defence mechanisms of which she may not, in theory, 'approve',

(vii) accept rejection by patients—some patients' need for privacy, and self-determination is stronger than that for assessment—orientated support.

She should possess a warm, outgoing personality. In addition, the following is a true reflection of her role: 'I do the best I can in the "here and now". Contrary to resistance, staff in their desperation usually welcome me. The need for my services is growing all the time—there could be three of me!'

CHAPTER 4

MOTIVATION

'What are you doing, my good man?'
'I'm dragging these ruddy stones from one place t'other.'
'And your workmate here, what are *you* doing?'
'I'm helping Sir Christopher Wren build St Paul's Cathedral!'

What are the *basic sources of power* behind human behaviour? What impels man to behave as he does? In dealing with human behaviour, we must answer these questions in a dynamic way, that is in terms of changing and active internal forces.

Motivation (Definition)

The original *internal stimulus* causing the mobilization of chemical, metabolic and physiological energy into a unifying force to achieve a goal is termed a MOTIVATION.

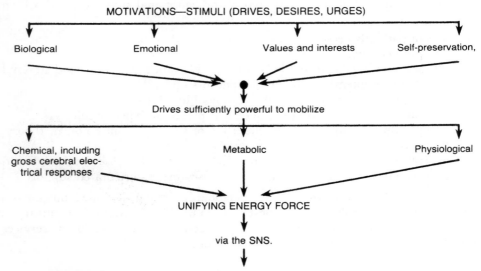

MOTIVATIONS—STIMULI (DRIVES, DESIRES, URGES)

Biological   Emotional   Values and interests   Self-preservation,

Drives sufficiently powerful to mobilize

Chemical, including gross cerebral electrical responses   Metabolic   Physiological

UNIFYING ENERGY FORCE

via the SNS.

via the Hypothalamus, certain parts of the Limbic System, the Sympathetic Nervous System and the Pituitary Gland

Tension energy

Goal-achievement*   (equilibrium: homeostasis)

These internal stimuli or basic motivations are named and classified according to the need or goal they aim to attain, eg:

the motivation to relieve thirst; or
the motivation to gain love and recognition.

In order to qualify as basic drives or motivations, these original energy stimuli must possess *three characteristics*, namely:

(1) INTENSITY: Absorbing and possessing the organism to the exclusion of other motivations, so that, at that time, nothing else matters.

(2) PERSISTENCE: The drives pertaining to a goal-object must persist, constantly recurring in mind until the goal is achieved.

(3) VARIABILITY: Motivations are, in general, variable in the sense that they may take a variety of forms, adapting themselves to many different contexts, and persisting intensely all the way, eg a person who is greatly motivated by hunger may think of *many kinds of food*, and many different ways of obtaining it.

Drives felt sufficiently intensely, persistently and variably to cause SNS mobilization of tension energy qualify as basic motivations.

In studying motivation, it is valuable to concentrate attention on the wide variety of circumstances which set off this vigorous response in the individual.

The four main varieties of motivation, drives or urges are:

1. *Biological drives*

The most elementary forms of energy mobilization arise from definite biological needs of the organism. Drives to relieve hunger, thirst, oxygen lack, fatigue, pain, the drive for defecation are some conditions giving rise to motivated action, or the exertion of mobilized tension energy.

A patient pre-operatively deprived of fluid is, for example, consumed by biochemically mobilized tension-energy designed by nature for the specific purpose of obtaining that fluid: in denying him satisfaction of this basic biological motivation we are placing him in state of powerful, environmentally blocked, unresolvable stress, in the face of which we must expect attempts at substitute tension release such as aggression, depression or desperate anxiety.

Similarly a patient driven by the biological motivation to defecate may be caught in the *conflict* between this basic drive and an equally strong emotional drive to protect himself from feelings of acute emotional shame and distress involved in using a bed-pan — a conflict of motivations causing a spiralling accumulation of suppressed tension-energy.

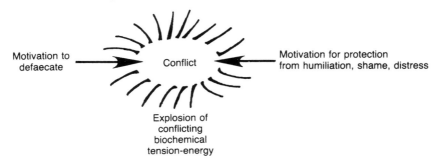

The motivation for physical *withdrawal from pain* is also primary and biological. There is a built-in individual point at which each person will involuntarily withdraw his body from exposure to a pain-producing stimulus. A classic experiment conducted by first-year psychology students counts the number and strength of painful pin 'jabs' at which each individual will involuntarily withdraw his hand.

The experiment shows a very wide deviation in this involuntary withdrawal point. Apparently each individual patient's ability to bear pain depends on the proportional development of his pain-interpreting brain centres, the number of afferent nerve endings in the pain-exposed area, childhood pain experiences, and many other factors over which the patient has no control. Ability to bear pain is thus dependent on anatomical structure, and biochemical activity level and early psychological experiences rather than on 'will-power'.

Attempts to persuade patients to 'hide' their pain reactions; to 'take it'; to 'be brave like Mr Jones', cannot change their organic organization and will only increase their guilt and tension.

More supportive nursing consists in getting a painful procedure over as quickly as possible, and letting the patient know we understand his pain and will help him 'see it through'.

2. *Emotions and emotional drives*

Fear, joy, anger, love, hate, disgust, desire for honour and recognition, curiosity, humiliation and embarrassment all *imply the presence of inner states leading to vigorous biochemical activity* as described on pages 24-30.

Because feelings ('affect') emanate from subjective personal experiences, definitions of emotion are understandably vague.

Accommodating physiological components of emotion, a relatively useful definition is submitted by Hilgard, Atkinson and Atkinson.*

Emotion: the condition of the organism during affectively toned experience, whether mild or intense.

The following are reasons for difficulty encountered in studying emotions:

It is sometimes difficult to distinguish the cause ⟷ effect relationship between physiological change and emotional experience. The two main theories on this sequence are:

(a) The Cannon-Bard Theory, maintaining that emotional process is conveyed *inwards* from the invironment.

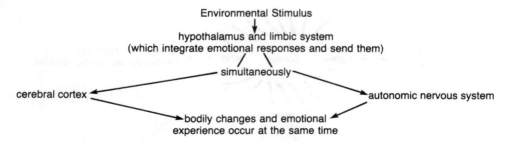

eg   a hypodermic syringe → fear
        an unjust accusation → anger

---

* Hilgard, Atkinson and Atkinson. *Introduction to Psychology.* 7 ed. Harcourt Brace Jovanovich.

This *inwards*-orientated concept maintains that generalized ANS alarm, anticipation or other physiological overactivity (pp 25-29) leads to:

→ paid
→ ander
→ desire, etc.

CANNON–BARD THEORY

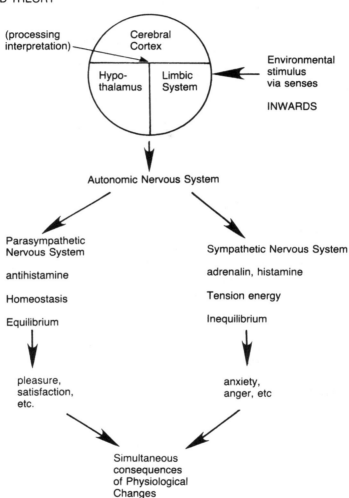

(b) The James Lange Theory, maintaining that in the light of experience the organism *learns to recognize,* from its *internal bodily changes,* the nature of its emotional life.

Emotion is thus an *outward, feedback experience* from physiological disturbance:

→ cerebral processing

→ emotional experience.

JAMES–LANGE THEORY. Feedback to the cerebral cortex of bodily responses interpreted as conscious emotional experiences. OUTWARDS

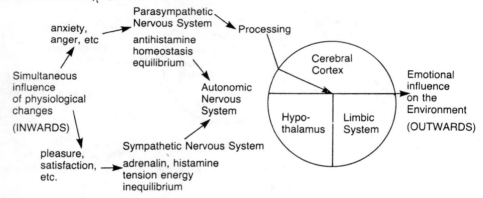

However, because

(i) the ANS bodily arousal symptoms (pp 25-29) do not differ much from one emotion to another,

(ii) internal organs are not well supplied with sensory nerves,

(iii) injections of adrenalin and other artificial inducers of tension-energy fail to produce feedback emotion,

this theory has met with little experimental reinforcement.

It is very difficult, and would, in fact, constitute an infringement of the rights of others, to subject them to laboratory-induced stimuli of painful emotions such as fear, anger and despair.

Conclusions

Irrespective of stringent experimental method, there is abundant evidence to show that:

1.   While we cannot identify the nature of an emotion from the *bodily sensations* it arouses, these *do determine the intensity of the experience.*

2.   Emotion is not a momentary split-second event, but rather an experience *taking place over a period of time.*

3.   It is the *individual's own*

sensory input, cerebral processing (pp 138 et seq), *interpretation,*

of the emotion-providing situation which will determine his emotional experience.

These in turn will depend on his:

(i) *Experience*

Although most emotions are innate,

eg *fear* of bright lights, noise, loss of balance
   anger at hunger
   search for the comfort and security of the mother figure
they are 'associated' 'conditioned' (pp 151-159) and amended by life events;
eg *Fear:* the burnt child dreads fire
   Safety, security: satisfaction in loving relationships: 'Mummy makes it better'
   Joy: in love returned.

(ii) *Innate personality and cognition*

   The more intellectually endowed and alert an individual, the higher his quality
of cognition (thoughts, knowledge, interpretation, understanding, ideational
processes and creativity), the wider, more astute and richer his reactions and
emotional predictions.

eg Chronological age 6 years is a peak period for expanding fears . . . animals,
    darkness, death, cripples . . . (pp 282-284).
    The more mature six-year-old is comforted by the knowledge that most will
    not materialize.
    The bright five-year-old may suffer acutely from premature fears before
    exposure to reassuring experiences. Conversely, simpler people are sometimes
    spared imaginative and anticipatory fears.

Certainly cognition is an important determinant of:

(a) the range, strength and persistence of emotions;
(b) the individual's ability to handle arousal and achieve coping skills, which help
       him to return to a state of psycho-physiological equilibrium (Homeostasis
       p 103).

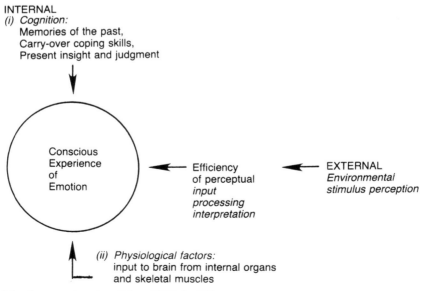

Individual stress levels of the ANS (p 30)
Hormonal reaction levels (p 27ff)

Experiencing Emotion

It is difficult to describe emotion, but experimentation has shown that, asked to do so, people present *the following sequence:*

1. Arousing circumstances → the cause.
   Environmental input which 'triggered off' reactions of, eg:
   > mention of surgery → fear;
   > an authoritarian tone of voice → anger;
   > praise → happiness;
   > necessity of defecating in public → humiliation.

2. Bodily reaction:
   > 'It made my stomach turn.'
   > 'I was goose-pimples all over.'
   > 'My knees turned to jelly.'

3. Difficulties in dealing with the emotion:
   > 'I was so embarrassed, I didn't know where to look.'
   > 'I wanted to get up and run.'
   > 'I itched to hit her — but I didn't dare.' (Stress aggravated by conflict.)

Certainly evidence points to the cumulative effect of these factors on the intensity and duration of emotional experience.

Classification of Emotions

Modern research considers efforts at complicated classification of emotions fruitless.

Only the following criteria are considered to serve a useful purpose:

1. *Pleasant*
   Stimulating advance, seeking activity:
   eg love, pleasure, joy, comfort, sexual fulfilment.
   (Satisfaction involves arousal of the Parasympathetic Nervous System.)

   Unpleasant
   Stimulating Fight-Flight attack or avoidance over activity.
   eg fear, anger, humiliation, disgust.
   (Effectiveness is dependent on arousal of the Sympathetic Nervous System)

2. *Intensity*
   On the continuum between:

eg *Mild*	*Intense*
pain	agony
displeasure	fury
sadness	grief
affection	love
distaste	hate

Search for limits to the concept of 'emotion' is less productive than the view that we are concerned with a whole range of affective experience.

Emotional expression is probably both innate and learnt

All over the world people weep when they are sad: laugh when they are amused.

As far back as 1872 Charles Darwin in his work *The Expression of Emotion in Man and Animals* postulated an innate evolutionary theory of emotions.

Impressed by the universality of emotional expression in animals, and even in the blind, he claimed that:

(i) the manner in which emotions are expressed is inherited.
(ii) Originally emotional expression had some survival value. (Indeed it still does! — Author.) In fear we tense our muscles for protection. Extreme disgust is expressed in mouth movements, which are primitively preparatory to protective vomiting of poisonous substances. (Learning Aggression pp 166-8.)

Modern experimentation, which included instruction to interpret photographs depicting facial expressions of happiness, anger, sadness, disgust, fear, surprise were administered to subjects from USA, Chile, Brazil, Argentina, Japan and New Guinea, all of whom easily identified the emotions depicted.*

On the other hand, while most emotional expressions are doubtless innate, many are modified by experience and exaggerated or inhibited by custom and mores:

> Samurai warriors laud the exaggerated expression of aggression.
> Teutonic races condition a stoic expression to hide fear.
> The British 'stiff upper lip' hides expression of grief (resulting, in psycho-analytic terms, in feelings of inhibited, and thus festering, debilitating stress).

Sometimes it is possible to mask facial expression, but sagging shoulders and bowed back reveal depression, defeat, disappointment: clenched fists or cold withdrawal betray anger (see Body Language, p 178ff.)

The Role of Emotions and Emotional Drives

The *distinction between emotions and emotional motivation* is not clearly defined and is, in fact, of academic rather than practical import.

Usual differentiation is as follows:

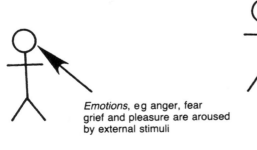

Emotions, eg anger, fear grief and pleasure are aroused by external stimuli

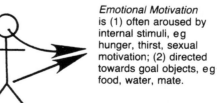

Emotional Motivation is (1) often aroused by internal stimuli, eg hunger, thirst, sexual motivation; (2) directed towards goal objects, eg food, water, mate.

* Ekman P, Friesen W V. *Unmasking the Face* Englewood Cliffs NJ: Prentice-Hall, 1975: 340,43.

Containable levels of emotions, such as

> anger,
> jealousy,
> the drive for honour and recognition,

in mobilizing the body's emotionally arouse Sympathetic Nervous System tension-energy (intra alia (pp 25-29, 88ff), stimulate a higher level of energy output. Hence desired goals are achieved and the balance of homeostasis restored.

However, when emotional drives, such as fear and anger, stimulate SNS Fight-Flight general alarm mobilization (p 32) the outflow of tension-energy may become *so intense* that its very purpose is impeded by the *disorganization of over-activity*.

Controlled free-flow of constructive action then gives way to *unproductive panic*.

Studies of soldiers under the intense Fight-Flight stress of combat show that only 15–25% can be relied upon to make the selective actions involved in firing their rifles.

Tyhurst* (1951) has shown that, in times of crisis and disaster, such as floods, fire and air raids, approximately

> 15% of those exposed thereunto show organized, effective behaviour;
> 70% show various degrees of disorganization, but are still able to function with some effectiveness, especially in routine, well-practised tasks;
> 15% are so disorganized that their panic results in random efforts at tension reduction such as screaming and aimless running around (see also p 566).

The Duration of Emotional Arousal

The duration of emotionally provoked tension-energy varies with individual personality differences and hence life experiences.

> anger . . . provoked by a personally diminishing senior nurse,
> fear of a serious illness,
> despair in any unhappy marriage,

may result in long-term unresolved conflict and frustrated tension-energy (p 55). Consequent unexpressed over-activity of body processes designed for Fight and Flight may be persistently channelled 'underground' and converted into psycho-somatic illnesses such as gastric ulcers, chronic hypertension, asthma (pp 29-31, 128-130).

Even mild, long-term unresolved pyscho-physiological stress may cause distress and impaired human relationships and mental efficiency.

3. *Values and interests*

At a more subtle and complex level, we recognize the energizing effect of the broad, non-biological group of drives which are called Values and Interest, eg a powerful need for religious or political fulfilment.

A girl, for instance, in whom the motivation for religious satisfaction is felt intensely, persistently and variably in all kinds of situations, may become a nun

---

* Hilgard, Atkinson, Atkinson. *Introduction to Psychology* 7 ed. Harcourt Brace Jovanovich.

and, in so doing, relegate to subsidiary positions many other motivations such as the need to love, to hate, to express anger, sometimes even the biological needs of eating and drinking.

The power of primitive biochemical energy mobilized by potent, deep-seated conscious and unconscious drives for religious satisfaction explains the otherwise inexplicable attitude of a parent who, through religious conviction, is prepared to allow his child to die rather than receive a blood transfusion.

Once the parent's body biochemistry is rallied to fill his organism with tension energy designed for the fulfilment of his all-engulfing religious drives, all logical reasoning is useless.

It is then necessary, in order to save the child's life, to turn without hesitation or delay to the legal machinery which, it is submitted, does exist for the purpose of safeguarding the life and welfare of the child thus affected. In the eyes of the law, the interests and welfare of a minor child are paramount.

First, an approach should be to the local magistrate who may, at any time, approach a judge of the High Court as upper guardian of all minor children for guidance and assistance. It is submitted that the court may decide to overrule a natural guardian of the child so as to *compel* treatment where such is shown to be necessary and essential.

The child's life would then be saved, and the parent, having been, if necessary, forcefully overruled, may yet experience religious satisfaction at having done his best to prevent treatment, thus being spared tension-producing guilt feelings.

4. Motivation for personal survival

Unclassifiable, because it contains elements of all three classifications, is the *motivation for personal survival* — often popularly described as 'the will to live'.

Freud believed the two basic energies governing our lives to be:

> *The Life Instinct* expressed in sexual behaviour
> *The Death Instinct* motivating the aggression of survival, but also of domination: killing and suicide.

Life and Sexual Behaviour are inextricably interwoven, and when one or the other drive is threatened, in reality or in phantasy, we encounter terror and depression and the search for sublimation, and compensation outlets (pp 111-114). Threatened by extinction, young soldiers (and indeed the terminally ill) frequently yearn for, and seek, survival through reproduction. Their progeny will live for them.

Frustration of sexual motivation, as in spinal-cord injury (p 508), or in the loneliness or institutionalization of the aged, is a serious percipitant of aggression or depression.

The interweaving of life, sex, death and aggression and their frustrated tension-energy, may explode in suicide, sexual violence or armed combat.

Understandably, in the face of great pain, depression, and sometimes overwhelming emotional stress, a person may lose 'the will to live'; he wants to 'finish it all off — to curl up and die'. And largely, to the nursing staff, falls the difficult task of 'fanning back to life' the motivation to survive and fight back to health.

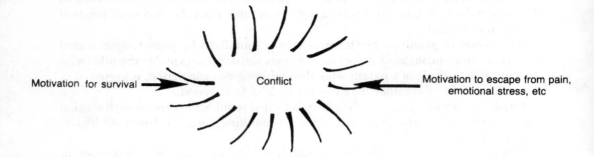

Motivation for survival ➤   Conflict   ◀ Motivation to escape from pain, emotional stress, etc

On the medical worker's side in this tug-of-war between the urge to live and the urge to 'get away from it all' is the fact that somewhere, *deep inside him, the patient wants to live,* and resists death with all his being. In what practical ways can the nurse assist that part of the patient's being that is striving for life, health and independence? Here are some suggestions:

1. Treatment procedures should be explained to the patient in simple language so that his anxiety, hostility and resentment, or hopelessness, may turn to calmer understanding. The very fact that he is treated with respect as a normal, intelligent individual, will increase his feelings of consequence and self-esteem. That he *matters* as an individual may help motivate a patient towards getting better. (However, because of the difficulty is bridging the gap between *intellectual* understanding and *emotional* acceptance, the nurse should not blame her patient, or herself, if the feelings of anxiety or depression persist.)

2. Clearly the attitude of the hospital staff is important. One should try to remember that the patient who hands himself over to others for treatment is, in Professor Gillis's words: 'very much in the situation of one who, although unable to swim, throws himself into the deep end of the swimming-bath and depends on the life-savers to pull him out.* Efficiency and caring enhance confidence.

3. Enhanced religious faith is important to many people, and a visit from a clergyman may give the patient the confidence to 'fight back'.

4. Lest he regress to passive, unmotivated helplessness the patient should be persuaded to do as much for himself as his physical condition allows. Again, to quote Professor Gillis: 'He should be made to feel that he is not just a passive piece of agonised and diseased flesh to which, and for whom people do things, but that he has a part to play in his own treatment, and that some, at least, of the responsibility devolves upon himself— thinking of the patient as a helpless invalid may incline him to share our view.'

Here is wise advice from Jill Brawley, a student nurse of sensitivity and intelligence, who won the Johnson and Johnson Writing Competition for her article 'The Aged Require Attention':†

'The patient's treatment can be broken down into short-term goals towards

* Gillis, Lyn. *The Emotional Problems of Illness. Faber and Faber.*
† *Curationis.* March. 1983.

which he can strive. Explain the procedures carefully so they do not seem something distant and hazy. By continually communicating about these goals of his care with the patient he will be more convinced that there is direcion and that others are concerned about his achievement. This prevents the patient from anxiously wondering what is happening and if things will ever improve. (One elderly lady, who was not told what was going to be done to her, was convinced, and kept saying so, that she was being kept there to die.) Goal setting will help the elderly person in hospital to gain a sense of purpose and achievement.'

(See also Regression, p 123 and The Elderly Patient, chapter 20).

5. Even, though to do so may disturb ward routine, patients should be encouraged to attend to their own personal functions as far as possible: to 'help' with ward duties, to read and study (even to a relatively late hour if, for example, an examination is at stake) and to keep alive contacts with the healthy vital, warm and moving world outside the hospital gates.

Before discharge it is the social worker's job to see that this world, familiar, or, of necessity, in some way changed, does welcome him back.

Medical personnel are sometimes deceived into supposing that a patient has abandoned the motivation to live, and is seeking refuge in death.

A pensioner suffering from multiple sclerosis verbalised thus:

'Doctor I know I am reaching the end of the road. Before me lie only helplessness and suffering. If this continues my wife will be sentenced to a proverty-striken old age. Please give me something to help me over the river.'

But his wise GP knew better. He realized that the man was in deep depression and his statement was really a plea for reassurance to the effect that he was, in truth, sufficiently important and loved to be kept alive.

The doctor prescribed standard anti-depressant medication, and at the same time contacted the appropriate branch of the Organization for the Welfare of the Aged to arrange for financial relief and inclusion in their social and recreational programmes. The motivation to survive was fanned back to life and the pensioner rallied to live out his admittedly short life-span in reasonably cheerful satisfaction.

Maslow's Hierarchy of Human Needs

Most Nursing Process Models are classified by goals rather than by the motivation tension-energy designed to achieve these goals. The meaning and impact of the motivation, tension-energy → goal-achievement relationship is, however, synonymous. Most Nursing Process Models are based on *Maslow's Hierarchy of Human Needs*. (See diagram on following page.)

Tension

Tension, as we have seen (pp 27-30, 25ff), consists in *mobilization of body resources* required to place the organism in readiness for an increased demand about to be made upon it, that it may preserve its life and fulfil its basic motivations.

When the fulfilment of these motivations is prevented, and the *expression of mobilized chemical tension-energy thwarted for relatively long periods,* then the organism is said to be in a state of *stress.*

Stress

Stress, as we have seen in chapter 2, classically results in conditions varying from mild psychosomatic changes to serious and pathological psychosomatic illness.

Max Halhuber, Medical Director of the Hoehenried Rehabilitation Centre in West Germany, reporting on 38 000 heart-attack patients who have passed through his hands in eight years, maintains stress to be 'the common denominator in most *heart attack* cases'.*

	SELF ACTUALIZATION	NURSING IMPLICATIONS*
	5. Self-fulfilment achievement is confined to adults, constitutes a goal of adolescents. Achieved only when a person aspires to that for which he is suited.	Implementation or restoration financial and social independence, creative satisfaction etc. Involvement in treatment choice.
Fulfilment → self-worth, healthy self-concept → contributor to society. Frustration → feelings of inferiority hopelessness → neurotic compensatory (sometimes anti-social) behaviour mechanisms.	4. ESTEEM —— For self-respect, recognition, honour, glory, status. Independence, freedom, appreciation, dignity.	Achieved by *Values and Interest* Drive Tension-Energy (p 88). Treat patient with respect. Preserve his dignity. Address correctly. Privacy.
When needs are unmet the individual feels unloved, rejected, friendless, abandoned and restless. This applies to 'rootless' and hospitalized children. Deprivation is core of maladjustment and psychopathology.	3. LOVE AND BELONGING NEEDS —— For a love partner—parents, family, friends and group relationships—expression and acceptance—aversion to isolation.	Achieved by *Emotional* Drive Tension-Energy (p 82). Assure presence of loved ones, communication (including tactile). Reassurance. Catharsis.
Safety needs dominate and are urgent in disasters, emergencies, war, disease and injuries; crime waves, hostage holdings, strikes, breakdown of authority.	2. SAFETY AND SECURITY NEEDS For physical environment free from threat and fear: Dependable social structure free from assault, wars, etc. Protection from germs, natural disasters; need for financial security.	Achieved by *personal survival* Drive Tension-Energy (p 89). Checking medication, sterilizing instruments. Apparatus in best working condition, etc.
Individual is dominated by physical needs. If one is unsatisfied (frustrated) all other higher needs recede eg no fluid, nothing else matters.	1. PHYSICAL NEEDS —— Air, food, fluids, sleep, rest, activity, elimination, stimulation, maternal response, etc. Sex not essential for individual but for group survival.	Achieved by *Biological* Drive Tension-Energy (p 81). When incapacitated nurse takes over, eg intravenous feeding, catheters, etc.

Left margin (vertical): 'Higher' needs emerge when physical and environmental needs are satisfied. When 'higher' needs are frustrated, the individual regresses to preoccupation with 'lower' needs. Realized as *healthy whole* results in realisation of maximal potential

From Maslow, A. *Motivation and Personality.* 1970. New York: Harper & Row.

* From Johnson & Davis (1975).

Hans Schaefer, the eminent Heidelberg physiologist, maintains that 'in addition to heart attacks, stress is responsible for three other major causes of death. These are *road deaths* which are very often the direct consequence of overstrain due to stress; *cirrhosis of the liver* from alcohol consumed in quantities to dissipate the agonies caused by stress; *lung cancer,* caused by excessive smoking which in turn is due to stress.'

Scientific investigators maintain that stress appears frequently in workers from whom too much is demanded, or whose work is too monotonous.

Of special import to Community Nurses are the following factors in modern living which, according to scientific investigators, precipitate *stress situations:*

(1) *cramped living conditions* — monkeys forced to live in cramped conditions show more stress symptoms than do controls living in more expansive conditions — especially is this so when the monkeys are forced to live with others whom they fear;

(2) *isolation,* which deprives the individual of stress release afforded by the adjustment mechanism of *identification. Group catharsis* also reduces long-term tension culminating in destructive psychosomatic stress symptoms;

(3) *the noises of civilization* because they

 (a) create long-term tensions unrelieved by periods of stress reduction, hormonal balance and homeostasis, and

 (b) seldom warn of real danger, but constantly place the individual in a state of 'false alarm',

are particularly precipitant of tension involvement.

Motor-car driving is considered to constitute an especially evil combination of four primitive stress precipitants, namely *fear, isolation, noise* and the *feeling of being chased.* This results in a high pulse rate, mounting blood pressure and dangerous generalized random over-activity.

Incidence of heart attacks is particularly high in truck-drivers as an occupational group.

Investigating stress

Wong and Shinn[*] have compiled the following abridged pointers whereby an interview or questionnare may be directed to identify and locate stress:

Perceived stress of combining job and parenting
(Source: Pearlin & Schooler, 1978; Quinn & Staines, 1979; Cook, 1978; Hall & Hall, 1979; Rapport & Rapport, 1976) 12 items $\alpha = 0{,}87$[†]

1. There's no room in my schedule for anything out of the ordinary (eg a transportation delay).
2. I have to impose on others to help with child care.
3. I have more to do than I can handle comfortably.

---

[*] Wong, Nora W, Shinn, Marybeth. Social Support and Resentment in Employed Parents: Appendix D. Presented at 94th American Psychological Association Convention, Washington DC, August 1986.

[†] α is a measure of *test reliability*. See chapter 1.

Poor mental health
(Source: Gurin, Veroff & Feld, 1960) 15 items α = 0,83

1. Do you ever have any trouble getting to sleep or staying asleep?
2. Have you ever been bothered by nervousness, feeling fidgety and tense?
3. How often are you bothered by having an upset stomach?

Poor physical health
(Source: National Health Interview Survey, National Center for Health Statistics, 1982) 3 items α = 0,61

1. In general, would you say your health is: excellent, very good, fair, or poor?
2. *During the last two months,* how many days did you stay in bed most or all of the day because of illness or injury?

Job distress
(Source: Caplan, Cobb, French, Harrison, & Pinneau, 1975; Pearlin & Schooler, 1978) 5 items α = 0,82

Here are some ways that people may feel. When you think about your experiences at *your job,* how much of the time do you feel these ways?

1. Bothered or upset.
2. Worried.

Family distress
(Source: modelled after job distress items) 5 items α = 0,84

When you think about *your family* how much of the time do you feel these ways? (Responses follow same format as job distress.)

Job satisfaction
(Source: Quinn & Staines, 1979) 3 times α = 0,84

1. Knowing what you know now, if you had to decide all over again whether to take the job you now have, what would you say?
2. If a friend of yours told you he or she was interested in working in a job like yours, for your employer, what would you say?

Family satisfaction
(Source: Campbell, Converse, & Rodgers, 1976; Quinn & Staines, 1979) 2 items α = 0,63

All in all, how satisfied would you say you are with each of the following:

1. Your children.
2. Your family life.

General life satisfaction
(Source: Campbell et al, 1976; Gurin et al, 1960; Veroff et al, 1981) 3 items α =0,72

1. All in all, how satisfied would you say you are with . . . the way you are combining working and parenting.

2.   All in all, how satisfied would you say you are with . . . your life as a whole.
3.   Taking all things together, how would you say things are these days? Would
     you say you're happy, pretty happy, or not too happy these days?

Frustration (Inequilibrium)

Definition: When an *internal conflict, impeding environmental barrier, or real or imagined inadequacy* constitutes an insurmountable obstacle on the way to the attainment of a desired goal, then tension-energy is said to be frustrated, and the individual in a state of *frustration.*

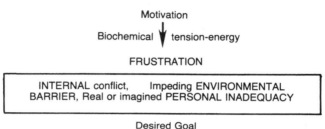

Nature demands that mobilized tension-energy finds expression of outlet, in order that the organism may return to a state of equilibrium.

This is known as the principle of *Homeostasis.*

Homeostasis (Equilibrium)

Frustration or inequilibrium brings into action the drive for homeostasis — *that compensatory adjustment by which an individual is driven to restore his physiological and psychological balance.*

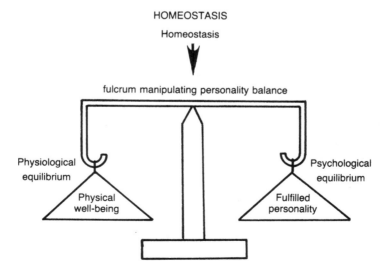

Homeostasis is that built-in self-regulating mechanism which inexorably and persistently makes every effort to restore psychological and physiological balance.

Selye, Harlow and other experimenters have shown that within the context of failure to achieve harmonic balance between the Sympathetic and Parasympathetic Nervous Systems, and thus the persistence of stress situations, there may well result a shortening of life-span. Apparently equilibrium or 'easing up' of the organism provides that essential recovery period without which an individual may well succumb to psychophysiological exhaustion.

When the *balance of personality is disturbed* by, for instance, denial of food satisfaction, exposure to fear or pain, threat to safety, an unfulfilled sexual urge or any other frustrated motivation, then the *urge for homeostasis* will act to drive the organism, through internal tension-energy, to restore fulfilled balance, or, if this is impossible, to seek alternative satisfaction through fight, flight, the constructive compromise or adjustment mechanisms described hereunder.

When the biological drive to escape from pain is rendered unattainable by an insurmountable environmental obstacle such as a plaster cast, nature demands that mobilized biochemical tension-energy finds an alternative pattern of expression in order that the organism may return to a state of equilibrium or adjusted repose.

States of extreme and persistent frustated tension-energy are described as 'stress'. How then does the organism under 'stress' cope with 'blocked off' tension energy which cannot be expressed or satisfied directly?

1. One may release tension-energy (and thus stress) by achieving homeostasis through therapeutic 'suggestion' or 'relaxation'therapy (see p 32 Behavioural treatment pp 499).
2. Another method of redirecting and expressing tension-energy is through physical activity such as sport.
3. The individual may handle pent-up tension by
    (i) taking to flight;
    (ii) fighting back;
    (iii) compromising;
    (iv) finding alternative outlet in a mental mechanism or 'adjustive reaction'.

Forms of Flight reaction to stress (see also p 26)

1. *Physical Flight.* Patients have been known to 'abscond' the night before surgery. Some, diminished by overpowering emotional or physical loss, may attempt to flee physically from their predicament.

2. An individual may seek *psychological Flight:* (a) for example, the patient who requires surgery may make *excuse* after excuse for avoiding admission. He may even convince himself of the genuineness of his excuses. (This, as we shall see, is termed *'Rationalization'.) (b) Withdrawal of attention and phantasy compensation 'day dreaming'* are other escape mechanisms.

'Make believe' is another form of flight. Small children often 'make believe' by pushing out of their minds the unpleasant fact they do not have much power over their environment, or that they are in other ways emotionally deprived.

Hospitalization frequently 'conditions' patterns of escape into the phantasy of being at home, free and healthy (see p 51).

When 'make believe' becomes a main adult activity, it is unhealthy, leading to inability to cope with the real demands of life, or else to complete withdrawal from reality.

Alcoholism, psychogenic loss of memory, refusal to eat and even suicide are flight reactions in extreme forms.

Refusal to eat may constitute a strong mechanism of flight or aggression.

The Fight reaction

In the battle between personal or group motivations, and the environment, the reaction is often to 'tear into' the problem and fight. The situation may, however, be thus damaged or even ruined. In war, for instance, the 'Fight' reaction may result in the collapse and suffering of both sides.

Atom bomb warfare is an extreme example of the possible annihilation of all peoples in the fight situation.

Criminals, in their aggressive behaviour, use the 'Fight' reaction constantly.

Arguments, refusal to co-operate, 'passive resistance', 'stubbornness' and 'nagging' are milder forms of the 'Fight' reaction. They are often the only forms of 'Fight' reaction open to sick people.

The acute, dependent, exhausting period of his illness now past, the previously overtly co-operative patient may, in *convalescence*, become argumentative, unco-operative and generally 'unpleasant' — this being his delayed *'fight' reaction* to the painful and humiliating procedures to which he was initially exposed.

Staff, feeling he should be 'grateful', are quick to take offence.

The Constructive Compromise or accommodation

The Constructive Compromise consists in *adjustment* to both the *motivations* of the personality and the *limitations* imposed by the environment.

This often entails *sacrificing* a little in the present, so that the future may be enjoyed more in the long run, eg giving up time to study now for the greater satisfaction of examination success. Maternally deprived children lacking patterns of sacrifice and reward find this especially difficult.

Compromises are often the essence of really 'grown-up' or mature behaviour.

The struggle between expression of the driving forces of the personality, and the restrictions imposed by the environment has been going on since birth.

Even in a small baby the personality makes demands which the environment cannot meet.

From the first struggles, one learns ways in which to react to these frustrations. These ways become set into *behaviour patterns*. These behaviour patterns in dealing with frustration of our motivations are called *mental mechanisms or adjustive techniques*.

CHAPTER 5

ADJUSTIVE MECHANISMS OR MENTAL DEFENCE MECHANISMS AND THEIR EFFECT ON HUMAN RELATIONS

Ego defence mechanisms or adjustive techniques *(Definition)*

The *mechanism by which one's ego or personality can defend itself against* insecurity, fear, anxiety, stress and the *frustration of mobilized tension energy,* is termed a defence or coping mechanism or an adjustive technique.

These reactions serve as one's first line of psychic defence. They *help the individual contain or cope with the tension energy emanating from anxiety, and the frustration of basic human needs.* Some mechanisms for coping with these frustrations are essential for mental health; others are signs of maladjustment, and even mental illness.

As coping mechanisms they do have drawbacks in that

(a) they operate at relatively unconscious levels; thus the individual has little control over their expression;

(b) they involve a degree of self-deception and reality distortion, thus hindering realistic efforts to cope with problems.

The nature of the mental mechanism unconsciously selected by an individual helps to define his personality and to determine his success *in adjusting his personal motivations to the requirements of society.* Mental mechanisms are thus important determinants of human relations.

(See also Suppression and Repression, p 61.)

Introjection

Introjection is that process by which one unconsciously absorbs unto oneself tension outlets, emotional attitudes, standards and ideals from the people around one.

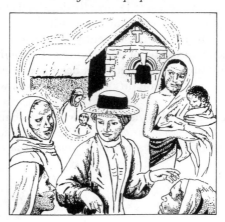

Most potent introjection is from one's familiar and earliest environment.

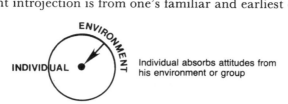

Individual absorbs attitudes from his environment or group

Thwarted in love, the individual who has grown up in an environment of physical aggression, violence, and generally uncontrolled physical tension outlet, may, in time of emotional crisis, automatically select that pattern of tension release which he has always seen around him, and slit the throat of his successful rival.

On the other hand, the individual who has grown up in an atmosphere of Christian gentleness, learning to return good for evil, to 'turn the other cheek', may, in the context of thwarted love, express his frustrated tension energy in youth-club activities, mission work, etc. One individual is no more blameworthy than the other — both are unconsciously taking unto themselves the crisis tension outlet pattern which they have always seen around them. Both are merely manifesting the mental mechanisms of introjection.

The patient who has grown up in an atmosphere of controlled long-suffering patience in the face of illness may well, in time of physical crisis, automatically present himself as the noble, courageous, self-sacrificing patient. On the other hand, he who has grown up in an environment characterized by panic, bids for reassurance, and generally uninhibited rebellion against pain, may well prove to be a demanding, complaining, disturbing, patient. Both are manifesting the unconscious mental mechanism of introjection. One is no more praiseworthy or blameworthy than the other. We should, therefore, refrain from branding one as a 'good' and the other as a 'bad' patient.

Introjected behaviour is so easily acquired that most of us find ourselves manifesting even those parental behaviour patterns of which we heartily disapprove.

Attitudes are introjected

'Attitudes are a more or less permanent state of readiness, of mental organization. They predispose an individual to react in a characteristic way to any object or situation',* thus constituting a 'guideline' to expected behaviour.

Attitudes are highly emotive feelings reflecting a person's state of mind towards a value — eg love of money, desire for fame, fear of racial groups, resentment of authority.

An individual is most likely to introject his attitudes from his earliest and most intense relationships such as his maternal, sibling, familial and community relationships.

Attitudes towards learning are of primary importance — if one's attitude is a positive one, learning is likely to be successful. *The attitudes introjected by the public are of great importance* in formulating the feelings of the individual and community

* John Sheahan *Essential Psychiatry*. Medical and Technical Publishing Co Ltd. p 48.

towards mental illness, therapy and mental health. Community education frequently arms to amend unfavourable attitudes through education — but this will not be effective unless a method of reaching people's *feelings* or emotional attitudes can be derived. Publication of optimistic case studies, films of emotional appeal, TV dramatizations may well afford the opportunity for positive identification and thus add *feeling* impact to intellectual information.

When attitudes are of an antisocial nature they may well constitute impediments to human relations — such attitudes are called *prejudices*.

Identification

Identification is the mental mechanism by which we associate or identify ourselves with a group or individual, sharing his emotions, 'feeling with' him, and putting ourselves in his boots.

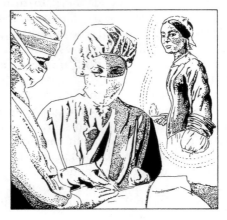

It is a device enabling us to bear, and express, tension-energy more easily in association with an individual or group than on our own.

Individual
moving from himself
to another individual
or group

When one joins a group one wants to be like the other people in the group, whether it be a Boy Scout group, a teenage gang, or a professional organization.

The pattern of tension expression adopted by a group governs the way its members are expected to express and adapt their personal motivations to the restrictions of their environment.

Nursing, being a profession fraught with special tensions, anxieties, restrictions, and personal frictions, has always utilized the security, fellowship, mutual support and group discipline inherent in identification of the individual with the group.

Uniforms, personal identification with the professional ideals and codes of nursing; identification with admired and respected nursing figures, such as

Florence Nightingale, or even an admired senior staff member, help nurses to express their own tensions, anxiety and frustrations in ways which relieve them without harming their profession or their patients. Hard work and professional pride are identification tension outlets.

Identification in the nurse-patient relationship

Identification may prove valuable in achieving happy and peaceful outlets in the hospital ward. When the nursing staff create a happy, confident and friendly atmosphere in the ward, individual patients will identify with them, directing their own mobilized tension-energy into positive outlets, such as a friendly conversation, helpfulness, and the creative pursuits of occupational therapy.

If, on the other hand, ward staff are unfriendly, rude, inconsiderate and aggressive, patients will identify in a negative manner, saying to themselves: 'If they can be like that, then so can we!'. While nurses usually derive considerable support and outlet by identifying with their own professional group, there is still grievous lack of identification with patients. Nothing arouses frustration, loneliness, anger and depression in a patient more than the sight of nurses identifying with each other, avidly participating in talk of their own social life, hospital routines and professional jargon to the exclusion of the patient, who lies as emotionally isolated as a sick sparrow among healthy cockatoos.

In her excellent address 'Nursing as a Profession', delivered at the 12th Quadrennial International Congress of Nursing, Dr Marie Jahoda MD, outlined the manner in which, since its inception, the nursing profession has taught the recruit to protect her emotional stability by preventing identification or 'feeling with' the mental and physical sufferings of her patient and his relatives. In order to do this, she has had to 'dehumanize' her patient, teaching herself to see him only as 'a case', as 'the gastrectomy in the side ward', 'the carcinoma in bed No 10'. But in so doing she has come very near losing her humanitarian role. In failing to *identify*, or *feel with*, her patient (and his relatives), she has failed to create the human bond by which he obtains the important comfort and support he needs as surely as his dressings and full-washes. In identifying with him she and he can, in fact, create a small supportive group. 'I will share the pain with you; I will hold your hand and see it through with you. It will come right for you as it has done for everybody else'.

If the nurse's role is to be more than that of a technician, she will have to learn to identify with her patient — 'to put herself in his boots' — while at the same time remaining reasonably optimistic, cheerful and personally well adjusted. In this she will herself require opportunity for identification and catharsis (the relief which comes with 'talking out').

While identification with the patient's suffering, frustration, grief is certainly the cornerstone of communicating caring involvement, the young professional may be trapped into over-identification with the overdependent, the psychopathic and the drug and alcohol addicted (pp 367–377). Excessive involvement may end with a disillusioned patient and a hurt 'burnt out' professional.

An example of over-identification lies in *'Medical Student Disease'* in which the student over-identifies with his patient's symptoms, introjecting them into his own psychosomatic mechanism so that he actually begins to *feel* the textbook syndrome. Nurses who are also at risk, should not hesitate to seek help in eliminating symptoms by achieving insight into psychosomatic anxiety symptomatology as well as catharsis and reassurance.

IDENTIFICATION WITHIN PROFESSIONAL STRATA

Vertical support between upper strata of the nursing hierarchy					
Horizontal peer support					Matron
					Sisters
					Junior sisters
	Matron	Sisters	Junior sisters	Nurses	Nurses

Nursing counsellors and group discussion therapy offer an important contribution in promoting nurse adjustment: but perhaps the nurse's most important source of support and outlet lies in *deeper-level identification* within the various strata of her professional group.

Identification with one's peers (horizontal identification) is not enough. Rather should mutual support also assume a vertical direction bringing together in their vocation sisters and 'juniors', staff nurses and matrons, not only in matters of discipline and instruction but also for purposes of mutual support, catharsis and joy in achievement.

Seniority brings maturity, tolerance, insight, a sense of proportion and experience which knows that 'tomorrow is another day'. Youth brings physical strength, young idealism, optimism and refreshing enthusiasm. In mutual identification comes vocational fulfilment.

Seeman and Evans (1961) have shown that:

inflexible stratification,
emphasis on hierarchy, rank and social distance,

reduce satisfaction and lower the standard of teaching and patient care. These factors are also responsible for detrimental staff rotation, negative identification and thus impaired ward or clinic atmosphere.*

---

* Seeman M, Evans J W. Stratification and Hospital Care. *American Sociological Review* 1961; **26**: 67-80.

That there is frequently positive value in identification to encourage, comfort and motivate patients who have suffered bodily loss has been shown by the achievements of self-help rehabilitation groups. Praiseworthy examples are the 'Lost Chord Club' (for those who have undergone laryngectomy), 'Reach for Recovery', (for women who have suffered mastectomy) and the post-colostomy groups. However, sensitivity and respect for individuality should monitor referral to self-help groups. Some 'private' and sophisticated people shrink from structured group participation.

Distress and resentment may result from well-meaning but misdirected, attempts to motivate inappropriate patients to participation in structured group rehabilitation. The lumpectomy patient, who has been spared the trauma of mutilating mastectomy, undergoes some degree of post-operative trauma. Most cancer patients she knows have, in the past, been subjected mastectomy, and she is fearful lest this unhappy fate may yet await her. In an effort to encourage her, the nurse may use words to the effect 'Look at Mrs Smith — she has had her breast amputated but she is up and about' — physically, at any rate. For Mrs Smith may well be hiding a gross emotional trauma, which she will feel free to manifest only when she returns to her own domain.

The last person the lumpectomy patient should identify with is the amputee. To encourage her to do so, is to encourage identification with her worst fears.

Many cancer patients want to run as far as possible from the disease, and feel better that way.

Although positive identification is a useful motivating factor, care should be taken to *avoid negative identification* with those whom the fearful patient feels to be in a worse condition than she herself.

For a deeper analysis of group dynamics the reader is referred to 'Group or Social Learning' pp 170-171; also Group Therapy chapter 26.

Sublimation

All of us are motivated to fulfil the love-hate swing of natural ambivalence.

When the direct fulfilment of love and hate outlets is denied us by the environment, then it becomes necessary to sublimate or rechannel frustrated tension-energy into alternative, socially approved love or forbidden hate outlets.

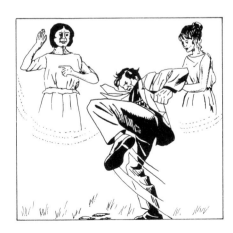

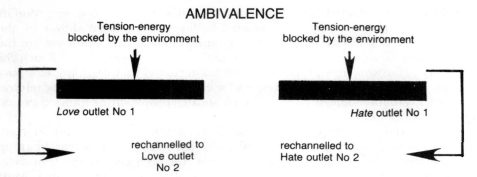

Because love expresses itself in thought and actions which are creative, and socially approved, love sublimation is fairly easy. A paediatric nurse may, for example, successfully rechannel the energy of her own frustrated maternal love-fulfilment drive into *love-fulfilment* in her relationship with her child patients. This is usually a successfully rechannelled love outlet, but attempts at sublimation can sometimes overreach themselves and adversely affect human relations. Driven by her own need of her patient's love and dependence such a nurse may come to resent natural parents, finding all sorts of unconscious excuses ('rationalizations') for keeping parents out of her ward thus denying the child the emotionally fulfilling support which only his own mother, by virtue of her special, longstanding relationship with him, can supply.

The rechannelling of the aggressive, destructive drives inherent in *hate fulfilment* is rendered especially difficult within the framework of our code of 'civilized behaviour'. The nurse who comes to hate her ward sister cannot find alternative hate-outlet satisfaction by murdering her room-mate.

A downtrodden son-in-law, consumed with enormous tension-energy, designed by nature for the specific purpose of killing his domineering, nagging mother-in-law, used each evening to go down to the bottom of his garden and kill slugs. In crushing each slug he would derive rechannelled alternative hate-satifaction by saying to himself 'that was my mother-in-law', 'that was my mother-in-law'. This rechanelling of his hate drive constituted a reasonably successful sublimation.

While direct individual satisfation of hate drives is usually denied us, rechannelled group identification in hating and killing (as in race riots, war, etc) is often lauded by society. The man who kills his next-door neighbour is hanged; the man who kills twenty fellow-men on the battlefield is decorated for bravery.

Many social psychologists claim that until mankind can find harmless outlets for personal hate feelings, the legitimized blood-bath of war will persist.

Humour is a socially acceptable form of sublimation — 'to laugh away one's troubles'.

Compensation

Compensation is the mechanism or adjustment technique mainly concerned with alternative satisfaction when motivations for recognition, honour and physical prowess are frustrated by real or imagined inadequacy within the individual (as opposed to the environmental blocks to be by-passed in sublimation).

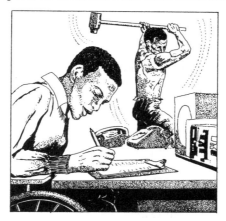

Compensation enables the individual to 'make up' for some real or imaginary emotional or physical inadequacy by success in different activity.

Patients are constantly obliged to seek alternative satisfactions in the face of changing physical circumstances.

The nurse and the occupational therapist are required to exercise considerable ingenuity in introducing compensatory satisfying activities — such as bridge to the patient who, having suffered a coronary thrombosis, is forced to quit the sportsfield with its previous satisfactions of honour, recognition and team companionship which he must now derive elsewhere.

Paul Brickhill's *Reach for the Sky* tells of the series of compensations which brought Douglas Bader, a young legless ex-rugby blue, from the pit of despair (in

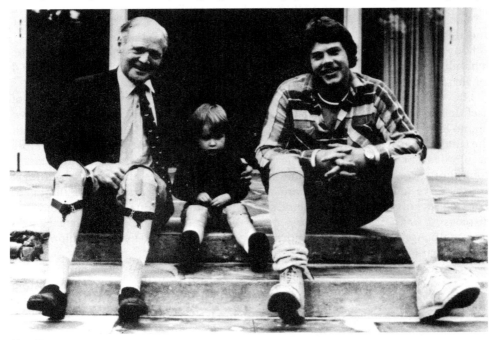

Identification and compensation.

the face of loss of all previous sources of honour, recognition, physical tension outlets and camaraderie), through the interim compensation-satisfaction of fame and honour as a war hero, to his ultimate satisfaction in inspiring others (by their identification with his hero image) to a new life. Here, in fact, we read of the near perfect compensation — for Bader's satisfaction in his compensatory behaviour in helping to rehabilitate others, eventually gave even greater satisfaction than his original role of sports hero.

Sometimes, as in the case of the blind who develop compensatory senses such as smell, hearing and taste, nature helps the thwarted patient towards compensation. But very often it falls to the nurse (who has the longest, most intimate contact with the patient) to *anticipate* his sense of loss, and thus introduce compensatory activities before the depressing 'rot' of uselessness, isolation and despair sets in.

Twenty-year-old Sally was an expert typist when she lost her right hand as a result of a car accident. When finally able to face her mutilated arm she was at first angry, and then became very depressed, lacking motivation for the effort required in learning new self-care skills. She would lie aimlessly in bed, remembering how she used to manicure her skilled fingers, and sob. 'What can a girl with an ugly, useless stump hope to achieve in life? Where will I find frienship and love? How will I earn a living?'

Then nurses noted Sally's caring involvement in the welfare of Peggy, who had been blinded in an industrial lab explosion. Staff Nurse Dean resolved to confront Sally:

'Why don't you become a social worker? You're so good with people needing comfort and support — your hand won't matter to them.'

'But I don't have A levels — how can I go to university?'

'You can upgrade . . . I'll ask our social worker to discuss adult education grants and things.'

Four years later Sally was back at the hospital as a professional member of the rehabilitation team, her satisfaction in rehabilitating others having compensated for her former secretarial accomplishments.

The *Community Nurse* should be particularly alert to the feelings of loss of usefulness, status, and love encountered by woman whose children, having grown up, no longer 'need her' in the same way; the active business man now faced with the small obscure domesticity of retirement; the old person daily encountering loss of physical prowess, independence and status. In counteracting such losses community workers should promote compensatory facilities such as social, cultural and creative activities for men and women of mature years, and for the aged. Lacking socially accepted compensation outlets, an individual is liable to develop displeasing *antisocial compensation patterns*. A frustrated nurse may unconsciously seek compensatory satisfaction in the power she tries to wield over her junior nurses and her patients.

A common source of antisocial compensatory behaviour results from excessive expectations on the part of teachers and parents who, by demanding the impossible from the basically non-academic pupil of 'dull' or 'low-average' IQ drive him to alternative antisocial status-seeking compensations such as:

(i) bullying, which compensates for feelings of intellectual inferiority by physical dominance;

  (ii) lying, which compensates for crippling feelings of inferiority and rejection by fantasy achievement compensation;

 (iii) stealing, which provides the compensation of tangible possessions to comfort him and to impress his peers.

In this context bullying, stealing, lying, etc are clearly *symtomatic* of inner feelings of inferiority, rejection, loss of love, guilt and anxiety tension, requiring some form of 'bolstering' alternative status symbol or comfort.

On the whole the mechanism of compensation is helpful, when personal loss or inadequacies seem to block the path one would ordinarily like to follow. New satisfactions and new interests can, of themselves, motivate a patient to mobilize his energy to achieve physical recovery. Without motivation (or internal drive) he will become so lacking in biochemical stimulation (adrenalin, blood-sugar, histamine, etc) that his body cells may atrophy and he may eventually die of depression.

Denial

Denial is that mental mechanism by which one attempts to defend oneself from painful and stressful experiences and feelings by denying their existence.

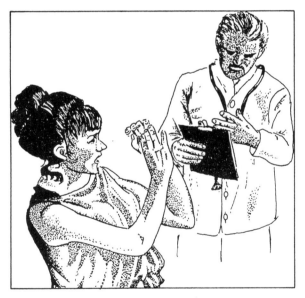

Medical staff may attempt to handle their guilt, anxiety and distress at the necessity to inflict pain by denying the existence of their patients' distress.

Relatives unable to bear the prognosis of death of a loved one may deny the diagnosis, pleading for one useless treatment after the other.

They may *need* to retreat to a state of denial, and even false hope, while gathering the inner strength which may lead to ultimate acceptance. (See Care of the Dying, chapter 23.)

At a simple level, most people tend to deny toothache before finally making a dental appointment.

Denial as a defence mechanism carries the disadvantage of alternating with distressing anxiety. In the long run it is usually better to face one's problems, tackling them in as constructive a manner as the circumstances allow.

Rationalization

Rationalization is a mechanism by which one unconsciously justifies (or makes excuses for) ideas and behaviour about which one feels guilty, inferior or anxious. As a method of safeguarding one's important self-image, self-respect and confidence, these 'reasonable' excuses fulfil a useful purpose.

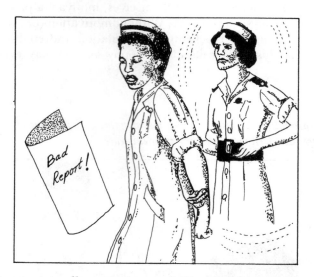

Were a junior nurse really to accept a ward report, declaring her to be 'stupid, unreliable, inconsiderate, useless and without any prospect of success' she would become seriously depressed; the shattering of her 'self concept' might destroy her self-confidence and even her mental health. So she unconsciously protects her emotional integrity and offsets her anxiety, by rationalizing aloud, or to herself, that 'It is just because sister's got it in for me'.

One can think of many nursing situations in which rationalization offsets anxiety, soothes and comforts.

A deteriorating chronic patient might, in a depressed mood, declare herself to be sure that her increasing pain will continue to grow and spread. To agree with this probability would be both unkind and unwise — rather would you 'rationalize' that her 'new drug always has this depressing effect' or that 'the weather is enough to make anyone feel that way'.

Sometimes, of course, rationalization, like most other mental mechanisms, may be unconsciously used to the detriment of the emotional needs of others.

A good case in point is again that of the paediatric sister who, sublimating her own love-needs in her devoted care of her little patients, and unconsciously resenting their 'real' mothers, might easily find herself 'rationalizing' or finding reasons (which she really believes) why it would be 'better for mothers not to visit'.

Unlike a lie or an excuse which has been purposefully 'cooked-up', rationalization is often an unconscious mechanism.

Reliance on rationalization can be damaging to real effort in tackling and overcoming life's difficulties. Often, however, rationalization, by offsetting real anxiety, preserves our confidence, self-esteem and mental health.

Idealization

Idealization consists in over-evaluating oneself or others. It is often a way of relieving tension caused by feelings of inferiority. Sometimes it is a healthy thing to do. If one does not take some pride in oneself and think oneself reasonably successful the chances are that one will not be. Anything you or your patients *think* you can do is a powerful incentive to achievement. We are all stimulated if we 'hitch our wagon to a star'.

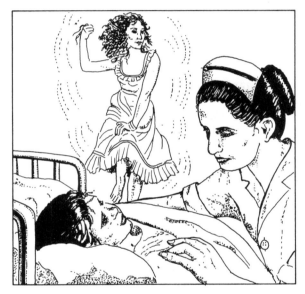

It is thus often helpful to idealize a patient scarred and disfigured, or lacking the confidence to try a new exercise.

If we tell an apprehensive post-operative patient, reluctant to take his first steps, we are sure that anyone as determined, strongminded, and courageous as he, will soon be walking strongly and confidently again, we are much more likely to inspire him to succeed than if we remark on his pale weakness.

However, idealization carried beyond the bounds of ability can impose feelings of inferiority, rejection, anxiety, guilt and depression.

Parents may, for instance, over-idealize the intellectual potential of a child whose IQ 95 presupposes success at fourth form level, insisting that he pass his matriculation certificate, for which attainment the minimum requirement is around IQ 105. Such inappropriate pressure will cause spreading feelings of inferiority, rejection, anxiety or hate, rebellion and recourse to antisocial status-compensation mechanisms such as bullying, lying and stealing.

Similarly, a nurse who over-idealizes her patient's ability to 'take pain' or bear anxiety will:

(a) impose feeling of guilt, anxiety and thus reinforced psychosomatic tension;
(b) deny him that direct tension outlet of weeping, fighting, or complaining which is a healthier reaction than inhibition or suppression of external reaction: for suppression channels tension energy underground into psychosomatic in-volvements or psychoneurotic behaviour patterns;
(c) deny him the opportunity fo find that reassurance, comfort and catharsis which his externalized distress would bring him.

The nurse who reproves her patient for not being 'brave like Tommy Smith' has failed to grasp the fact that every patient has his or her own afferent nerve distribution, cerebral pain-centre structure, life story, personality, and thus individual threshold for stress and pain. To over-idealize patients to equal standards of courage, patience, etc is to deny them the tension outlet, comfort and support that are intrinsic to true nursing.

Reaction formation

Reaction formation is a way of offsetting a very strong, unconscious, guilt-laden drive or urge by doing the opposite in one's conscious behaviour. For example, a woman who has been brought up to feel guilty, and thus anxious, about her natural basic sexual motivations may, in an effort to delude herself that she does not have this 'forbidden' urge, 'bend backwards' in her disapproving protest against the sexual motivations of others. Such a person may well develop into a chronic newspaper letterwriter, constantly protesting against the allegedly sexually provocative clothes and behaviour of modern youth; or into the village 'Mrs Grundy' taking upon herself responsibility for preserving public morality.

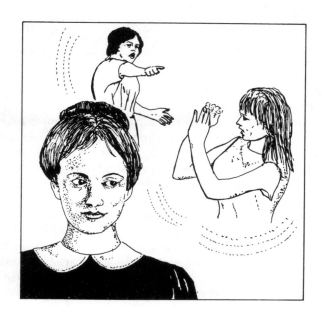

Another example of reaction formation can be seen in the over-fussy, over-meticulous, compulsively clean housewife or nurse who is deeply disturbed by every speck of dust or evidence of casual untidiness.

As babies such people were not bothered by dirt — they did, in fact, derive a certain natural, primitive, spontaneous satisfaction from contact with 'dirty', 'gooey' often 'sensuous' media.

In the process of growing-up they have *learnt,* through excessive 'pressure' for conformity and cleanliness, *to feel guilty* about these tactile pleasures, and about their pleasure in relaxed, casual 'sloppiness'; but their *unconscious enjoyment of 'dirt' remains so strong* that the 'conscience' can control their inner conflict only by bending backwards towards painful perfectionism in an effort to offset forbidden unconscious urges.

Shakespeare described *reaction formation* very neatly in Hamlet's analysis of his mother's strong, guilt-laden denial: 'Methinks the lady doth protest too much.'

Obsessive compulsive symptoms may take *many forms* of wide-ranging severity and frequency. Some in fact are recognizable by most of us when under pressure and stress. Frequently encountered are, for instance, repetitive checking of doors and windows, lights and taps; redundant, repetitive adding of columns of figures; touching every third lamp-post or every fourth crack in the pavement; oft-repeated, time-consuming hand-washing to the point of damaging one's skin; cleanliness compulsions which prevent the handling of 'dirty' money, 'infected' doorknobs or bus rails; ruminative, repetitive, painful or blasphemous thoughts, especially in the minds of people who believe they should be religiously perfect; constant worrying about the 'meaning of life'; continual checking for dreadful repetitive fears of performing some dreadful action, such as the nurse who fears to give medicine lest she leaves broken glass in the container. Checking dosage is laudable, but *one should distinguish between excellence in a high degree of efficiency as against neurotic wastage of work-power.* Constant eating and smoking may also constitute compulsive-neurotic symptoms. Most of us, when under stress, suffer some form of neurotic symptom. This form of mental suffering is so common as almost to be termed 'normal', should one wish to use so meaningless a term; for in the wide kaleidoscope of human personality there is no real 'norm'.

However, when a person's (i) job efficiency, (ii) participation in normal social intercourse, (iii) ability to give and accept love, (iv) peace of mind, are engulfed by his neuroses, then he may be headed for disintegration in worthwhile living.

Obsessive compulsive neuroses

In an effort to relieve guilt feelings and resultant painful stress, or to prevent catastrophe the patient feels compelled, against his will, to perform set acts, or to think certain painful thoughts. Even though the emotion or impulse behind the ritual may be recognized as absurd and unproductive, it insistently intrudes into conscious awareness. The compulsion may serve as a guilt-reducing, ritualistic penance but it feeds upon itself. *The subject hopes to achieve peace of mind by 'bargaining' emotionally or physically painful ritual with the 'powers that be'.* Painful obsessive rituals even extend to self mutilating actions such as slashing wrists and face; picking flesh until it bleeds; pushing foreign bodies such as cigarette stubs into open wounds — especially those resulting from mutilating surgery.

'I must have done something terrible to deserve this punishing mutilation. I must do something painful to myself, lest I be punished further.'

Sometimes loss of body image and inturned punitive anger are important operant factors.

When the painful compulsion is complied with there is sometimes a certain lifting of tension, and thus temporary relief — but in a personality so predisposed, it is not long before the next painful or irresistible impulse occurs. (See 'body searching compulsions in cancer' p 520-523 and AIDS p 347) *Because he is neurotic rather than psychotic, this patient has isight* into the irrationality and fruitlessness of his ritual-impulse, which he usually recognizes with a feeling of anxious dread. Like Lady Macbeth, wringing her hands fruitlessly on the parapet before hurling herself to death, the sufferer knows all too well that 'all the perfumes of Araby will not sweeten this little hand' even though, unlike Lady Macbeth, his own guilt may be imaginary.

Psycho-analytic interpretation claims that when one encounters guilt-laden aggressive drives, and shame associations too painful for self ('Ego') recognition, the Unconscious ('Id') attempts to achieve expression by tricking the censorship of the Conscience ('Super Ego'). In order so to do forbidden drives split off from the original threatening stimulus, to reattach themselves to an apparently harmless situation. This *new substitution guilt stimulus* now triggers off the necessity for performing a compulsive act with no *apparent* connection with the original aggressive feeling. The connection may be only subtle or symbolic. Substitution attempts to protect the patient's self-image or 'super ego' by hiding from him the real original aggressive and thus guilt-laden source of his feelings, as illustrated, for example, in the following diagram:

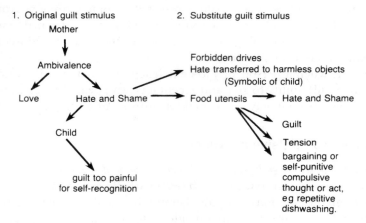

Here a mother, feeling guilty about the strength of her natural ambivalent aggression-swing towards her child, has developed compulsive dusting and washing rituals when handling his food utensils, having transferred to them her feeling of anger and guilt. Her constant banging and rough repetitive washing of the pots and pans is really an attempt to purge herself of her own unacceptable emotions towards her child. Were the aggression and guilt feelings to remain attached to the original stimulus, *child abuse* may result.

There is about obsessional neurosis a strong element of *reaction formation*. It is as if the ambivalent mother is seeking *to deny* her destructive feelings towards her child by *'bending backwards' in her need to protect* her baby from her own involuntary conscious and unconscious aggressive thoughts. She is internally driven to repeat the ritual of, for instance, washing and checking for broken glass in the bottle over and over again as a 'small price' to pay for her baby's safety from destruction by her hand — or indeed, through any other punitive agent.

Freud maintains that in order to achieve that emotional-level *feeling involvement* necessary for successful psychotherapy, *interpretation and reliving experiences in respect of this splitting off process are indispensable.* The patient must face, acknowledge, re-experience and deal with her own *original* ambivalence, aggression and guilt feelings as pertaining to her child.

In *psychotherapy*, in order to achieve effective *emotional or feeling level* (as distinct from intellectual level) *insight*, it is desirable to embark on a chain of *'symbolic undoing'*. For instance, the nurse who may have had an urge to put ground glass in her patient's cup *should be helped to return and face her original aggression towards her patient as felt at the time she was tending him.* By therapeutically regressing to the orignal hostility-wish on handling the medicine container, she should be helped to verbalize (and to feel), 'I take that thought back. I am freed of (imagined) guilt'.

This therapeutic stage, while essential to success, is a painful and difficult one, in that it requires *support in facing up to the original 'shameful' destructive wish* suppressed by the 'Super Ego'. Psychotherapy gives the patient opportunity to find relief in 'taking back'. It is as if she is saying, 'I disown it — please do not punish me by withdrawing your loving acceptance of me'.

Displacement

Displacement is a means of transferring the emotion concerned with one person or thing, to an unrelated, usually weaker, person or object. Anger is taken out on unexpected, innocent people.

A nurse may be angry with her ward sister, but, because she dare not reveal her true aggressive feelings to the sister, she displaces them, or *'takes it out'* on her patients in domineering behaviour, aggression or unkindness.

The tension-energy created by unexpressed anger at a real or imaginary injustice may, for instance, find an unconscious outlet in a forcefully plunged hypodermic needle or a dressing ripped away with unnecessary force.

Patients, of course, also find tension outlet in displacement. A patient injured by a drunken motorist may be tense with inhibited aggression towards the offending motorist. Unable to find direct relief in appropriate physical attack upon the driver, he may displace his tension-energy by aggressive behaviour towards the nursing staff, especially towards the junior nurse whom he senses to be in a particularly weak position, and thus most at his mercy.

In patients the displacement of aggression towards healthy people occurs frequently.

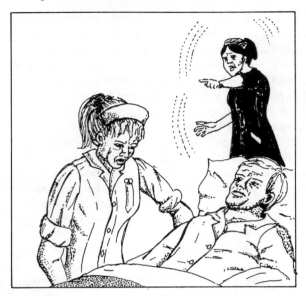

Aggressive behaviour aroused by the demands of an unreasonable employer may well be 'taken out' on innocent family members on the employee's return home: conversely the hen-pecked schoolmaster may displace the aggressive behaviour he dare not show at home by unconsciously victimizing his helpless pupils.

Cruelty to animals is a common form of displacement. Mother, resenting the interference of influential mother-in-law, stifles her anger, but later, in disproportionate temper, lashes out at noisy, shouting Tommy. Tommy, frightened to direct his anger at mother, kicks out at his dog.

Although displacement is not always avoidable, we shall find it easier to accept and tolerate such behaviour in ourselves, and in others, if we understand the mental mechanism involved, and do not take such aggression, when displaced, upon ourselves, personally.

Projection (see also Transference pp 64-65)

Projection is a device for consciously or unconsciously attributing to others guilt-laden, tension-fraught and thus unacceptable wishes or actions which one will not, or cannot, claim as one's own.

This mechanism is used diagnostically by psychologists as a technique in which patients are asked to tell or act out stories, pictures, etc about people in various significant situations. These *projective techniques* reflect the subjects' own feelings and experiences attached to impersonal figures.

In order to offset one's own feelings of guilt, allay anxiety and preserve one's important self-concept, one may *unconsciously disown certain ideas or aggressive wishes by attaching them to somebody else.* We find an example in the nurse who, desperate to get off duty punctually by 19h00 in order to meet her boy friend, is suddenly inundated with delaying duties. She asks her colleague to help her and, on being told this is impossible, accuses *her* of 'just wanting to dash off to the boy friend'. Clearly, in order to offset and disown her own guilt feelings she is projecting

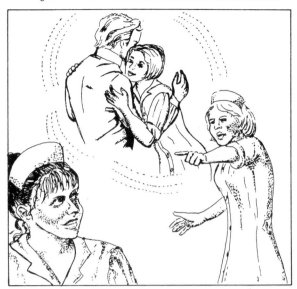

them upon her fellow nurse. (Similarly, a child who has himself been 'cheating' at school is quick to accuse his neighbour of so doing.)

As a maladjustment, this mechanism is seen in people who habitually blame everyone else for their own troubles and shortcomings.

Regression

Regression is a way of avoiding a tension-fraught situation by reverting to a behaviour pattern which belongs to an earlier phase of development. Often this behaviour pattern is selected (usually unconsciously) because, in the past, it did bring protection, security and comfort.

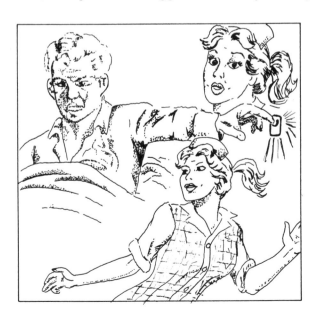

Sick people regress to childish patterns of behaviour which in the past afforded them mother love, relief and comfort. A sad example is that of an old lady of 93 who, on the night she died, kept calling for her mother in a desperate effort to return to an earlier source of solace and support.

Old people regress in many ways — even to childish satisfaction in contact with faeces and similarly texture material.

Regression in the face of emotional and physical shock can, of course, prove very trying in a busy ward, but should be recognized as a desperate signal for solace and support.

One is familiar with the adult patient who is continually demanding more than his share of attention and comfort. He is fractious, apparently 'selfish', temperamental and 'cowardly'. He is unnecessarily helpless by day, and he 'sits on his bell' all night.

To tolerate him, let us understand him. Emotional shock and an inability to face, perhaps, months of discomfort and helplessness, have caused the patient instinctively to revert to a childish level of behaviour which, in the past, brought comfort and reassurance. In a way the nurse is called upon to take unto herself the personification of the mother figure; by accepting his need of dependence and support she establishes a motherlike relationship with him which, at a later stage, because he has come to value her praise and approval, may well provide incentive for his conformity, and the sacrifices involved in adopting more adult behaviour patterns.

Patients in Intensive Care Units are able to indulge their need to return to helpless dependence in their relationship with efficient and comforting mother-nurse figures.

On removal from the Intensive Care Unit they are apt to carry over this regressive pattern to the ordinary ward. They resent, and even fear, removal from the safe protection of the unit, and in the ward may well require tapering off of individualized and special attention.

Caution: Regression can, if allowed to persist, lead to a *permanently dependent state*. The more helpless the patient is, the more dependent he is on others, the more he is liable to regress. Indeed, that very acceptable of routine personal care which causes him to be praised as a 'good' patient is liable to encourage regression. His acceptance of a dependent or sick role hampers his readjustment to the rough and tumble of normal life. Social workers know only too well that lack of fight and initiative which renders discharged long-term patients all too ready to accept permanent dependence on public support.

It is thus important, after initial support, to encourage the patient to do as much for himself as possible, even though to do so may sometimes slow down procedures and disturb ward routine.

Some nurses thrive on the mother-role. They should, however, be on their guard lest their own mothering needs hamper their patients' return to independence.

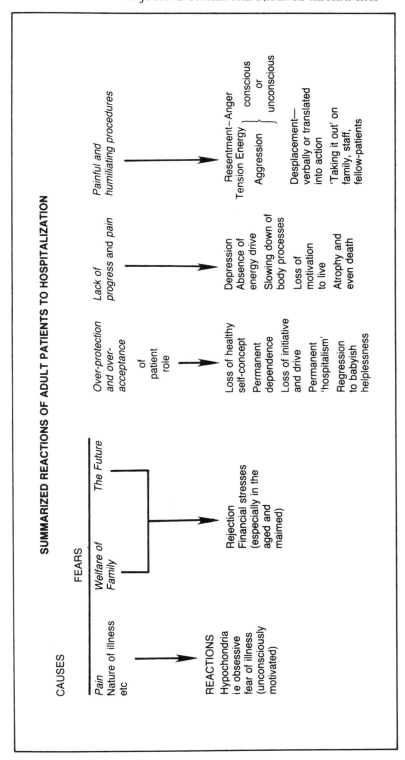

SUMMARIZED REACTIONS OF ADULT PATIENTS TO HOSPITALIZATION

CAUSES

FEARS

Pain	Welfare of	The Future	Over-protection	Lack of	Painful and
Nature of illness	Family		and over-	progress and pain	humiliating procedures
etc			acceptance		

of
patient
role

REACTIONS

Hypochondria
ie obsessive
fear of illness
(unconsciously
motivated)

Rejection
Financial stresses
(especially in the
aged and
maimed)

Loss of healthy
self-concept

Permanent
dependence

Loss of initiative
and drive

Permanent
'hospitalism'

Regression
to babyish
helplessness

Depression
Absence of
energy drive

Slowing down of
body processes

Loss of
motivation
to live

Atrophy and
even death

Resentment–Anger
Tension Energy } conscious
Aggression } or unconscious

Desplacement—
verbally or translated
into action

'Taking it out' on
family, staff,
fellow-patients

Older persons often bitterly resented the lack of privacy, the depersonalized care, the hustle and bustle, the procedure-based approach and know-all attitudes of young doctors and nurses in the urban hospitals. It is clear that these human beings, insecure and afraid, far from the support of family and community, find it difficult to accept the unknown terrors of the hospital. The result is that treatment is rejected and the unfortunate person flees to the security offered by the traditional healer who personalizes his care, ensures his privacy, devotes time to his care and provides spiritual support by bringing him closer to his ancestors. Prof. Charlotte Searle, *Nursing RSA/Verpleging* Vol 1. No 10. (See also Chapter 21, Emotional Reaction to Illness.)

Conversion

Conversion is the mental mechanism whereby emotional tension is converted, via the Sympathetic Nervous System, to physical symptoms.

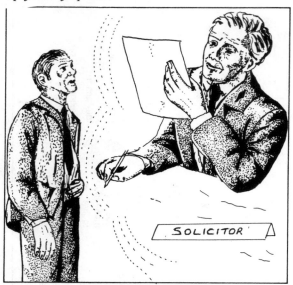

As we saw in chapter 1, the biochemical, and eventually cellular, changes resultant upon this cycle of:

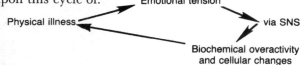

constitute the basis of *psychosomatic medicine*.

A typical example of a psychosomatic stress symptom is afforded by the case of a student nurse who suddenly developed acute gastric discomfort and painful abdominal muscular spasms.

Primary organic etiology having been excluded, several psychodiagnostic interviews revealed that the onset of these most distressing symptoms coincided with the death of an elderly male carcinoma patient, hostility to whom she was eventually (but very reluctantly) able to verbalize.

In the course of further interviews she associated this patient with her own grandfather to whom he had borne a certain physical resemblance, and who had died of the same condition at the same age.

The grandfather's death had actually removed much stress and emotional deprivation from the familial situation. The little girl's behaviour had revealed appropriate satisfaction, but her mother's reproaches had inhibited expression of tension relief, thereby associating the grandfather-figure with suppressed guilt and anxiety tension.

The death of the disliked patient, and the involuntary 'forbidden' relief following thereupon, had associated back to, resurrected, and reinforced the nurse's original suppressed feelings of guilt and anxiety pertaining to the grandfather. She now relived her relief, but also her guilt and anxiety, at both associated deaths, with resultant accumulated emotional stress. SNS stimulated biochemical change, tension-energy, over-activity of the involuntary circular abdominal muscles and inhibition of gastric juices, and consequent painful psychosomatic symptoms.

Intensive psychotherapy, consisting of reliving traumatic experiences, emotional level interpretation, reassurance, catharsis and the establishment of new reaction patterns, was required in order to relieve the cause of her psychosomatic conversion symptoms.

Dr George Pollock, director of the Chicago Institute for Psychoanalysis, and Dr David Sackin, chairman of the Department of Psychiatry at Milwaukee Children's Hospital, are currently working to develop a profile of the organic and psychological factors contributing to the development of peptic ulcers in children.

Because of reluctance to diagnose this condition in childhood, few statistics exist. Pollock & Sakin report peptic ulcers in children as young as 4 years, but the condition is more common in school-aged children and presents in all socio-economic and racial groups.

Blood type O is probably associated with vulnerability, the condition being precipitated by the *projection* of the mother's problems upon her child.

Ever since birth, the mother has felt the child to have some defect — such as intellectual dullness, a speech defect or a club foot; or she may have preferred a child of a different sex.

The mother then *identifies* herself with the child's real or imaginary imperfections, giving the child the impression that he has to 'prove himself' by 'bending backwards' to overcome his handicap. *(Reaction formation.)*

To quote Dr Pollock:

> 'The burden then falls upon the child . . . the child tries harder and harder to prove himself an adequate person. He engages in "phenomenal acitivity" and strives for top grades . . . The children are frightened for failure. They "churn and churn inside", get ulcers, haemorrhage, even have ulcer perforations and end up in hospital for surgery. Many of these children are extremely capable, but the more they can do the more they feel they have to do.'

There is much statistical research to suggest that psychosomatic conversion conditions, such as coronary thromboses and gastric ulcers, occur with significantly greater frequency among business executives, lawyers, politicians and other emotionally involved groups who are forced passively to bear the long-term stress involved in major decisions and responsibilities, than in manual labourers. These less afflicted groups, as long there is some variety and satisfaction in their work,

(a) are free from the long-term tension involved in major decisions and responsibilities;

(b) are able to express their tension energy directly through primitive physical activity, as originally designed by nature, in the Fight-Flight reaction.

Owing to the mistaken stigma which is still attached to troubles of the mind, patients feel that a physical symptom is much more 'respectable' than a more direct symptom of emotional stress. Thus, often unconsciously, they seek expression of their emotional tension at a physical level, or else they wait until the physical complications of their emotional tension necessitate, or even 'make an excuse for', seeking professional help.

Hospital beds and out-patient facilities are often overwhelmed by patients with physical conversion symptoms, which, though no less painful and frightening, and even physically dangerous, are nevertheless emotional in origin.

It has been estimated that one-third of patients in hospitals under Britain's National Health Service suffer from psychosomatic illnesses. (See presentation Table p 29.)

General practitioners are, of course, most aware of the suffering emanating from conversion symptoms. Most surveys indicate that the incidence of 'emotional disorders' (including psychiatric disorders) ranks second only to upper respiratory conditions.

It is, of course, easy and serious to err in the opposite direction, classifying a primarily somatic or physical condition as one of emotional origin.

All of which goes to show that there is no substitute for good clinical medicine, or for the approach which aims to investigate the patient as a whole individual and not just 'the gastric ulcer in the side ward' or 'the coronary in the corner'.

Of course, everybody develops stress at times. When you are under emotional stress, some physical distress should not disturb or frighten you. Again it is a matter of degree. When people are faced with a difficult or frightening situation they react, via the Sympathetic Nervous System, with everything they have — brain, emotions, internal organs, skin, blood vessels — the whole organism!

Hysteria

Hysteria a special conversion symptom resulting in paralysis or loss of function of a particular part of the body without appropriate organic cause. Conversion disorder).

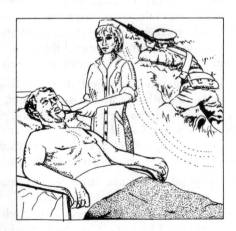

Tension-energy aroused by deep-seated mental conflict, guilt or anxiety, is habitually channelled (by an as yet unknown physiological process) to overcome the voluntary function of a particular organ. Usually the inability of this organ to function relieves the individual of environmental stresses, guilt and anxiety.

During World War I, Sigmund Freud, father of the pscho-analytical school of psychology, worked with German soldiers suffering from organically groundless paralysis of the legs. Often using techniques such as hypnosis (which relaxes conscious control), he came to the conclusion that deeper levels than consciousness contain unrecognized by dynamic motivation for self-preservation. Prussian socio-cultural standards interpreted this normal motivation as 'cowardice'. The soldier was thus caught in a conflict between motivation for self-preservation on the one hand, and honour on the other, with consequent tension-energy.

By an involuntary, as yet unknown physiological process, this tension-energy was channelled to the leg, overcoming voluntary movement. The soldier's leg rather than he himself was blamed for 'cowardice'. In other words, painful guilt was displaced, impersonalized or *dissociated* from the individual. The consequent paralysis, removing the soldier from his conflict, his guilt, and his environmental stresses was unconsciously reinforced, the pattern of leg paralysis firmly established.

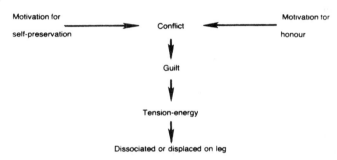

More religious soldiers from Southern Germany who felt guilty about satisfaction derived from killing, 'punished' the arm that did the deed and avoided their emotional conflict in arm paralysis.

The location of conversion is varied and flexible. Among the commoner forms of hysteria are:

(i) hysterical blindness;
(ii) motor paralysis;
(iii) hysterical deafness;
(iv) amnesia (loss of memory);
(v) areas of spontaneous cutaneous anaesthesia; usually in the shape of a stocking or a glove; such anaesthesia is quite incompatible with anatomical nerve distribution;
(vi) trance states;
(vii) 'globus hystericus' (the sensation of having an unswallowable blockage in the throat);
(viii) wild, uncontrolled behaviour.

The hysteric is often of lower than average intelligence and highly suggestible. This suggestibility helps determine the seat of his conversion symptoms. Whatever he has heard, seen or imagined he reproduces (at an unconscious level) in a fairly accurate facsimile.

An illustrative case is that of a child of below average (but not 'handicapped') intelligence who had been exposed to the explosion of a large firework near his ear. His temporary, but nevertheless real, deafness immediately after the explosion created a sensation in the neighbourhood. For the first time this highly suggestible, formerly emotionally neglected and rejected non-academic child found that he was of import, irrespective of his school failures. In spite of all medical reassurance to the effect that no organic damage had resulted from the firework incident, the deafness had persisted for six months before admission to hospital. Only under dilute sodium pentothal (in which state of semi-sleep the repressive power of the conscience is reduced) was he able to hear.

Investigation by the team psychologist revealed his sub-normal, 'borderline retarded' IQ 75, together with inappropriate and tension-producing home and school pressures, many of which were relieved by his deafness, which condition was thus unconsciously reinforced. Only when environmental pressures were reduced by sound social casework was the patient able, at an unconscious level, to dispense with his hysterical deafness.

It is particularly tempting to 'blame' the hysterical patient for his 'weakness of will', 'malingering', 'self-concern' and 'irresponsibility', but to do so reveals lack of insight into the fact that he is essentially a sick person).

His behaviour, socially displeasing as it may be, attempts to express and 'work out' a pressing problem he is trying to solve. Far from deceiving, he is, in reality, seeking to express his problem and his need for help. Most hysterics have, in the past, been denied the attention, warmth and protection for which their symptom is now pleading.

Dissociation is the mental mechanism by which certain tension-fraught activities and situations escape from the conscious control of the individual.

The anxiety of a guilt-laden stress area, constituting too heavy a burden, is 'split off', fragmented, disowned and dissociated in order to preserve the self-concept.

A murderer for whom violence is an unaccustomed behaviour pattern may be so appalled by the realization of his deed, that he may 'dissociate' or disown the episode in the oblivion of a genuine amnesia (loss of memory).

Sometimes to protect itself the psyche or mind 'splits off', the individual seeing himself as from outside his body.

Dissociation is frequently an element in hysteria.

A keynote of <u>stress reduction</u> when human relations are 'snarled up' or 'side-tracked' by devious mental mechanisms is tactful confrontation, often by a third party. Here the mediator or 'facilitator' confronts the parties (alone or in association) with their real feelings;

> 'It seems to me that the anger between you two nurses is really displacement of the understandable anger you both feel about the unresolved pay dispute. Realizing this may assist you in finding a less destructive outlet for your pent-up stress'.

When a mental mechanism, due to its inability to relieve

tension
stress
anxiety

becomes

> persistent
> repetitive
> unproductive
> maladjustive

it becomes a neurotic disorder (eg involuntary cleanliness compulsion, psychosomatic illness, compulsive thoughts).

CHAPTER 6

PERCEPTION, LEARNING, MEMORY, FORGETTING

PERCEPTION

Perception is the process by which sensory cerebral areas receive, organize and interpret patterns of stimuli

> from inside the body, or
> from the environment

in order that the individual may be made aware of present data.

> Organization **+** Interpretation → Perception

The human brain is composed of some ten to twelve billion specialized cells called *neurons*, the basic units of the nervous system. It is postulated that these neurons hold the secrets to learning and mental functioning.

We know they are responsible for the *transmission* and *co-ordination* of nervous impulses, but we are just beginning to unravel their more complex functioning in learning, emotions and thought. It would appear that:

> *resistance* to or *ease* of transmission in the *synapse* containing the axon of one neurone and the dendrite of the older, determines the ease or sluggishness of message transmission.

Main neuron function divides into four broad categories, namely

1. *Stimulus input*
2. *Perceptual processing association*
3. *Interpretation input*
4. *Motor output—behaviour response*

(1) Stimulus input

The *stimuli* consisting of *messages* of sight, sound, temperature, pain, pleasure, etc are conveyed to the cerebral sensory areas by *afferent* nerves.

Stimulus input is the process by which information about

(i) the environment and
(ii) one's own body,

originating in specialized cells in the sense organs, muscles, skin joints, etc is conveyed to the *cerebral cortex*, the grey, walnut-shaped upper layer of the brain. The cortex is a thick layer of grey nerve cell bodies and unmyelinated fibres in which *all complex mental activity takes place.*

The cerebral cortex is divided into two hemispheres by the deep, longitudinal cerebral fissure.

Each cerebral hemisphere contains areas responsible for important functions which are intimately associated with

Sensory awareness—internal feelings—parietal;
Visual—occipital;
Auditory—temporal;
Reasoning, learning and self-control—frontal lobe;
Output behaviour—a response or reaction set in motion
                  by the motor co-ordination area: motor neurons.

The cortical system controls the level of consciousness and thus perceptual impact. The area and weight of the cerebral cortex increase with evolutionary development, being much larger in man than in any other animal.

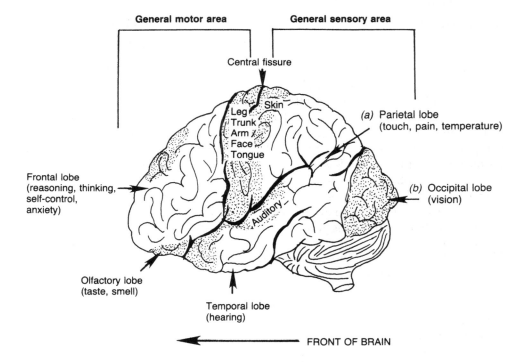

Grouped in the cerebral cortex, posterior to the central fissure and the 'Alice Band' of motor neurons, are the *sensory areas* where messages brought up via the afferent nerves, through the brainstem, cerebellum, medulla, thalamus and inner white cells are processed.

The sensory areas consist of

(a) the *parietal lobe* or *somato-sensory area* where sensory experiences involving body-sense such as heat, cold, touch, pain, body movements and placement sensitivity are received, organized, integrated, and (in the light of experience, gained and stored in the frontal lobe), interpreted.

Dysfunction of the partietal area due to trauma, infection, etc may lead to dangerously reduced sensitivity—for example to temperature change or pain—inaccurate body image and impaired balance.

Similarly certain benign drugs such as painkillers may cause reduced sensory and interpretative accuracy in the cerebral somato-sensory area.

Kephart has demonstrated the necessity for a good 'body image' if the individual is to attain adequate perception of space. 'As used here, body image refers to the child's awareness of his body and its capabilities. It includes the answer to four major questions: What are the parts of my body? What can they do? How do you make them do it? What space do they occupy while doing it?'

(b)   The visual (occipital) area:

At the back of each occipital lobe lies the visual cortex.

Through studies of the electrical responses of single cells in the visual cortex of cats and monkeys, investigators have proceeded far in mapping the site and function of this area. When in the course of brain surgery under local anaesthetic, this area is stimulated locally, the patient 'sees' flashes or spots of light.

When appropriate electrodes were implanted in the visual cortex of two blind subjects, and stimulated electrically, the subjects experienced patterns of visual sensation crudely approximating real sight. Here is an area of hope for the blind.

The functions of the occipital area include not only the *registration* of vast and complicated light-visual patterns but also the *inversion, synthesis* and *sequencing* of pattern parts into *visual syntheses* that are interpreted, through the experience of the frontal lobe, as objects, letters, words, etc.

Impaired visual concepts impede accurate frontal lobe interpretation of spatial relationships, resulting in poor patterning and drawing, impaired insight into design and shape—including letter shape and synthesized word shapes. Clearly damage to cortical visual areas may result in reading disability (sometimes termed 'dyslexia'). In spelling there is a disproportionate reliance on phonetics, the word-shape appearing distorted, eg seme for seem, hten for then. Such children are unable to profit appreciably from emphasis on 'look-say' reading teaching. Failing to recognize word-shape, they are obliged to sound words anew each time they are encountered.

Dysfunction of this area may well result in misplaced, inverted, incomplete or incorrectly sequenced stimuli such as letters, numbers, etc, or in a reduced ability to synthesize letters and syllables into a visual word-image even where the actual eye mechanism is perfect.

Because we mainly *perceive objects rather than their individual component features*, we *perceive objects as stable and enduring*. However, this stability depends on various constancies of:

brightness,   size, and
colour,   location
shape,

Clearly we cannot accommodate a house on the retina, our visual relay screen. The size of the retinal image subtended by an object is indirectly proportional to its distance from the lens of the eye. Thus a matchbox close to the eye would subtend the same size image as a skyscraper far away from the eye. Size perception represents a compromise between the size of the object and the image on the retina. The more familiar the object, the easier it is for us to perceive its real size.

A basic principle of visual perception is *figure* and *ground*. Irrespective of familiarity, we recognize patterns as figures against the anchor of their background.

Because our visual configurations change in time and space so does our perception of stimuli. *Perception therefore involves an innate and active search for the best integration and interpretation.*

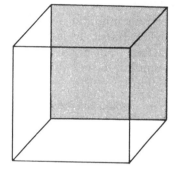

The Necker cube illustrates an illusion devised in 1832 by the Swiss naturalist, L A Necker. One notes that the tinted surface can appear as either the front or the rear surface of a transparent cube.

The potent factors in visual interpretation are

    figure and ground,
    perceptual grouping and patterning,
    visual illusions, and
    analysis and synthesis,

providing information about size, shape, depth, distance, movement, etc.

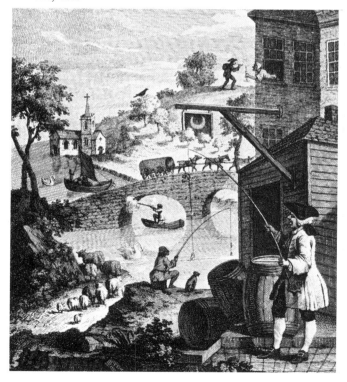

Engraving entitled 'Satire on False Perspective' after William Hogarth (1754). At first glance, the picture appears sensible, but closer inspection indicates that the scene could not appear as depicted. Note the many ways in which the artist has misused depth cues to achieve unusual effects.

Effects of visual deprivation

We shall now discuss an experiment designed to examine the effects of visual deprivation.

To obtain a controlled experimental situation, animals were raised in various degrees of light deficiency and then tested for visual ability.[*]

But nature rebelled at experimental imbalance. It was discovered that experimental chimpanzees had suffered neuronal deterioration, suggesting that a certain minimal amount of light stimulation is necessary for normal neuronal development. In later studies, translucent goggles were attached to monkeys and kittens from birth to around 1 to 3 months of age. The goggles did allow light stimulation, but this was diffuse and unpatterned.

Thus:

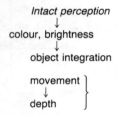

Intact perception	*Impaired perception*
↓	↓
colour, brightness	*Inability to*
↓	
object integration	(i) Follow a moving object with the eyes,
movement ⎤	(ii) discriminate forms such as a circle and a square
↓ ⎬	(iii) perceive depth
depth ⎦	

Conclusions

While admitting to the possibility of deteriorative changes, and the development of compensatory skills, it would appear reasonably justifiable to draw the following conclusions.

Our perceptions develop gradually from primitive generalized visual experiences dominated by

figure—ground—brightness—colour
↓

through *learning* to
↓

more accurate, detailed perceptions increasing in their freedom from parietal-sensory dependence—an observation consistent both with Gesell's theory of development from the general to the specific (see p 261) and Piaget's basic Sensory-Motor Stage (see p 264), setting the stage for later more intellectualized *cognitive learning*.

An interesting experiment investigating the effects of *visual deprivation* on human beings, involved the comparison of

Euro-Canadians raised continually in a 'carpentered' environment featuring vertical and horizontal contours,

---

   * Risien, A H. 1965. 'Effects of Early Deprivation of Photic Stimulation', reported in Osler, S & Cooke, R (eds). *The Biosocial Basis of Mental Retardation* Baltimore: Johns Hopkins University Press. 146.

and

> Cree Indians, whose lifestyle alternates between rounded summer tents and linear winter lodges.

Results

The Euro-Canadians exhibited a higher acuity for vertical and horizontal than for diagonal orientations.

The Cree Indians showed no difference in perceptual efficiency as applied to directional orientation.

In the absence of genetically determined differences, one concludes that the wider visual experience of the Cree Indian resulted in increased perceptual efficiency.

(c) *The auditory (temporal) area,* situated on the surface of the temporal lobe, is responsible for the reception, organization and synthesis of sound. The area sensitive to high notes is different from that sensitive to low ones. Because both ears are represented in the auditory areas on both hemispheres, the loss of one temporal lobe has little effect on the hearing.

To investigate the relationship between the auditory area and behaviour, Miller, Moody & Stebbins (1969) report an experiment in which electrodes were implanted in the auditory cortex of monkeys who were trained to press a key in response to a tone.

Response: When the tone was turned on, and its sound conveyed, via afferent nerves, to the auditory-temporal cortex, the animal required 20 milliseconds to respond.

From direct temporal stimulation (eliminating afferent nerves), the response took place in 5 milliseconds. One is thus justified in concluding that the time required for the nerve impulse to reach the auditory cortex was 15 milliseconds.

The primary auditory receptive area is located in the transverse temporal gyrus.

In processing auditory material the auditory receptive area is responsible for

> loud–soft discrimination,
> sound sequencing as in syllables, words, etc,
> sound integration, ie from individual sounds to words, phrases, etc.

If the auditory receptive area is damaged or impaired auditory stimuli may lose sequence or come from the *incorrect direction* (the child seeking the speaker, music, etc in inappropriate places) or appear inappropriately loud or soft.

Auditory stimuli may be misinterpreted, the pupil being unable to distinguish, for example, the sound of a racing car from that of a whistle, or a teacher's voice from the sound of a passing lorry. The pupil *cannot associate letter shape with letter sound* or *synthesize* sounds into words. Thus he encounters reading difficulties. In spelling, word shape approximates requirements, but internal sound synthesis is inaccurate, eg vun for fun, light for eight, damidge for damage.

Contemporary research reinforces observation to strengthen the premise that autistic children, grossly lacking in normal emotional responses, may well be brain-damaged.

(2) Perceptual processing: association

The Association areas are not directly concerned with the sensory input or motor output processes, but rather *integrate inputs from more than one channel* via *associate fibres*.

Examples of common area combinations are

visual–motor ('doing' movements);
visual–temporal (seeing–hearing) + learning experience in frontal lobe → reading;
parietal–temporal (internal feeling–hearing) + learning functions in frontal lobe → sport, music, etc;
visual–motor (seeing–doing) + learning function in frontal lobe → typing.

To the naked eye the two halves of the human brain look like mirror images of each other. *Yet the function of the two sides is not identical.* For one thing, we know that nerve tracts cross so the right side of the brain governs the left side of the body, and the left side of the brain governs the right side of the body. Furthermore post-mortem examination reveals certain asymmetries, one hemisphere, usually the left, being larger than the other—even in fetal brains. It appears that these anatomical differences are related to a deviation in function between the two hemispheres.

In 1932, Jackson introduced the idea of a *leading* hemisphere:

'The two brains (hemispheres) cannot be mere duplicates if damage to one alone can make a man speechless. For those processes, of which there are none higher, there must surely be one side that is leading.'

The *left* cerebral hemisphere is specialized in the use of *language* and *logic*.

The *right* hemisphere is specialized for mental imagery and the understanding of spatial relationships, and would, for example, be the source of an artist's creativity. However, it should be noted that this theory is based on generalized findings and does not always apply in individual cases.

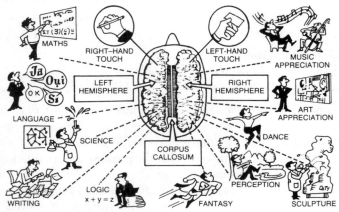

How the brain divides its work

Research indicates that different functions are specialized in either the left or right hemisphere. This figure presents a very speculative attempt to summarize research findings; cerebral locations for some of these abilities are not yet firmly established by research.

As early as 1861, French anthropologist Paul Broca conducted a post-mortem examination on the brain of a patient with speech loss. He found damage in an area of the left hemisphere just above the lateral fissure of the frontal lobe. This region, now known as Broca's area, is involved in the control of articulatory organs and thus of speech. A person who suffers trauma in the left hemisphere is more likely to show language impediment than one whose damage is confined to the right hemisphere. In fact, about 60% of language functions lie in the left hemisphere.

An interesting application of Broca's finding involved the treatment of stutterers. A tape recorder feeds high-frequency sounds into the right ear, stimulating activity in the left hemisphere, seat of the main speech centres. Recordings before and after high-frequency treatment showed a quite dramatic improvement.

Disorders of dominance are frequently associated with disorders of visual-motor organization, hearing, speech and reading.

It has long been recognized that pressure upon a child whose brain is structured for left-hand dominance (ie whose right hemisphere is dominant) to achieve artificial right-hand dominance, may well be accompanied not only by clumsiness but also by stammering and other speech defects.

In 1937 Orton presented the view that stammering resulted from *a failure to develop complete dominance of either hemisphere*. He presented the hypothesis that in naturally left-handed children inappropriate pressure to use the right hand results in *failure to develop* complete right-hemisphere and thus efficient *left motor dominance*. This gives rise to artificial *mixed dominance*, the artificially dominant right hand attempting to lead from left to right, while the naturally governed left eye attempts to lead from right back to left—this, he contended, contributes to the dyslexic's difficulty in reading. The pupil is unable to develop a consistent habit of scanning written material in the left→right direction. Orton's was the first presentation of the implications of incomplete dominance in the left hemisphere accompanied by lack of substitutory power in the right hemisphere. In Western writing the child's natural left-handed and left-eyed lead are not allowed to become dominant (p 519).

In 1945, Brain emphasized that the left hemisphere in many is usually the major hemisphere for controlling speech and eye–hand co-ordination. If the left hemisphere is not dominant, and the right hemisphere is not allowed to develop dominance, then difficulties in both speech and eye–hand co-ordination will result.

Observation of the number of dyslexics who are left-handed or who have mixed dominance, obliges us to consider dominance in reading problems.

The two important areas in which the teacher or nurse may help a patient to achieve purposeful and spontaneous dominance are:

(i) As an accurate observer—it is important that as many details relating to dominance as possible be collected.

(ii) To provide practical help—if it has been clearly established through the teacher's observation, confirmed by the neuropsychologist, that the child is, in fact, left-handed, *every effort should be made to turn him into a proficient left-handed writer.*

Similarly there exist special teaching techniques to overcome reading and writing difficulties encountered by left-eyed children in coping with Western left→right-directioned reading and writing (see p 519 et seq).

(3) Interpretation input

Integration of stimuli

Only under the most unusual circumstances are we aware of a single stimulus such as a pure musical note in a soundproof room. As a rule, we rather hear words or tunes instead of pure notes, and see pictures instead of light spots. *We react to integrated patterns of stimuli rather than to their isolated component parts.* The finished product, like a completed jigsaw puzzle, is quite different from its individual parts—a contemporary scientific observation utilized by the impressionist painters, who use complicated patterns of coloured dots brought together in such a way that they project familiar and real objects such as people, flowers, rivers, etc.

The theoretical significance of the 'pattern of stimuli', introducing a perceptual experience, is the corner-stone of *Gestalt psychology*. Gestalt, a German word, has no exact English translation, though 'form' 'configuration' or 'pattern' approximate the German denotation.

According to the Gestalt school there is a reciprocal relationship between whole leading to parts, and parts leading to whole, through the process of *perception*:

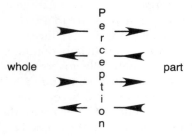

Perception thus acts to draw sensory data together into an holistic pattern or Gestalt.

The most complex patterns in our perceptual experiences relate to *vision*. Vision, our preferred spatial sense, gives us varieties of pattern, form, colour, in one, two and three dimensions. Because we see in a succession of configurations, vision gives us the perception of *change*, of *movement* and *time*:

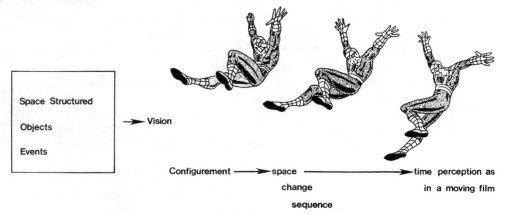

Audition consists of the synthesis and integration of *Time* and *Sound*. Audition provides a simultaneous experience of many sounds coming from different locations in subtle combinations. Spatial patterns do not feature much in audition, which is primarily *a time sense*. In listening to an orchestral concert we can certainly experience a strong, astutely timed sound combination without seeing the performers. The predominant patterns in audition are *succession, change* and *rhythm*

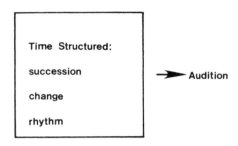

Because auditory stimuli are so time-oriented, they are *transient stimuli*, persisting for much shorter periods than visual stimuli.

Visual perception, on the other hand, usually being of *much longer duration* and also providing *the medium through which we see our body in its environment and objects surrounding us, provides that relative constancy of perception* that renders this medium more stable, enduring and measurable in psychological discussion.

However, this stability depends on various constancies of shape, form, and size, background and foreground, time, etc.

Because the retina is small and visual configurations change in time and space, our perceptual interpretations represent a compromise in size, distance, and foreground–background.

The role of learning in perception

The results of scientific experimentation lead to general agreement concerning the phenomena of perceptive organization and the interpretation of

movement and depth
constancy and change, etc

But the question *whether our ability to organize and interpret—in fact to perceive aspects of our environment—is learned or innate is still unanswered*. This is another instance of alleged conflict between *heredity* and *environment*, an 'argument' dating back to the philosophers of the seventeenth and eighteenth centuries and, in fact, a dispute probably as old as mankind.

The *nativists*, favouring the hereditary domination of the perceptual processes, include Descartes and Kant, who argue that we are *born* with the ability to perceive as we do.

The *empiricists* or *environmentalists*, including Berkley and Locke, maintain that we *learn* our ways of perceiving through more fundamental *life experience* with objects in the world around us.

Again we ask the useless question: 'which blade of a pair of scissors is the more important?'

Most contemporary psychologists agree on the fruitful integration of these two viewpoints. Of course, appropriate *anatomical perceptual equipment must be inherited*. But there is no doubt that *practice* and *experience affect* perception. This is the cornerstone of the *learning process* through which

   perception intake and
   behaviour output

are modified by experience, provided the material to be learnt is focused by *attention*.

Attention

Definition: *The focusing of perception, leading to a heightened awareness of a limited range of stimuli, is termed 'attention'.*

Clearly a process of filtering stimulus input is required for efficient cerebral processing.

That stimulus range upon which cerebral input focuses is termed the *attention range* or *attention span*. Attention enables us to *select* certain stimuli for processing, and to discard others. The brain is thus able to *avoid constant bombardment* by a wide range of irrelevant stimuli. It is thus possible to select stimuli that are pertinent to the task in hand.

The filtering process is amongst the responsibilities of the *reticular formation*, an internal chamber of sinus linking the perceptual association areas.

When psychoneurological dysfunction extends to the reticular formation, there is reduced ability to select relevant perceptions, and the cortex is indiscriminately 'bombarded' with sounds, visual perceptions, kinaesthetic hypersensitivity and even irrelevant odours.

Attempts to cope with all these sensations may result in marked involuntary distractability, inability to concentrate and, to the onlooker, that irrelevant excessive behaviour termed *hyperactivity*. An extreme instance is that of the autistic child who, most authorities agree, may well prove to be a child with a subtle cerebral dysfunction.

Sometimes visual and auditory impulses may become so distorted that the child is confused and frightened by them—this is often apparent in the terrified reaction of the young child trying to cope with what appears to him the sound–sight onslaught of his peer group. All too often he tends to retreat or 'take flight' into lonely and sad withdrawal.

Tranquilizing medications, such as Reserpine either alone or in combination with Carbamazephine, appear promising in counteracting the disturbing effect of unfiltered perceptual impulses.

Sometimes Ritalin is found to increase the *inhibitory powers of the frontal lobe in overcoming bombarding stimuli* which would otherwise result in over-excitability and hyperactivity.

Many workers who handle the brain-injured child on a long-term basis find phenobarbitone disturbing and over-stimulating rather than soothing in its influence.

During consciousness one is never totally unaware of one's surroundings. It would appear that the *reticular formation monitors peripheral stimuli without conscious direction*. The *efficiency of intake* of peripheral material depends upon its *familiarity*. In the case of more difficult and unfamiliar material the subject rarely recalls or holds unattended messages that require a more concentrated attention focus. For instance if one is talking to a friend while passing through unfamiliar terrain, one is unlikely to remember landmarks.

Attention mechanisms

What factors determine the strength of competing stimuli?

The physical characteristics of the stimulus: size, colour, aesthetic appeal, contrast, movement, the strength of emotions aroused; the extent to which they satisfy goal needs—all these determine the strength and effectiveness of attention focus.

Thus, in seeking to focus attention on a *primary health preventive information programme*, one would seek stimuli consistent with cultural problems, interests, motivation and goals. Display of size, colour, movement, contrast, will focus attention on key points.

Stimulating reflexes which enhance stimulus focus:

Somato-sensory (parietal) stimulus focus involves classic body adjustments and movements. Thus *associated bodily movements enhance input efficiency*, eg in teaching personal hygiene, bodily movements (mime) focus increased awareness on washing one's clothes and person, cleaning one's teeth, breathing exercises, etc.

To facilitate visual field intake

→ turn head
     turn eyes→
     pupils dilate to let in more light
→ image falls on retina
→ less muscles work
→ focus on stimulus;
To enhance faint auditory intake
→ cup hands: turn ear.

Stimuli arousing emotions pertaining to survival, reproduction and the satisfaction of basic goals motivate:

dilation of cerebral blood vessels,
constriction of peripheral blood vessels,
increase in gross electrical responses of the brain (EEG),
changes in muscle tone, heart rate and respiration→facilitate the reception of stimulation
preparing the organism for a quick response
in case *Fight* or *Flight* tension-energy is needed

THE ORGANISM IS NOW IN OPTIMUM PREPARATION FOR MAXIMUM LEARNING EFFICIENCY

THE COGNITIVE FUNCTIONS OF THE FRONTAL LOBE

Cognition consists of an individual's thoughts, interpretation, knowledge, understanding and creative ideas: his cognitive processes during perception, thinking and learning.

The quality of his cognition must, in turn, depend upon the quality of his own inborn intellectual potential operating in the frontal lobe.

Intelligence is the capacity to meet a novel situation by improvising a novel adaptive response; the insight to meet and solve new situations and problems quickly and successfully.

Is intelligence a unitary general factor (G in terms of factor analysis)?

Pioneer research psychologist Charles Spearman postulated that all individuals possessed, in varying quantities, a general intelligence factor which he called G. His first serious challenger was Louis Thurstone (1938) who applied the statistical technique of 'factor analysis'. By testing and retesting correlations on many test results, Thurstone extracted from G the following seven factors which, showing very low inter-correlations, he presented as independent or primary abilities comprising general intelligence.

Ability	Description
Verbal comprehension	Measured by vocabulary. The ability to understand the meaning of words and ideas associated with them.
Word fluency	The ability to think of words and their meanings rapidly, as in solving anagrams or thinking of words that rhyme.
Number	The ability to work with numbers accurately and quickly.
Spatial reasoning	The ability to visualize space-form relationships, as in recognizing the same figure presented in different orientations; includes two to three dimensional switch.
Memory	The ability to recall verbal stimuli, such as word pairs or sentences.
Perceptual speed	The ability to grasp visual details quickly and to see similarities and differences between pictured objects.
Reasoning	The ability to find a general rule on the basis of presented individual instances, as in determining how a code is constructed after being presented with only a portion of the series: to use abstract rules to solve a classification of problems e g Archimedes principle.

Source: Thurstone and Thurstone (1963)

Certainly, the last word on the components of general intelligence has still to be spoken. Research claims to discover new component abilities, and there is still search for the isolation and measurement of *original and creative thinking.*

Perhaps personality factors such as motivation to achieve, independence of judgment, initiative, ability to accept ambiguity, and unknown factors; to accept failure and start all over again, are aspects of creativity which cannot, as yet, be objectively measured.

Most modern standardized *intelligence tests* are constructed from subtests measuring these primary abilities. Binet (the Stanford University Intelligence Scale, 1937) constructed subtests measuring these abilities for each Chronological Age level up to year XVI.

The subject's successes at each age level are added up to give his Mental Age.

$$\frac{\text{Mental Age}}{\text{Chronological Age}} \times 100 = \text{Intelligence Quotient}$$

In constructing his highly regarded tests of Adult Intelligence, David Wechsler (1946 and 1958) devised, and applied to a standardized American population, tests measuring the seven primary abilities.

Average scores on each subtest were taken as *norm scores*. Individual Verbal, Performance and Full IQ scores are derived from tables comparing the subject's scores with norm scores and translating these differences (above or below age group norms) into IQ scores.

This scale, which may be administered and evaluated only by a registered clinical psychologist, comprises:

Verbal Scale

    Information—general knowledge
    Social Comprehension and verbalization
    Arithmetical Reasoning
    Similarities (abstract reasoning)
    Digit Span (rote memory: attention span)
    Vocabulary (general learning ability: range of ideas: memory)

Performance Scale

    Digit symbol (speed of new learning: directionality and retention of spatial constellations)
    Picture Completion (observation of detail: discrimination in practical situations)
    Kohs Block Design (analysis and synthesis of patterned configurations: spatial-creative ability)
    Picture Arrangement (insight into social sequences: synthesis: cause–effect relationship in practical situations)
    Object Assembly (observation of detail: visual-spatial analysis and synthesis for tangible configurations).
        Verbal Scale IQ + Performance Scale IQ = Full Scale IQ

The Intelligence Quotient is a measurement of intelligence on a standardized scale. Relative to statistical norm 100 (range 90–110) IQ scores for a given standardization population fall into a bell-shaped distribution curve termed 'Normal' or 'Gaussian'. Most cases fall near the mean. The further scores deviate from the middle, the more remote their classification from Normal or Average.

INTELLIGENCE QUOTIENT DISTRIBUTION

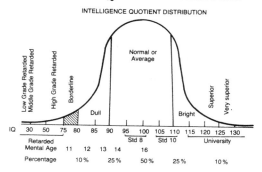

In this type of symmetrical distribution the scores distribute evenly on either side of the middle.

The mean—arithmetical average, ie the sum of all scores divided by their number. The median—the score on the middle case when arranged in order of size of scores. The mode—the most frequent score in a distribution, or the classification containing the greatest number of cases, all fall together.

This is not true of an unbalanced or 'skewed' distribution, where scores distribute unevenly on either side of the middle, as would pertain where bus timetable departure scores (including rush hour) to be thus distributed.

IQ scores, like any other diagnostic instrument, should be evaluated within the whole context of the case presented. In experienced hands *individual tests* are of diagnostic value, revealing the subject's intelligence classification, attack on problems, his response to frustration and the qualitative tone of his thought processes.

They may be particularly revealing of disturbed thought processes in mental illness.

However, in assessing the intellectual potential, aptitudes, interests and scholastic attainment of large numbers it may be necessary to apply *group pencil and paper tests*. Such tests focus on ability to use previously acquired skills to solve new problems. Group tests require careful observation of candidates' understanding of instructions, motivation and concentration.

Is a person's intellectual ability stable throughout his life span?

Since Wechsler's large-scale research on this subject in the late nineteen forties, it is accepted that measurable intellectual ability:

(i)   continues to rise steadily until approximately Chronological Age 16;
(ii) flattens at its highest level (approximately 35 years);
(iii) gradually falls off thereafter.

The fall-off becomes increasingly conspicuous after CA 60, this being due to significant loss in abilities involving speed, new learning, recent memory, unfamiliar spatial concepts and flexibility of thought processes.

Abilities dependent on experience and long-term skills, such as vocabulary, social insight, detail and familiar practical tasks, do not show comparable fall-off. People whose careers depend on established learning in these spheres, such as skilled professionals do not show the same fall-off.

The earliest age when, by virtue of maturation of:

(i) testable skills
(ii) reasonable attention span and co-operation levels,

intelligence testing becomes useful, is around two years. However, due to

(i) limitations in abstract verbalization and thus undue dependence on tangible visual-motor tasks,
(ii) insufficient time for individual differences in maturation of component skills,

pre-school intelligence test results constitute indices rather than reliable measures of intellectual potential.

From Chronological Age 7 years, however, correlations between original and retest scores reach and exceed $r = 0,71$ all the way up to CA 18, which high reliability score confirms that, in experienced hands, IQ scores on well-constructed and standardized tests do not change radically all the way into adulthood.

Wechsler and others have confirmed by well-validated research that after approximately 35 years, and to an increasing extent after 60 years, mental abilities measuring speed, new learning, recent memory and flexibility of thought processes, especially those involving spatial concepts, do fall off, and are thus termed *'Don't Hold' abilities*.

By a formula comparing scores on these 'Don't Hold' abilities with those on *'Hold' abilities* measuring general knowledge, vocabulary, social comprehension and insight, observation of visual detail, psychologists are able to calculate a *Deterioration Index*. This may be of importance in cases of cerebral insult, senility, etc (see p 529ff). Which is the more important determinant of intelligence . . .

HEREDITY OR ENVIRONMENT?

Heredity/Genetics

Summarizing research findings Hilgard, Atkinson and Atkinson[*] present the following correlation coefficients between the IQ scores of:

parents	
natural children	r = 0,50
adoptive parents	
adopted children	r = 0,25
fraternal twins	
(from separate eggs)	r = 0,55
identical twins	
(single egg)	r = 0,60–0,90

Conclusion:

'In general, the closer the genetic relationship, the more similar the tested intelligence. . . . Most probably, intellectual ability is determined by a number of genes, whose individual effects are small but cumulative[†]. (See experimental statistics p 13.)

Environment

1. The IQ correlation coefficient for: individuals living in different environments r = 0-0,30; living together r = 0,1-0,40.
2. The IQ scores of adopted children resemble those of their natural parents more closely than those of their adoptive parents.

Nevertheless the IQ scores of adopted children are higher than those predicted on the basis of their blood-parents' scores (Scarr and Weinberg 1976.[‡]

'Even though intelligence has a genetic component, environmental conditions are extremely important.[§]

The interdependence of heredity and environment was stressed in chapter 2:

'Heredity may be compared to a liquid contained in the bottle of environment.'

In the case of intelligence:

heredity sets the innate *reaction range* of intellectual ability, ie defines upper and lower limits (see diagram p 148).

environmental influences determine where, within the individual's innate intellectual range, his IQ will function eg from IQ 90 to IQ 110 within Average or Normal range.

* Hilgard E R, Atkinson R L, Atkinson. *Introduction to Psychology* 7 ed. Harcourt Brace Jovanovich.

† Wechsler D. *The Measurement of Adult Intelligence; The Measurement and Appraisal of Adult Intelligence.* Williams and Wilkins, 1958.

‡ Scarr S (1977) Testing Minority Children: why, how and with what effects? *Proceedings of the National Conference on Testing Major Issues* Nov. 1977. New York Center for Advanced Study in Education 273.

§ Weisman S. Environmental and Innate Factors and Educational Attainment. *In*: Meade J E, Parkes A S. eds. *Genetic and Environmental Factors in Human Ability.*

In an effort to overcome the persistent haggle between the roles of heredity and environment in intellectual presentation, psychologists have, in recent years, evolved the concepts of 'Fluid Intelligence' and 'Crystallized Intelligence'.

Capacity to Learn

'FLUID INTELLIGENCE' refers to the biologically based, probably genetically determined, constitutional *capacity to learn to solve problems and to acquire the skills needed to adapt to the demands of one's environment.*

Achievement

'CRYSTALLIZED INTELLIGENCE' refers to the *amount of knowledge acquired or achieved.* It is viewed as the product of fluid intelligence and the background history of experience and training.

Fluid or genetically determined intelli- **+** History or experience of training
gence

Produce→Crystallized Intelligence

(Jersild's Inborn Maturation pattern p 255ff)

(Jersild's Opportunity for learning p 255ff)

Crystallized Intelligence

ACHIEVEMENT (Jersild's Growth p 255ff)

'It seems reasonable to assume that people differ in their capacity to learn, (their fluid intelligence), so that some persons are easily able to excel, while others are deficient and are unlikely to learn more than the most rudimentary survival skills, regardless of the amount or quality of the tutelage they may receive.'*

Because it has not yet been possible to devise an intelligence test free of environment, experience and training, all existing intelligence tests must be viewed more meaningfully as measures of 'crystallized intelligence' or achievements.

If it were possible, by the structure of environmentally free 'new tasks' to measure a child's pure 'fluid' intelligence', such a measure would be largely genetically determined and constant, in spite of cultural and environmental stimulation and nurture.

Because this is not currently possible IQ test scores may, within the limitations of the test used, change with the passing of time and the amendment of environments.

'From a clinical standpoint it is useful to conceive of a child's current level of intellectual functioning, as assessed by an intelligence test, to be the outcome of multiple interacting circumstances.*

Thus

1. Both genetic and environmental factors significantly influence intellectual level as reflected in overt behaviour.
2. Genetic and environmental factors interact at all levels to produce observable behaviour.

---

* Friedman, Kaplan and Sadock. *Comprehensive Textbook of Psychiatry* Baltimore: Williams and Wilkins.

So of course do a child's

> cerebral status.
> sensory status.
> motor status.

The work of Piaget (pp 264-5) has emphasized the integration of sensorimotor development into generalized intellectual processes. Certainly, without

1. sound cerebral structure and efficient sensory and motor equipment for communicative efficiency (often impeded in cerebral palsy)
2. a reasonably well-integrated and motivated personality
3. stimulating environmental status

intellectual potential cannot be fulfilled.

Sadock and Kaplan present the following diagram* illustrating operation of multiple interactive determinants of intellectual functioning.

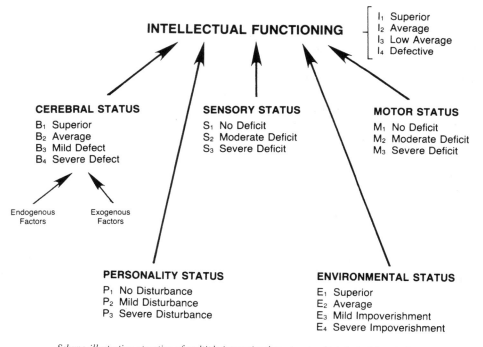

Schema illustrating operation of multiple interactive determinants of intellectual functioning.

The Intelligence Quotient is a scale unit used in reporting intelligence test scores and is calculated on:

(i) the ratio between the Mental Age and the Chronological Age expressed as a percentage

$$\frac{\text{Mental Age}}{\text{Chronological Age}} \times 100$$

* Ibid.

The decimal point is omitted so that the average IQ for children of any one Chronological Age is set at 100.

Clearly, the higher his innate capacity:

(i) the greater the individual's potential for environmental enrichment
(ii) the more he has to lose from an unstimulating, depressive environment.

ie an adverse environment has its greatest negative effect on children of above average ability. Hence the need to cater for gifted children as well as subnormal children (Weisman 1966).*

Environmental factors determining intellectual potential include:

Nutrition,
Environmental stimulation: a loving, rewarding family life,
A community atmosphere feeding back high value on intellectual effort and achievement.

Many studies show that IQ differences between children of low and high socio-economic status become greater in the pre-school years. *It would thus appear that environmental differences accentuate innate intellectual differences* (Bayley 1970). †

In 1965 the United States Congress voted funds for projects providing enriching learning experiences for two- to five-year-olds in their own homes. Special teachers visited deprived children in their homes, engaging in stimulatory activities such as building blocks, matching colours and shapes, interpreting pictures, experiencing concepts such as rough–smooth, noisy–quiet, up–down . . . in fact providing those perceptual and intellectual experiences usually available to middle and upper class children.

Results:

1. Children who have experienced these enrichment programmes score 6 to 10 IQ points higher on the Stanford–Binet Intelligence Test and Wechsler Individual Scale for Children when they enter school than those who have not participated.
2. The experimental children tend, on entering school, to be more self-confident and socially competent.
3. Follow-up studies show lasting gains.

Conclusion

Changing their environment from 'deprived' to 'normal' enables children to move towards the upper limits of their innate intellectual ability or 'reaction range'.

Learning

Definition: Learning is the process by which perception and behaviour are modified by experience.

---

* Weisman S. Environment and Innate Factors and Educational Attainment. *In*: Meade J E, Parkes A S, eds. *Genetic and Environmental Factors in Human Ability*. London: Oliver and Boyd, 1966.

† Bayley N. Development of mental abilities. *In*: Mussen P ed. *Carmichael's Manual of Child Psychology*. New York: Wiley I: 363, 367, 1163-1209.

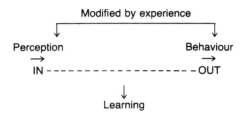

Learning processes are seated in the *frontal lobe*, seat of memory, cognitive (creative) reasoning, inhibition and that learned anticipation of consequences which is the basis of anxiety.

By specifying that learning is the result of *experience* changes due to maturation, disease or physical damage are excluded.

Learning is basic *understanding* behaviour. It involves much more than reflexes and technical skills. Motivations, goals, emotional reactions and personality behaviour patterns, all are *learned by introjection and other experiences*. Children learn by perceiving the world around them, and by *identifying* with parents, peers and the social goals which control their behaviour in accordance with accepted social norms.

Certainly the effect of learning does much to modify *personality* or the *total person*. (See chapter 4.)

William James pictures the world of the infant as a 'big booming, buzzing confusion'.

Intelligent, adaptive behaviour becomes possible as we organize this confusion. We learn to perceive objects, relate them to one another, anticipate what they will do to us, and what we can do to them.

Motivation and *attention* select from this complex totality those things we wish to differentiate out from the confusing whole.

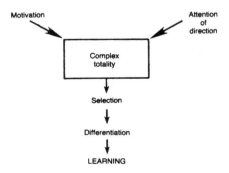

In a baby, for instance, those things that he wishes to differentiate are those which move, sound, taste good and carry danger. These stimuli or goal objects attract his attention and fulfil his motivations. By extending his experience with these stimuli his *perception intake* and his *behaviour output are modified* and *learning takes place*..

(4) Motor Output—Behaviour Response

The effect of learning is measured by the subject's response or behaviour reaction, set in motion by the *Motor co-ordination area* (motor neuron).

Response Behaviour consists of

 (i) Gross Efferent Behaviour visible to the observer, eg withdrawal from pain, pleasurable smiling, speaking, writing, etc.
 (ii) Internal physiological activity, eg accelerated heartbeat, increased blood sugar which may be ascertained by instruments, chemical tests, etc.
(iii) Conscious experience, described by the subject in terms of thinking, seeing, hearing, sorrowing, etc.

When these responses are modified or changed by experience *learning* has taken place. Because behaviour can usually be measured with reasonable accuracy, such investigations are conducted on a scientific experimental basis.

Psychologists very partial to this type of experimental psychology are termed Behaviourists (see p 3 above).

Prominent amongst the Behavioural school are Watson, Pavlov and Skinner.

Learning by conditioning

Conditioning takes place when a response formerly evoked by one situation is now given to a new situation which did not previously evoke this response.

The simplest form of learning may be defined as 'the process of combining or associating at least two experiences which occur *in close proximity in space and time*'.

Learning constitutes a large part of human education and training, eg a child learns to associate his mother with pleasurable food:

Food (primitive stimulus or goal object) → Pleasure
Mother + Food → Pleasure
(Stimuli together in time and space)
Mother → Pleasure

Because

 (i) the food has the primitive ability to produce pleasure in the child,
 (ii) the mother has become associated with the food.

→ Now the mother also has the ability to produce pleasure in the child.

The pleasure constitutes a *reward* by which a positive 'approach' response to the mother figure is *reinforced* or strengthened. If, however there is a long time-lag or space deviation between the presentation of the two stimuli to be associated, or between the stimuli and their effect, one encounters difficulty in learning the association.

For example, the mother who props the feeding bottle on a cushion and then wanders away (space deviation) for the major period (time-lag) of the baby's feed will not easily be associated with pleasure, and thence with love and security.

While a pleasurably learnt association results in a positive or 'approach' attitude towards the stimulus, a painful or unpleasant association results in a *negative* or *avoidance* reaction: 'A burnt child dreads the fire.'

Stove + Pain → Fear
Stove → Fear
          → Avoidance

The pain constitutes a *punishment* by which a *negative or avoiding* reaction is established.

However, were a significant time-lag to occur between the occurrence of the pain and the child's recognition of the stove as the cause of it, the stimulus impact of the stove would be reduced and associative learning would not take place.

To make things clearer, a more elaborate example follows.
Jane was not afraid of white coats.

One day Jane received a painful injection. (Stimulus No 1.) She experienced fear at the same time as she was treated by a doctor in a white coat. (Stimulus No 2.)

Now each time Jane sees a white coat she associates it with pain and fear and reacts accordingly.

A previously irrelevant fear of pain has now become attached to the white coat. (Stimulus 2.)

Response A (fear) was originally initiated by pain stimulus No 1 (hypodermic needle).

As a result of a *simultaneous presentation* of stimuli numbers 1 and 2, stimulus 2 (white coat) now results in the same fear response A.

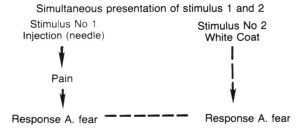

Simultaneous presentation of stimulus 1 and 2

Stimulus No 1
Injection (needle)

Stimulus No 2
White Coat

Pain

Response A. fear — — — — — — Response A. fear

This process of *reaction transference* by a virtually simultaneous presentation is called the *conditioned response*.

Both stimuli having occurred together, they now share a common response.

Learning and remembering are closely related processes, but in terms of time, learning must be prior to memory.

Learning has been described as the process of 'impressing' or forming 'traces' in the nervous system.
↓
Memory or *retention* is the persistence of the new impression.
↓
Forgetting is the decline of the initial impression made by learning.

Through careful experimentation, research workers have been able to measure the *relative strength* of some factors involved in associative learning.

Findings show the following factors to be of importance in determining the speed and persistence of learning and effectiveness of Behaviour Modification Therapy (see "The Psychiatric Nurse" Chapter 26).

1. *Frequency*

Grice showed that accuracy and strength of association increase with the frequency of exposure of the stimulus to be absorbed, eg the more frequently a student goes over her work, the better she learns it.

2. *Continuity*

It was Aristotle who first pointed out that learning takes place most easily when stimulus and response are associated closely in time and space,

$$Stimulus \rightarrow Response \quad SPACE$$
$$\rightarrow LEARNING$$
$$Effort \rightarrow Reward \quad TIME$$

eg a child who is rewarded promptly with a small gift for co-operating in physiotherapy will learn the habit of co-operation in this situation more quickly than the patient who is given only the long-term reward of eventual recovery.

3. *Recency*

Generally speaking, we remember recent happenings better than those in distant time.

Certainly most successful students find it necessary to 'go over' or 'swot', the syllabus in immediate preparation for an examination.

4. *Familiarity*

Studies of the speed of learning nonsense syllables, as opposed to familiar words, indicate that familiar material can be organized into a memorized list more rapidly than unfamiliar items. Hence the advisability of becoming familiar with examination material prior to 'swot week'.

5. *Similarity*

It follows that if learning task B involves items which resemble those in task A, the learning of task B is facilitated.

It is easier to learn to set one sterile tray once a previous tray has been learnt.

6. *Intensity*

Experimenters have found that, within limits, intense stimuli such as brighter lights, louder voices, and increased rewards speed up both human and animal learning.

Certainly the effectiveness of intensity is reflected in successful advertising.

7. *Functional isolation*

Isolated material stands out. It is perceived more easily and learned more efficiently. By its very nature, the episode of hospitalization stands out in the patient's mind as being far removed from the ordinary run of his life. Unhappy incidents occurring during this period quickly result in the learning of adverse avoidance associations.

8. *Duration*

The effectiveness of stimulus–exposure diminishes after reaching maximum effectiveness.

How much should one try to learn at any one time?

Long learning assignments are characterized by 'output valleys' or drops in efficiency.

At a certain point an increase in the length of a task requires more than the proportional increase in time and effort to make elongation worth the while.

That extra study hour late at night may not be worth the loss of sleep entailed.

Distribution of practice

Is it better to spend four hours of one day on a difficult task, or one hour on each of four consecutive days?

Many studies confirm the view that distributed practice is better than massed practice. In fact, for complex learning tasks the 24-hour spacing of trial learning periods seems to give optimum efficacy.

In problem-solving, such as research where one needs time to find submerged relationships, massed practice may help, but one may also 'get stuck in a rut'. A time interval between trials may be advantageous. If, however, the time intervals are too long, the process of forgetting impairs the prior learning experience. It is fruitful to return refreshed, but after not too long.

Thresholds for learning

Low threshold for learning

When the above factors 1–8 are favourable to learning, a subject is said to have a *low threshold for learning*.

New material, finding few obstacles, achieves easy entry into associative learning.

High threshold for learning

When the above factors are rendered unfavourable, especially due to fatigue, a lack of stimulus interest–impact (reduced intensity) or the presence of powerful, diverting extraneous stimuli (poor functional isolation) a subject is said to have a *high threshold for learning*.

New material thus encounters resistance to achieving associative learning.

Conditioned response or conditioned reflex

A conditioned response may be either simple, or elaborated through a 'chain reaction' of many simultaneous presentations.

In a famous series of experiments on dogs, the Russian scientist Pavlov illustrated the manner in which this associative 'conditioning' proceeds.

Using special apparatus he put meat in front, but out of reach of, a dog. At the same time a bell was rung and the dog's saliva measured.

In the second phase he merely rang the bell, eliminating the meat altogether. On careful measurement, the dog's salivary reaction was identical to that obtained in the second phase in which the meat was also presented.

In fact, the dog had learnt to react to the bell in the same way as to the meat, ie conditioning had occurred, the salivation reaction having been transferred to a previously unassociated stimulus, ie the bell.

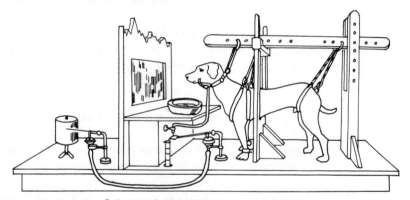

Collection of saliva in Pavlov's early experiments
Observe that the drops of saliva, as they fall upon the platform above the calibrated glass tube, activate a recording mechanism which makes a scratch for each drop on a moving smoked drum. (From Yerkes, R M & Morgulis S. 'The Method of Pavlov in Animal Psychology.' *Psychological Bulletin* 6; 257, 1909.)

The experimental process can be illustrated thus:

(1) meat   .... → saliva
(2) meat and bell .. → saliva
(3) bell   .... → saliva.

It is interesting to note that 'graduates' of the Pavlovian school of conditioning or 'behaviourist' science, provided the space dogs 'manning' the early Russian satellites.

An interesting application of the principle of conditioning in psychosomatic therapy has utilized a primitive intermediary stimulus (a buzzer) to condition the enuretic patient in whom the sensation of a full bladder was not sufficiently strong to elicit the response of constricting the urinary sphincter muscle.

Using a device which causes a buzzer to sound as soon as urination takes place, research workers found that through simultaneous presentation with a primitive stimulus sufficiently strong to cause waking (buzzer), patients began to awaken before the sound of the buzzer showing that they were now giving to the weaker sphincter sensation the same response as they had previously given to the strong buzzing sound.

BUZZER ————————→ WAKING
Weaker sphincter sensation + first few drops + buzzer ——→ WAKING
Sensation alone ————————→ WAKING

The child has now learnt to associate the sphincter sensation of a full bladder with awakening.

Experimental extinction

Experimental extinction is the method whereby the subject is taught not to respond by the removal of the primitive unconditioned stimulus (goal–obect: meat) which originally aroused motivation. Thus the chain of activity aimed at tension relief will be broken.

Referring back to Pavlov's experiments on the learned salivary responses of dogs, one is led to ask 'What happens if we ring the bell and give no food?' The dog appears to have established an expectancy that the bell will be followed by food. If we now ring the bell but fail to feed him, he continues to salivate for a number of trials, but the quantity of the saliva decreases until he eventually secretes no saliva at the sound of the bell.

Because we have removed the primitive unconditioned stimulus or goal object, namely food (which originally set up the learning chain), his motivation is removed. As a result of this 'negative' experience he has learned *not* to respond.

All our learnt reactions are built up by the interwoven patterning of learning, and elimination by extinction. However, extinction seems less durable than the original conditioning, some learnt memory tending to persist.

Learning by reinforcement

Behaviour modification (operant learning)

Behaviour modification applies the findings of behavioural science to human subjects:

desired constructive behaviour is *rewarded* and thus reinforced by praise, privileges, token payments, etc;
negative, destructive behaviour is *punished* and thus extinguished by reproach, loss of privilege, token penalty, etc.

Learning by reinforcement, as demonstrated by Pavlov's classic experiment, required *no voluntary action* by the dog in order to condition his new response.

Meat + bell → saliva
(unconditioned stimulus + conditioned stimulus → response)
Bell → saliva

Rather did the bell elicit *normal canine activity*.

B F Skinner was concerned with the ability to learn a *new voluntary behaviour previously unassociated with natural behaviour*, eg to teach a dog to sit up on his haunches in order to earn the reward of a titbit.

This could only be done by rewarding desired behaviour *after* it had been elicited.
Here the sequence is reversed:

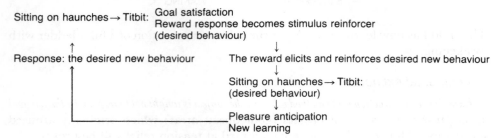

The dog was required to *do* something in order to establish new learning.

The two essential elements of behaviour modification are

(i) Voluntary purposeful behaviour operating upon the environment:
The dog sits on his haunches in expectation of his rewarding stimulus, ie titbit.

(ii) The order of learning is reversed, the reward becoming the reinforcing stimulus.

Experiment: 'The Skinner Box'

In a box, bare except for a protruding bar and a food receptacle beneath it, Skinner left a rat. The animal's random movements reached the protruding bar, which, when pressed, activated a food magazine, delivering a seed pellet. Henceforth, every time the rat pressed the bar, he was rewarded and his newly reinforced behaviour pattern speeded up.

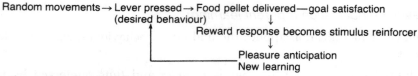

Most voluntary behaviour is operant.

Classical conditioning (Pavlov)
The animal is passive. It merely waits for a natural response to the new stimulus

Meat	+	bell	→	saliva
↑		↑		↑
unconditioned	conditioned		new learnt	
stimulus	stimulus		response	

Operant conditioning (Skinner)
The animal must actively *do* something in order to earn his
(i) pleasure achievement or
(ii) avoidance relief.
These latter goal satisfactions constitute the reward reinforcers linking back to the newly learnt desired behaviour.

Scientific measuring instruments underline the *orderliness, efficiency and speed of operant learning*.

Skinner showed that a pigeon who had learnt that pecking a lighted disk-mount would deliver a peanut (stimulus reinforcer), continued to peck some 6 000 times an hour although he had only been rewarded 12 times!

Behaviour Modification Therapy (BMT) seeks to reward acceptable social behaviour by tokens (food coupons, privileges, etc). BMT converts these rewards into conformity reinforcers,

```
e g   standing patiently in line    sweet coupon
      at canteen (ie desired        ie reward
      behaviour response)           ← reinforcer
```

Social training of psychopaths relies heavily on BMT.

> '. . . Behaviour modification is an effective treatment modality for alleviating human problems, among which are psychiatric disorders. Although behaviour modification has not yet been proved to be the treatment of choice for strictly intrapsychic conflict, it can help to alter those behaviours which result from and exacerbate such conflict. Strictly behaviourally orientated therapists, for example, are not likely to treat a client who is experiencing a significant loss. These clients would benefit more from evocative or insight psychotherapy.*

Factors strengthening the efficiency of the reinforcer

1. Generally speaking *the more powerful the reinforcer,* ie the value placed on the reward, *the more often it is sought and experienced,* the greater its efficiency and reinforcing power.
2. *The closer the conjunction in time* the more efficient the reward reinforcer.

Delaying the reward (or indeed the punishment) may interfere with the learning of that new desired behaviour which one seeks to reinforce (see Behaviour Modification Therapy, p 607). The most appropriate choice of reward reinforcer is of course determined by personal situations and preferences. In 1953 Olds, investigating the reticular system of the rat brain, using micro-electrodes implanted near the hypothalamus, found subjects experienced sensations so rewarding and pleasurable that the animals pressed the bar an average of 2 000 times an hour until they collapsed with exhaustion!

Clearly

(i) so acute a sensation may lead to exhausting overreaction,
(ii) being impersonally administered, and lacking the secondary reinforcers of intimate relationships and warmth, this type of new behaviour may be eliminated sooner than more generalized reward stimuli.

Reinforcers may be either

(i) POSITIVE, *reinforcing* learnt behaviour by the provision of stimulatory, pleasurable reward experiences such as food, money, praise; or

* Stuart & Sundeen. *Principles and Practice of Psychiatric Nursing.* Mosby & Co. pp 589-90.

(ii) NEGATIVE, increasing a certain behaviour by the elimination of a particular stimulus. A rat placed in an electrified cage will learn to press the right lever to eliminate the electric shock: thus a new behaviour (pressing the appropriate lever) has been learnt by removing a painful stimulus (the electric shock). Thus the elimination of pain becomes a reward reinforcer.

Absence (a negative approach of *not* happening) is thus, in the short term anyway, reinforced.

Punishment, such as beating, delivered every time the subject expects a reward, is a simple form of conditioning that associates undesirable behaviour with pain, thus decreasing the probability of the particular behaviour.

The undesirable behaviour is associated with pain and is therefore avoided.

There is considerable evidence to show that *switching from positive reward reinforcers to punitive negative reinforcers* results in conflict, anxiety, tension and thus increased likelihood of undesirable behaviour.

Psychological experiments provide evidence that—

1. Because it temporarily *suppresses* a response but does not weaken it, punishment is often less effective than reward.

2. While prolonged and severe punishment may be effective:

    (a) it often forces the individual to *select alternative*, even more undesirable behaviour designed, consciously or unconsciously, to <u>imperil a relationship</u> already impaired by the infliction of pain.

    (b) because the response is *suppressed and not unlearned it may later reappear, even in the form of maladjusted behaviour* such as over-activity, neurotic withdrawal, aggressive displacement (p 121) behaviour towards other children or animals. The attitude 'I suffered and learnt at the end of a cane—now it's your turn' constitutes a typical aggression displacement pattern imperilling relationships which should provide support and constructive example of satisfying life patterns.

Punishment, or the association of undesirable behaviour with unpleasant or painful negative reinforcers, does sometimes constitute *an emergency, 'on-the-spot' learning elimination* experience in the following circumstances.

1. Where alternative responses are available which may constitute *alternative reward reinforcers*: Experiments have shown that rats who had learned to take a shorter path in response to the reinforcing reward stimulus of food quickly switched to the longer, pain-free path if shocked at the end of the shorter one. Where, however, the rats were not provided with an alternative path, they soon resorted to random, neurotic and purposeless behaviour.

2. Fear of punishment does often constitute an effective signal *to avoid punishment*. Fear of a speeding ticket may teach one to slow down, which activity by reducing anxiety itself becomes a reinforcing reward stimulus.

3. Punishment which follows *the normal course of events may be informative*. When a child touches a hot pan he learns to avoid cooking utensils. Natural-consequence punishment, where it is not dangerous, does provide an impersonal lesson, allowing the parents to rush in and comfort the child, their relationship intact.

Even 'informative' punishment becomes more effective when the experience shows ways of *redirecting behaviour to an alternative stimulus-reward situation*, as would apply in a teacher's rebuke accompanied by suggestion of alternative more acceptable and praiseworthy behaviour output.

A real danger accruing from the infliction of painful punishment, especially by a feared, or admired and powerful 'senior' or authority figure, is the development of *masochistic, pain-seeking satisfaction*, the loss of self-esteem and substitution of abnormal goal motivation.

Perhaps the most dangerous consequence of behaviour control through infliction of physical pain is the manner in which it conditions the impression that human conflicts can be solved by aggressive behaviour. Patterns of problem solving by physical violence, in varying forms, *legitimize aggressive behaviour*, and may well, within the context of frustration, reduced self-control through alcohol abuse, grief and tension, *slip into child abuse, wife battering, mob violence, etc.*

Certainly *rewards* of love, praise and privilege, especially within the context of meaningful, individualized relationships do constitute a more lasting and civilized way of establishing patterns of self-control and conformity.

The socialization processes we would hope to pertain in human relations emanate from a satisfying mother–child relationship. Where this relationship is imperilled by association with pain, it can no longer constitute the most important incentive to those sacrifices entailed in conformity (pp 48-50).

Conclusion

Within the context of a warm, loving or admiring relationship, visible approval by the loved one provides a more effective and lasting reward reinforcing learning experience than punishment. In this way patterns of self-control and socialization are effectively established.

Systematic Desensitization (a technique developed by behaviour therapist J Wolpe)* may be understood as an 'undoing' or 'deconditioning' or 'counter-conditioning' process. The procedure may be effective in eliminating fears or phobias. It is based on the *incompatibility of antagonistic states*.

For example an individual cannot be
   relaxed and anxious
         (vs)
at the same time. Because these two states cannot coexist, by strengthening or reinforcing relaxation we must eliminate anxiety.

This process is known, in behaviourist terminology, as *reciprocal inhibition*.

Deviation from behavioural norms, whether personally painful or socially disruptive, may have been learned and *reinforced* by some sort of immediate stress-relief, usually stalling off fear of rejection.

Elimination of the painful or disruptive behaviour may take place by a relearning process described by Wolpe *as reciprocal inhibition*. The patient is taught to inhibit his painful (and destructive) behaviour by substitution of a more satisfying long-term

* Wolpe J. *The Practice of Behaviour Therapy*. New York: Paramedical Press, 1969.

adaptive behaviour pattern ie by presenting simultaneously, mutually antagonistic states.

Behaviour modification through reciprocal inhibition has been especially favoured in attempts to eliminate persistent and painful obsessional behaviour.

In treatment the patient is taught *to relax by*

(a) alternatively contracting and relaxing, first specific, and then more generalized muscle groups, until he feels his whole body to be heavy, floppy, relaxed.
(b) associating muscular relaxation with a soothing, dissociative thought: 'You are floating gently towards the sunset.'
(c) in some cases, complementary hypnosis or drugs are used to achieve relaxation.

The patient is then asked to construct a *hierarchy from her least to her most painful and dreaded fear stimulus*, eg a patient suffering from nexophobia (an excessive, illogical and disproportionate fear of dead bodies) may list seeing a dead body in an open coffin at a graveside at the top of hierarchy.

```
most painful and
dreaded stimulus—dead body in open coffin at graveside
        ↑           closed coffin at funeral
                    cemetery
least painful and   hearse
dreaded stimulus—hearing about a death
```

When the patient has learnt to relax, she is asked to close her eyes and imagine the least fear-provoking scene described in her therapist's feedback. When the patient can imagine this scene without any increase in muscle tension, the therapist proceeds to describe the next least fear-provoking stimulus.

When the fear encounter results in anxiety-tension, the scene is repeated until relaxation neutralizes anxiety.

This process of relaxation countering fear continues upwards until the formerly most feared situation elicits only relaxation. The patient's fear of dead bodies has now been desensitized by strengthening the antagonistic and incompatible response of relaxation.

Comment

1. Overcoming fears in phantasy is clearly less effective than successful encounters with the reality situation in a series of graduated steps. However when the reality encounter may prove traumatically destructive, or impossible, phantasy desensitization may reduce crippling fear.
2. The source of the phobia being still operant, anxiety may be channelled into other even more crippling phobias.

Desensitization by positive reconditioning

By presentation of a feared stimulus simultaneously with a *strongly* desired stimulus, it is possible to desensitize or attach a new and pleasant association so that the fear reaction is eliminated.

Desensitization constitutes repetitive exposure to a feared situation, each experience teaching that the situation is not, after all, potentially dangerous.

A doctor, who through the infliction of pain, has himself become a conditioned fear stimulus, might approach his child patient with an ice-cream in his hand. If he has no further occasion to hurt the child, the ice-cream may be substituted as a primitive unconditioned stimulus attaching pleasurable experience and thus positive approach reward.

Doctor + Pain → Fear
(Feared stimulus)
Doctor + Ice-cream ———→ Pleasant reward situation
(Substituted desired stimulus)
Doctor → Pleasant reward situation

A new pleasure association having been built up linking the doctor and the interposed ice-cream, the child's response to the doctor may eventually become a happy one.

This remedy should, however, be used with discretion lest the fear response to the doctor be so strong as to be transferred to the ice-cream, causing the child to scream every time he sees ice-cream:

Doctor + Pain → Fear
Doctor + Pain + Ice-cream → Fear
(stronger stimulus)
Ice-cream → Fear

Positive conditioning and overcoming fear

Many fears are overcome in the normal process of growth. Many apprehensions wane as *experience* extinguishes fears and *maturity* gives the child his own built-in weapons of overcoming fear.

A fundamental principle in dealing with fear lies in seeing beyond specific symptoms to underlying precipitating circumstances. If, for instance, a child has been surrounded by an atmosphere of uncertainty, insecurity, excessive demands, threats, severe punishments and intimidation, it is clearly more important to look for ways of relieving these environmental pressures, rather than merely to tackle surface symptoms of general tension.

As long as underlying difficulties are pressurizing the child, the extinction of one particular expression of fear will soon be substituted by other disguised fear outlets stemming from the same generalized anxiety situation. By pushing anxiety underground, symptom treatment merely forces alternative (perhaps even more painful) tension-outlet expression. Shaming a child for showing his fear of a painful treatment, may enable him to hide his fear: attempts at fear extinction may appear to rob the treatment of some of its terror, but tension may well be diverted into a psychosomatic ailment such as asthma or urticaria.

A child's fear of being abandoned in hospital by his mother may be inhibited by teasing or by 'firmness' on the part of the nursing staff, tension-energy only to reappear in other guises such as anorexia nervosa, fear of the dark or night terrors. Clearly effective reduction of fear of abandonment lies in opening wards and welcoming mothers on a broader basis.

Practical techniques of reassurance

Studies by Hagman, Jersild and Holmes demonstrate that the method of overcoming fears used most frequently by parents is the intellectual approach—trying to 'talk the child out of his fears', endeavouring thus to convince him, at an intellectual level, that his fears are groundless. Where the child has unusual confidence in the adult, some emotional-level acceptance may be achieved, but this approach seldom relieves the child's fears at deeper emotional levels. To be effective, verbal reassurances must be well within the child's comprehension, and must really deal with those aspects of a situation which frighten him.

Some constructive applications of learning principles in overcoming fear

1. It is sometimes helpful for adults to set an example of fearlessness. Such an example may bolster the child's confidence in the protection afforded by the adults in his life.

In identifying with the adult, the child may begin to feel in control of the situation.

The adult may—

  (i) herself carry out the suggested feared actions, proving the safety thereof,
 (ii) illustrate techniques for handling the feared situation,
(iii) set a standard of courage for the child.

The example of fearlessness, is, however, unlikely to succeed if it uses abilities and techniques which are beyond the child's understanding and experience. Nor will an example of courage succeed if it implies that the child is, by comparison, cowardly.

2. In some cases the example of overcoming fear set by other children serves as a booster—however, again care should be exercised in avoiding inhibition of fear thus encouraging the emergence of alternative compensatory fear situations or psychosomatic symptoms. Also comparison should not leave him belittled.

3. 'Positive reconditioning' (as described above). The presentation of the feared stimulus (eg hypodermic syringe), simultaneously with a desired stimulus (such as a chocolate bar) may serve to attach a pleasant reward situation, thus eliminating the feared response. The dangers inherent in this method have already been discussed.

4. The most effective method of dealing with a fear is to help the child, by degrees, to come actively and directly 'to grips with' the situation that scares him; to aid him in acquiring familiarity and experience with the fear stimulus and to help him find skills which are of value in coping with the feared event.

Dr Arthur Jersild, who has made a special study of children's fears, writes:

> 'Although skill may fail to root out fear, in general it may be said that, other things being equal, the child who has acquired the widest range of competence and the best array of skills is likely to have the fewest fears.'*

* *Child Psychology* by Dr Arthur Jersild, Teachers College, Columbia University, New York.

Such skills include not only proficiency in motor activity such as opening doors and switching on lights but also the social skills involved in getting along with people, and intellectual skills involving insight, foresight and a wide experience range.

Frequently, in the context of a good adult relationship, a child will exert himself to improve his competency in coping with a feared situation.

A nurse on night duty in a children's orthopaedic ward had committed the serious offence of threatening a restless child with the words 'see that dark little room down the passage . . . there's a spook in there, and if you cry once more I'll lock you in there with the horrible spook'.

A new duty-nurse found the child in an anguish of fear as soon as the sun began to set. Forming a friendly relationship with him, she learnt the cause of his terror. Together they worked out a plan of action to extinguish his fear by overcoming fear stimuli. First she switched on the light and stood holding his hand in the 'spook room'. Then she held his hand while he switched on the light. Then she stood in the doorway waiting for him. Further extinguishing the fear, she waited for him in the corridor. Night after night, the room becoming increasingly darker, she repeated the process until the child, having been supported in facing and coping with the fear situation, was able to eliminate his fear by experiencing that his fear was without reality or power.

One notes that part of the value of this technique lies in the fact that, in the process, the child benefits from the companionship and participation of a trusted adult. In *identification* the burden of fear is shared and thus more easily overcome. In a positive relationship he is actually *experiencing* that he need not feel ashamed, guilty, afraid, defenceless and alone.

Many of the techniques useful in overcoming fear may be adapted to counteract stimulus power before the event, thus preventing fear. Steps taken to forewarn may forearm, the child being gradually prepared before a sudden painful happening. *However, while one can prepare a child at an intellectual level, one cannot always prepare him effectively for the emotional involvements of a painful and frightening experience.* If, therefore, in spite of the nurse having taken the trouble to prepare a child by explanation and reassurance, he still fears the pain stimulus and cries, fights and resents treatment, she should try not to feel disappointed or annoyed. Even adults experience difficulty in bridging the gap between intellectual and emotional acceptance. *The externalization of fear and distress is healthier than inhibition.* The best she can do in these circumstances is to comfort and soothe the child, trying to divert his attention, as soon as treatment is completed, to more pleasant things.

Assertiveness training applies where the patient's anxiety emanates from disturbed interpersonal relationships marked by anxious *inability to stand up for one's own legitimate rights.* In therapy the patient defines his usual behaviour pattern, and is led into role play and other situations where he practises reactions of increasing assertiveness, self-esteem and self-control and is rewarded for so doing by the therapist's approval. (See also Role Play, chapter 26.)

Aversion Therapy consists in associating negative behaviour with the punishment of a painful shock. Desired behaviour thus becomes associated with a pain relief reward stimulus (p 161). Patients who accept this kind of therapy choose it as being preferable to the extent of emotional pain caused by their obsessive behavioural pattern.

Behavioural therapy has been criticized as authoritarian, endangering self-decision and resembling indoctrination and brainwashing. There is certainly some justification for distrust of imposed learning at the hands of the unscrupulous, the maladjusted, the brutal and intellectually limited. Control and protection in the application of Behaviour Modification Therapy is specified in the U.S. Developmentally Disabled Assistance in Bill of Rights Act.

Psychotherapy and counselling should take cognisance of the individual's multi-faceted personality and individual needs, approaches and methods complementing each other.

Aggression as a learned response

We have learnt (chapter 4) that when goal achievement is blocked by an internal conflict, an impeding environmental barrier or personal inadequacy, equilibrium or homeostasis is disturbed and frustrated tension-energy seeks an alternative outlet. Physical discomfort (as in the case of illness) has been demonstrated as an arousal which places the subject particularly at risk to a tension-energy outlet in the form of aggression. There is considerable experimental evidence to show that aggression-eliciting stimuli such as aggressive role models and TV film identification create a strong need for letting out aggression tension.

Imitation of aggression

Nursery-school children who observed an adult expressing violent forms of aggressive behaviour towards a large inflated doll subsequently imitated many of the adult's actions, including formerly unknown aggressive behaviour patterns.

Does the letting out (release) of aggression provide constructive catharsis? Scientific evidence suggests this is not the case.

It would appear that participation in aggressive activities either increases aggressive behaviour or maintains it at the same level. The Nazis, for example, found that concentration camp inmates who were forced to shock an immobilized person with increasing strength became increasingly punitive and aggressive as the experiment proceeded.[*]

Loew in 1967 demonstrated that subjects who are angry become more punitive in successive attacks than subjects who are not angry. Indeed, if aggression were cathartic, angry subjects, through aggression, would become less angry.[†]

Is there a 'significant' (statistically meaningful) *relationship between viewing violence* in real life, on film and on TV on the one hand, *and aggressive behaviour* on the other?

The results of experiments contra-indicate the claim that watching violence discharges the aggressive impulses of the viewer: on the contrary, social learning theory maintains that a state of *arousal, or anger* may be *reduced at least as efficiently through non-injurious vicarious displacement* as would occur while watching a game of rugby.

---

[*] Buss, A H. 1966. 'Instrumentality of Aggression Feedback and Frustration as Determinants of Physical Aggression.' *Journal of Personality & Social Psychology* **III**: 153–62, 326.

[†] Loew, C A. 1967. 'Acquisition of a Hostile Attitude and its Relationship to Aggressive Behaviour.' *Journal of Personality & Social Psychology* **5**: 326, 335–41.

An important longitudinal study, tracing TV viewing habits over a ten-year period during which more than 800 children were studied in relation to viewing time, the type of programmes viewed, family characteristics, and personal aggressiveness as rated by schoolmates, presented the following findings:

> Boys who preferred programmes with considerable violence were much more aggressive in their interpersonal relations than those who preferred programmes with little violence.

Ten years later, more than 400 of the original subjects, now aged 18 to 19, were:

> interviewed concerning their TV programme preferences, given a test measuring their delinquency tendencies rated by peers as to the aggressiveness of their behaviour.

Findings

1. A high exposure to violence on TV at CA 9 is positively related to aggressiveness in boys at CA 19.

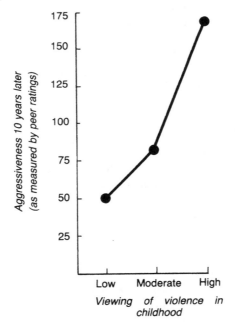

Fig. 7 Childhood viewing of violent television and adult aggression

Preference for viewing violent TV programmes by boys at age 9 is positively correlated with aggressive behaviour at age 19. (Plotted from data by Eron, Huesmann, Lefkowitz & Walder, 1972.)

2. The relationship between girls and TV violence was not so marked—but one wonders about the influence of current aggressive TV dramas in which female models are participating as policewomen, female super-sleuths, tough spies, etc.

3. The majority of studies leads to the conclusion that *viewing violence does increase interpersonal aggression*, particularly in young children (eg Leyen & others, 1975; Park & others, 1977) in the following ways:

(a) By teaching aggressive styles of conduct.

(b) By increasing anger and aggression arousal.

(c) By desensitizing people to violence.

(d) By reducing restraints on aggressive behaviour.

(e) By providing a 'legitimate' opportunity for introjecting patterns of violent outlet.

(f) By distorting views about conflict resolution—on TV or the movie screen, physical aggression is the most common pattern of conflict 'resolution'. Watching the 'good guys' triumph over the 'bad guys' by violent means, increases the acceptability of physical aggression. Even adults may find their view of conflict resolution distorted by TV and films. Research shows that 'heavy' adult viewers of television are more distrustful than 'light' viewers, that they overestimate their chances of being criminally assaulted, and are more prone to buying locks, guns, etc (Gerbner & Gross, 1976).*

4. On the other hand, programmes showing more positive ways of problem-solving have been shown to reduce interpersonal aggression (Leiffer, Gordon & Graves, 1974).†

Behaviourist vs Cognitive Education

Behaviouristic learning leans heavily on automatic, unconscious association. However, this type of learning over-emphasizes piecemeal activity and gives too little attention to organized relationships and meaning. Teaching by automatic association results in too much meaningless drill and rote memorization, irrespective of the child's organization of thought processes or understanding of the work being learnt. Later (see p 263) we shall read of that educational 'rethink' on the part of Western educationalists that followed Russia's first Sputnik in 1957. There was a realization of the *importance of the dynamic cognitive process*. A new emphasis on concept formation, languages, techniques of problem-solving, and creativity brought to the foreground of child development Piaget's cognitive theories. Modern child development attempts to find guidelines for encouraging the maturation of intellectual understanding and the ability to generalize and to think creatively.

Fruitful learning requires reasoning, insight and an understanding of many facts in complex relationships.

Although most modern educational systems do pay at least 'lip service' to the importance of cognitive reasoning, some still lean heavily on a degree of automatic learning such as memorized tables, rote spelling, etc. Some authorities will see in

---

* Gerbner, G & Gross, L. 1976. 'The Scary World of TV's Heavy Viewer.' *Psychology Today* **9**: 41–5.

† Leiffer, A D, Gordon, N J & Graves, S B. 1974. 'Children's Television: More than Mere Entertainment.' *Harvard-Educational Review* **44**: 213–45.

such automatic learning a threat to human individuality as well as to meaningful, motivating and rewarding teacher–pupil relationships.

Individualized learning

For centuries teachers and lecturers have stood in front of classes imparting knowledge which students, on examination, try to regurgitate. Only at Oxford and Cambridge did the 'one to one' tutorial arrangement apply, and this has now been modified to the more economical teacher–class arrangement.

The 1950s saw a 'breakthrough' in the form of a 'teaching machine', utilized in the computer-assisted learning (CLA) framework devised by B F Skinner.* The most important feature of computerized instruction lies in the degree of *individualization*. Students can proceed at their own pace, following the curriculum in a programme edited to suit their own interests and abilities.

Paradoxically the 'teacher computer' can deal with thousands of students simultaneously, and yet individually.

Stanford University presents a particularly sophisticated computer-learning programme: Each student's station consists of a cathode-ray tube, a microfilm-display device, earphones and a typewriter keyboard. The teacher's transient auditory message is complemented by longer visual display, the pupil responds by operating the typewriter keyboard or touching the surface of the cathode-ray tube with an electronic pencil. The response is fed back into the computer and evaluated. A student whose tempo is faster than his peers is able to branch out into special materials, while those encountering difficulties may be branched back to review earlier material.

The message may be simplified down to grassroot-learning, both stimulating and rewarding the pupil on an individual basis.

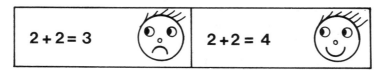

Advantages of individualized instructional procedures

1. Active participation, realizing Dewey's 'Learning by Doing'.
2. Information feedback with minimal delay, allowing immediate correction and thus appropriate association. The immediate reinforcement of correct responses produces faster learning on both animals and human subjects.
3. The individualization of instruction catering for individual differences and varying potential fulfillment.

Criticism

Some authorities foresee in this teaching system a threat to human individuality, as well as to meaningful, motivating and rewarding teacher-pupil relationships.

---

* Skinner, B F. 1978. *Reflections on Behaviourism & Society.* Englewood-Cliffs, N J. Prentice-Hall.

It would appear that, as in most human situations, an eclectic or all-embracing approach is the *most fruitful*.

Group or social learning

Social learning emphasizes the reciprocal interaction between

It stresses the constructive ways in which the individual can learn to cope with his environment.

Behaviour patterns are *learnt or modified through direct experience, or by observing the behaviour of others*. Behaviour earning peer group praise is usually reinforced and that 'punished' by group reproach eliminated.

> Patterns which are successful → are reinforced.
> Patterns which are unsuccessful → are discarded.

Group learning combines Behaviourist responses with cognitive processes.

> Responses that lead to social acceptance and recognition
> or
> symbolic thoughts that lead to social acceptance and recognition
> } are rewarded by a group acceptance and thus reinforced.

Those experiences that *anticipate* non-acceptance or rejection are discarded. Within the context of conditioned experience + insight + *introjection* one should not have to wait and see, through trial and error, that rudeness or selfishness will lead to rejection.

Group development

Groups like individuals, possess an innate capacity for growth and development. They also possess the vulnerability to regress and to resist work and growth. Tuckman has summarized the various phases of group development as:

forming; storming; norming; performing.

Phases	Definition	Task activity	Interpersonal activity
Forming	Group members are concerned with orientation	To identify task and boundaries regarding it	Relationships tested; interpersonal boundaries identified; dependent relationship with leaders, other group members, or pre-existing standards, established
Storming	Group members resistant to task and group influence	To respond emotionally to task	Intragroup conflict
Norming	Resistance to group overcome by members	To express intimate personal opinion concerning task	New roles adopted; new standards evolved in group feelings; cohesiveness developed
Performing	Creative problem-solving done; solutions emerge	To direct group energy toward completion of task	Interpersonal structure of group becomes tool to achieve its task; roles become flexible and functional

Modified from B Tuckman. 'Developmental sequence in small groups.' *Psychol Bull* **68**: 384. 1967.

Vicarious (second-hand) learning

This is learning by observation and *identification* with the feelings, behaviour patterns, failures and success of others. Both behaviour patterns and emotions may be learnt vicariously. Often fear is learnt by watching the pain and discomfort of others, as would apply in traumatic hospital experiences. One learns especially easily from copying the behaviour patterns of role models in whom one has an emotional stake, such as one's parents, sports heroes, film stars and teachers.

The group situation does, of course, provide the advantages of

>*reassuring identification*: through the realization that similar learning difficulties are encountered by others, the student feels reassured;
>
>*obtaining new ideas for tackling a problem*, especially within the context of wide opportunity for intellectual and cultural 'cross-fertilization';
>
>*co-operative rather than individual research*, affording an opportunity for pooled knowledge and extended research;
>
>*instilling hope* by giving new members successful role models.

Nurses often encounter groups brought together for mutual support in illness and distress, for the purpose of support problem-solving education and comfort (see Mutual Support Groups, chapter 26, p 613).

Five common groups which either potentially, or actually, provide therapeutic help for their members are the family group, informal groups, training groups, self-help support groups, and psychotherapeutic groups.

Dr Irvin Yalom has described some of the positive forces characteristic of group dynamics.*

>imparting information,
>instilling hope,
>universality,
>altruism,
>corrective re-enactment of a primary family group,
>development of socialization techniques,
>imitative behaviour,
>interpersonal learning,
>existential factors,
>catharsis, and
>group cohesiveness,

which developments do not occur in isolation, but interact in different circumstances.

Lieberman, Yalom & Miles think of cognitive learning as resulting from the introjection of group information or insight that is of value to oneself.

Cognitive group learning is a frequent nursing activity from the earliest days of training until retirement, and even beyond. *For nursing is not a job; it is a shared way of life.*

---

* Yalom, I. *The Theory & Practice of Group Psychotherapy*. 2 ed. New York: Basic Books Incorporated, 1975. 320–7.

MEMORY

Without memory life would consist of a series of fleeting, unrelated experiences. If we did not remember our thoughts, we could not communicate them. The very concept of 'self' depends on continuity.

Memory processes, like learning and cognitive reasoning, are located mainly in the *frontal lobe*.

The weight and size of the frontal lobe in monkeys approaches that of man. Experiments have shown monkeys to be capable of remembered learning, thus illustrating basic memory processes.

Method

The monkey watches while food is placed in one of two cups, which are then covered with identical objects.

An opaque screen is placed between the monkey and the cups. After a specified time (5 to 60 seconds) the screen is removed and the monkey is allowed to seek food in one of the cups.

Normal monkeys 'remember' the correct cup after delays of several minutes, but monkeys with frontal lobe lesions cannot solve the problem if the delay is more than a second or two. This *delayed-response deficit following brain lesions is unique to the frontal cortex*.

It is a feature of frontal lobe brain damage in human beings that they can perform some intellectual tasks normally, including delayed-response problems. However, lacking the ability to shift in amending the learning process, they *perseverate* and remember old-established tasks better than those 'traced' after brain damage.

Psychologists distinguish three stages of memory:

1. encoding—information brought in by sound or light waves is encoded into a form (eg an auditory or visual mental arrangement acceptable to the memory);
2. storage;
3. retrieval—material is recovered from storage.

The processes of memory can be illustrated in the following way:

'Good morning, nurse, this is Mrs Thomas. Last night she had the bad luck to be involved in a motor accident and has a compound fracture.'
(That afternoon) Nurse: 'Good afternoon, Mrs Thomas, how does your leg feel now?'

Here the following processes occurred:

(i) encoding—sound waves = physical phenomenon: corresponds with **name** and **ailment** coded for memory storage
(ii) storage—short-term memory am–pm **name; ailment**
   long-term memory—months, years
(iii) retrieval—the nurse has successfully recovered **name** and **ailment** from her memory storage.

Memory can fail at any stage—so you might, in the afternoon, remember the *ailment* but not the *name*, retreating to the diminishing escape of calling your patient 'the compound femur in Bed No 10'.

Causes of memory failure

Experiments suggest that these three stages of memory do not always operate in the same way, and the *time lag between input and stimulus recall* is an operant factor. It appears that *short-term memory* is comparable to *conscious knowledge*, while *long-term memory* is comparable to the *psychoanalytic concept of subconscious knowledge* stored in a vast reservoir, only a small part of which is active at any given moment. (See above, pp 5ff and 60ff.)

The *Cognitivist* concept of memory (see p 4) differs from the psycho-analytic concept in the former's belief that material in long-term 'cold storage' is

(i) passive rather than disturbingly active,
(ii) *memory* storage will contain only that which is *selected*, so that much of what we are exposed to does not even enter memory, is gone for ever, and hence can never be retrieved.

Also, according to the Behaviourists, non-selected memories cannot cause unconscious suffering. The crucial criterion is the importance, the usefulness, and thus the attention focus applied to the facts.

Short-term memory

Short-term memory: usually from a few seconds to a few hours.

Long-term memory

Long-term memory: involves information retained for intervals as brief as a few minutes to as long as months, even years or decades, as in old people's childhood memories. However, most researchers have used much shorter intervals. This area is of interest to students in that it is intimately involved in *study input* and *examination retrieval output*.

Is there a biochemical basis to long-term memory storage?

There is growing scientific evidence to suggest a positive answer to this question.

DNA never leaves the cell nucleus, but its 'assistant' product, ribonucleic acid (RNA), does move out into the cytoplasm, where it controls essential functions of the cell.

Flexner (1967) showed that when mice that had learned to avoid shock in a maze were injected with a known RNA inhibitor, they lost their memory of the maze. Clearly RNA was active in the learning process.

Hyden (1969) investigated mice who had been taught to balance on a thin wire—a skill involving vestibular nerve cells. These cells were then found to contain increased RNA of a different composition.

Even more dramatically, McConnell *et al* (1970) trained planaria (small waterworms) to respond to a mild shock and light passed through their aequous beds, with a muscular contraction (Group I).

The shock stimulus was conditioned to a neutral light

to which the worms learned to respond with the same muscular contraction.

RNA extracted from the bodies of the trained flatworms was injected into untrained planaria (Group II).

Muscular contraction conditioning training was then applied to flatworm Group II which *learned* this new conditioned response more rapidly than a control group injected with RNA of 'untrained' worms.

Conclusion: RNA extracted from the conditioned group carried the memory of that training to a subsequent group.

However, this experiment has never been replicated and we are still far from learning Mathematics or Greek by injection or a pill.

References:
Flexner, L. 1967. 'Dissection of memory in mice with antibiotics.' *Proceedings of the American Philosophical Society* **111**: 343-6; Hyden, H. 1969. 'Biochemical aspects of learning and memory.' *In*: Pribram K (ed). *On the biology of learning*. New York: Harcourt Brace Jovanovich. 233; McConnell, J V, Shigehisa, T & Salive, H. 1970. 'Attempts to transfer approach and avoidance responses by RNA injections in rats.' *In*: Pribram, K H & Broadbent, D E (eds). *Biology of memory*. New York: Academic Press. 233.

FORGETTING

The learning process moves in two directions:

> We advance through *association*;
> We retreat through *forgetting*;

We acquire new response patterns, but these do not always remain with us.

Forgetting is the negative phase of this process. Several studies have investigated the rate at which we forget and, at times, this rate of forgetting is dismayingly rapid.

Ebbinghaus, having devised the 'nonsense syllable' as a learning task, used this technique in his momentous study of memory.

Among other observations, Ebbinghaus found that

(1) forgetting is continuous,
(2) forgetting is most rapid in its early stages.

The amount forgotten in the first twenty-four hours may be as great as in the succeeding five days. After the first few days the decline in learning is very gradual.

There thus emerges the desirability of reading over one's syllabus, albeit briefly, on the day preceding an examination.

Students seeking examination success, may well ask whether, by varying certain external conditions, it is possible to slow down the rate of forgetting. Apparently it is not only the *passage of time*, but what *happens in time*, that determines the rate of forgetting. A new learning activity tends to displace memory of immediately prior learning. In preparing for an examination the following day, it is important to avoid interposing a new learning activity which may push important material to the background.

It is therefore apparent that one forgets least where there is nothing to follow and thus 'eclipse' material awaiting expression. The best way to avoid usurping follow-up activity is to interpose a period of sleep.

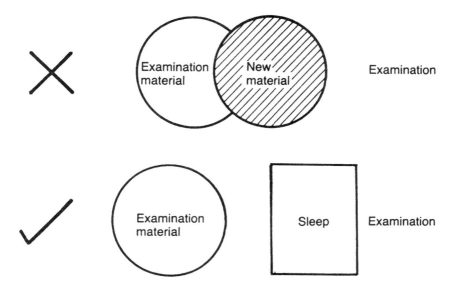

In order to ascertain the *effect of sleep upon the rate of forgetting* Jenkins & Dallenbach (1924) instructed their subjects to memorize nonsense syllables at different times during the day.

Results showed a decisive difference in favour of the protective barrier of sleep. The protection of memory offered by one hour's sleep was small, but by eight hours the difference in favour of the sleep barrier was statistically 'significant'.

The advantage of studying just before going to sleep is thus apparent.

Is forgetting merely a passive process of disuse and decay, or does it present an active function?

It appears that negative experiences, can actively teach a subject *not* to respond.

Do emotional factors reinforce forgetting by protective inhibition?

Freud's concept of memory inhibition

An important operant in forgetting may lie in Freud's repression hypothesis (see pp 6, 56 above). In order to protect ourselves from memories so traumatic, so painful, so shameful that they would overwhelm us with anxiety or distress if we allowed them to enter Consciousness or Super Ego

consciously *suppresses* or
unconsciously *represses*

'forbidden' material into the unconscious Id.

It is this mechanism of *active blocking that distinguishes suppression and repression from all other forms of memory failure.*

In the psycho-analytic model such material may be disinhibited by the relaxation of the censor role of the Conscience by accident, when the Super Ego or Conscience relaxes in sleep and 'forbidden' material slips through into Consciousness in dreams, in delirium, in successful psychotherapy and in hypnosis.

By contrast, in some instances, emotionally charged situations can actually be of value in memory encoding, for example the Christmas gift list.

The very emotional aura surrounding these situations endows a quality of *functional isolation* (see p 155 above). Certainly they are more emphatic than neutral learning situations. Distressing hospital experiences are thus deeply engrained.

Emotionally exciting memories such as those surrounding a fire, a special treat or honeymoon are usually remembered in very vivid detail. However, strong excitement may slip into anxiety, triggering off disorganizing tension-energy designed for Fight or Flight (see, inter alia, pp 27, 104). Soon signs of panic appear.

When one first enters an examination room, words formulating the questions may appear as an incomprehensible jumble. Operating on the limited mental-content of the 'Conscious' one's mind seems a 'blank'. Over-reactive physiological resources render it impossible to isolate and focus mental resources on specific memory associations. Panic spirals. Extraneous thoughts flood the mind. Attention wanders.

'I'm going to fail for sure—I'll let my parents down—What will people think of me?'

These extraneous thoughts interfere with the delicate process of memory-retrieval, exposing the student to anxiety-provoked memory failure.

Now is the time to *breathe deeply*—there is *involuntary relaxation in exhaling. Then sit back and allow link-back association processes into the stored contents of the mind. As long as the material is there, organized and meaningful, you will retrieve it!*

CHAPTER 7

COMMUNICATION:
THE NURSE–PATIENT/CLIENT
RELATIONSHIP

'I find it is the small, intangible things that make the biggest difference . . . the smile, pat on the arm, word of praise, compliment, held hand, conspiratorial wink and, yes, even the shared tears in this day when "heaven forbid one should lose one's professionalism." For me, nursing is just another word for caring.'*

Communication consists in the establishment of a relationship. In human relations communication involves a reaching out, an interflow between individuals, that they may become involved, one in the other. Two individuals communicate when they establish a common 'wavelength'; when, in contemporary language, they encounter matching 'vibes'.

'*Communication may be defined as the transmission of meanings by the use of symbols.* When men interact by means of symbols they are engaged in communication. The sender and receiver of symbols have communicated, however, only if they *identify themselves* with each other's situation.'†

Meaningful definitions of communication emphasize the necessity of exchanging a *message*.

Because the nurse is presumed to be the healthy and relatively unstressed communicant in the nurse–patient relationship, the initiative for establishing contact-messages is usually hers.

MODES OF COMMUNICATION

Mechanisms of communication

Verbal communication is the process of achieving interflow of subjective states such as ideas, sentiments, beliefs, by means of language.

Lower animals and primitive man established lower forms of communication through emotional cries, bodily movements and other signals.

Thus patients in fear or pain tend automatically to *regress* to communicating distress by crying out, lashing out, gesticulating, etc.

Communication by writing enables man not only to share his experiences with members of his group but to record and preserve these experiences, and their accompanying ideas, sentiments and beliefs.

Thus different groups of men have developed specific communication patterns. The culture, society and class into which one is born, structure, in part, the kinds

---

* Melissa H. Johncox, RN, Upjohn Health Care Services employee, Baltimore, Maryland, June 10, 1981.

† Lundberg, G A, C C Schrag & O N Larsen *Sociology* (New York: Harper and Brothers, 1954). 360.

of information *intake*, cerebral *perception* and *interpretation* to which group members become conditioned. Jews frequently communicate by gesture.

Indians are more perceptive of minute physical differences among individual Orientals than of Caucasians; some ethnic groups discriminate more finely than others among varieties of sound or pain. This observation pertaining to differing perception, or message intake-sensitivity, is of particular importance in nursing varying racial groups.

Physiological communication relates to the organs with which human beings transmit messages in the form of words, gestures, tactile contact, facial expressions, smell, taste, pain.

These media are combined in the concept of *Body Language*—the *transmission of a message by body position or movement*; eg a stiffened neck, closed eyes, clenched hands or head turned away, may well convey that the person does not wish for intrusion on her privacy.

There is no limit to subtlety and combinations of body language. In fact research claims that only 7% of communication is verbal. Dr Denise Bjorkman, specialist in non-verbal communication, states

> 'Parents can discover whether their children are distressed, frustrated or lying by examining the molecular or micro-responses.
>
> These are the involuntary movements such as eye-blinking, voice tone, pupil dilation, touch (the skin is the most receptive and neglected organ in the body) and hand-sweating, which cannot be controlled to deceive others about our feelings.'

In that she is often *obliged to communicate by the infliction of pain, the nurse may encounter special difficulties in establishing warm, trusting relationships.* She is thus obliged to establish strong bonds through alternative media such as a smiling, friendly facial expression, warm tactile gestures, association with pleasant tastes and odours and eye contact when wearing a mask.

The vehicles of *societal communication* include gossip, public speeches, town meetings, pamphlets, newspaper publication, radio and TV broadcasting, etc.

Mechanisms of interpersonal communication

Psychologists believe that *all behaviour communicates something*. Every message involves an 'actor' (sender) and an observer (receiver).

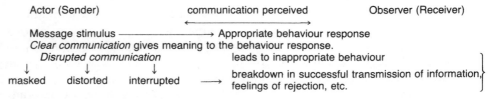

Transactional analysis

Seeking the purest elements of human interaction, delegates at a San Francisco Transactional Seminar in the early 1960s structured the 'intimacy experiment' in which experimental pairs

were seated close together,
retaining 'eye-ball' to eye-ball' contact while talking
'straight to each other' for a period of 15 minutes.

Finding

Any two people really looking at and 'talking straight' to each other can, under appropriate conditions 'attain intimacy always' (as far as these and other similar 'encounters' go), and end up liking each other.

Hence, reason the experimenters,

dislikes result from
   1. 'people not really seeing each other';
   2. 'people not really "talking straight" to each other'.

The greatest preventive of intimacy seems to be a critical parent and, next to that a child rendered incapable of 'straight' communication.

'Ego states' are the result primarily of an individual's conditioning, but also his *introjection* pattern and *genetic programming*.

According to Berne, 'each individual is three different persons, all pulling in different directions . . .'.

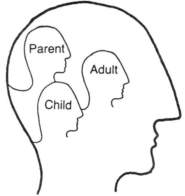

'The *"Parent ego state"* is characterized by parental behaviour, which presupposes a certain authority and even superiority—"parents know best". This "ego state" is partially conditioned by the experience of raising children, but it is also learned during childhood as one observes, and seeks to emulate, one's own parent.'

The Parent 'ego state'

'represents someone in the individual's head telling him what he ought to do, and now to behave, and how good he is, and how bad he is, and how much better or worse other people are. In short, the Parent is a voice in his head making editorial comments, as parents often do, on everything he undertakes. You can tell when your Parent or Parental "ego state" is talking, because it uses words like "ridiculous", "immature", "childish", and "wicked" . . . The parent has another side however. It can also be affectionate and sympathetic, just like a real parent, and say things like "You're the apple of my eye", "Let me take care of it" and "Poor girl".'

The parent can be comforting and wise, but also overbearing and dictatorial.

The *'Adult ego state'* is characterized by rational objectivity and self-control.

> 'It works like a computer, taking in information from the outside world, and deciding on the basis of reasonable probabilities what course of action to take and when to take it . . . The Adult tells you when, and how fast, to cross the street, when to take a cake out of the oven and how to focus a telescope. . . . The Adult ego state is careful, whenever possible, to preserve your dignity. . . . You can tell when your Adult is talking, because it uses expressions like "ready", "now", "too much", "not enough", "here not there".*

The *'Child ego state'* enriches adult objectivity by adding spontaneity and enthusiasm, but is also characterized by a lack of emotional control and a shortened attention-span.

When the Child ego state takes over, the person acts in the childlike way which characterizes the individual at a certain specific age.

> 'The Child is not there to be squelched or reprimanded, since it is actually the best part of the personality: the part that is, or can be if properly approached, creative, spontaneous, clever and loving, just as real children are. Unfortunately, children can also be sulky, demanding and inconsiderate or even cruel, so this part of the personality is not always easy to deal with.'†

Hence, apart from the anger and distress aroused by treating patients as children, the nurse increases her own burden.

> 'Since your Child "ego state" is going to be with you for the rest of your life, it is best to acknowledge and try to get along with it. . . .'‡

All three ego states coexist within the generalized ego of the individual. They constitute deeply engrained conditioned behaviour and response patterns. Each possesses the potential to dominate temporarily the individual's psychological state as his mood changes.

Adults are expected to behave differently from children, and the process of growing up is a transition to the Adult 'ego state'. The Child 'ego state' is not eradicated, however—it coexists with the Adult and the Parent, albeit in a diminished form.

Each individual tends, to some degree, to shift involuntarily or unconsciously from one 'ego state' to another, the personality tending to 'regress' to the 'Child State' more frequently in illness, pain and stress and with the physical degeneration of age.

---

* See also Eric Berne. *The Games People Play*, Penguin Books.
† Eric Berne. *Sex in Human Loving*. Penguin Books.
‡ Ibid.

Examples of Ego State Transactions

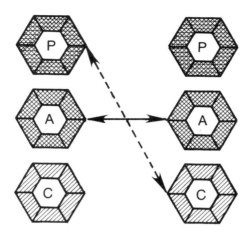

Switching in to a Mutual Ego State
This diagram also illustrates the old authoritarian Nurse–Patient concept
(Parent→Child), as opposed to the new co-operative and mutually responsible
Adult→Adult communication goal.

Sometimes, in order to achieve meaningful communication, it is necessary that one communicator assists the other in switching in to a mutual 'ego state', as would apply when a mother interprets to an adolescent her fears regarding the sexual implications of dating an older man. In this case 'the Parent' seeks to provide information facilitating *identification with the Adult or Parent 'ego state'*:

'I want to speak to you as a friend.'

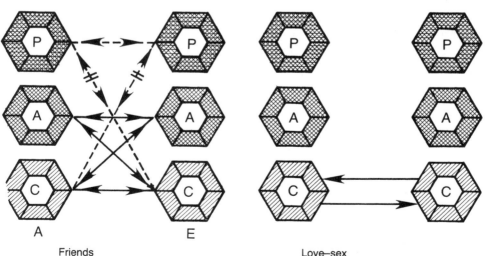

Friends

Love–sex
'Intimacy is a candid Child-to-Child
relationship with no games and no mutual
exploitation.'

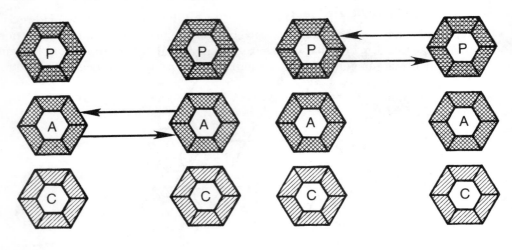

Adult⟷Adult
e.g. Work colleagues

Parent⟷Parent
Committee members and administrators

In order to achieve insight into particular behaviour–communication patterns, one should identify and accept each component and, since they are all there to stay, seek the most productive and personally fulfilling integration.

Freud divided the psyche into different parts. Berne's 'Ego states' are not parts but rather phases.

The ego states of two individuals engaged in communication or *transaction* may be the same, in which case messages can be sent and received with minimal distortion—or they may be out of phase with each other, sometimes leading to disrupted communication.

Complementary transactions occur when the message is directed from one ego state to a listener who receives it in a similar ego state. For example

Sender A: 'What do you think of inflation?'
Receiver B: 'I think the government must reduce money supply.'

This is an Adult-to-Adult exchange, two people communicating on the same level. It can be diagrammed (as in 'work colleagues' above):

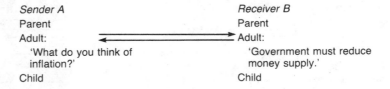

The transaction might continue as follows:

Sender A: 'I disagree with that.'
Receiver B: 'Let's discuss it.'

This would be a continuation of an Adult-to-Adult exchange of views. However, Receiver B might instead feel threatened by disagreement—his emotional reaction might take the form of 'What you are really saying is that I'm stupid, and I resent that'. He is reacting in his Child ego state, as if he were a child being rebuked by a 'superior' parent.

Many communication problems arise when *transactions are crossed:*

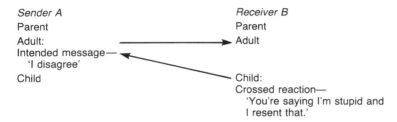

Or, similarly, from Nurse (Sender) to Patient (Receiver): 'Here is your lunch. The dietitian has substituted saccharine for sugar for nutritional reasons, but the pudding will taste just as good.'

This is a straightforward Adult-to-Adult transmission of information—but, in stress, the Patient may react as a surly, rebellious Child: 'You're forcing me to eat what I don't want, and I won't do it.'

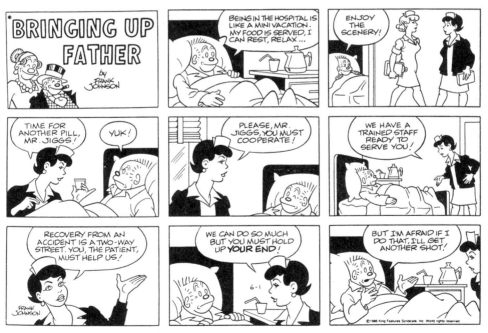

Reproduced by kind permission of King Features Syndicate.

This type of *cross transaction* is frequently encountered in hospital situations, as the patient's feelings of diminishment can easily reduce him to a Child ego state. This 'regression' can manifest in excessive passivity and relinquishing of Adult responsibility, or as above, in illogical resistance, leading to communication blockage and so-called deviant behaviour.

Similarly, because of her tendency to assume the Mother role, there is a danger that the nurse will too often relate to patients in her Parent ego state. This is a natural response, as the vulnerability of patients can arouse the desire to nurture or comfort. At the same time, the dependence of patients can evoke feelings of superiority in the nurse which she is not aware of. Her behaviour may be overbearing, and patients may interpret it as a lack of respect for their human dignity.

Crossed transactions and resultant interpersonal tensions lead to deterioration of the nurse–patient relationship, exerting a negative effect on rehabilitation.

It is vital that the nurse cultivate self-awareness in this regard. There may be 'difficult patients' in every ward, but all too often the difficulties arise, not from the patient as an individual but from the breakdown of communication between patient and staff. Such difficulties can and should be avoided.

Double Bind Communication features confusing inconsistency between verbal: (Parent: 'You should be polite to others') and non-verbal messages: (P herself presents with ill-mannered and inconsiderate behaviour).

Addressing the biennial Congress of the American Nurses' Association (New Orleans, June 1984) a spokesman for the National Council on Patient Information and Education criticized the customary:

| Active Parent | passive, unchallenging Child |
| role of the Doctor | role of the Patient/Client |

Because the patient fails to confront his doctor on equal 'adult–adult terms' studies show that up to 50% of prescription drugs are not taken properly.

'Asking the following five questions is a good start. But don't stop there. Keep working with your health care practitioners. They are partners in your drug treatment. They want to help you use your medicines properly.

1. What is the name of the drug and what is it supposed to do?
2. How and when do I take it—and for how long?
3. What foods, drinks, other medicines, or activities should I avoid while taking this drug?
4. Are there any side-effects, and what do I do if they occur?
5. Is there any written information available about the drug?'*

The NCPIE presented medicinal drug information combining communication impact by colour, sound, repetition, movement in video-tapes, illustrated self-correcting, packaging, etc.

---

* Pamphlet *Get the Answers!* Produced by the National Council on Patient Information and Education, a non-profit organization representing health care professionals, consumers, pharmaceutical manufacturers, government agencies, and other health-related organizations. To order copies of this brochure and/or participate in the 'Get the Answers' campaign, write to:
  NCPIE Campaign
  PO Box 1080
  Purcellville, VA 22132-1080, U.S.A.

The games people play

(i) *Introjection* of social and parental taboos and inhibitions, causing conflict between:

> the need for privacy and personal achievement
> versus
> the need for belonging, and merging, in a love relationship, and

(ii) certain basic genetic programming'

provokes Berne's claim that 'Most human relationships (at least 51 per cent) are based on trickery and subterfuges, some lively and amusing, and others vicious and sinister. It is only a fortunate few, such as mothers and infants, or true friends and lovers, who are completely straight with each other.'

Even the broody hen is tricked into her maternal role: Certain glandular influences which overheat her to the point of discomfort, drive her to seek the comfort of her cool eggs.

In transactional games

> *the bait*, which seems like one thing, but is really intended for something else, is called a *con*.
> The *payoff* is the outcome.
> The *weakness* or *need* of the other player, which makes him respond to the con, is called a *gimmick*.
> The *surprise ending* is called the *switch*.
> The formula for all transactional games, then, is:
> > con + gimmick = response → switch → pay-off.

Amongst Berne's many examples of 'game' subterfuge is the 'Let's Make Mother Sorry' pattern in response to the mother who has consistently frightened, thwarted and manipulated her daughter through an obsession about virginity (the Need). In order to punish (the Pay-off) her mother whose indoctrination has prevented her from enjoying heterosexual relationships, the daughter 'makes mother sorry' (the Switch) by becoming promiscuous or getting pregnant, causing a neighbourhood scandal, and perhaps ending up in a Juvenile Court.

> 'The boy (the Bait) serves merely as an instrument, and the girl may never see him again once he has done the job on mother. . . . Variations with increasing age are "Let's Make Girlfriend (or Boyfriend) Sorry", "Let's Make Husband (or Wife) Sorry", or "Let's Make the Social Welfare Department Sorry".'*

'Making Someone Sorry' (MSS) works particularly well if aimed at a person or organization functioning as a Parental 'ego state' harping on the theme 'I'm Only Trying to Help You', for example the nurse or hospital. 'Passive resistance' may arouse guilt and anxiety in staff.

Such relationships are well illustrated by Dr Stepehn Karpman's Drama Triangle, which shows the manner in which 'the game' switches each of the

---

* Eric Berne. *The Games People Play*. Penguin Books.

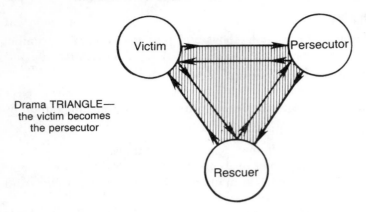

Drama TRIANGLE—
the victim becomes
the persecutor

players from one role into another. The victim (the patient) becomes the persecutor, while the 'rescuer' (the nurse) becomes the victim. It will be noted that the pregnant daughter, in spite of her overt social predicament, through astute handling—conscious or unconscious—holds the initiative. This type of 'game' may be the only self-assertion available to the physically diminished.

The Alcoholic can turn his nagging wife who is ostensibly trying to help him into the victim by physically beating her, or by turning his would-be 'rescuer' into his 'persecutor', 'always picking on me':

'Parental programming is not the "fault" of parents—since they are only passing on the programming they got from their parents—any more than physical appearance of their offspring is their fault, since they are only passing on the genes they got from their ancestors. . . . Therefore a parent who wants to do the best for his children should find out what his own script is, and then decide whether he wants to pass it on to them. . . . If we want things to be warm and straight later, we've got to stop being cold and crooked now.'

Berne's advice in counteracting harmful 'games' is to observe two basic rules:

'The first rule is to spend your time spotting your own games instead of other people's. The second rule is to try not playing long enough so your favourite players will realize you have stopped, and they may stop too. Then see what happens. If things go well, you'll get your reward in good pay-offs instead of bad ones.'*

Watzlawich† classifies the following disrupted communication patterns:

(1) There is an effort *not to communicate*, which is self-defeating because it is impossible.
(2) *Inconsistent levels of communication*: the focus may seem to be on the content of the message, but actually involves the relationship between the communicators.

* Eric Berne. *The Games People Play*. Penguin Books.

† Watzlawitch, P, J H Beavin & D O Jackson. *Pragmatics of Human Communications* (New York: Norton & Co, Inc, 1967).

Nurse: 'Visiting hours are over—it is time for your boyfriend to go home so you
can get some rest.'

Patient interprets communication: 'You're just jealous of our relationship and
want to assert your authority.'

When the sender makes a statement about himself the receiver may confirm, reject
or deny it. Disconfirmation denies the reality of the message. At times there is
considerable conflict between the communication needs of patients and staff—
usually to the detriment of the former. Commenting on ward rounds, Professor S
Saunders spoke thus at a congress 'Future of the Nursing Profession' (1976):*

'I would think that the most alarming and adverse effects of a ward round arise
out of thoughtless words or gestures on the part of the people at the bedside.
Such comments as: "He could have died with that injection!" "He looked
ghastly." "His blood pressure was in his boots!" "He had an *enormous* infarct!"
"He was breathing like a steam engine."

I was looking at a patient's fundus when somebody at the bedside said: "Mr
Jones died last night." The patient's eyes immediately started moving rapidly.
Another voice said: "It was expected." The patient's eyes moved even more
rapidly and a voice in the background said: "Who was Mr Jones?" This
thoughtlessness and this expression of the anonymity of the patient in the
hospital plainly greatly upset my patient.

It is not only the words that are said, but also gestures, which can be
alarming to the patient. Furthermore, lack of language and lack of
communication on a ward round must be very alarming and there are many
of us guilty of inefficiency in communicating with people in the language of
their own choice.

If more than two people attend a patient, one of them, preferably the one
ultimately responsible for taking the decisions, must come back subsequently
and talk to the patient alone, to sustain and comfort him, and to discuss things
which can only be discussed in private, between the patient and his doctor.'

(3) *Imperviousness*: the sender and the receiver both assume reciprocal understanding which does not really exist, leading to confusion.

(4) *Discrepancies of punctuation* occur when one party has less information than the
other, but does not know this, leading to different perceptions of reality.

Surgeon: 'We are going to remove an obstruction in your bowel—you'll be fine.'
The Receiver (Patient) perceives his post-operative body image as an
unimpeded, functional bowel. The reality, however, will be replacement of
normal function by an externally opening bag for the retention of faeces.
Little wonder at his horror!

(5) *The self-fulfilling prophecy* is exhibited by the Receiver who introjects (see p 61)
the picture of himself he expects to arouse in others, thus reinforcing his
(usually negative) self-concept. 'I know they'll think I'm a fool, so I might as
well act as one.'

---

* Details available from the author.

Patients may well intercede communication between doctor and nurse, *introjecting* or taking unto themselves messages of alarm or depression.

Because communication depends on efficiency of information intake via the sense organs, and interpretation thereof in the cerebral perceptual areas, lack or impairment of communication equipment, resulting in impaired sight, sound, smell, taste, touch or pain, will result in impaired communication. As Helen Keller has demonstrated, however, nature often compensates for such losses, enabling the handicapped to 'see' through *compensation* development of other senses and perception areas.

It frequently falls to the nurse to alert the patient to the possibility of such *compensation* development, and to help him persevere in achieving such compensation skills.

In order that our feelings of *identification* with the patient may support and comfort, it is necessary that we be able to convey our involvement to him.

Some people possess an extroverted behaviour pattern, an easy warmth facilitating the establishment of meaningful relationship communication, either endogenous to their personality, or engendered therein by easy-going, warm parental relationships. Others find difficulty in establishing meaningful communication bonds—they describe themselves as 'shy'—their patients may describe them as 'aloof', 'stuck up', 'unapproachable'.

Very frequently their inability to communicate lies in their own anxiety lest they be rejected, lest they convey some ignorance.

Some nurses attempt to *deny* their own normal feelings of anxiety and inadequacy by *rationalizing* that their services are more valuable to poor and simple people, than to 'middle class' more sophisticated patients whose questions and self-assertion they fear and resent. Classically, their fear arouses *hostility towards 'better-off', 'private patients'*, many of whom have contributed heavily in taxes, and worked long and hard in order to pay for private facilities. The more affluent and sophisticated patient feels fear and pain as intensely as his poorer brethren, and is equally deserving of efficient and compassionate nursing. Over-familiarity is not necessary, but the ability to 'be with' patients, to become involved in their welfare, is the keynote of a meaningful nurse–patient relationship.

It is true that sick and nervous people do create a tense and sometimes frustrating environment for others, but it is important that the nurse learns to deal with her own anxieties.

Techniques facilitating communication

(1) *Real listening* is a difficult, active rather than passive process, involving the nurse's full attention. Obviously one cannot listen when one is talking. Listening involves *suspension of one's own experiences and problems*: 'Listening is faster than speaking. The endings of most sentences can be guessed before they are completed. In this situation we should listen attentively to the end of each sentence rather than guess or assume what will be said.' (Murray and Zentner, 1979: 77). When effective, listening encourages and reinforces the patient's verbalized information.

(2) *Broad openings* confirm the patient's presence and encourage him to select

topics, eg What shall we discuss today? What's been happening since our last meeting?

Acceptance responses, eg I understand—What happened then?

(3) *Restatements* indicate the nurse's attention and reinforce something important. They consist in the nurse's repeating to the patient the whole or part of the main thought he has expressed: 'You are convinced that your boss dislikes you.'

(4) *Clarification*: the nurse attempts to restate in simple, concise words the patient's sometimes indirect and vague explanation of his ideas, thoughts and feelings.

These verbalizations are frequently intrinsically important; also response thereunto emphasizes the nurse's full attention. Because they usually attempt clarification of subjective thoughts, these openings should be tentative rather than adamant. 'Do you mean that . . .? Can you explain to me more precisely what you mean?'

Clarification of his thoughts provides a direct link with the patient's actions.

(5) *Reflection of content* serves not only as a stimulus to further communication but also

  (a) validates the nurse's impression,
  (b) recapitulates,
  (c) gives the patient an opening for negation or affirmation of the nurse's impression,
  (d) reflects feelings of respect, insight, understanding and empathy, thus increasing nurse–patient involvement. For example, 'I get the feeling that. . . . My impression of what you say is that . . .'.

(6) *Focusing* helps the patient become more specific and reality orientated. By avoiding abstractions and generalizations he is brought to his 'gut feeling', setting the stage for problem analysis. Focus on anxiety-producing topics may necessitate 'on-site' psychotherapy (see pp 61-64, 609).

'Try to tell me what you felt about. . . . Was that one of your strongest experiences. . . . Now when exactly did that happen?'

(7) *Silence* may convey support, understanding and acceptance to a depressed non-vocal patient—as long as he knows the nurse is listening, the latter being indicated by an appropriate sound. Sometimes a sympathetic involved silence is more effective than repetitive questioning such as 'why', or questions which can be answered by a simple 'yes' or 'no'. Excessive questioning robs the patient of initiative and discourages free thought exploration.

(8) *Humour* restores a sense of proportion, tempers aggression and teaches free expression of pent-up emotions. However, humour which meets only the nurse's needs may well be destructive and frightening in the nurse–patient relationship.

(9) *Suggesting* presents an alternative when the patient, having analyzed a problem, is seeking other coping or adjustment mechanisms: 'Some people have tried . . . do you think it might work for you?' (see p 127). Used too early in a therapeutic relationship, however, it may stifle self-exploration and assumption of personal responsibility.

Communicating respect may be achieved in many ways:

(a)   by sincere listening,

(b)   by sitting silently, and perhaps holding the hand of a patient who is weeping,

(c)   by respecting a request not to share an experience; by apologizing for a tactless statement and admitting one's own inadequacies,

(d)   by a genuinely shared joke,

(e)   by avoiding patient dependency,

(f)   by avoiding imposition of decisions.

Diminishing treatment is humiliating and anger-provoking in all patients.

African culture lays down special requirements in preserving the dignity and self-image of its ageing, and thus more vulnerable, members. Strict procedure defines the *necessity for treating anyone who has reached one's parents' age with the same formal respect as one would extend to one's parents themselves*. In fact one may call such a 'senior' 'Mother' or 'Father'. Thus it is particularly offensive for an elderly black patient to be rudely 'pushed around' by a young nurse. Rather than be spoken to brusquely and without decorum, stripped of his clothes and relegated to baby-status by one young enough to be his child, many a patient will choose to deprive himself of the benefits of Western scientific medicine.

The custom, in out-patient departments, of standing in the middle of the assembly and yelling out the patient's name, is particularly hurtful, arousing a strong need to protect oneself from diminishment at the hands of impersonal bureaucracy!

The professional interview

The above 'techniques facilitating communication' are brought together in the professional interview consisting of *structured* 'person-to-person' communication designed to:

(i)   establish, reinforce or extend a relationship;

(ii)   provide opportunity to—
    collect data
    identify problem areas (assessment: diagnosis)
    mutually decide on a plan of action to eliminate or relieve problems (planning)

    execute and amend
    motivate   ⎫
    reassure   ⎬ implementation
                          ⎭
    evaluate—feedback to evaluate progress in alleviating problem

The interview is divided into three phases:

(i)   opening;

(ii)   body of the interview;

(iii) ending.

Bennett (1976)* stresses the need for sensitivity in both verbal and non-verbal aspects of the interview, which should of course be recorded by some medium for purposes of diagnosing, implementing and assessing case development as well as interdisciplinary communication. Summarizing the professional role:

1. *Opening*

Establishing rapport and data collection.

non-verbal: a smile, a handshake, a warm and concerned tone of voice, a comfortable friendly room. The client's body language (p 178) is of import throughout the interview.

verbal: greeting—'How do you do, Mrs Jones? My name is Mary Smith. I am the community nurse for your area.'

Communication techniques facilitating the opening Data Collection phase of the interview within the Nursing Process are:

Open-ended questions: 'Would you like to tell me about your problem?'

Probing questions: 'Tell me more about your mother-in-law.'

Direct or closed questions requiring a direct answer: 'Do arguments seem to precede your headache?'

Clarification: 'Am I correct in assuming that you believe your headaches to be caused by anxiety and frustration?'

Translation or Interpretation: Patient: 'I get all worked up.' Nurse: 'Worked up—what do you mean—frightened or angry or . . .?'

Indicating understanding: 'I can understand that.'

Evading questions in order to 'put the ball in' the patient's 'court': 'What do *you* think about it?'

Accepting ideas: 'That's a sensible idea.'

Accepting feelings: 'I don't blame you for becoming so upset . . . and emphasizing empathy: 'I'm sure I'd feel the same way.'

Uncovering feelings: 'I get the impression that you are anxious/angry/depressed.'

2. *Body of the interview*

Closed questions designed for specific answers: 'Have you got room for your mother-in-law? Yes or No?'

Leading questions: 'Did you have the headache when your mother-in-law went on holiday last year?'

Echoing: 'She thinks I am a bad housewife.'
  Nurse: 'A bad housewife? What does she regard as a bad housewife?'

Reflecting: 'Do you think I should encourage her to join a Seniors' Club?'
  Nurse: 'Do you think that involvement in community facilities will help solve the problem?'

Challenging or Confronting: 'Do you really mean that you have *never* lost your temper with her?'

* Bennett A E, ed. *Communication between Doctors and Patients.* Oxford: Oxford University Press (Nuffield Provincial Hospitals Trust), 1976.

3. Ending: Closure

Summarizing: 'I am going to sum up the position as I see it. Please correct me if I am wrong.'

Feedback—assessing client's comprehension and involvement: 'Well, what do *you* think are the main causes of your headaches?'

Conveying information/professional opinion (in words the client will understand): 'I think your headaches may be caused by your body's physical reaction to your anxious and angry feelings about your mother-in-law.' (It is important to gauge the client's understanding of your information.)

Reassuring: 'You are doing nicely—we are certainly over the worst.'

Directing or advising: 'Remember to take your medicine twice a day—after breakfast and after supper.'

Enlisting—defining the client's active, participatory role: 'I am sure that if we work together, you and I will alleviate your pain.'

Continuing programme: 'Remember, we are always here to help.'

Many people find it *difficult to end the interview*. Over-dependent and anxious clients may be reluctant to 'let go' of the professional's presence and support. The last sentence or turn-about at the door often reveals the client's conscious or unconscious innermost needs.

'So you are confident it is not a brain-tumour?'

Non-verbal signals such as standing up and escorting the client to the door, laying down a pen or looking at a watch, signal to the client that the interview is coming to an end.

Tangible reassurances, such as a letter, a drawing, or a tape recorder, may facilitate separation from the professional (p 522).

Impediments to a fruitful interview consist in:

Rejecting the client's ideas: 'How could you be so silly!'

Rejecting his feelings: 'I don't want to hear such nonsense.' 'I am sure you can do better than that.'

Evading questions: 'We don't have to go into that.'

Not listening (p 188).

In a multicultural and -language population *an interpreter* may be required creating a *'communication triangle'*, a situation which may be fraught with misunderstanding and misinterpretation. It is important to know that the interpreter is comfortable in the language and cultural patterns of both professional and client.

Launer 1978* presents the following guide to the *trans-cultural interview*:

Greet the client in order to establish personal contact.

Check the interpreter's understanding of professional jargon and his understanding of the information you wish to convey.

Keep questions short.

Do not allow the interpreter to 'censor' communication in either direction. What he considers nonsensical or irrelevant may prove just the opposite. In order to

---

* Szaz T S, Hollender M H. A contribution to the philosophy of medicine: the basic models of the doctor–patient relationship. *Archives of Internal Medicine* 1956; 97, 585–92.

check the validity of the translation it is wise to ask important questions in different ways.

Give very special attention to the client's non-verbal communication while she is both speaking and listening.

In order to establish empathy it is important that the professional learn ways of showing and expressing concern which are appropriate to the culture. (Refer to the traditional healing framework to which a client may be accustomed.)

Communication triangles are often complicated by the *'interpreter's' acute emotional involvement*. Typical situations include a sick baby and an anxious mother; an angry hurt parent and a rebellious teenager; a stressed adult and a senile parent; marriage counselling. Sensitivity, tact and careful listening to both parties are of primary importance.

The role of the interviewer may be that of a *neutral observer; an articulate clarifier* of many-faceted problems; a guiding defusing 'umpire'. Observation of interactions and relationship dynamics are of primary importance. The interviewer should respect any solution or programme suggested by any participant. Solutions emanating from clients themselves are often most specific to their problems and needs.

The nurse–patient relationship

The innately aggressive, exploitary needs inherent in the theory of 'Narcissism' (p 61) slant and spike the communication mechanisms of both client and nurse.

Szasz and Hollender (1956)[*] classified the following three types of client–professional relationships namely:

(i) *Activity–passivity*
   The professional is active, the client passive, a framework emanating from the emergency care situation where the patient is helpless, requiring medical 'take-over' of his basic needs (Berne's Parent–Child transaction).

(ii) *Guidance–co-operation*
   The patient's awareness renders him capable of exercising judgement and following directions, but still dependent upon the professional's unquestioned decisions.
   Verbalizations such as:
   'I have faith in you—tell me what I should do and I will co-operate.'
   This transaction is comparable to Berne's Parent–older Child transaction.

(iii) *Mutual participation*
   This relationship is typical of preventive medicine and the management of chronic illness such as diabetes mellitus and arthritis in which the client assumes major responsibility for his care, with appropriate professional guidance and support. The professional's role is to monitor progress and help the patient to help himself. As this relationship is Adult to Adult, it is gaining favour in the world of consumer-orientated medicine. It does, however,

* Launer J. Taking Medical Histories through Interpreters: Practice in a Nigerian Out-Patients' Department. *British Medical Journal* 1978; **2**: 934–5.

require amendment in communicating with the mentally defective or full-blown psychotic.

Some clients present with personality features so resistant, aggravating or demanding as to seriously impede the mutual setting and attainment of goals.

Groves (1978)* describes four classes of clients precipitating in care-givers strong feelings of dislike, aggression, guilt, anger, frustration and rejection.

Clients' arousal of such strong feelings within the helping professions is, in psychoanalytic terms, defined as 'counter-transference'.

CLINGERS present with bottomless, inexhaustible need for repetitive reassurance and support. Their insatiable need can eat away at care-givers' emotional and even physical resources.

Handling:

(a) Acknowledgement of limit in the care-givers' skill, knowledge and patience,
(b) setting firm limits to the opportunity and time allowed for repetitive reassurance and support,
(c) insight into, and reasonable resistance to, the client's utilization of flattery, gifts, emotional seduction, etc

all help structure a more fruitful relationship.

The DEMANDERS resemble clingers, but instead of manipulation they utilize intimidation, threats, criticism and guilt induction to place the helper in the role of inexhaustible and constantly obtainable support. This client insists on getting every attention to which he is 'entitled'.

Handling:

Acknowledgement of the client's rights but re-channelling of his motivation into a co-operative treatment plan. This patient may be helped by active inclusion in the nursing process.

Manipulative HELP-REJECTORS hide their need for support and comfort behind a screen of proud or angry rejection. In fact, their rejection constitutes 'reaction formation' (p 118) as a defence against fear of diminishment, loss of self-determination and personal disintegration. They seem blessed with endless emotional energy in their disguised bid for the sympathetic involvement of care-givers. In spite of their repetitive rejection of help they repeatedly return to report that treatment has not helped. Such patients use symptoms as a lever to an intense therapeutic relationship.

Handling:

The care-giver should firmly convey that her client will not lose his identity and self-determination in the treatment programme. He will receive a fair share of involved attention. Healthy areas in his life-pattern should be used as a vehicle for compensation and self-esteem enhancement.

The SELF-DESTRUCTIVE DENIER is the man who cannot stop pedalling his bicycle perilously near the edge of the precipice. He may, in fact, present with unconscious self-destructive, suicidal behaviour. An example is the chain-smoker

---

* Groves J E. Taking Care of the Hateful Patient. *New England Journal of Medicine* 1978; 298, 883–7.

with chronic bronchitis. In reality such clients are deeply dependent. Having abandoned hope of need fulfilment they defy 'significant people' to show love and involvement: 'Much you'd care if I drank myself to death!'

Handling:

> Check for depression—endogenous or reactive (pp 587–90). Prove that the client will not be abandoned—but neither will the care-giver become trapped in her client's self-destructive behaviour.

In Transference the client attaches painful and destructive learnt attitudes to his therapist, working through them in the therapeutic relationship
Counter transference: Professional's reactions to the burdens imposed by "Difficult" "Disliked" Patients

In their response to such clients, care-givers are burdened by their own feelings of hate, anger, aggression, guilt, anxiety and frustration. Because these negative emotions are inconsistent with their own self-images they attempt to displace them on their clients.

'This patient is always full of anger and hate.' Care-givers may be helped by realization that these clients do, in general, arouse negative feelings about which there is no need to feel anxious or guilty.

This having been said, care-givers should remember that such 'hateful' behaviour is embedded in fear of illness, diminishment, helplessness, mutilation, death and personal integration. It is a plea, a last-ditch protest, against fear and suffering. Assuming the care-giver to be the healthy partner in the care-giving relationship, it falls to her to use insight and tolerance and rally resources to meet her client's hidden needs. The keynote is the ability not to take 'hateful' behaviour personally.

In her inaugural lecture (1 June 1982), Professor Paddy Harrison chose as her subject 'Nursing: Essential Expression of Human Endeavour':

> 'My students have expressed their concern at the apparent lack of interest of certain staff towards THE PATIENT AS A HUMAN BEING, with feelings of fear and anxiety over his or her illness.
>
> Long and earnest discussions will take place at the foot of the bed over the clinical problem before them. Furrowed brows and solemn voices, and an incomprehensible vocabulary—but no attempt at reassuring the patient, or treating him as a rational being.'

Professor Harrison said a *balance between humanism and science* was essential to the concept of health care: 'This should be the grass-root approach of all nursing education. . . . The nurse should have an opportunity to cultivate the God-given gift of concern for human suffering under the many guises of pain, loneliness, frustration and failure.'*

The nurse–patient relationship embodies a special intimate and subtle content, *a rich communication interflow* described as EMPATHY. Empathy consists in the ability to view the patient's world from his own internal frame of reference . . . to creep under his skin. Within the nurse there is a two-way process involving

(a) Inward: the nurse's sensitivity to the patient's current feelings and

---

* Further details available from authour.

(b) Outward: the cerebral, facial and tactile ability to communicate this understanding in a language attuned to the patient.

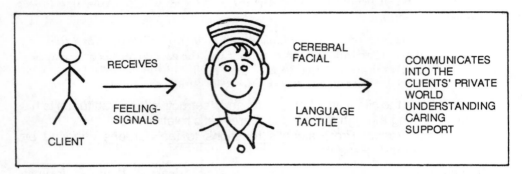

Empathic understanding consists of a number of stages:

(1) If the patient <u>allows the nurse to enter his private world</u>, if he communicates his perceptions and feelings to her, she must be ready to receive this communication.

(2) In order to understand this communication the nurse must be able to *identify* with her patient. She must then be able to step back into her own role and communicate her understanding.

Factors contra-indicating empathy

Concentration on 'facts' rather than the patient's current feelings and experiences; sermonizing and advice-giving; the nurse's tangent private thoughts; all set up barriers.

> 'The nature of the nurse–patient relationship is characterized by the mutual growth of two individuals who "dare" to become related, to discover life, growth and freedom. It is an I–thou relationship, or an authentic relationship between two people who are in the process of "becoming". The uniqueness of each is valued, and there is respect for differing values. There is mutual satisfaction derived and the world of each is enlarged and enriched by the other.*

We shall see, in our consideration of the Nursing Process (chapter 9) that psychosocial aspects of the *implementation* stage are largely dependent upon the existence of a strong, positive therapeutic nurse–client relationship. This in turn is dependent upon the nurse's empathic understanding. The nurse–patient relationship is essentially a *mutual* one, focused on the *needs of the patient*. Emphasis is on respect for the patient's own innate strength and dignity as a person, and his growth potential. The patient, being an active participant, is asked for a feedback about effectiveness of the total nursing plan. Amendments thereunto result from patient–nurse collaboration.

---

* Buber, M. *I and Thou* (New York: Charles Scribner's Sons, 1958).

Non-compliance

'When I first suspected I had cancer, my mind went woolly. After that it ran in several directions at once. In fact, I was a prime example of the classic patient who appears in all the textbooks—the non-complier who avoids medical treatment which could save his life.

Not only did I avoid the treatment, I also avoided thinking about it.

Several specialists sampled, prodded, tested and scanned, in the process giving me an insight into the role of patient I had never possessed before.

In my medical career I had always thought myself fairly empathetic towards the needs of patients. Perhaps I was, but my recent experience taught me much about a whole new world of waiting, hoping and fearing.

As it happened, I had a reprieve. Fate said not this time, perhaps next time.'
    —Chris Barnard Heart Transplant Pioneer Surgeon 15 October 1984.

'One of the underlying assumptions of all professionals is that patients will adhere to the treatment that has been proposed, eg taking medication, following a diet, relaxing or taking exercise as directed, and keeping appointments as requested. Forget it! . . . up to half the patients that present for help do not comply with the instructions given and, in fact, set up maladaptive "games". Such patients are called "non-compliant" and phrases like "not motivated" and "treatment drop-out" are used. They trigger feelings of concern, anger and despair in professional medical staff, as in all crossed transactions.*

What factors trigger 'non-compliance'?

On the client's part:

1. *Immaturity.*
2. *Denial of illness* as a defence mechanism.
3. *Unpleasant side-effects.*
4. *Disturbed judgement* as in schizophrenia or senile depression impairs ability to carry out a given task.
5. Especially in *transcultural situations involving guilt feelings and punishment by a wrathful supernatural power* there is a tendency for fatalistic acceptance of suffering inconsistent with Western medical realities.

On the professional's part:

1. *Emotional detachment*, lack of involvement and preoccupation with personal thoughts.
2. *Failure to identify* with a client's socio-economic or cultural situation.
3. *Vague generalizations* such as 'Watch your diet' rather than a specific dietary programme.
4. The assumption of an *authoritarian 'parent–child'* communication model.

Certainly the *relationship between professional and client* is of primary import in motivating implementation of a treatment programme.

---

* Nash, Stoch, Harper. *Human Behaviour*. David Philip, 1984.

'In order to improve co-operation you need to apply all your understanding of human behaviour, and *your belief in the power of medical care*. Treatment is a *collaborative matter*, so that the goals of treatment need to defined by the professional team together with the patient. These should be discussed in a language that the patient can understand.*

(See Nursing Process Phase 3: Planning, p 230 pertaining to *mutually set* goals.)

Factors triggering the search for medical help and thus patient 'compliance' are, according to Mechanic (1968):*

(i) exceeding the limit of tolerance—pain, confusion, weakness, anxiety concerning symptoms, problems in living, inability to earn a living, to maintain relationships;

(ii) administrative requirements such as a medical certificate or insurance medical examination;

(iii) preventive care programmes' eg antenatal checking.

In order that she may assess and control her own role in the therapeutic patient–nurse relationship, Stuart & Sundeen commend the following self-analysis of nurse participation.

Do I label patients with the stereotype of a group?

Is my need to be liked so great that I become angry or hurt when a patient is rude, hostile or uncooperative?

Am I afraid of the responsibility I must assume for the relationship and do I therefore limit my meaningful contacts?

Do I cover feelings of inferiority with a front of superiority?

Do I require sympathy, warmth and protection so much that in *projecting*, I err by being too protective towards patients?

Do I fear closeness so much that I am indifferent, rejecting or cold?

Do I need to feel important and keep patients dependent on me?

In order to 'let their patients go' nurses should have different sources of satisfaction and security in their non-professional lives . . . if this is not the case, they should be aware of the danger of impeding the patient's independent growth to self-actualization.

The unique nature of the nurse–patient relationship

The nursing profession is unique in that one is frequently *allowed into* the lives, the worlds, of 'strangers' who, hopefully, become friends. This privilege calls for sensitivity, tolerance, trustworthiness. It also imposes unique responsibilities and stresses.

'We must be able to understand, and deal helpfully with, our own reactions to change and with new experiences; to contact with tragedy, death, severe mental disorders, operations which have deep emotional significance, eg hysterectomy, abortion, breast amputation, or serious illness in children. Then there are situations involving colleagues or other members of the health

* Mechanic D. *Medical Sociology*. New York: Free Press. 1968.

team in which, for instance, loyalty is divided between the patient and one's colleagues, or prestige and dignity are lowered by a reprimand from a senior in front of patients or junior staff.'*

The greater part of the contents of this book attempts to convey to the nurse that knowledge of human needs and human behaviour by which she may achieve insight into the fundamentals of the *nurse–patient relationship*; what she needs to impart in order that she may fulfil her important and many-sided role, not only as skilled healer but also as emotional supporter and comforter.

She should acquire insight into such important facets of human behaviour as

(a) the individuality of personality,
(b) the indivisibility of mind and body,
(c) gradations of human development based on the all-important mother–child relationship,
(d) deeper levels of emotional functioning,
(e) universal ambivalence, guilt feelings and anxiety,
(f) the difference between intellectual and emotional acceptance,
(g) her role in catharsis or the relief that comes with talking out,
(h) the needs of patients and their families in times of pain, fear and death, and
(i) above all the sufferer's need of the nurse's identification and emotional-level support.

Sometimes the many-faceted demands upon the nurse result in her retreating defensively into an uninvolved, 'touch me not' emotional detachment. This withdrawal pattern will do little to solve her own problems or those of her patient.

Sometimes a nurse who has been downtrodden in her formative years may seek to *compensate* by communicating an authoritarian discipline; a nurse who has suffered parental withdrawal of love, or rejection, may, unconsciously, elongate her patients' dependence upon her, thus encouraging *regression* and delaying patients' return to healthy independence.

Insight into mental or adjustment mechanisms (chapter 5) should equip her for a reasonable level of patient and self-understanding, that she may avoid common pitfalls in that communication which is basic to a comforting, supportive and thus, in a wider sense, *feeling* nurse–patient relationship.

The nurse–patient relationship, while fundamentally supportive and comforting, is also conflicting.

The patient needs the loving efficiency of a *mother-figure*; he also needs to maintain his *own dignity and independence*. He requires the opportunity for catharsis, but also respect for his privacy. He requires to mourn the results of mutilating surgery, but also guidance in the achievement of compensatory satisfactions.

In order to fulfil her role in the nurse–patient relationship, the nurse requires the insight and imagination to assume the mother role, but also to share it with his true-life family support. She requires an all-encompassing tolerance for human beings in their agony of physical and mental suffering. She also requires the personal adjustment allowing her 'to let go of' her patient, that he may find his way back to a dignified and personally fulfilling life. *The nurse must also be careful not to make the error of treating her patients like children.* These are heavy demands.

---

* Lynn Gillis. *Human Behaviour in Illness* (Faber and Faber, London).

Stress in the healing professions

The specific demands peculiar to her profession expose the nurse to particular risk of occupational stress.

Vincent (Canada, 1983) presents the following stressors in the healing professions:

disillusionment,
stagnancy of ideas and creativity: 'visionlessness',
rigidity and ineffectiveness in the face of change,
bitterness,
resignation to boredom and despair; awaiting pension,
reactive depression.

Specific contributors

1. Those very qualities which make a good nurse, namely:

competence,
confidence and conflicting humility,
concern,
conscientiousness, so easily turned into obsessiveness within the stressful 'life and death' situation

constitute *an emotionally 'tough situation'.**

2. Most nurses enter the profession inspired by bright-eyed idealism, but experience often brings *disillusionment* engendered by:

emphasis on isolated, routine procedures, rather than inclusion in integrated patient care,
personal diminishment,
lack of patient-involvement by senior members of the team,
the realization that suffering, palliatives and death often predominate over cure,
the realization that people who are angry, mutilated, diminished, in pain or frightened are seldom grateful, loving or lovable . . . in fact, the nurse is often the 'whipping boy' for other—sometimes less dedicated but more powerful—members of the team, and for an unkind fate in general.

3. The nurse who spends long hours in intensive communication with suffering, frightened and demanding patients is often the team member exemplifed by *Jung's archetypal concept of 'the wounded healer'.*

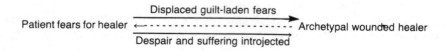

Displaced guilt-laden fears
Patient fears for healer ← - → Archetypal wounded healer
Despair and suffering introjected

---

* Nash, Professor Eleanore. *The Impaired Doctor.* Inquiries to author.

Seeking within her patient his 'healing core', the empathic nurse enters an intensive two-way relationship. *She* encounters and often *introjects his despair and suffering. He in turn is burdened by guilt fears* that, in 'displacing' upon her his suffering, he has contaminated and endangered his protector and healer . . . which is often an inner truth.

With mounting 'contamination' she becomes at risk to 'burnout'. Just as, physically contaminated, she fears lest she infect her own loved ones, so, emotionally contaminated, she calls upon them to share a role of suffering so burdensome that it may result in disrupted family life.

Presentation

Frequent mistakes may constitute a significant index.

The more sensitive and conscientious the nurse, the higher her investment in work achievement, the more she will blame herself when things go wrong, often regressing to reactive depressive illness (p 591). She is trapped in conflict between the dutiful demands of her damaged ego, and her urge to 'flight'.

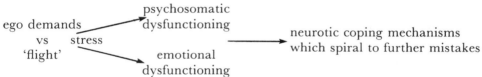

Thus she becomes, in varying degrees, an 'impaired' nurse, unconsciously seeking refuge in non-productive, *neurotic coping mechanisms*, including:

> guilt and shame: 'I should have been able to manage; it's all my fault'
> 'denial' of need for help: 'There's nothing wrong with me . . . it's this set-up that's wrong'
> reaction formation: 'I've never made a mistake in my life'
> anger: 'Mind your own business and get on with your job'
> obsessive perfectionism: 'If I sterilize the forceps 5 times, Heaven will take mercy on me, and he'll recover'
> flight from fear of mental illness: 'They're driving me mad, I must get out of here'
> clinging to the protective professional role: 'You don't have to tell me . . . I'm a registered nurse'
> erection of barriers to her suffering: 'I'm going to push it out of my mind'
> fantasizing that she's immune: 'I'm not weak like the others—I don't need help'
> self-diagnosis of her own condition and formulation of her own treatment: 'There's no need for anyone to interfere. I know what's wrong with me and I can handle it. All I need is a hot bath and an aspirin and a good night's sleep.'

Taking 'rationalization' a step further, she may seek refuge in:

Suicide

As pertaining to the ultimate 'flight' of suicide, figures for nurses are not to hand, but Pitts et al (1979) estimate that the rate for male doctors in the USA is 1,5 times as high for the general age-group male population. The rate for unmarried woman doctors over 25 is 4 times that of the general age-group female population.

Alcohol and the nurse's tempting solution of the *drug cupboard* are also professionally loaded escape mechanisms.

How can she be helped?

1.   Constructive confrontation and firm holding to the etiology and symptoma-tology presented. 'I know you have been taking drugs from the cupboard. We must discuss your problem and the reasons for it.'
2.   Motivation to seek professional help, preferably on an outpatient basis, and as far from her work-base as possible.
3.   Reduction of work stress and increased support by colleagues. This involves considerable understanding, tact and firm guidance by senior administrators. Confidentiality must be guaranteed. If her vocation is worthwhile, it should be profitable to 'nurse the nurse'.
4.   Reassessment of either career choice or direction.

Who is especially at risk?

Especially vulnerable to professional impairment is:

the introverted, withdrawn nurse who takes refuge from intimate colleague and patient involvement in sluice room and lavatory;
the nurse who manifests her anxiety and disorganization in
'cut off' behaviour, dissociation,
reaction formation, bending backwards to prove to herself and others that she is coping,
obsessional behaviour,
frequent mistakes followed by 'denial',
abject guilt-feelings and depression;
the socially isolated nurse;
the nurse who seeks structure and support by 'flight' into abstract philosophies and extremes of religious cult;
the nurse who lacks a sense of humour;
the nurse who is always in friction with authority;
the nurse whose financial and domestic affairs are always in chaos;
the nurse who seeks escape, courage and comfort in alcohol and drugs;
the student nurse who, in addition to the above warning signs, in part or in toto
has tried several training programmes,
studies too little or too much,
is often absent from class or fails repeatedly.

(For particular risks of burnout in psychiatric nurses see p 600.)

The emotional demands made by her vocation upon the nurse from her late adolescence, through the peak of her womanhood to her menopause, and thereafter, are indeed heavy. Yet her profession offers inner-need satisfactions which are unique in the field of human relations. In order that she may achieve these satisfactions, and at the same time fulfil her role in the important, intense and essentially dynamic nurse–patient relationship, she herself must find within the structure of her professional hierarchy that emotional-level tolerance, support and identification which should suffuse all ranks of the profession (p 108).

In many Western countries patient-care is becoming a consumer commodity. The emerging role of active patient participation is giving rise to the concept of the *'nurse–client relationship'* within the Nursing Process.

> 'The client does not need to earn approval or liking by expressing some desires and suppressing others, by portraying certain attitudes or beliefs and denying others or by being one type of person and not another.'*

---

* Yura, H & M B Walsh. *The Nursing Process* (New York: Appleton-Century-Crofts, 1978).

CHAPTER 8

LEADERSHIP,
PREJUDICE AND CONFLICT*

Nurses should never be regarded merely as workers but accepted as human beings with:

(a) strengths and weaknesses;
(b) a need for understanding, support and recognition;
(c) the opportunity for personal and occupational development.

If the individual perceives himself as important and worthwhile, his job satisfaction and loyalty increase. Ultimately the patient and the community, who are the reason for the nurse's existence, must benefit.

Leadership is an interaction between the leader and his followers, as applied to the personality-environment relationship. Leadership describes the position of one or, at the most, a few personalities whose will, feelings and insight direct and control the pursuit of a joint objective.

Research into the nature of leadership, that magic ability to motivate individuals, groups, even nations to hurl themselves unquestioningly through 'blood, toil, tears and sweat'† to their glory or their destruction, received great impetus after World War II.

Sociologists, psychologists, statisticians and physiologists translated into technical terminology their quest for some solution to the burning question in the minds of all thinking men:

How could nations, old in culture, history and human experience, so-called 'civilized' nations, be moved to accept as their leaders, and follow to victory, even to defeat, leaders such as Hitler and Mussolini?

It would be naïve to postulate that the mass of the German people did not support Hitler in his dramatic rise to power, and in the achievement, within a few years, of what was nearly global conquest.

What makes people follow leaders who are clearly maladjusted, even perhaps mentally sick? What is it in man that responds to war cries, slogans, gimmicks, clearly destructive or, at best, deceptive? What is it within one man which calls forth in his fellow-men an acceptance of sacrifice, suffering and motivation for great and laudable ideals and achievements?

What powerful magic is common to personalities as diverse as Churchill and Hitler, Napoleon and John F Kennedy?

In what way are they able to reach, and set aflame, the basic frustrations, dreams, fears and ambitions of millions of men and women they have never met?

---

* The author wishes to acknowledge the contribution made to this chapter by Beatrice Goodchid-Brown Dip Gen Mid Nursg Admin, BA (Soc Psych).

† Winston Churchill in a speech delivered in 1940.

Indeed, in their millions, such men and women are prepared even to forgo their own lives at the bidding of these leader-giants.

If mankind is to survive the atomic age it is essential that this magic be probed and revealed—only if leadership to negative goals of aggression, cruelty, false ambitions and hate is to be prevented, will mankind survive.

Clearly types of leadership vary according to group needs.

Research has set forth two main interacting approaches in establishing the etiology of leadership.

Trait approach

1. Carlyle's 'Great Man Theory' is based on the observation that the leader has the same traits as his followers, but the strength of the leader's traits exceeds that of the followers in quantity and quality. For example, if the rank and file are aggressive, their leader is more aggressive. If they are enthusiastic, exuberant and impulsive, their leader is the more so.

Carlyle in his book defines leader traits as aggressiveness, dominance, intelligence, confidence, initiative, enthusiasm, participation.

Other traits predominating in strong leaders are said to be extroversion, selfless dedication, fortitude, the power of persuasion, the ability to identify with the hearts and minds of followers. Intellectual endowment, economic and social status are also leader determinants.

However, since traits are loosely organized habits and attitudes, they do not constitute the sole or the most satisfactory method of isolating leadership function.

2. Kretschmer and others postulate that the leader is the executive, the planner, the most experienced, the purveyor of reward and punishment.

Because the leader is the father-figure, the scapegoat, one of us, the best of us, the most of us, his followers welcome him as a substitute for their own unfulfilled individual responsibilities.

It would appear that the leader projects an image reflecting those traits his followers universally admire, and would like to possess, but don't.

Through *identification* with his leader, the cowardly man can find courage and acknowledgement; the puny man strength and virility; the inadequate man stature; the poverty-stricken man affluence and influence.

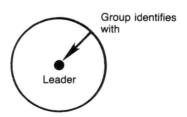

In the ward situation the inadequate, physically plain, frightened and embarrassed nurse, through identifying with an appropriate sister-leader, achieves a measure of success, confidence, achievement, dignity and hence even a feeling of increased physical attractiveness.

The situational approach

This approach to leadership involves more subtle interactions of the group and its leader.

The leader is able to assess the fears, needs, resources and *goals* of his group, introjecting them unto himself.

What do the followers want?

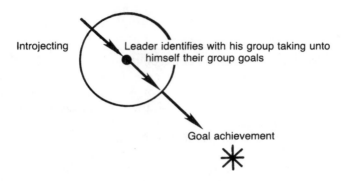

Introjecting

Leader identifies with his group taking unto himself their group goals

Goal achievement

These having been defined, he is able to *arouse in himself*, and thus to reinforce in the rank and file membership, *those personality traits and situational manipulations which will lead to mutual goal-achievement*, thus further entrenching his acceptability as leader.

In order to achieve those aims which the leader and his group hold in common, it is often necessary that the leader be able to motivate or *'inspire' increased group activity and effort, and reduced self-interest*, thus ensuring socio-emotional stability and maximum effort output. For example, in the situation pertaining in good ward management, the ward sister is able to assess and further those aims which she shares with her group—by motivating her followers to increased group activity, reduced self-interest, tolerance, compassion and efficiency.

Types of situational approach

Syntality

The proposition of Moreno and Jennings involves 'star group choice'.

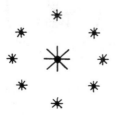

The 'star' personality is chosen for the strength of his influence on, and his contribution to, the project in hand.

This method of leadership-choice results in some individuals being over-chosen and some under-chosen. These latter, unless steps are taken to draw them into the group, will become isolated. In the context of their feelings of rejection, anxiety and inferiority they may well seek to compensate through negative activities such as group or individual destruction.

The choice of a head nurse is usually a syntality choice, having been made by reason of the strength of her influence and contribution.

Formal organization

Here leadership function is subdivided to achieve greatest efficiency, but all within the context of a shared overall goal.

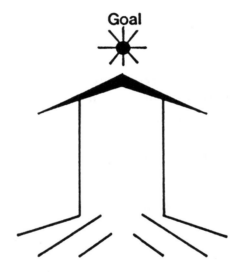

Within the living whole formal organization, each leader has a specialized function, eg the Cabinet constituting the government; within the ward situation, individual units.

It is usually easier to motivate individuals within smaller groups, where some rudiment of the individual and his needs still pertains. (Thus some student nurses do better in smaller training hospitals.)

The human being finds it intolerable to adjust to large groups in matters of more intimate need-satisfaction. Thus more manageable groups are formed, each with a leader, or number of group-leaders coming together, to account to a higher policy-making authority.

The psycho-analytic approach

The leader ascertains and then exploits the personality needs of his followers.

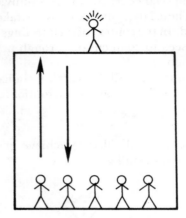

Psycho-analysts believe these personality needs to be, in the main, *universal and contradictory* in their apparent conflict within the individual.

It is in the nature of man that he is motivated by *alternating or ambivalent* needs for:

(a)   dominance on the part of the leader: submission on the part of the follower,
(b)   freedom on the part of the leader: protection on the part of the follower,
(c)   the parent role on the part of the leader: the child role on the part of the follower,
(d)   The need for recognition, honour and glory on the part of the leader: the need to lose identity in the group on the part of the follower.

The individual may experience either need-swinging in differing circumstances, sometimes as leader, sometimes as follower.

Jung, follower of Freud, extends the leadership role to the assumption of recurring group symbol roles, eg

(a)   the authoritarian father figure,
(b)   the embracing, comforting mother-figure,
(c)   the soldier warrior-figure,
(d)   the king-figure,
(e)   the god-figure,
(f)   the fairy-queen figure.

To all these leadership figures the individual will respond, by virtue of his own inherited group-conscious life.

Role-analysis

The leader is he who initiates most action. He is the best idea-giver, the provider of most effective guidance an protection.

Kurt Lewin's field theory

By virtue of his intellectual endowment—his ability to generalize, to foresee the results of his actions, to recognize and define choice possibilities, man is exposed to a diverse, ever-changing, dynamic field of goal choice. Frequently his motivations are in conflict, and the *necessity to make decisions* exposes him to unbearable tension, anxiety and distress.

Most people cannot tolerate conflict, anxiety and tension (which prevent the attainment of homeostasis) and will do almost anything to escape the distress entailed in them.

Lewin claims that the leader is he who can consistently make the correct choice for the well-being of the greatest number of the group.

Certainly individuals and groups appreciate, welcome and follow he who can solve painful conflict-choice, or achieve reconciliation between conflicting motivations and their goal achievements.

Examples of conflicting motivations are:

Avoidance—avoidance: vacillation between two negative goals. Which is the lesser of the evils?

– ———?——— –

Approach—approach: vacillation between two positive goals. Which of these offers is the most tempting?

+ ———?——— +

Approach—avoidance: the choice between a positive and a negative goal. Which will be the wisest course of action to follow?

+ ———?——— –

Lewin, Lippit & White present the following leadership classification:

(a) The authoritarian leader is aggressive, aloof, commands and dictates, eg Hitler. His followers are inclined to become dependent, hostile, apathetic, eg Third Reich.

Because they are ruled by force and fear, rather than by co-operation in attaining mutual goals, their fear leads them to seek scapegoats to absorb the wrath of the leader when inevitable failures occur, eg the Jews.

In a ward ruled by fear, senior nurses use juniors to absorb the wrath of the sister. Unaccustomed to the assumption of responsibility, followers begin to lose initiative and may develop into permanent 'drones'.

Temporarily or partially bereft of leader-influence, they are unable to function effectively.

(b) The 'laissez-faire' leader does not believe in asserting active direction, preferring a more passive permissive role.

Unless his followers identify very strongly with his goals, and are markedly intelligent and highly socially evolved, their production will be chaotic and their lack of team cohesion, will lead to frustration and aggression.

(c) Democratic leadership. Here the keynote of leadership organization is consultation, discussion and delegation.

Responsible opinion is discussed and weighed, the most constructive suggestions being integrated into leadership policy.

Being strengthened and endorsed by group or team identification, democratic leadership is relatively secure and effective. The followers are apt to work well in co-operation, exert maximum effort, criticize less, and thus realize higher potential.

Democratic leadership is certainly favoured in theory—however, within the essential 'committee' situation, valuable time may well be lost in debate. Also too much weight may be placed on the decision of a less intellectually endowed or experienced majority.

In addition the airing of strongly maintained individual opinions may lead to serious long-term dissension within the ranks.

It would appear that *different situations demand different types of leaders.* Different personalities of necessity adopt a particular leadership-style best suited to themselves, their followers and the situation pertaining.

Whereas the democratic leadership approach may be advisable in planning a surgical operation, the debate situation may well prove fatal in the theatre.

The famous *Mayo experiment*, designed to reveal the most powerful single stimulant to increased productivity, studied the effect of many variable motivating situations.

The most powerful stimulant, the experiment revealed, was that of *management interest and recognition*.

Recognition and honour bestowed by management appeared to constitute a more valuable reward, and thus a more powerful motivating factor, than shorter hours or increased pay.

The experiment thus emphasizes the power of effective leadership.

Norms and leadership

The effective leader is *he who conforms most strictly to group norms or standards*, thus facilitating identification by his followers. He has usually achieved a high rank by virtue of the fact that he represents group norms. For a leader to rise, and to stay in control, it is essential that his adherence to group norms be genuine and sincere. If he pays merely 'lip service' to group norms, he no longer sincerely represents the feelings of his followers, who then find it difficult to identify with him.

For cohesion and stability of an organized hierarchy, it is essential that subgroup norms adhere to those of the larger, more comprehensive whole. The closer a subgroup norm resembles that of the whole, the higher the social rank of the subgroup.

Thus, unless leader and group identify in the sharing of norms, standards or goals, the leadership situation is not a reality.

Thus, had not her band of nurses fundamentally identified themselves with her ideals, Florence Nightingale's Scutari campaign would not have been a success.

Leadership power

Power can be

(a) reward power,

(b) coercive power—involving punishment for non-compliance,

(c) expert power—the power exerted by he who possesses the highest degree of knowledge and skill.

(d) referent power—because the leader upholds and represents the values held by his followers, he possesses the power, and the right, to direct and influence the others accordingly. His actions are backed by the power of his group. Because his beliefs are their beliefs, he exerts their mandate for the expression of their power. Because people with power are imitated by others, their influence is both direct and indirect.

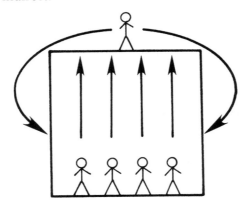

Authority and leadership

Leadership which is approved by the group is termed 'headmanship', eg elected class leader.

'Ascribed authority' is that in which the leader is the appointed head of an organization, eg class leader appointed by school principal.

Achieved leadership occurs where the leader is considered 'a superior being', eg class leader on grounds of highest academic attainment.

McGregor's X and Y theory

In the past the X theory predominated, viz man is inherently lazy and disinclined to work—he must be coerced, punished and pushed in order to perform his tasks.

Modern research favours the Y theory: work is as natural as breathing; all persons want to achieve.

There is a basic universal motivation for self-realization and, when stimulated to do so, and provided with a task within his ability, every man will give of his best.

It is important that the leader instils in his followers a healthy self-concept. The follower will live up, or down, to the self-worth image which the leader has instilled in him.

The attributes of a good leader

There is, of course, no fixed pattern for perfect leadership—nevertheless the following qualities do emerge complementary to the specific leadership theories enumerated above:

interest in the task in hand
superior knowledge and skill
ability to grasp essentials and organize elements
ability to guide effectively
insight
ability to share knowledge
ability to reconcile conflicting interests
ability to stimulate the best in others
to avoid partiality or favouritism
to utilize various leadership styles and techniques
to recognize superior knowledge and experience
to be approachable
to work with all types of people
to co-operate without unjustified opposition
to give of one's energy to others without undue selfishness
to lead by example
to possess integrity
ability to identify, to feel with, to be a good listener (catharsis)
ability to inspire confidence
ability to achieve good communication
knowledge of education techniques
ability to make decisions
ability to achieve a democratic rule
to integrate persons and tasks
to refrain from exploiting the weaknesses of others
possession of acceptable attitudes
inclination to spurn abuse of power
ability to inspire loyalty and to be loyal
to protect, guide and reward followers
to adapt to the individual situation pertaining
to orientate others to new tasks
to see different points of view

Application of leadership functions in the specific nursing culture

(a) It is important to seek, and to recognize, the possession of any *positive traits indicative of leadership material*.

(b) *Nursing education*. The aim of nursing education is to promote

(i) intelligent participation,
(ii) self-realization,
(iii) enhancement of promotive, preventive, curative and rehabilitative health services in the community.

Modern nursing education thus seeks to encourage self-activity methods preparatory to the assumption of leadership.

The student nurse should be trained not only to be an efficient follower but a potential leader. It is important that she assume positive attitudes towards professional ethical standards, a philosophy of life, human relations, acquisition of technical knowledge and a high standard of nursing care and administrative skill. For the achievement of such attitudes she herself will require to recognize maturity criteria in herself and in others.

Because knowledge is a powerful leadership force, it is beholden upon the academically orientated nurse to achieve post-basic qualifications.

The strength of a profession rests on the proportion of its exceptionally qualified stratum.

A profession which relies on a relatively small proportion of exceptionally qualified members runs the risk of monopolistic autocracy.

In order to preserve its professional status, it is essential that nursing education receive the benefit of academic influence at university standard.

The existence of post-graduate educational centres broadens the field of both leaders and followers.

(c) Leadership in nursing administration. The nursing profession should utilize developments in the new science of occupational (managerial) psychology. This eclectic science seeks to utilize the valuable contributions of many professional disciplines in achieving professional efficiency.

It is important for leaders to remind themselves that *life is too short to learn merely from one's own experience.*

It is beholden upon the modern professional woman to continue learning through formal educational programmes throughout her career.

(d) Leadership in psychological fields. By virtue of the *wide spectrum* of people with whom she comes into contact during her professional life, and of the *unique intensity* of her contact with people in pain, suffering and that appreciation of new values that comes with regained health, the potential influence of the nurse on the public is a very special one.

She can do much to promote healthy interpersonal relationships, and to prevent that alarming increase in personality disorganizaton which is the hallmark of this century.

(e) In fields of *sociological leadership*: rural to urban shift, the changed age structure of society, pollution, are areas where her specialized knowledge and active participation may well make an appreciable contribution.

(f) As a *health educator* the nurse-leader actively participates in improving standards within her total environment.

(g) As a *member of the comprehensive health team* both nurse-leaders and nurse-followers should take their rightful position in the collective contributions and decisions made by medical practitioners, social workers, physiotherapists, ministers of religion and family units in working towards the total physical, social and psychological welfare of the patient.

(h) Because nursing science is concerned with *diagnosis, prevention, health promotion, curative* and *rehabilitative services* in all situations and conditions, the nurse-leader should work actively in all these fields.

Because of her wide experience in all sorts of human relationships, and her specialized education, the nurse has much to *contribute by active participation in spheres outside the nursing culture*. She also has *much to learn* from such activities in the achievement of a balanced and productive personality.

While it is certainly of the utmost importance to draw the young nurse's attention to the wide range of her future leadership potential, it is also necessary to stress her future importance in the role of ward sister.

It is important that she *projects an image* with which both nurses and patients would wish to *identify*. If she herself shows compassion, tolerance, conscientiousness and efficiency she can expect to instill these qualities in others.

If on the other hand she projects an image of indifference, lack of personal involvement and inefficiency, she will give licence to similar negative qualities in all those with whom she comes into contact. The effectiveness of her leadership role will depend upon both her innate potential for positive influence upon others, and the extent to which she is able purposively to project an image that others admire, with which they would identify, and which they would seek to emulate.

The nurse administrator

Delegating leadership functions

In order to operate freely within this quality-structure it is necessary to overcome a fear of delegation.

This fear is as old as mankind:

> 'And Moses' father-in-law said unto him, the thing that thou doest is not good. Though wouldst surely wear away; both thee and this people that is with thee, for this thing is too heavy for thee; thou art not able to fulfil it thyself alone . . .'*

Factors aggravating a fear of delegation are:

(i)   generalized feelings of insecurity and anxiety,
(ii) shaky self-esteem projected on to others, and resulting in a lack of faith in their ability.

Clearly, each trainee-administrator should have a clear picture of her role per se, and the complementary manner in which it fits into the 'administrative jigsaw puzzle'. Subordinate administrators are entitled to opportunity for development, set times for training projects, thorough information and clear instructions. For precision in duty allocation there is necessity for job analysis to correspond with administrator skills.

The process of delegation does not involve a loss of authority but rather the increased confidence that comes with alert efficiency.

Evaluation

Placing the patient at the focal point of this learning process, one's evaluation of it should pose the following questions:

---

* Exodus 28, 17–18.

Does the plan satisfy the patient-client?
How does the patient feel about the care he receives?

Prejudice and conflict

Prejudice: pre-judgment. Preconceived opinion, bias, injury that results or may result from some action or judgment. Latin root: prejudice lit. before judging.

At this particular moment in history, people are engaged in *war in virtually every country on earth.* Many of these are civil wars, fought bitterly by ordinary civilians, and many have been raging for several decades. Sikhs and Hindus in India, Jews and Muslims in the Middle East, Armenians and Russians in the U.S.S.R., Protestants and Catholics in Northern Ireland—the participants in the conflicts and the places in which conflict occurs seem unrestricted by geographic and ethnic boundaries.*

Of course, there are less extreme forms of hostility between groups than war. The prejudiced attitudes among certain Americans in Florida toward immigrant Cubans, the employment practices in many European countries which excluded women from certain types of jobs until very recently; are a few examples of *subtler conflict.* It is the extreme cases that catch our attention. Few of us are aware of the many *stereotypes* we use in our everyday dealings with other people, but many of us will never forget the slaughter of two English soldiers by a crowd of Irish funeral-goers in early 1988. Few of us too, are aware of the extensive presence of *prejudiced attitudes in our everyday lives, or of the destructive effect that these attitudes have on the people at whom they are aimed.* A famous psychological experiment, in which black and white children are presented with pairs of black and white dolls, for example, shows that black children identify with, and prefer white dolls at relatively early ages. White children, in contradistinction show no such misidentification or reverse preference.† This experiment suggests that disadvantaged children introject a poor self concept from environmental diminishment. They would rather be somebody else. Social Psychologists have long been interested in these phenomena, and have accumulated a body of research of substantial interest. Two questions in particular have received extended treatment:

what are the causes of conflict (and prejudice)?
how can the conflict be lessened?

Causes of intergroup conflict.

There are roughly speaking, two types of psychological theory about the causes of intergroup conflict.

* This section is contributed by Colin G Tredoux, M.A.

† These results stem from the early work of Clark & Clark (1947)*. There is some evidence to suggest that the pattern of these results is changing (positively). Nevertheless, a recent study observed and reported the same negative pattern in second generation West Indian children living in London.

*Clark, K B & Clark, M P (1947). Racial identification and preference in Negro children. In T M Newcomb and E L Harley (Eds). *Readings in Social Psychology*. New York: Holt, Rhinehart and Winston.

EXPRESSIVE THEORIES

These theories see conflict as the result of prejudiced attitudes held by certain people, and these attitudes are hypothesized to be an *expression of the personality of the people who are prejudiced.*

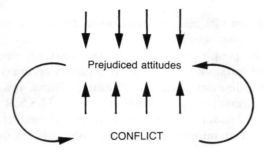

Prejudiced attitudes

CONFLICT

introjected from the environment of the prejudices, but claimed by them to be the expression of personal attributes of those prejudiced against them. My dad says: "The Scotch are stingy and they are!"

These theories claim that ethnic (or intergroup) hostility stems from a personality structure <u>that group members share</u>.

The group is brought and bound together by individuals with similar personality patterns—traits, goals and beliefs. The group is thus the product of its similar component patterns.

AUTHORITARIANISM

NEED TO DOMINATE | NEED TO BE DOMINATED

obsession   anger
feeling of deprivation

The group is brought and bound together by individuals with similar *personality patterns* — traits, goals and beliefs. The group is thus the product of similar component patterns.

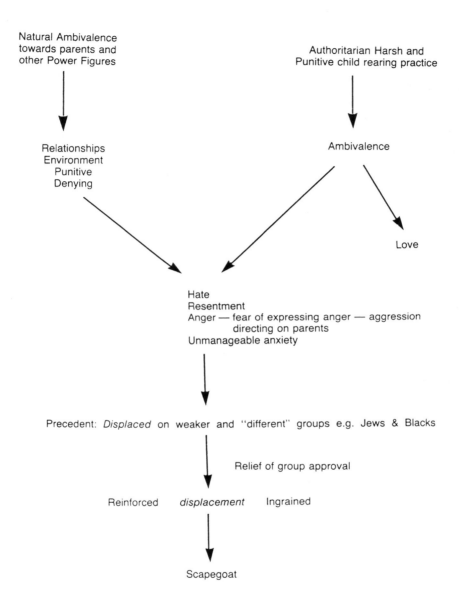

Natural Ambivalence
towards parents and
other Power Figures

Authoritarian Harsh and
Punitive child rearing practice

Relationships
Environment
Punitive
Denying

Ambivalence

Love

Hate
Resentment
Anger — fear of expressing anger — aggression
              directing on parents
Unmanageable anxiety

Precedent: *Displaced* on weaker and "different" groups e.g. Jews & Blacks

Relief of group approval

Reinforced   *displacement*   Ingrained

Scapegoat

It is not difficult to see that there is at least some truth in this contention. *Bigots all over the world bear a striking resemblance to each other.* Nazis and members of the National Front show the same kind of rigid, obsessive thought as members of the Klu Klux Clan. They have similar goals, similar ideological beliefs, and tend to be extremely authoritarian, 'patriotic', and militaristic in their conduct. They also make a point of reproducing their ideology in their children.

The best known of these theories is the so-called <u>Authoritarian Personality Theory</u>, which was developed after the Second World War as an attempt to explain the extraordinary dominance of Hitler and his racist ideology over the German people. This theory which has strong ties to Freudian psychoanalysis, postulates that prejudiced attitudes stem from particular childrearing practices. These practices are authoritarian and harsh in nature, so that the child builds up a virulent resentment towards the parents (which itself builds on the ambivalent feelings the child already has towards the parents as a natural consequence of development). The effect of this resentment is complicated by the punitive, denying environment the parents create for the child: the child may not vent his/her anger (or anxiety) at the source of the resentment (the parents), and so the anger, or anxiety, is displaced (see Defence Mechanisms, chapter 5). The effect of the displacement is to partly shape the child's personality, by creating a precedent for the displacement of unmanageable anxiety. In later years the displacement, which becomes ingrained as a way of dealing with anxiety, often takes on the form of <u>scapegoating</u>: people or groups, who are seen as weaker than the bigot, are chosen as the targets of displacement.

Thus, Jews are blamed for the economic woes which beset countries from time to time, blacks are blamed for the high crime rate, and so on. Much of the time there is not even a rationalization of the scapegoating. <u>In all cases, the prejudiced attitudes are hypothesized to serve the function of displacing unmanageable anxiety.</u>

Proponents of this theory have attempted to support it by exploring and measuring the <u>relationship between authoritarianism</u> (the central feature of the bigot's personality) and prejudice, empirically.

● Authoritarianism → ? ← Prejudice, Bigotry ●

Attitude scales (a special type of questionnaire) were developed to measure both authoritarianism and prejudice, and have been administered frequently in many countries to a wide spectrum of people.

There is some empirical support from these studies for the theory of the Authoritarian Personality. The hypothesized relationship between authoritarianism and prejudice holds, but not universally, and the relationship is generally not as strong as the theory claims.

There are many <u>grounds on which to criticise expressive theories</u> of prejudice. Two are worth singling out here.

1. The first is that while personality factors may play some role in the development and expression of prejudice, their role is not always important. In some instances, as we have seen, they are not present at all. A more important determinant may well be the sociocultural ethos (ie the ideology and history) of the group in which the prejudice occurs. This is thought to be the case in South Africa.

2. The second is the fact that *intergroup hostility is an historically specific phenomenon*. Anti-semitism is much stronger in particular historical eras and in particular geographical loci; racism, which flourished in the heyday of colonial history, is currently combatted in many countries in the world. This suggests that one looks to the material and historical bases of prejudice for an explanation, as well as to psychological factors.

<u>GROUP BASED THEORIES</u> are preferred by most contemporary psychologists. These theories see conflict as the outcome of intra- and intergroup dynamics. The basis of these theories is the observation that *people assembled in groups often tend to behave in a manner which obscures their personal, individual identity, and enhances their group identity.*

The group is thus the product of people submerging or transforming their own different personality patterns into a new group entity.

Think of two opposing groups of soccer fans (the flag waving, the chanting, the jubilation when one of the teams wins). *They respond to each other in terms of their group identity, and not in terms of their individual characteristics.* You're either Liverpool or you're Everton—that you're John Smith and not Reginald Dworkin is irrelevant. Many social psychologists believe that behaviour of this sort *cannot be reduced to the psyches of the individuals* that constitute the group. An explanation that takes the group as a unit is required.

There are several theories which attempt to explain conflict in terms of the processes that occur within groups and between groups.
These theories draw heavily, in one sense or another, from <u>Realistic Group Conflict theory</u>, which was developed by an American psychologist, MUZAFAR SHERIF.*
Sherif proposed that *conflict between groups is a consequence of real, objective differences. These differences concern the distribution of salient resources* and are postulated to be *sufficient to bring about conflict.*

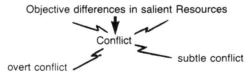

Objective differences in salient Resources

Conflict

overt conflict

subtle conflict

The way in which these differences enter the dynamics of the relationships *within* the groups, and *between* the groups, is quite specific. If the differences in the *distribution of resources are taken to be important,* then the Out-group will compete with the In-group to swing the differences in its (Out-group's) favour. This competition may become quite intense to result in *overt conflict,* or may take *more subtle* forms, depending on the situation.

INTRA-GROUP relations are also strongly affected.

When differences are great enough to impoverish one side hierarchical group structure, with dominant (often aggressive) leaders and subordinates is formed, and the nature of the intra-group relations becomes rigid and stereotyped, producing cohesion and boosting morale. If the differences are not perceived to be very important on the other hand, and if the respective groups need to cooperate to obtain a superordinate goal, then the intergroup relations may become much less hostile, and the intra-group relations much more fluid.

---

* See for example Sherif, M (1966). *Group Conflict and Co-operation.* London: Routledge and Kegan Paul.

Sherif explored his theory in a series of famous field experiments, which he conducted in the 1940s and 1950s on WASP (White Anglo Saxon Protestant) boys in summer camps. He manipulated an environment shared by different groups of boys in such a way as to produce *objective differences* between the groups, and carefully recorded the consequent behaviour of the opposing groups.

He found convincing evidence for his theory. The boys (many of whom were previously friends) soon formed tightly knit, hierarchically arranged groups, and the campsite began to resemble a battlefield rather than a holiday camp!

Sherif also orchestrated incidents in which the boys had *to cooperate to attain important, superordinate goals.* In one of these, he arranged for a truck to break down during a much awaited trip to a nearby lake. The truck could only be coaxed back into action by being towed, and the only possible method in which this could be achieved was by both groups of boys combining and pulling the truck with a tug-of-war rope. The groups successfully combined their efforts, and as predicted by Sherif, became

  (i) much less hostile towards each other
 (ii) far more fluid within, admitting members of the other group to their ranks.

The nub of Sherif's Realistic Conflict theory is that REAL DIFFERENCES BETWEEN GROUPS ARE NECESSARY IN THE PRODUCTION OF CONFLICT BETWEEN GROUPS.

The Minimal Group Experiments

European psychologists have taken Sherif's theory several steps further. They claim that *real differences* between groups are powerful, but *not necessary* in the production *of conflict* (see Tajfel (1982), and Brown (1988)* among others). Their evidence for this claim lies in a series of experiments called the 'minimal group experiments'. These experiments appear to demonstrate an <u>alarming fact: it is simply the division into groups, and not the basis for the division, that produces conflict.</u> No matter how arbitrary, or 'minimal' the groups, intergroup hostility is always present between them.

Simple, minimal, random division into groups
(without objective divisors)

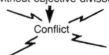

Conflict

Let us consider one of these 'minimal group' experiments to see where this claim comes from. In the experiment *schoolboys are divided into groups randomly.* The boys neither know who is in their group nor who is in the other group. Following this, the boys are required to play a game in which they are *to allocate money in a series of trials to one of the two groups.* They are not told how to allocate the money; they are simply told that they have to allocate the money. The results of the experiment show that group members tend to *maximize the difference between the amount allocated* to their group and the amount allocated to the other group (*in the favour of their group*).

Many of these so-called 'minimal group' experiments have been conducted, using different experimental scenarios and different subject populations. In essence they all show the same thing: that <u>merely categorizing people into groups is sufficient to bring about ethnocentric behaviour</u> (which is an important precondition for conflict).

---

* Tajfel, H (1982). *Social Identity and Intergroup Relations.* London: Cambridge University Press. Brown, R.J. (1988). *Group Processes.* Oxford: Blackwell.

INTERGROUP DYNAMICS

Real objective differences:
If intergroup
distribution
of salient
resources
is too lopsided

↓

Conflict

↙   ↘

Overt   Subtle

↓   ↓

Designed to swing distribution
in favour of 'Out' group

IN

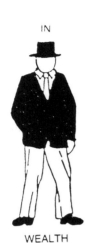

WEALTH

OUT

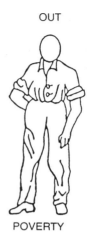

POVERTY

INTRA-GROUP DYNAMICS

If Differences are important enough to strongly disadvantage the 'Out'-group:

IN GROUP

e.g.
immovable
capitalists

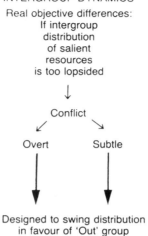

'Out' structure
becomes tough.
Leaders are
hierarchial,
rigid.
   Followers are
organised,
aggressive,
motivated for
revenge.
e.g. militant
trade unions.

e.g. immovable capitalists

ECONOMY PLUNGES

Less important, reconcilable differences

lead to
↓
Co-operation:

Outwardly
Co-operative

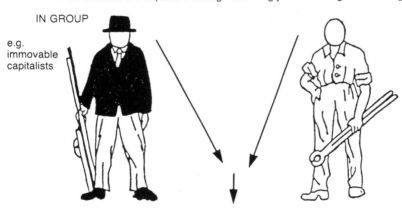

Inwardly Fluid.

Mutually Important Goals
↓
NATIONAL WEALTH
ECONOMIC GROWTH

How do psychologists explain this phenomenon? The most satisfactory explanation of the phenomenon is rendered by HENRI TAJFEL (late of Bristol University), and is known as Social Identity Theory. Unfortunately, the theory is a little too complex and lengthy to discuss here. Suffice it to note the following brief aspects of the theory. The chief assumption of the theory is the rather reasonable proposition that people are motivated to achieve and maintain positive self concepts. Since each person's identity (or self concept) is constituted in part by his/her social identity, which derives from the groups the person belongs to, each person will tend to evaluate his/her group positively, thus improving his/her individual identity. According to Tajfel, this evaluation takes place through 'social competition', in which the in-group is positively evaluated at the expense of the out-group.

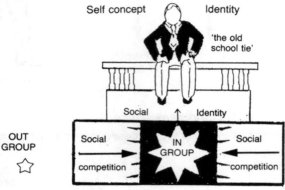

Lessening intergroup conflict

Intergroup conflict, as we have seen, is a widely prevailing phenomenon in the modern world. We have explored several theories that attempt to explain the origin of this conflict. We come now to the interesting (and inevitable) sequel to the previous question: *in what ways can conflict (and prejudice) be lessened?*

Of a number of social psychological answers to this question, perhaps the most interesting is the one suggested by Sherif in his summer camp experiments (see above). You will remember that Sherif found that contact between groups in the attainment of a superordinate, mutually important goal ● may serve to lessen conflict and reduce the exaggerated group dynamics characteristic of situations of intergroup conflict. Sherif's answer to the question, then, is that by intervening an overwhelmingly important (superordinate) mutual goal, contact between groups, under certain conditions, may lessen conflict.

The contact hypothesis

Sherif is not the only person who prescribes contact for intergroup maladies. In the U.S.A., for example, public policy for many years reflected this belief: the forced "bussing" of black children into white areas and schools is a poignant reminder of the ways in which social contact was engineered in the 1960s. This notion that contact between groups serves to lessen intergroup conflict is a popular one, and is known in psychological literature as the 'contact hypothesis'.

In the lay person's conception of things (and indeed, in many psychological theories), contact is presumed to work for the following reasons.

(i) Prejudice is thought to be the result of *inaccurate, stereotyped perceptions* (ie women drivers aren't really any worse than men drivers; Jews aren't really money diggers). It is in effect pre-judgment.

(ii) Contact exposes the prejudice for what it is: by meeting <u>members</u> of the group we ordinarily show prejudice against, <u>we come to realize that our perceptions of them are sorely mistaken, and that they are, in point of fact, remarkably similar to us.</u> In this way our mistaken impressions correct themselves, and hence, eliminate the basis for the prejudice.

<u>But is contact really such an effective antidote to prejudice and conflict?</u> Social psychologists have examined the contact hypothesis in some detail over the last 30 years, submitting it to a number of empirical tests. *The answer* that emerges from this work *is a qualified yes*. Yes, contact does reduce prejudice, and yes, contact may lessen conflict, but only under certain highly specific circumstances (and sometimes perhaps not even under any circumstances).

The *circumstances that favour the effectiveness of contact* are as follows:

(i) the parties in contact must be of equal status socially,
(ii) they must share common goals,
(iii) they must need to co-operate in order to achieve their mutually chosen goals.

Unfortunately in some contemporary scenarios contact is specifically and purposefully robbed of its healing power by the prevention of the above criteria.

"No man is an island, entire of itself; every man is a piece of the continent, a part of the main. Ask not for whom the bell tolls: it tolls for thee." John Donne, 1573-1631. Dean of St. Pauls.

When will we learn?

Nurses are especially blessed by their vocational role in helping create in their communities those conditions by which prejudice may be overcome.

No-one wants pain. Everyone wants a good healthy life for their children and themselves.

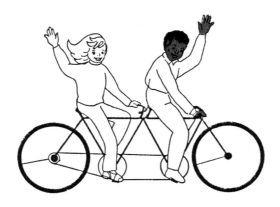

CHAPTER 9

THE NURSING PROCESS: PSYCHOSOCIAL ASPECTS

THE NURSING PROCESS

'The nursing process is a designated series of actions intended to fulfil the purposes of nursing—to maintain the client's wellness and, if this state changes, to provide the amount and quality of nursing care his situation demands to direct him back to wellness, and if wellness cannot be achieved, to contribute to his quality of life, maximising his resources as long as life is a reality. Inherent in these purposes is the fulfilment and maintenance of the integrity of the human needs of the person.'*

Psychosocial aspects

Stuart & Sundeen declare that the aim of nursing care is to 'maximize the patient's positive interactions with his environment, promote his level of wellness, and enhance his degree of self-actualization'.†

In the past, much learning and devotion were compounded into the nursing vocation. Professional practice, however, sometmes lacked scientific method and sequence, and there were those who failed to see patient-care as a dynamic patient-centred process.

The nursing process seeks to bring the nursing profession in line with other *mulitfaceted scientific processsesses*, by structuring a methodical model in which the nurse is obliged

(1) to consider her patient as a total entity, with his own individual psychosocial-emotional needs, limitations, and growth potential.
(2) to see his progress as a purposeful continuum from admission in illness to discharge at his maximum potential.

The nursing process is comprised of five essential phases:

(1) Data collection;
(2) Nursing diagnosis (Assessment);
(3) Planning;
(4) Implementation;
(5) Evaluation.

These phases may well overlap and are complemented by validation.

The following elucidation of nursing process stages is extracted from the *Standards of Nursing Practice*, published by the American Nurses' Association, Kansas City, Missouri.

---

* Yura & Walsh. *The Nursing Process.* Appleton-Century-Crofts.

† Stuart, G W & Sundeen, S J *Principles and Practice of Psychiatric Nursing.* Mosby, 1979.

Phase 1: Data collection

The collection of data concerning health status is systematic and continuous, being accessible, communicated and recorded. It emanates from formal question-naires and history taking, informal conversation, observation and general alertness.

It includes biophysical status, emotional status, cultural, religious, socio-economic background; daily-life patterns, copying patterns, personal interaction patterns, patient perception of health status; physical, social, emotional, vocational goals; material and human resources, as collected from patient, family, health-care personnel, individuals within the immediate and extended community.

Of importance in achieving patient-centred quality-care through a systematic approach to nursing is knowledge of a patient's *'ego strenghts'* as manifested by the effectiveness with which he has, in the past, handled the demands and challenges of everyday life.

> Bellak et al (1973)* classify 'ego strenghts' as:
> intactness of the senses (sight, hearing etc);
> intelligence (problem solving), use of language;
> motivation to regain health;
> capacity to face reality, to assess, to judge and to plan on a reality-basis independent of phantasy;
> stability of mood;
> ability to control impulses such as anger and sexuality, to exercise some self-discipline;
> maturity of 'ego-defences' (chapter 5, pp 106-8);
> capacity to accomplish age-appropriate life tasks, eg study, responsibility for others;
> recovery history in previous illness;
> capacity to make and maintain friendships and other relationships;
> evidence of a 'core value system', eg religious philosophy, purpose in living, etc.

The nurse should not be discouraged by incompleteness of 'ego-stength' structure. It is almost impossible to achieve positive presentation in all these areas.

Comment

This is indeed wide-flung and intensive scrutiny. One must surely question acceptability to the patient of adding to the many inroads on his person and privacy occasioned by medical examination. He may well interpret such investigation as exhausting, impertinent and diminishing. There may be justification for in-depth scrutiny in psychiatric nursing care, in long-term rehabilitation programmes such as those pertaining in spinal injuries or in care of the terminal patient. However, exposure of the patient entering hospital for a fractured wrist or rhinoplastics to pap smears, questions concerning marital relationships and job difficulties may provoke indignation, or cause diminishment. Most patients enter hospital for

* Bellak L, Hurvich M, Gediman H K *Ego Functions in Schizophrenics, Neurotics and Normals.* New York: John Wiley, 1973.

specific procedures, and their main goal is to get out with as much speed and dignified privacy as possible.

Yura & Walsh maintain that 'the goal of the formalised data collection process is to gather information from which to formulate a plan for bringing about change in the patient'.

Most patients wish to bring about change by reduction of pain and discomfort. For the nurse to assume the advisability of other change may seem presumptuous. Indeed, achieving 'change' in others is a task at which the most skilled multi-disciplinary team may well balk! No doubt, in the fullness of time and experience, data collection will be tailored to apply specifically to

(i) the life-area in which the patient has sought treatment;
(ii) the creation of a hospital atmosphere and life pattern as litte deviant from the home situation as possible, thus reducing to a minimum unfamiliar environmental stresses, and facilitating a speedy return to a useful and full life in the community.

Phase 2: Nursing diagnosis (assessment)

This involves assessment of the extent to which the patient's health status deviates from the norm.

Assessment factors:

(1) The patient's health status is compared with the norm in order to determine whether any deviation from it may validly be termed 'abnormal'.
(2) The patient's capabilities and limitations are identified.
(3) The nursing diagnosis is related to, and judged within the context of, diagnoses made by other caring professionals.

The nursing diagnosis concerns

(i) aspects in which the patient's health may need to be promoted;
(ii) areas in which the patient requires help in adapting to, and overcoming biopsycho-social stress in attaining his own individual goals.

Most nursing diagnosis are based on the deviation between the client's resources and his goal-attainment in terms of Maslow's Hierarchy of Human Needs (see p 100).

Stuart & Sundeen* caution: Inexperienced nurses often feel pressurized to identify nursing problems quickly, and feel confused and frustrated by the private or non-communicative patient who does not participate in the relationship, and does not share his thoughts or feelings (with staff). In this case the primary nursing problem may be the nurse's attitude. There is a mistaken tendency to attempt to break into this withdrawn state. Instead, one should enter sensitively, and with supportive rapport.

---

* Stuart, G W & S J Sundeen. *Principles and Practice of Psychiatric Nursing.* St Louis: Mosby. 1979.

Phase 3: Planning (in accordance with goals derived from the nursing diagnosis) **the contract**

The client's response to, and participation in, Planning reflect and confirm the *type of contract* existing between him and his care-givers.

Criteria of acceptable goals:

(i) they should be *mutually set* by consultation with the patient. Programming should include goal identification and timing. Goals should be stated in terms realistic to the patient's own limitations and resources.

They usually centre on the alleviation of his physically and mentally painful and disturbing symptoms, which should constitute the pivot of planning. The nurse should avoid the temptation to overlook the patient's goals, *projecting* her own into the care plan.

(ii) Goals should be consistent with other planned therapy.

Procedure

Agreed goals are recorded specifically and explicity for the purpose of long-and-short-term reference and implementation. Areas in which goals are sited and planned are:

physiological: related to specific nursing problems, physical care procedures, etc.

psychosocial: pertaining to emotional welfare; adjustment to permanent disability; motivation for rehabilitation; parental participation in the illness; community participation; group identification and harnessing of community resources.

Clearly the *delegation of goal priority* is of import to both nurse and patient. While lifesaving procedures carry highest priority in most situations, the patient's physical comfort, his emotional peace of mind, together with support of the family may well take precedence in care of the terminally ill.

Phase 4: Implementation

Frequently goals are recorded to one side of the page and the planned therapeutic techniques for their fulfilment on the other. For Example:

Goal	Planned Therapeutic Techniques
Immediate reduction of patient's emotional isolation.	Unrestricted visiting by loved ones: staff to establish relationships by spending time keeping the patient company, discussing matters other than his illness, telling him about their own lives and interests; provision of a telephone, radio, television, etc.
	Introduction, with patient's permission, to others suffering from similar conditions who have managed to adjust to a reasonably acceptable lifestyle.

No new patterns will be learned unless the motivation to acquire them is greater than the motivation to retain old ones. An authoritarian attitude will merely provide the stimulus for more anger and resistance. As in most areas, the nurse's warm, friendly, respectful and empathizing *relationship provides the most powerful incentive* for the sacrifices involved in meaningful goal achievement. (See *inter alia* Goldfarb, Harlow, chapter 2.)

The development of and advantages pertaining in a truly healing nurse–patient relationship feature throughout this book. Their definition and summary comprise the contents of chapter 7.

A person's adjustment patterns (see pp 106-108), adaptive and maladaptive, have been built up slowly throughout his life. Although the nurse may disapprove thereof, some may serve for him a real and protective purpose. *Patience, caution, respect for privacy and a self-questioning modesty should characterize the approach of anyone presuming to intervene between an individual and his life pattern.*

Caution: Intellectual-level insight may serve to break down protective mechanisms, causing anxiety and anger.

In order to avoid regression to even more maladaptive coping mechanisms, it may be necessary to help a patient by locating real areas of emotional trauma, reliving painful experiences, providing catharsis, and emotional-level guidance. (See Psychotherapeutic Process, pp 63 et seq.)

Phase 5: Evaluation

This is the 'feedback' phase. Together nurse and patient assess progress, or the lack of it, as measured by his current human need attainment.

In the patient's opinion, are nursing actions improving, in the long or short term, the quality of his life?

Are timing expectations reasonable?

Have the patient's needs changed?

Has the nursing process presumed to extend beyond the area relevant to the patient's problems?

Is lack of progress due to poor data collection, behavioural analysis, nursing diagnosis, patient–nurse relationship?

Patient and nurse should both be generous in their assessment of any improvement, any step nearer goal-achievement in that long and difficult path which we all encounter in the journey towards reasonable mental health. Evaluation is a mutual patient–nurse appraisal of progress towards previously mutually identified goals; it is a continuous dynamic (active) process beginning with the initial phases of this relationship and present throughout its development and fruition to, ideally, 'optimum self actualisation'.

Case example:
Psycho-social Rehabilitation within the Nursing Process

Case presentation: Jane, aged 19, below-knee amputation resultant upon motor-car accident.

Three weeks after surgery Jane is depressed, angry, and has chosen the protective mechanism of isolated withdrawal. She is indifferent to the rehabilitative efforts of the multidisciplinary team.

Phases of the Psychological Nursing Process
Phase 1: Data collection

Visual and auditory observation: Jane's face is expressionless. She stares fixedly ahead, or lies motionless, eyes closed, refusing food. She tolerates her parents without response, but has refused all other visitors. Her only arousal is insistence on the privacy afforded by the curtains surrounding her bed, and occasional scathing comments to the multidisciplinary rehabilitative team: 'You cannot grow me another leg, so go away and leave me alone.'

Jane responds monosyllabically to essential questions. Her speech is flat and expressionless. She has refused radio, TV and reading material.

Tactile: There is no response to nursing procedures or to friendly efforts at tactile communication.

Interview information as presented by parents:

Janes's parents divorced when she was 8 years old—both are remarried and her relationships with them have always been reasonably conforming although not intimately involved. Jane was at boarding school throughout her senior years where she enjoyed a few friendships rather than wide peer popularity. She was always a proud girl, and since going to boarding school her relationship with her parents was politely dutiful rather than intimate. Her school progress was always satisfactory and her major source of satisfaction and achievement was on the sports field.

At the time of her accident she was a second-year student majoring in physical education. She had recently, at his insistence, broken her relationship with her boy-friend of 2 years' standing. The driver at the time of her accident was a first date.

Phase 2: Nursing diagnosis (assessment)

Goal-achievement deviations (see Maslow's Hierarchy, p 100)

Physical survival goal: threatened at time of accident.

Safety-security goals: threatened by accident trauma, loss of mobility, mutilation and loss of body image.

Love and belonging goals: long-term threat by familial break-up. Rejection feelings reinforced by break-up with boy-friend. Loss anticipation reinforced by conviction of rejection by normal physically intact peers.

Esteem goals: specific unsightly mutilation by accident, and anticipation of categorization as a 'cripple' relative to peer group. Fear of loss of feminine identity values.

Self-actualization goal as physical educationist rendered unattainable by mutilation.

DIAGNOSIS

Jane's response of acute and all-permeating psycho-physical *depression* is basically a *normal* (reactive) one requiring a customary individualized long-term rehabilitative programme.

Maladaptive adjustment is reflected in selection of the withdrawal isolation mechanism, which will deprive Jane of the motivating power to participate in the rehabilitative programme, thus serving further to isolate and depress.

Phase 3: Planning

Long-term goal-fulfilment (within three months)

Jane's participation in the establishment of compensation areas capable of rebuilding her self-concept to the point of goal-satisfaction approximating her pre-accident life situation (see p 114). This will include a personalized vocational guidance programmed—tests of aptitude, interest and personality.

Return to participation in personal, social and community activities (ideally, at least) as satisfying as those pertaining pre-accident.

Re-establishment of goal satisfaction in areas of physical safety, love and belonging, esteem and self-actualization.

Short-term fulfilment (within three weeks)

Establishment of a meaningful client–nurse relationship with an initial focal Nurse A.

Nurse A to sit beside Jane knitting, and occasionally remarking on the difficulties client is encountering; expressing empathy with her feelings of anger, isolation, diminishment, etc. To talk about things other than her accident, keeping her company and occasionally telling her of nurse A's own life and interests. Nurse A to 'go along' with Jane, accepting her displaced aggression and thus resistance (see p 114).

3rd week: Utilizing in any client response, verbalize empathy and then suggest more profitable ways of handling problem. By the end of two weeks the nurse–client relationship will *it is hoped, lead to some sort of mutually agreed goal-attainment plan*, for example:

(i) moving Jane's bed to the window to initiate at least distant contact with the outside world;

(ii) motivation towards some sort of pleasant goal reinforcement such as watching TV, selecting pleasurable food, using a wheelchair for personal toileting, etc prior to initiating introduction to prosthesis;

(iii) agreement to stimulate some *joie de vivre* motivation by alleviating depression with anti-depressant medication;

(iv) initiate therapeutic discussion with the aim that Jane will achieve insight into her selection of extreme isolation avoidance mechanism. Extension of this therapeutic process into discussion of traumatic experiences, catharsis; trial selection of other coping mechanisms and revised patterns of human interactions;

(v) specifically mutually agreed goal direction of tension-energy towards adjustment to a prosthesis and development of satisfying, loving relationships, esteem and actualization goals.

Priority and amendment of goals will be by mutual agreement.

Phase 4: Implementation

In the realization that the *nurse–client relationship* constitutes the vehicle via which the client is motivated, supported and in a sense rewarded for the effort, the physical and mental pain, the anxiety and distress involved in participating in the nursing process, this became the *priority area*.

The therapeutic contract

Meaningful communication inherent in empathy having been established, Jane and her nurse drew up an implementation programme.

Within six weeks Jane will try the prosthesis for short periods, concentrating on those specific voluntary movements which have replaced natural walking.

By ten weeks Jane will be prepared to bear the stress involved in wearing her prosthesis for two hours at a time, and will attempt short outings with Nurse A.

Within twelve weeks Jane will consider going to the movies with another girl.

Within fourteen weeks Jane will begin to achieve the goal of feeling the prosthesis to be part of her own body. By this time she will have embarked on a vocational guidance programme designed to achieve her ultimate potential, and most satisfying and profitable compensation areas.

Phase 5: Evaluation (i)

Jane is now staying with her mother, with whom she is communicating more intimately than before her accident. She is able to discuss her childhood, her exboy-friend, the accident, her feelings about the prosthesis.

She does not yet feel it part of her body, and is frequently offended by its appearance and the feeling that it is a mockery of her former self. She is however beginning to experience its advantages.

She is beginning to go out with girl friends, but takes to emotional flight at the thought of boys, and sex, in relation to her diminished body image.

She is beginning a secretarial course, being interested but not enthusiastic. Jane and Nurse A agree that she is making progress but still requires support and guidance in achieving her *physical* safety, *love and belonging, esteem and self-actualization needs*. In preparation for the *termination phase*, they agree upon a further sub-implementation programme to extend over the next two months.

Evaluation (ii) (three months hereafter)

Jane has come to recognize the essential therapeutic nature of her relationship with Nurse A, together with a growing need for independence and freedom.

Having begun to accept her prosthesis as an extension of her own body, her *physical-safety needs* are well on the way to fulfilment.

Feeling a closer union with her family, the love of her parents and friends and, having established a growing friendship with a young man in the rehabilitation programme, Jane is beginning to experience, in some ways, *more fulfilment of her love and belonging needs* than before the accident. Having completed a condensed secretarial course, she has enjoyed promotion, an increase in salary and status employment which set her well on the way to achieving *esteem and self-actualization goals*. She is thinking of moving into a small flat near to her mother.

Three-monthly sessions with Nurse A would, within the next six months, give way to the mutually agreed termination of regular sessions.

ADVANTAGES

(1) The nursing process structures a methodical model in which the nurse is *obliged to consider her client as a total entity*. The individual's physical, psycho-social-emotional and sexual needs, limitations, and growth resources must be seen as a dynamic continuum, pre-illness, during illness and post-illness, and the nurse must care about him as a *total human being*.

(2) Data collection provides information required to minimize home and hospital discrepancy. By providing familiar home comforts, both physical and emotional, stress of exposure to the foreign 'sterile' hospital environment may be considerably reduced.

(3) In that all health disciplines know, understand and use the model, client-care is scientifically orientated, co-ordinated and total, guiding the client towards maximum fulfilment of his own chosen life goals.

CHAPTER 10

NURSING IN THE COMMUNITY

Community nursing

The community is composed first of the individual, and then the family unit.

In considering personality formation we have seen, in chapter 2 (especially pp 47 et seq), how the socialization process in healthy development emanates from the mother–child relationship. The ability to make those sacrifices necessary for the maintenance of long-term human relations and the assumption of social responsibility spreads out from:

the mother–child relationship–family relationships
→ peer, usually same-sex, relationships in childhood and early adolescence
→ protection by group-identification-assumption of social norms and heterosexual relationships in later adolescence.
→ marriage partner and parenting group
→ sub-group and communal identification.

In chapter 5 Erikson's Maturation Theory emphasizes the role of Introjection (p 106) and Identification (pp 108-111) in resolving life's developmental crises.

The importance of *group identification* in individual and communal growth and achievement is very clear. Thus *the role of group or social learning* in understanding the reciprocal interaction between

individual and group behaviour⟷Man's control over his environment (pp 170-1) is very pertinent to the structure and function of the community.

In understanding that behaviour patterns are learnt or modified through *direct experience* or *vicariously* by observing and identifying with the behaviour of others, we begin to understand the cumulative effect of co-operative or communal experience. Within the high-powered hierarchy of modern living, each generation *identifies* with, *introjects* from, and builds upon the efforts and achievement of his forebears and peers. On page 170 we learnt that group development takes place through the conciliatory and often sacrificial merging of the individual with his group in

forming,
storming,
norming,
performing.

Insight into the cycles and plateaux involved in:

task identification,
the arousal of emotional stimulation,
the overcoming of individual resistance,
creative problem-solving and the motivation of group energy,

should impress upon the community worker the need for insight and patience in achieving social change. (See Leadership, pp 204-224.)

A *community* is a locality whose residents enjoy a fairly complete social life, a feeling of local unity and an ability to act collectively.

The behaviour of individuals within the community, and the community itself, is governed by:

norms or conventional, expected behaviour upon which a particular society depends for cohesion and organization,

mores, the ideas of right and wrong which the community attaches to certain behaviour. Mores forbid certain acts such as murder and incest but require one to pay one's bills.

values are passed down from generation to generation until they assume an almost sacred character to be accepted and obeyed unquestioningly.

Folkways, which are literally the ways of the folk, norms, mores and values, emerge gradually from the social life of a community or a nation, and represent its conclusions as to what practices are beneficial or harmful to its people.

The American sociologist William Graham Summer said 'Mores can make anything right and prevent the condemnation of anything.' In other words, right and wrong become whatever the members of a society agree is good or bad for people. An example is the mutilating practice of female circumcision in many areas of North Africa.

The role of the community worker in the elimination of such destructive practices, and the motivation of new norms and mores, does indeed call for intense and impressive group communication through:

> motivation of emotional drives, values and interests (p 90),
> reconditioned learning (pp 156ff),
> co-operation with strong leadership figures operating through Role Analysis and the Trait, Situational and Psychoanalytic approaches (pp 205-209).

Role analysis

Kurt Lewin's Field Theory maintains that the leader is he who can consistently make the correct choice for the well-being of the greatest number of the group (p 209).

> 'I know what they want and I'll lead them to attain it.'

This too is a difficult, conflicting task for the most effective leader is he who conforms most strictly to group norms or standards.

> 'I keep my fingers on the pulse of my people's dreams and goals, making them mine. Thus I can make the correct choice for them.'
> But what when the group choice is no longer appropriate?

The community worker is faced with the *necessity for motivating that change in group norms or conventions which will enable an effective leader to bring about change.*

> 'I must introduce a new norm-goal which can be seen to provide greater happiness and fulfilment that that to which the community's group-effort is currently directed.'

Demonstration that a new technique does indeed work by improving the quality of life, is of course a very strong reinforcement agent in new learning. Demonstration of the effectiveness of immunization against childhood diseases certainly facilitates the adoption of new norms.

Identification with the fears, hopes, dreams and emotional needs of a group resulting in goal-achievement such as a lower infant mortality rate, certainly facilitates the establishment of new childbirth and mothercraft norms.

Attention and interest *facilitators*, such as size, colour, aesthetic appeal, movement, contrast and appropriate goal satisfaction, are detailed on pp 142-3. Examples are large, brightly coloured posters and teaching videos, especially where goals, satisfactions and humour are similar to those of the population at which they are aimed.

The *role* of the Community Nurse is a relatively new one, as yet unformalized even by professional workers themselves. It certainly goes beyond education.

A role consists in the *expected behaviour for one in a certain state*. Roles are thus tasks defined by society, each possessing a set of social norms or expectations.

Roles are either:

> *ascribed* by virtue of birth, sex, kinship, age, or other unalterable factors, eg hereditary royalty,

or

> *achieved* through education, experience, demonstrated achievement, and are thus attained by choice or effort, eg Hospital Superintendent.

The role of the bedside nurse is that of skilled care-giver and healer; that of the policeman, law enforcer.

In the *role network*, role identification and function are especially complex in multiracial, multilingual, multitraditional societies. Each individual is required to adapt to both *traditional* and *modern* roles, as well as those transferred from *rural* to *urban* society; from, for example, a middle eastern culture with its learned patterns of *group* acting, feeling and thinking introjected from, and shared by, a deeply rooted social system, to an intricate society based on *individual responsibility*. Adjustment may be further complicated by differing *ethnic characteristics*, standards, privileges and restrictions. Culture shock is indeed a reality.

The extent of *role conflict* in any given multicultural community is reflected by the Community Nurse's differential role within

communities requiring predominantly primary or 'grassroots' health care, such as immunization and water purification, as opposed to those

more affluent and sophisticated societies demanding specialized, individual supportive services and the fulfilment of personally determined health, educational and legal expectancy goals.

The Common Denominator:

All strata of society see *the nurse* as a respected and efficient *comforter and healer*. There is justification in those authorities who believe *her role in community health* can only develop within the context of a *complementary curative role* in which the goal of healing or sustaining people out of hospital is achieved. The healing role is a valuable passport into the community.

Clearly the attainment of community health goals requires motivation, achievement and maintenance, through the action of organizations termed *institutions*.

Social institutions designed *to cope with the functions and problems of society* include stable families, schools, banks, hospitals, clinics, churches, universities and law courts which meet the needs of both the individual and society. Organizations are characterized by the following attributes.

the allotment to each person of a specific task or group of tasks,
a hierarchy of authority,
administration by recorded rules and regulations,
officials specifically trained for individual roles.

Usually those at the top of the hierarchy exercise discretion while those at the bottom are allotted specific procedures. All participants identify with the general norms of the organization, institution or group brought together by common interests, needs and goals.

The organization of health-care institutions has been studied in different contexts:

 (i) the micro-context of professional–patient interaction,
 (ii) the meso-context of the institutions, eg hospitals, clinics, etc,
(iii) the macro-context of the health-care system as a whole.

There are several schools of thought as to *optimum motivation units* within a work structure.
According to McGregor's somewhat outdated X and Y theory of organized goal motivation (p 211):

X Theory characteristics predominate. Man is predominantly lazy, disinclined to work and must be coerced, pushed and punished in order to achieve.

There is still a tendency to project this X image on lower-strata organizational participants, while those in higher echelons are usually attributed with:

Y Theory characteristics of basic motivation for self-realization in order that they may give of their best.

The community nurse, in order to achieve her goal of motivating maximum physical and mental health in all community members, will operate on the wise theory that *the average person seeks responsibility*, and those endowed with average intelligence, imagination, ingenuity and staying power will contribute towards the growth and fulfilment of community goals.

Even in Britain the pattern of socio-economic stratification results in a mixed and contrasting disease profile.

Among the more affluent the diseases of civilization, ie chronic and degenerative disorders and psychiatric loss, predominate.

By contrast, the poor and underprivileged present with predominantly social diseases, such as infections and nutritional disorders. The diseases of poverty are associated with inadequate housing, poor sanitation, insufficient food and ill-balanced diet, environmental hazards, insufficient work, low income, migration, and 'culture shock', aggravated by escape to drugs and alcohol.

Community Nurse Peg Anderson introduces her community and her efforts to promote 'optimum reaction between man and his environment in order to improve overall quality of life':

'Daily life in our Merseyside slum clearance project is tough. Problems are never-ending. So many homes have to deal with alcoholism or drugs which in turn bring unemployment. Next year we want to start support groups for alcoholics, and hopefully get as many as possible to agree to rehabilitation. Often pressures are placed on men which they can't deal with, and they turn to drink. The trouble is, our people have been used to living in tenement rooms . . . when they move into flats they find it difficult to meet extra expenses. They want furniture and curtains and get caught up with hire-purchase which they cannot afford.

Drink leads to assaults, which have become a daily occurrence. This morning I attended a woman, four months pregnant, who had been assaulted by her husband. She can't leave him because she has nowhere to go. That is what women put up with because they have no alternative.

Residents don't want to go out into the streets anymore. They stay home most nights because it's not worth the risk of being assaulted or robbed.

I am desperately motivating support from people who run special service clubs such as Rotary. Perhaps they will help us start projects for our youth, and help provide sportsfields or other facilities.

St John Ambulance has organized First Aid and leadership courses for many of the youngsters and has started a youth band to keep them off the streets.

Many ex-gaolbirds try hard to keep a clean record, but they find it hard to get jobs. We've had success placing a few of them at a shoe factory, but many are unemployed and sometimes revert to crime.

Frail and elderly people who are housebound often find themselves in debt to hawkers. Too infirm to walk to the shops, they buy fish, meat, vegetables on credit. The traders keep their pension books as a safeguard against mounting debts.

As much as we struggle against problems, we feel we are making some headway. Voluntary workers counsel families in their homes and provide support in times of crisis.

Another of our projects is to encourage schoolchildren to fight malnutrition, and to learn about food values, by planting vegetable patches around school buildings. The vegetables are used for soup for lower form pupils.

A nursery school has been started for pre-schoolers. A mobile maternity and child welfare clinic and a TB diagnostic centre operate in the area.'

The *effectiveness* of all community programmes *emanates from*

(i) research,
(ii) mobilization of resources,
(iii) a tolerant, accepting, encouraging, involved and supportive professional–client relationship.

Because hers is an eclectic training embracing medical, social, psychological and educational planning the Community Nurse constitutes the pivot of the community health programme.

Because the Community Nurse comes into contact with the client in his natural environment, be it family, clinic, or place of work, it is important that she familiarizes herself, and indeed identifies with the *definition and fulfilment of physical and mental health goals specific to her community*. In Hampstead, seven people living in a three-bedroomed house may be termed 'overcrowded'; in Brixton such housing distribution may be deemed 'privileged'.

In preparing this book the author was tempted to assemble relevant material in a special chapter. But realization of the client's holistic physiological, emotional and social unity soon led to reaffirmation of the *indispensability of integration*. Within the whole gamut of personality development, human relations, developmental psychology, applied sociology, stands that precious entity — the dignified Individual.

Where the specific functions of the Community Nurse can be separated and emphasized, this has been done within relevant chapters. (See also Index under 'Community Nurse'.)

'Local authorities and Community Nurses execute their responsibility during the *maintenance phase* in the family and in the community. Thus it would appear that to the Community Nurse, pivot of community health services, falls responsibility for *less dramatic, more long-term rehabilitation* as would pertain in conditions such as paraplegia, limb loss and mutilating surgery. She is also responsible for long-term *planning* and *implementation* in common, burdensome and debilitating conditions such as diabetes, hypertension, circulatory diseases, genetic diseases, breakdown in mental health and the problems of ageing and terminal illness.

Clearly in order to fulfil her multiple functions it is necessary that she motivate and co-operate with allied health professions, voluntary organizations and, often at grassroot level, with individual community members.

Hospitals and other residential institutions do not, Heaven be praised, constitute man's natural environment. In fact, in the health of the nation, their function is rapidly contracting to the highly technical investigations and intensive short-term care usually associated with surgery, acute illness and trauma. Indeed, the underlying attitude, conscious or unconscious, of some hospital units is 'Get better or die—your bed is needed for more acute (and, frequently, medically more interesting) cases'.

The key functions of the Community Nurse may be classified as: preventive; promotive; curative and rehabilitory.

A. Preventive

The preventive function includes the motivation, organization and administration of prophylactic clinics; the dissemination of preventive information; the removal of anxieties and prejudices causing 'flight' from, rather than attraction towards, preventive and community therapeutic procedures.

'Health for all by the year 2000' is the global social goal accepted by WHO in 1978 in the form of the *Alma Ata*. Primary health care is considered the key to this target.

> 'Health for all does not mean medical repairs by doctors and nurses for everyone in the world for all their existing ailments. It means that health begins at home, in schools and working places and that people will use better approaches for preventing disease and alleviating suffering.'

APPLYING THE NURSING PROCESS MODEL TO COMMUNITY NURSING

It is possible to apply the Nursing Process model to the community by:

1. **Collecting data** as to population, boundaries, socio-economic status, cultural origin, mores, goals, resources, frustrations, homogeneity, etc.

2. **Diagnosis** of deviation of the community and its internal strata from the achievement of their goals—do most urgent and widespread *goals* pertain to Maslow's

   physical needs—to the attainment of fresh air, adequate nutrition, housing, etc

   safety and security needs—does the community yearn for freedom from crime, from primary illnesses such as malnutrition, diseases of childhood, TB, etc?

   love and belonging needs—family support and guidance, divorce rehabilitation, extended family substitutes—religious, social, cultural and recreational groups.

   esteem and status needs—through higher education, social and political opportunity, status housing and the fulfilment of social aspirations.

   self-actualization goals—search for fulfilment through the achievement of self-help community cultural and creative facilities; pride in community service, a reputation for a high standard of living for all age groups.

3. **Planning** community facilities to achieve specific community goals—through the use of questionnaires, opinion surveys and professional sources to plan priorities, needs and preferences, for example

   provision of family planning, antenatal and mother-and-child clinics; nutrition groups—preschool care facilities; or

   geriatric clinics, social groups, retirement housing schemes, mobile clinics, home-care networks, etc,

   all in accordance with community composition, age, financial resources, mores, etc.

4. **Implementation:**
   Community and state action to provide these facilities.
   Information and utilization plans to the target market.
   Transport.
   Staffing, maintenance and expansion of community facilities.
   Expansion or amendment of goals in accordance with the extent to which faclities are utilized, discarded, approved or rejected.

5. **Evaluation** of the effectiveness of community services. Quantitative and qualitative assessment of feedback on goal-achievement. Were the selection and timing of facilities productive of optimum service?

   eg Have crime rates fallen?
   Have unwanted pregnancies decreased?
   Is there less depression and isolation amongst the aged?
   Has the Nursing Process extended beyond relevant areas?
   Have the community's needs changed?
   Are community goals progressing on Maslow's hierarchy from those connected with physical survival, safety and security through to feelings of belonging, participation, community pride in achievement, to self-actualization in communal goal-service and -achievement?

Barriers

There are many barriers to attaining health for all including adequate environmental health, overpopulation, maldistribution of health manpower and the state of the world economy. The most vital resource is manpower—and there is ample manpower—because there is a large, and largely unexploited workforce for health—the community itself.*

Reinforcing the importance of community involvement and motivation, Miss Muriel Skeet, International Health Services Consultant, maintains:

'Unless a health programme develops from within the body of the community and is of the community, it will not succeed. Health care should entail a long-term programme involving the basic principles of identification with the community; the sharing of ideas and decisions; and recognition of the influence of past culture, as well as current trends.'†

The Community Nurse's relationship with her community

The Community Nurse *must know and respect the cultural structures and traditions* of her community. Within her own soul-searching she should be sure that what she has to offer is better than that which prevails.

The effectiveness of her communication will depend upon the establishment of meaningful communication or rapport—often earned in spheres of personal contact, communal projects, recreation etc, far removed from her more formal preventive, promotive and curative roles.

If roles can be reversed so that her community is able to help *her* in some personal way, so much the better for the community's self-image.

Only when one is known and liked for oneself, can one inspire feelings of faith and confidence at an emotional level. In order to motivate that *emotional-level faith* which is necessary for *acceptance of the unfamiliarity and risks inherent in what she has to offer*, the Community Nurse would be well advised to consult established community leaders. Long-term, deeply ingrained faith has endowed them with a reassuring aura of reliability and security.

Certainly common courtesy, compassion and consideration help condition positive attitudes to primary health care. Hammond M and Collins R in their article 'Maternal and Child Health Services—A Nurse's Perspective' (1986) write thus:

'Have you ever heard people complaining like this about health workers?

- "They are always so rushed with me . . ."
- "They are so rude and uncaring . . ."
- "They never take the time to explain things properly . . ."
- "They seem more interested in filling in my card than in listening to me . . .".'

B. Promotive

The promotive function consists in promotion of that multifaceted, holistic and

---

* See also 'That our children may not die'.
† National Community Nursing Symposium 1980.

integrated communal functioning which constitutes the individual's most effective defence against distress and isolation.

The motivation of *promotive facilities* such as maternal and child-welfare clinics, school clinics, youth clubs, mobile treatment centres, psychogeriatric clinics, old folks' clubs—all of these fall within the promotive sphere of the Community Nurse. (See Leadership, especially p 212.)

C. Curative and rehabilitory

Miss Nourith Ben Dov, Director of Nursing Services, Israel, maintains that a *home-care network* by professionals and volunteers is fundamental to

(i) any realistic plan for keeping people out of hospital;
(ii) the role of the nurse as healer and teacher—her traditional association with pain-relief, physical succour; her personal involvement and specialized knowledge endow the nurse with special prestige;
(iii) an intimate knowledge of community, family and individual assets, liabilities, goals and needs.

Curative and rehabilitatory services include those *self-help groups* within which people with common problems may come together in order to enlighten, support, comfort and work for facilities to improve their situation. They constitute a key to curative communal medicine. They are not, however, always as easy to handle as one may suppose. (See Support groups, p 613ff.)

Among the members a *delicate ambivalence between personal and group needs prevails*: we are all human. *Pre-existent feuds*, resentments and competitiveness often cut across common problems. Confidences revealed within the cathartic group are not always honoured and may be held against members. People who 'live in each others' pockets' are often tempted to resort to using confidences as ammunition. There may well be *negative identification* of lower standards, anxieties, resentment, fears and distrust. Clients seeing others in more advanced stages of their own illnesses are much more distressed. By bringing people together into highly emotionally charged situations, the nurse may be playing with fire.

While the curative role of the hospital is primarily specialized and specific to a particular illness, there are many *long-term, chronic conditions* which allow for a productive, happy, spiritually and emotionally fulfilling life only when treated within the community.

Conditions such as diabetes mellitus, rheumatism and arthritis; mental retardation and psychiatric maintenance; long-term malignancy and terminal illnesses — to name but a few — are least traumatically and most happily handled within home and community environments, complemented by periodic visits to specialized investigatory and curative palliative facilities. Provided the Community Nurse carries out home nursing procedures or teaches these to volunteers, to her client or his family, she performs the very valuable and usually popular service of keeping people out of hospital. (See also The Community Nurse's role in caring for the aged, pp 456 et seq; in Terminal illness, pp 546 et seq.) In addition, her specialized knowledge of nursing procedures, emotional and social needs, community facilities, etc, *enriches the functions of maintenance agencies such as self-help residential groups of the disabled and neighbourhood Seniors' residences.*

The Community Sister should feel au fait, comfortable and confident in her role in *communal, familial and personal disasters and crises*. Her intimate knowledge of

clients' personal and familial difficulties, resources, etc;

existing long-term relationships;

techniques for providing 'hot' on-the-spot and thus especially effective crisis intervention, before attitudes of anger, hopelessness, guilt and anxiety solidify;

render her a particularly important member of the crisis intervention team. (See Crisis intervention and disaster, chapter 24.)

Any *rehabilitation* that is worthwhile must take place within that community and familial situation in which the client is to find his ultimate quality of life. The Community Nurse (refer to chapter 22, 'Rehabilitation', especially pp 511-12) is reminded of the necessity of working with the professional team (ie Occupational Therapist, Social Worker, Orthopaedic Technician, Physiotherapist) in adjusting the client, his home circumstances, and his familial situation to his specific needs. Only thus can optimum independence and restored status in both the family and the community be achieved. Role reversal (pp 506, 511) should be carefully avoided.

The big, unstructured, grown-up world of the Community Nurse is a turmoil of hating and loving; self-indulgence and self-deprivation; continuous battling and rushed struggle for survival. This is the stamping ground of her 'patient', now more surely evolved to her 'client'. The nurse is now, at best a skilled healer, a welcome guest; at worst, an 'inquisitive', 'interfering', officially designated 'do-gooder'. Her professional skills must pass from safe, tangible catheters and thermometers to her own abstract knowledge, insight into human relations, flexibility, ingenuity, self-direction . . . and the magical quality of empathy.

Antibiotics may cure pneumonia, but only long-term, concerted and highly motivated family insight, support, compassion and tolerance will control a juvenile delinquent or contain a demented granny.

Whereas the veteran District Nurse could rely on the sustained co-operation and involvement of the old-fashioned, 'consanguineous' extended family, the young Community Nurse must depend on the integrity of the nuclear Western family, precariously held together by one 'romantic' marriage relationship.

The record of this key to her 'preventive', 'promotive' and 'curative' goals is not encouraging. The first of these 'independent' generations moved away from intense responsibility for parents; the second has sought to free itself from responsibility for spouse and children.

It would seem that among the first tasks of the Community Nurse is the motivation of positive goals for the ailing family, the strongest bulwark of the community.

New developments highlight the key role and increased responsibility of the Community Psychiatric Nurse. Experimental services auguring well are as follows:

Littlemore Hospital, Oxford conducts a maintenance service for identified chronically ill patients, mostly schizophrenics but including the mentally retarded and geriatric.

The service is the responsibility of a Senior Nursing Officer and operates thus:

	Senior Nursing Officer	Community Nurse
Community psycho-geriatric cases are in the care of 2 charge nurses	Work rehabilitation; execution of vocational guidance recommendations, job placement; industrial liaison is the responsibility of 1 charge nurse	2 'halfway house' hostels, 32 group hostels accommodating former in-patients who cannot live independently. These facilities are the responsibility of 4 charge nurses

Four additional charge nurses are responsible for miscellaneous psychiatric community services, such as out-patient departments, day group-therapy centres, and the interesting concept of *'general practitioner clinics'*. In these clinics Psychiatric Community Nurses, social workers and occupational therapists join with local general practitioners in the conduct of maintenance psychiatric clinics within the community.

The Barnett General Hospital conducts a 24-hour community service for *on-the-spot 'hot' treatment of psychiatric crises*. As a result it claims reduction of admissions to 'a bare minimum'. Research shows the main necessity for admission to depend on the reaction of family members to the patient's difficult behaviour. 'On-the-spot' crisis support frequently enables the family to weather the crisis without institutionalizing the patient.

Crisis teams consist of general practitioners, Community Nurses, and social workers who remain on duty one night in every four.

The organization claims an ability to reach any home in the Oxbury–Barnett area, catering for 200 000 people, within one hour of any emergency call.

Within 24 hours the Community Psychiatric Nurse follows up referrals to specialist agencies. She also regularly visits police stations from which originate many of the crises presented. From her (or in many cases his) community work, the Psychiatric Nurse prepares a consultative *register of persons 'at risk'* for psychiatric illness, mental deficiency or geriatric attention.

Bromley, Kent psychiatric community services have reduced the need for institutional care by extensive use of *nurse–therapists* who are trained in general psychotherapy with special emphasis on behaviour therapy.

Isaac Marks, the psychiatrist responsible for the area, speaks very highly of the competent skills displayed by nurse–therapists especially in dealing with neurotic illnesses.

Throughout, it is readily admitted that delegation of increased responsibility to psychiatrically qualified community nurses has made possible the existence of these important community services. Many nurses operate with only 'remote control' by a psychiatrist.

Nevertheless in the United Kingdom, according to year-round data collected by 'Crisis at Christmas' and published in *Crisis News*, 50% of overnight shelter facilities for the homeless are taken up by the mentally ill. This figure compares with 4% a few years ago, when patients were not prematurely turned out into the community.

Recommendations by the Griffiths Report include:

 (i) the appointment of a government Minister for Community Care;
 (ii) provision of a 'key' worker for each patient — the 'carer' being shared by a defined patient group;
 (iii) one 'leading' social welfare agency, preferably the local health authority, to be responsible for community care in each area.

Emotional support and 'on-site' therapy: Mental Health is every nurses responsibility

The communal role of the psychiatric nurse:

 (a) Essential ability to *identify with the feelings* of patients and relatives stimulates appreciation of the acute emotional suffering which accompanies hospitalization. Indeed, fear of mutilation and depression accompanying surgery often constitutes the patient's major distress area. Failure to provide surgical nursing would be unthinkable, yet succour for emotional suffering is frequently uncatered for or left to chance. Community preparation and support for surgery reduce resistance and suffering.

   'Mental health is every nurse's responsibility. The coronorary thrombosis of today may be the psychiatric patient of tomorrow. Forty per cent of patients in your hospital today could also be classified as suitable for psychiatric hospitalization.'*

 (b) Provision of a 'screening' and psychotherapeutic service, gauging the severity of emotional disturbance, based on assessment of the potency of
   inner personal resources (intelligence; personal philosophy and religious faith; flexibility, optimism, etc.)
   and
   outer resources (familial, hospital and community, financial) available to the patient. Assessment includes reference to the patient's *own image of himself.* At this level the Psychiatric Nurse may either

   (i) request referral to specialist facilities, or
   (ii) 'reach out' to patient and family, rendering assistance at an emotional level meaningful to them.

In this capacity the Psychiatric Nurse intervenes directly, acting as a primary therapist, assessing, planning, implementing and evaluating within the *nursing process.*

---

* Brüwer, Anna Marie. Further inquiries to author.

CHAPTER 11

COPING WITH LIFE'S CRISES—
ERIKSON'S MATURATIONAL CRISES

Definition of crisis

When the strength of frustration blocks is so great that no established adjustment mechanism can contain or channel off biochemical tension-energy, uncontainable anxiety and distress engulf the personality (see p 103ff). Homeostasis is impossible, and the individual is said to be in a state of crisis.

A crisis is thus an internal disturbance or loss of equilibrium resulting from an actual, overwhelmingly stressful event, or a stressful set of circumstances, seen as such a threat.

Typical precipitating events are associated with loss, or threat of loss, including the death of a loved one, divorce, the loss of a job, illness, mutilating surgery, etc.

Crises may be divided into three types, namely: maturational; situational; adventitious.

Erikson identified eight specific stages of development in the human cycle, for each of which he describes a 'psycho-social crisis' marked by conflict between the two poles of the following diagram:

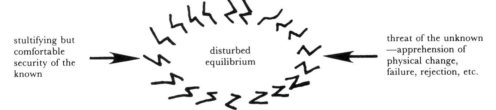

stultifying but comfortable security of the known → disturbed equilibrium ← threat of the unknown —apprehension of physical change, failure, rejection, etc.

Only the resolution of each developmental crisis can lead to that confident and integrated self-image that Erikson calls 'ego identity'.

Maturational crises of infancy and childhood

The following table extracted from Stuart & Sundeen *Principles and Practice of Psychiatric Nursing** summarizes the first four of Erikson's eight developmental stages: Infancy, Toddler years, Early childhood and Middle childhood, and relates them to Havighurst's arrangement of the specific developmental tasks for each stage.

Developmental stage	Erikson's Conflict Crisis Summary	Havighurst's Developmental Tasks
Infancy	*Trust vs mistrust* 1. Oral needs of primary importance 2. Adequate mothering necessary to meet infant's needs 3. Acquisition of hope	1. Learning to walk 2. Learning to take solid foods 3. Learning to talk 4. Learning to control elimination of body wastes

* Stuart, G W & S J Sundeen. *Principles and Practice of Psychiatric Nursing.* 1979. p 108.

Developmental stage	Erikson's Conflict Crisis Summary	Havighurst's Developmental Tasks
Toddler years	*Autonomy vs shame* 1. Anal needs of primary importance 2. Father emerges as important figure 3. Acquisition of will	5. Learning sex differences and sexual modesty 6. Achieving physiological stability 7. Forming simple concepts of social and physical reality 8. Learning to relate oneself emotionally to parents, siblings, and other people 9. Learning to distinguish right and wrong and developing a conscience
Early childhood	*Initiative vs guilt* 1. Genital needs of primary importance 2. Family relationships contribute to early sense of responsibility and conscience 3. Acquisition of purpose	
Middle childhood	*Industry vs inferiority* 1. Active period of socialization for child as he moves from family into society 2. Acquisition of competence	1. Learning physical skills necessary for ordinary games 2. Building wholesome attitudes toward oneself as a growing organism 3. Learning to get along with age-mates 4. Learning an appropriate sex role 5. Developing fundamental skills in reading, writing, and calculating 6. Developing concepts necessary for everyday living 7. Developing conscience, morality, and scale of values 8. Developing attitudes toward social groups and institutions

Identity formation is the 'capacity to synthesise successive identifications into a coherent, consistent and unique whole'.*

Erikson maintains that the *vehicles* by which the eight stages of internal synthesis are reached consist in

(i) *Introjection*—that process by which one unconsciously absorbs unto oneself goals, tension outlets, emotional attitudes, ideals, optimism or pessimism from the people around one (op cit 64).

When the mother–child relationship is felt as secure, supportive, reliable and mutually satisfying, the child develops the *optimistic self-concept required to reach out and take unto himself* those 'love objects' he has introjected from his mother;

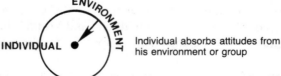

Individual absorbs attitudes from his environment or group

(ii) *identification*, by which the child associates or identifies himself with the goals, standards and attainments of admired parents, and hence, admired peers, teachers and folk-heroes. Through examples set by these 'role models' the individual develops the confidence to reach out and *follow the paths* of personal, social, emotional and sexual fulfillment he has watched them tread.

* Stuart, G W & Sundeen, S J. *Principles and Practice of Psychiatric Nursing.* 1979. p 108.

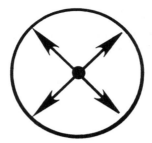

identifies outwards to be absorbed into parental, peer, pupil, social, vocational role models

In each identification he fulfils a particular role as seen from within by himself, and from without by others. At each developmental level his growth task consists not only in achieving

    introjection and
    identification

but also in *bringing together and synthesizing all his roles into a coherent, consistent and unique whole, a process known as identify formation.*

Through a process of *introjection*, interwoven with *identification*, and *role synthesis*, the child who has been allowed to reach out from his mother–child relationship into identification with other love objects, broadens and expands that sense of self which should ultimately develop into 'ego identity'.

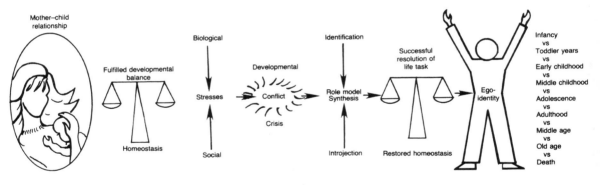

Failure to overcome and reconcile a growth crisis results in a *fixation* (Freud's terminology) or persistent 'hangover', *freezing a specific developmental task in a previous life-stage*, eg a youngster in middle childhood who is still anxiously fixated on defaecation has failed to reconcile Erikson's Autonomy-versus-Shame conflict of the toddler years.

Mastering each developmental task is essential for the successful solution of each maturational crisis. As one proceeds through each life-stage from infancy to death, social and biological *pressures and stressors disturb one's equilibrium*, prevent homeostasis and *precipitate choice crises.* Resolution of these crises imposes *life tasks* which, for an acceptable *'ego identity'*, must be worked out within acceptable *role-models.*

Infantile stressors impeding the formation of self-esteem

Because the infant initially views himself as an extension of his parents, he is very responsive to their own *self-hate* or any *perceived feelings of hatred and rejection* towards himself.

Parental rejection →	uncertainty of self and others	Failure to be → loved	impaired self-love, inability to reach out with love to others
Lack of evidence of recognition and appreciation as a → valuable and important individual	Feelings of inadequacy, discouragement, impaired motivation for independence and responsibility	Over-possessiveness, over-permissiveness, → over-control	Feelings of unimportance, lack of self-esteem
Harsh criticism, punitive behaviour patterns; → unfavourable comparison with a sibling rival	Early feelings of frustration, defeatism; → destructive sense of inadequacy and inferiority; feelings of hopelessness	Internalization of failure as proof of personal incompetence and hence unwillingness to try again	

Sexual identity consists of the image one has of oneself as a male or a female, and one's conviction and satisfaction concerning membership of either sex.

'What does it feel like to be a girl?'
'Do I like being a boy?'

The answers to these questions are built up gradually, from infancy, as the result of

a child's feelings about the female-mother and the male-father; society's ideals of masculinity and femininity, and the advantages of disadvantages pertaining to those ideals →
good, bad, inferior, superior, desirable or undesirable feelings about sexual identity.

These introjected attitudes are passed down from generation to generation and from culture to culture

These identity feelings and society's introjected pattern of inter-sex relationships plus hormonal and genetic differences

→ eg the assertive authoritative 'superior' self-image of the male;

the passive, obedient, dependent image of the female.

Only when the individual has accepted himself as a unique, esteemed personality, apart from, and yet strongly related to others, can he achieve that sense of *healthy identity* that will enable him to participate in genuinely intimate, mature and successful relationships.

Maturational Crises of Adolescence (See also chapter 15)

Because adolescence is essentially a *period of transition*, and thus of internal conflict, it constitutes a critical developmental period for upheaval, change, anxiety and insecurity.

Crisis conflict pivots on decisions regarding ones

Occupation: 'Am I good enough to succeed?'

Peer groups and personal and sexual relations: 'Should I become part of this group or that?'

'Will they accept me?'

'Am I attractive enough to arouse sexual interest?'

'Will I be chosen and succeed in marriage?'

'Do I have the courage of my convictions to stand out as an individual apart from the crowd, yet remaining a member of it?'

'Am I a leader, a follower, or a coward?'

'Am I satisfied with the roles thrust upon me and with those I have chosen?'

The adolescent stands on the threshold of life, one foot in childhood, one in adulthood; the conflict is clear and intense.

It concerns the *establishment of his identity versus the ability to diffuse this identity beyond self and family into the peer group, society, and an intimate, lasting heterosexual relationship.*

	Erikson's Conflict Crisis Summary	Havighurst's Developmental Tasks
Adolescence	*Identity vs identity diffusion* 1. Search for self in which peers play important part 2. Psychosocial moratorium is provided by society 3. Acquisition of fidelity	1. Accepting one's physique and accepting a masculine or feminine role 2. New relations with age-mates of both sexes 3. Emotional independence of parents and other adults 4. Achieving assurance of economic independence 5. Selecting and preparing for an occupation 6. Developing intellectual skills and concepts necessary for civic competence 7. Desiring and achieving socially responsible behaviour 8. Preparing for marriage and family life 9. Building conscious values in harmony with adequate scientific world picture

In self-protection the adolescent becomes involved in a conflict between his search for group acceptance, as opposed to his intolerance of his friends and peers. Group membership comes at a high price, including the submergence of his own identity in ferocious conformity

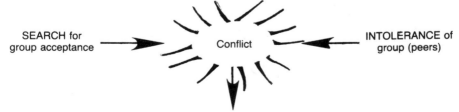

Submergence of own Identity in ferocious conformity

Sexual identity achievement is impeded by →
fears and doubts pertaining to the transition from a same-sex group to heterosexual identity → long-term, intense heterosexual relations

Body image (the way one sees and experiences oneself): *Deviation* from group identity such as small stature in males, and fatness or plainness in girls (danger of anorexia nervosa); advisability of plastic surgery, etc →
physical changes of adolescence symbolize the end of childhood and increase the anxiety accompanying the transition.

'The concept of body-image is central to understanding the *relationship between one's body and one's ego identity*.' The intimacy of this relationship has important implications in the assessment, diagnosis, implementation and evaluation that comprises the Nursing Process.

Typical developmental stressors include:

constant parental intervention which interferes with adolescent choice and exacerbates conflict-stress, disrupting Nature's growth pattern. In our society the necessity for lengthy academic and vocational training elongates this period of parental authority. By comparison, only three or four generations ago our forefathers were marrying in their teens;

parents' own middle-age crisis conflict often evoking distrust in themselves, which, introjected by the adolescent, aggravates his anxiety and distrust of his own decisions →
belittlement of his self-concept → indecision, feelings of nothingness, exasperated impulsiveness.

loss of respect for parents →
the adolescent conflict is aggravated by disagreement on significant issues such as war, peace, race and religion.

peer group stressors, including rigid standards of behaviour →
the adolescent's need to immerse himself in the behaviour and language of his group. But the group's own conflicts and anxiety create a cruel testing ground that may be rejecting and hurtful.

Concept of self → *self-esteem* → *ego-identity*

The frequency with which an individual attains his goals, or alternatively the frequency with which they are frustrated, will determine the structure of his self-esteem and ego-identity.

Maturational Crises of Adulthood

As the individual matures towards adulthood, the self-concept should stabilize, maturity providing a clearer self-picture.

Erikson maintains that conflict-crises of adulthood pivot on the conflict between

Motivation for privacy and independence of decision ——→   vs   ←—— Motivation for intimate association

Developmental stage	Erikson's Conflict Crisis Summary	Havighurst's Developmental Tasks
Adulthood	*Intimacy vs isolation* 1. Characterized by increasing importance of human closeness and sexual fulfilment 2. Acquisition of love	1. Selecting a mate 2. Learning to live with spouse 3. Starting family 4. Rearing children 5. Managing home 6. Getting started in occupation 7. Taking on civic responsibility 8. Finding congenial social group

The adult has learnt to tolerate and accept his own self-deficiencies, and build on his self-strengths. A poor 'ego structure' based on *persistent stressor hangover in previous identity-crises* will inhibit the self-esteem that is necessary for vocational, social and sexual fulfillment.

Typical maturational stressors of adulthood

Stressors upsetting psycho-physiological equilibrium include the loss of a loved one, an unwanted pregnancy, the deaths of parents, illness, marital conflict and divorce, all of which may cause a loss of emotional support and familial role reversal . . . such as the necessity for the wife to assume the breadwinning, decision-making role or the ill husband to assume the passive, dependent role.

Adventitious crises in response to overwhelming environmental stressors (see p 419) include war, floods, etc.

A common stressor in the maturational crisis of adulthood is the persistent 'hangover' of an inability to achieve a *healthy sexual body-image, a strong sexual identity* and a satisfying self-image in the heterosexual relationship. Often specific *sex therapy* is required in order that one may come to feel comfortable and good about one's body. Increased tactile contact with one's body, an educational medical examination of the sex organs, advice concerning techniques for sexual arousal and fulfillment and, above all, an ability to communicate one's sexual needs, problems, satisfactions and pleasures, are all inherent in sex therapy.

Maturational Crises of Middle Age

Most crises of maturity are aggravated by hormonal changes, a decrease in physiological strength, the 'empty nest' and other loss syndromes, threats of emotional isolation, fears of financial insecurity and, as old age looms ahead, death.

	Erikson's Conflict Crisis Summary	Havighurst's Developmental Tasks
Middle age	*Generativity vs self-absorption* 1. Characterized by productivity, creativity, parental responsibility, and concern for new generation 2. Acquisition of care	1. Achieving adult civic and social responsibility 2. Establishing and maintaining economic standard of living 3. Assisting teenage children to become responsible and happy adults 4. Developing adult leisure activities 5. Relating oneself to one's spouse 6. Accepting and adjusting to physiological changes of middle age 7. Adjusting to ageing parents

Specific Stressors of middle age consist in

(i) the transition from physical strength
→ the reduced physical power of the menopause, both

	Male	Female
possible aggravating stressors: →	reduction in sexual potency	hysterectomy
	prostatectomy	breast cancer

→ changes in body size, shape, appearance
→ threaten the body image
diminish the self-concept

(ii) transition from emotional and physical focus of the family constellation to a less central role, necessitating relinquishing of the central nurturing role;
→ 'empty nest' syndrome—feelings of uselessness, isolation;→ threat to ego-identity.

See also below 'The Climateric—The Middle Years' pp 433 et seq.

Maturational Crises of Old Age

	Erikson's Conflict Crisis Summary	Havighurst's Developmental Tasks
Old Age	*Identity vs despair* 1. Characterized by a unifying philosophy of life and a more profound love for mankind 2. Acquisition of wisdom	1. Adjusting to decreasing physical strength and health 2. Adjusting to retirement and reduced income 3. Adjusting to death of spouse 4. Establishing explicit affiliation with age-group 5. Meeting social and civic obligations 6. Establishing satisfactory physical living arrangements

At this developmental stage physical factors constitute a grave threat to the body-image, self-esteem, and ego-identity.
Stressors include:

fear of loss of self-determination,
forced regression to the child role,
emotional isolation,
financial diminishment, and
physical incapacity,

all of which present real and often justified apprehension in the individual.

This is especially true of potentially threatening medical or nursing procedures such as enemas, catheterization, suctioning, dilatation, surgery and restriction of movement. (Fear of Mechanical Invasion of the Body, p 471.)

Above all, when the aged person faces the overwhelming fear and separation of *imminent death, he faces a life crisis without solution!*

Although he chooses seven rather than eight life-stages, no-one since has described the life-roles into which our lifespan forces us better than Shakespeare:*

>   All the world's a stage,
> And all the men and women merely players;
> They have their exits and their entrances;
> And one man in his time plays many parts,
> His acts being seven ages. At first the infant,
> Mewling and puking in the nurse's arms;
> Then the whining school-boy, with his satchel
> And shining morning face, creeping like snail,
> Unwillingly to school. And then the lover,
> Sighing like furnace, with a woeful ballad
> Made to his mistress' eyebrow. Then a soldier,
> Full of strange oaths, and bearded like the pard,
> Jealous in honour, sudden and quick in quarrel,
> Seeking the bubble reputation
> Even in the cannon's mouth. And then the
>   justice,
> In fair round belly with good capon lin'd,
> With eyes severe and beard of formal cut,
> Full of wise saws and modern instances;
> And so he plays his part. The sixth age shifts
> Into the lean and slipper'd pantaloon,
> With spectacles on nose and pouch on side;
> His youthful hose, well sav'd, a world too wide
> For his shrunk shank; and his big manly voice,
> Turning again toward childish treble, pipes
> And whistles in his sound. Last scene of all,
> That ends this strange eventful history,
> Is second childishness and mere oblivion;
> Sans teeth, sans eyes, sans taste, sans everything.

* *As You Like It* II, vii

CHAPTER 12

PRINCIPLES OF CHILD DEVELOPMENT

(with special reference to motor, intellectual and cognitive development)

Among pioneers in the methodical, scientific study of child development were Terman, Merrill, Goodenough, Gesell, Jersild and Piaget. It was their work which provided the initial data for the construction of reliable developmental scales based on the *norm or average attainment* in various skills at each age-level.

A developmental skill which could be successfully completed by 50% of the standardization group was accepted as the norm for the task in question.

An important scientific pioneer in the field of child development was Dr Arnold Gesell, late Professor Child Development at Yale University, who is the 'patron saint' of child development. His careful, scientific study of thousands of children in his famous glass-walled 'one-way vision rooms', in their homes, schools, playgrounds, led Gesell to the presentation of a comprehensive set of norms. These norms indicate the various age levels at which the mythical statistically 'average' child reaches significant 'milestones' in:

Motor Development, eg at 2 years 50% of the sample showed central nervous system myelination sufficient to achieve voluntary control of bladder and bowel sphincters.

Personal Social Insight, eg it was not until 12 months that 50% of Gesell's sample realized themselves to be mentally and physically separate personalities from their mothers; it was not until 5 years that 50% of his sample could play co-operatively at the kindergarten level.

Language Skills, eg at 3 years 50% of the sample had begun constructing sentences from separate words.

Adaptive Behaviour, eg at 12 months 50% of his sample realized that in order to reach a raised object it was necessary to adopt a standing position.

Over the years Gesell's norms have encountered considerable criticism from those who feel that strict adherence to fixed standards does not allow for normal *individual differences* in development, causing unnecessary anxiety and burdensome pressure for conformity.

A mature, balanced appraisal of norms allows them to have both *uses* and *abuses*.

Use of norms

1. To gauge readiness for new activity, eg at what age a child is ready to start feeding himself.

2. To reassure parents that while certain attainment may seem slow to them, it is well within Nature's normal range.

3. To re–orientate those parents, teachers and nurses who, by expecting too much, are putting undue strain on children. Norms, sensibly used, should enable us to avoid efforts to force the child's development, or to impose tasks and obstacles

which, being beyond his powers, may produce irritation and resistance. In contrast, at a later stage, these tasks would be undertaken with interest, eg realization that most children are not ready to achieve daytime urinary sphincter control until at least 20 months avoids premature pressure, frustration and rebellion, allowing for a favourable attitude at the appropriate developmental stage.

Abuse of norms

The development of too rigid a set of expectations: norms should be interpreted in a wide sense. There are wide individual differences within the norm. Provided a child's development in most spheres is not far outside normal limits there is no need for the mother or nurse to become anxious.

Specific Principles of Child Development

1. *The developmental milestones of each child vary relative to the group*, eg one child learns to walk at 12 months, another at 18 months. Both lie within the wide limits of a sensible norm. By 2 years they will be equally skilful, the observer not being able to distinguish which child walked first.

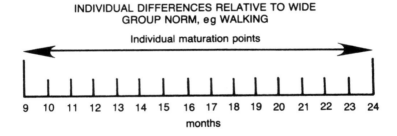

INDIVIDUAL DIFFERENCES RELATIVE TO WIDE
GROUP NORM, eg WALKING

Individual maturation points

9 10 11 12 13 14 15 16 17 18 19 20 21 22 23 24
months

Within the broad limits of the norm, each child has his or her own individual rate of maturation in each skill.

'*Maturation* denotes the process of ripening, of moving towards complete or mature development. It denotes not only change in physical characteristics, but also in function, in the capacity to perform or behave, that becomes possible through changes in the physical characteristics of any part of the organism' (Jersild in Child Psychology). Prentice-Hall, New York).

The child does not become ready for a given activity at one particular day or hour; rather his behaviour is influenced by many variables such as physical strength, stimulation, opportunity to develop and learn, awakening interest, etc.

Given opportunity for learning, each skill will blossom forth spontaneously at its own maturation point.

2. *The developmental milestones of each child vary relative to the child's own individual, inborn ability pattern*, ie each child has within him his own inborn pattern of development for each skill; and these skills vary one unto another.

He may, for instance, be relatively quick to learn to talk, but slow to learn to feed himself.

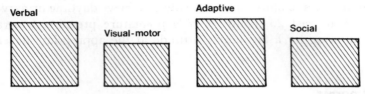

It is only when the majority pattern is depressed that the possibility of pathological development requires investigation by specialists in this field (paediatricians, neurologists, clinical psychologists, etc).

3. *Throughout development two factors are at work, namely maturation and learning.* Both are interdependent, being separable only for academic discussion.

Growth depends largely on:

(a) The child's own inborn pattern of readiness, or his maturation pattern. The process of growth is linked with the spontaneous blossoming forth of each skill in accordance with individual genetic programming.

The blossoming of maturation point for a particular skill is the optimum moment for exposing the child to:

(b) Learning, ie stimulation, encouragement and opportunity for practice.

Thus learning nurtures nature's inborn maturation pattern and growth can only take place in the presence of both maturation and learning.

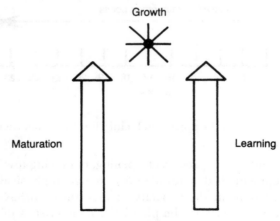

Until the relevant blossoming point in the child's maturity pattern is reached, stimulation and encouragement will be of no avail. Similarly *repression of learning* opportunity *at the time of blossoming* misses nature's optimum learning point and inhibits growth.

At maturation point the child is motivated by an internal drive to concentrate all his efforts on acquiring a new skill. Later, at a point where nature has designed the organism for concentration on the maturation of some other skill, attempts to artificially introduce a formerly stifled skill may meet with emotional resistance due to lack of interest on the part of the child, and clumsiness due to his having 'overshot the mark' and reached an inappropriate stage of co-ordination. His body is now designed for the learning of some other skill. It is easy for the 4-year-old to learn to swim, but difficult for the 12-year-old, whose body is poised for another stage of development. We should thus be careful not to hamper the sick child's development of skills.

The 1-year-old, right-handed child who, for orthopaedic reasons, must have his right hand immobilized at just that time when nature has decreed that he is ripe for learning to feed himself, will encounter difficulty in acquiring the same skill at 3 years old. His interests and muscular co-ordination are now mobilized for skills other than eating. It is thus wise, especially in the case of long-term hospitalization, to try to gear ward activities to patients' maturation points and opportunities for the practice thereof, rather than to irrelevant, merely time-saving ward routine.

4. *Development is cyclical; it does not proceed in an uninterrupted upward gradient.*

Cyclic Development

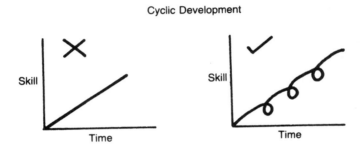

Thus a child may 'improve' in a skill for a few days and then 'backslide', before achieving permanent progress, eg a child may achieve urinary sphincter control for a few days, and then appear to 'lose' this skill before showing more reliable control. Clearly children (and parents) should not be made to feel guilty or anxious about inevitable backsliding; rather should they be reassured that nature, and not 'laziness', is responsible for the cyclical character of the eventually upward developmental gradient.

5. *As the child develops there is a spontaneous impulse to put into use, to practise to perfection, his newly learnt skills,* eg when the mechanics of creeping have been established, he will creep of his own accord, even if there is nothing external, such as a toy, to lure him from one spot to another. Once he starts, there is an impulse to go on practising his new skill over and over again until he has reached perfection. This can be an irritation, especially in the hospital ward, as in the case of the child who insists on practising his newly found skill in drawing faces all over the bed-linen and wall above his head. Clearly one should work with nature, giving him plenty of paper and crayons as an acceptable substitute medium for the expression of his inborn need to practise to perfection.

To stifle this inborn urge is to interfere with the unfolding of nature's developmental pattern. Constant interference with these patterns, usually for the sake of expediting ward routine, is one cause of that general retardation of growth in hospitalized children to which reference has been made in chapters 2 and 13.

6. *Development proceeds in a cephalo-caudal, ie head to tail direction*, eg in propelling himself along the floor the child's shoulders and hands have become efficient and strong, but he still drags helpless legs and feet behind him.

By a year he may be able meaningfully to verbalize several words, while still having no control over his urinary and anal sphincters.

Because the cells comprising the sacral area of the central nervous system only become myelinated, and thus voluntary, from about chronological age 18 months, 'toilet training' before this time is both fruitless and ill advised. Premature and *pressurized 'toilet training'* may well disrupt the important mother-child relationship. The child may either—

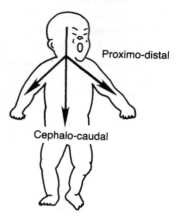

CHILD DEVELOPMENT

Proximo-distal

Cephalo-caudal

(a) become resentful, angry, hostile and un-willing to please his mother by confor-mity, or

(b) he may 'give in'.

Lacking anatomical equipment for anal and later urinary control, and thus unable to please his all-important mother figure, he may feel anxious and guilty. In an effort to 'win back' mother's approval, he becomes *anxious and obsessive about cleanliness*. He may even reach the stage where, in tense anxiety to avoid contact with those 'dirty' faeces which 'disgust' mother, he is not even able to relax sufficiently to defecate in, and thus 'dirty' the 'potty', with resultant distressing toileting accidents. He over-denies normal sensuous satisfactions. In his anxiety to win approval by cleanliness, he may develop the obsessive traits inherent in reaction formation (see Mental Mechanisms chapter 5). 'Bending over backwards' to prove himself absolutely clean 'in thought, mind and deed', he may grow up into the type of person who is continually compelled to wash his hands, disinfect, indulge in ritualistic, perfectionist procedures, demand perfection in himself and others, carrying though his life the heavy burden of cleanliness and perfection compulsions.

7. *Development process in a proximo-distal (from central outwards to extremeties) direction*, eg the centrally placed mouth is skilled at birth, long before fingers become reliably co-ordinated. Thus a verbally quick 6-year-old may be talking, reading and adding efficiently, yet be unable to execute those finer, more delicate, smaller finger movements involved in wielding a pencil.

Ignorance of this developmental principle often leads teachers to misinterpret nature's pattern as voluntarily dirty, grubby and untidy pencil work, thus stifling self-expression and developing fearful avoidance associations to the school situation in general.

8. *Perceptual and motor reactions proceed from the general to the specific.* The neonate experiences hunger-pain as a generalized pain, and the pleasurable sensation of his mother's caress as generalized pleasure—it takes several years for perceptual and motor experiences to 'specialize out' into specific isolated reactions.

In fact, even in adulthood, one tends under stress of strong sensation or emotional disturbances to regress to inability to isolate out and thus deal constructively with feelings of pain, anger, fear, etc. Regressing, he is swamped by pain. (See Pain, chapter 21.)

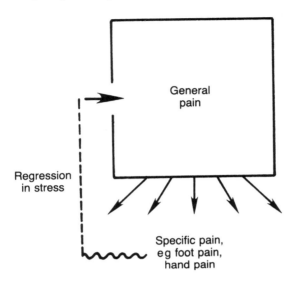

9. *'Every hurdle a hazard, every gain at a price.'* A gain in power does not always mean a gain in composure. The more a child can do for himself, the more there is for him to do. This leads to added frustration in the hospital ward. However, every effort should be made to move with the child's development, thus avoiding artificial, but permanent thwarting of his personality. (See Erikson's Maturational Crises, chapter 11.)

Sometimes this conflict between security and gain demands considerable ingenuity and flexibility of ward routine. In the past, one often encountered long-term patients who had not passed school examinations because the ward staff had not made provision for the expression of increasing intellectual development. In order to acquire an arbitrary 10 or 11 hours' sleep, children in Form II or III were required to put off the lights at 19h30. There being no facilities for night-time homework or examination 'swotting', these children almost invariably failed their examinations and lost their incentive and drive. Physically handicapped and intellectually stunted, they were doomed to a marginal existence based on the pattern of passive behaviour they had learnt during long-term hospitalization.

10. *Persistence of immature behaviour patterns.* It sometimes happens that a youngster, instead of progressing according to his inborn pattern of development retains, like cumbersome excess luggage, an old, outworn way of behaviour, even though a new 'streamlined' way would be more appropriate, eg a child who has undergone long-term orthopaedic treatment, and thus been over-protected, may retain the habit of dependency appropriate to a younger chronological age, shrinking from an effort to strike out for himself.

A child who feels (due to lack of contact with mother during his hospitalization) that she has deserted him in his time of need, may cling to her like a frightened baby at that stage when he should be ready to leave her side to start kindergarten.

Developmental stressors encountered in the first years of life

Probably the most important features of the first years of life are:

(a) The child's phenomenal physical growth, with corresponding dramatic increase in adaptive, co-ordinative, verbal and social skills.

The average new-born child is about 50 cm long. During the first year his length increases by over a third, and by the age of 5 years he will have doubled his birth length.

At no other time in his life-span will his proportionate physical development approach this 'all-time high'.

(b) The enormous pressure brought to bear upon him to realize that he is no longer a happy little parasite, but just one of the human community. He must learn to postpone the pleasures of eating, eliminating, continual fondling, dawdling and many other self-gratifications.

In the normal hustle and bustle of even a well-organized household, it is often the all-important mother figure who is obliged to deprive him, causing him to develop real feelings of *hate* towards her: but in the love periods of his *ambivalence* (love-hate swing) he may feel guilty and anxious about his hostility towards her. He dreads lest, as a punishment, she will abandon him. So, seeking reassurance, he clings to her and, at 2 or 3 years, responds especially bad to separation in hospital.

At best, even in the context of easy-going, reasonably graduated demands, and a loving, rewarding and supportive mother–child relationship, he will sometimes find these frustrations hard to bear and burdensome. His reactions being naturally primitive and generalized, frustration-tension will sometimes explode in temper-tantrums. However, in the long run he will learn for himself that personal frustration is an evil necessity if one is to receive the greater rewards of love and acceptance. A temper tantrum is a natural, developmentally appropriate tension outlet that is better ignored than punished.

At worst, in the context of harsh, rigid demands, punishment, a cold, unresponsive mother figure, or no mother figure at all, he may come to hate the world and everyone in it.

As Goldfarb, Harlow, and others have shown (see p 47), having no incentive to conformity, he may grow up void of patterns of conformity, irresponsible, insecure, without love and gentleness. Much research has shown the first few years of life are very important to later development. The child subjected to unreasonable developmental demands may grow up hating and resenting his fellow creatures, unable to make the sacrifices involved in conformity and doomed to a life of emotional isolation, rejection and regrets.

Every child wants to grow up—he wants to be good, accepted and successful. Within the context of reasonable parental example and a developmentally orientated, stimulating, loving, accepting environment, he can usually be trusted to develop healthy in mind and body, free of need for Fight-aggression, or

Flight-escape into fantasy, alcohol, or drugs or reaction formation in crippling obsessions.

It would appear that much truth lies in the old Yorkshire adage on child-rearing: 'Have them, love them, and leave them be.'

Specific development in the first two years of life

In that it is difficult to conceive of improving upon them, the classic developmental tables compiled by Dr Arnold Gesell at Yale University are quoted below in full. Readers wishing to study Years III to V are referred to Gesell's book *The First Five Years of Life* (Harper).

THE ONE-YEAR-OLD

Visual-motor and intellectual (adaptive) development	Verbal	Social	Emotional
Milestones: *Head* erect— 12–16 weeks. *Hands:* By 1 year. Can hold cup himself. Likes to eat with his fingers. Starting to spoon feed himself. *Bowel* control may sometimes occur, but may resist potty. (Should not be forced.) Likes to practise *walking* with hand held. 12–18 months —standing unaided. 18–24 months —walking unaided. Can handle single 'fitting-in' toys and enjoys put and take games with an adult. *Eyes:* ±4 weeks eyes begin to focus to moving objects; 0–12 weeks sees inverted and blurred. 12 weeks, vision upright.	By 1 year correctly says 'Mama' and 'Dada' and a few other words.	Beginning to realize that he is a separate personality apart from his mother. Defining his individual status by saying *no* even about things he really likes. Likes to watch other children playing but not yet ready to play with them. Social inter-course with familiar adults, e g being chased, hiding. Suspicious of strangers at first meeting. Warms up gradually if not rushed.	The world is beginning to make its demands upon him. He must endure post-ponement of his satisfactions. Attempts at bowel control may add to feelings of frustration. He requires support, approval, love which make him a more self-sufficient person. Too much stress or over-protection lead to aggression, undisciplined behaviour, bullying *or* undue submission, excessive docility. In any case child must learn to adjust to his ambiva-lence towards his mother. Guilt feelings may lead to dreadful fear of desertion or withdrawal of love.

THE TWO-YEAR-OLD

Visual-motor and intellectual (adaptive) development	*Verbal*	*Sexual*	*Social*	*Emotional*
Still wet in the morning even if 'picked up' during the night. Day-time bowel and bladder control fairly reliable —occasional stool. Finger paints, clay, etc possible legitimate substitute, outlet for sensory satisfaction.

Dressing:

Can put arms into armholes, feet into socks. Likes to imitate mother. 'Helps' in the housework, runs errands etc.

Play:

Builds tower of 6–7 cubes. Likes to play with action toys, trains, toy telephones. Likes rhythmic patterns. Enjoys painting, clay. Likes to feed himself, still spills a lot. Helps wash himself in bath.

END OF 2nd YEAR:

Achieving elimination control. (Proud of success, upset by failure.) Girls may achieve night dryness. | Vocabulary growing rapidly, Refers to self by name. Uses 3-word sentences. Recites short rhymes, sings parts of songs but little sense of tune. Likes to point to and name objects in picture books.

By end of 2nd year can stand on one leg, cross feet on demand. | In investigating his body, is discovering anatomy of sex organs. If mother is pregnant it is wise to tell child baby is growing inside her. | Continuing efforts at self-definition. May say *no* to almost every request. Occasional temper tantrum. Enjoys playing *near* but not with another child. Relishes rough and tumble play. Grabs other children's toys but refuses to share his own. Some children find it hard to be with both parents at once. Finds it hard to separate from family at night, and hard to fall asleep. Many demands. May come out of his room. | Very affectionate towards mother. Frequently whines and clings to her. Upset if member of family (especially mother) is absent for a few days, or if family moves to another place. Relishes water play—probably a relief from demands of toilet control. Both jealous and loving towards new baby—ambivalence. |

Of special interest to nurses is the 'Stormy Six-Year-Old'. Year VI is a year of rapidly developing powers and new horizons. The 6-year-old is learning of danger situations more quickly than experience can eliminate corresponding fears. Thus Year VI is marked by anxiety, fear of death, hypochondria and conflict between participation in the adventure of living and the search for retreat into mother's arms. (See Erikson's mid-childhood growth conflict, p 246.)

Latest trends in child development

The emphasis of modern developmental psychology, indeed its greatest scientific strength, has been objective observation, description and measurement.

The undoubted master of this approach was Arnold Gesell of Yale. As a reliable 'rule of thumb' guideline and source of reassurance to over-ambitious and otherwise anxious mothers. Gesell's developmental charts are unsurpassed.

However, they *lack that dynamic quality, those answers to the 'whys' and 'wherefores'* which the fast developing science of child psychology has demanded with increasing insistence during the past twenty years.

Age trends are valuable but not enough.

The evolution of World War II was a great social tragedy, the Nazi régime representing the most terrible regression to barbarism which has ever befallen mankind. The international 'soul searching' and new evaluation of human relations which followed this holocaust contributed to the post-war predominance of research into socialization and personality—to the work of Bowlby, Spitz, Levy and Goldfarb. These studies, as later epitomized by Harlow, continue to constitute valuable and fruitful areas of research and practice.

In 1957 scientists of the West were 'caught on the wrong foot' when Russia's Sputnik blazed new trails into space, technology and man's vision of the universe. The financially powerful public of the Unites States now joined pioneers in psychology and education *in questioning the utilization of their country's intellectual resources.* Public and educational bodies began an intensive drive to improve educational and social facilities for the culturally deprived. New plans for educational programming provided incentive for better understanding of the dynamic *cognitive processes*—perception, learning, thinking, language ability, concept formation, techniques of problem solving and creativity.

Of major importance were the questions of *deprivation* and *stimulation* of these cognitive processes. Investigations have gained in breadth, scope, rigor, system and ingenuity.

In an effort to release and exploit these *innate* intellectual qualities, United States educationalists (the recognized spearhead of Western child psychology) are swerving away from confining emphasis on learning-theory and psycho-analytic explanations, in which *environmental* events are the main determinants of response. The work of Piaget and other cognitive theorists who believe that psychological development is primarily *self-generating*, being set in motion by inborn drives towards overcoming the challenges of the intellectual and concrete environments, is now attracting attention.

The work of Piaget, eminent contemporary Swiss developmental psychologist

Piaget, who died in 1982, believed the child's future does not depend on what happens *to* him but rather on his *own activity* within his environment.

Of primary importance is stimulation of the child's own curiosity, searching and problem solving. He must interpret his environment in his own way.

CHANGING DEVELOPMENTAL CONCEPTS

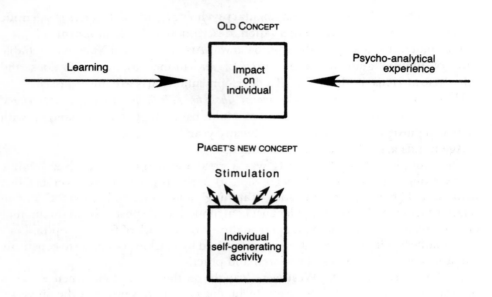

How does his innate development proceed? Is his developmental pattern continuous by gradual regular increment, or discontinuous, in sudden jags and jumps or is it 'sticklike', divided into stages, initiated by dramatic growth spurts?

Piaget favours *the stage pattern* established by other schools of thought.

Each stage involves a period of:

1.　Formation.
2.　Genesis.
3.　Attainment.

This process is characterized by *progressive organization* of *cognitive ability*.

Stage No 1: Sensorimotor Stage

(Chronological Age 0–18 months)

The infant learns and expresses himself through sensory-motor experience.

This stage occurs prior to language usage when intelligence is manifested in *action*; eg a 1-year-old, desiring to hold a toy placed on a rug, will pull the toy to him. This is interpreted by Piaget as a sign of intelligence in the form of an *action-concept or a generalized response* to the variety of problems to be overcome.

Assimilation is the incorporation of a new stimulus or object into an existing schema (or mental image), interpreting it in relation to something he already knows; eg the new concept of a train may be assimilated into the original concept of a car. There is no significant difference between the train and the car.

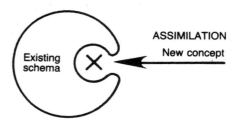

New conceptions or new knowledge may thus be distorted in order to fit into the child's existing organization of his world.

Accommodation, in opposition to assimilation, is the tendency to amend, change, or accommodate a schema in order that it may meaningfully cater for the new object.

ACCOMMODATION

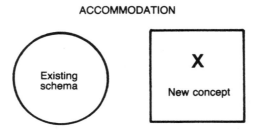

For example, a 2-year-old, exposed for the first time to a telephone, will in the first place try absorbing it into his established schemata, acting towards it as towards a familiar object, attempting to taste, bang, bounce or throw it. However, once he realizes the unique properties of the telephone he will develop a new schema of action to cover the concept of telephones.

The resolution of tension

The resolution of tension between

Assimilation using old response systems for new situation, and

Accommodation acquiring new concept systems to fit new stimuli

constitutes intellectual growth or adaptation to new situations

(See Erikson's growth conflict theory, p 245 et seq.)

Stage No 2: The Pre-operational Stage

(Chronological Age 18 months to 7 years)

Because by this stage the child has language, he is now able to handle not only overt physical actions and things, but he also understands *meanings* of objects and events.

His schema now consists of a *symbolic unit—one object* standing for a similar *object*. He is able to use the box as if it were a lorry, moving it around to an appropriate carlike noise.

Piaget presents an illustration of a child treating a doll as if it were a living baby.

One should, however, note that although the child is now using one object as a symbol of another, he is *still essentially dealing with objects*. Objects and their symbol-units cluster around the child's *personal usage* rather than around their own classification 'set'. Involuntarily, he is the centre of his object universe. He cannot symbolically visualize or classify the world, the room, the toy, as organized and conceptualized by another person; thus Piaget describes the pre-operational child as 'egocentric' in his perspective.

Still bound to individual objects (and their individual symbolic units) he is as yet unable to categorize or classify. Definition of common characteristics comes later.

Stage No 3: The Stage of Concrete Operations

(Chronological Age 7-12 years)

The child now begins to be 'operational'. He now possesses:

(1) *Mental representation of a series of actions*. It is true that our 5-year-old could walk three blocks from his home to the shop. However, he was not yet able to map his path with a pencil and paper.

He remembered a series of concrete actions but he was as yet unable to carry an *abstract mental representation of the entire integrated sequence*. Thus mental representation appears for the first time at CA 7 to 12 years.

(2) *Conservation*. He now knows that objects *conserve* their characteristics in different forms and that the measurements are constant for different objects. The child now knows that solids and liquids undergo a shape transformation without changing volume and mass. He knows that the same piece of plasticine can be used to make a sausage or a potato. The quantity of plasticine is *conserved*. He can verbalize that the sausage is wider, but thinner. 'Look', he says, 'I can make the potato out of the sausage again.'

He also realizes that

$$6 = \begin{matrix} 00 \\ 00 \\ 00 \end{matrix} \text{ or } \begin{matrix} 000 \\ 000 \end{matrix}$$

(3) *Relational terms*. The *'operational'* child has insight into relativity—he understands such terminology as prettier, dirtier, sister of, cat of.

    degree: pretty, prettier, prettiest
    space: left of
    consanguinity: cousin of.

(4) *Class inclusion*. He can now reason simultaneously about part and whole, eg four white balls and six green balls make a total of 10 ball objects. He now knows that both number concepts refer to the classification 'balls'. Balls now belong to their classification rather than to his centrifugal world.

(5) *Serialization*. He now possesses the ability to arrange objects according to a quantity dimension such as weight, size or length, eg blocks of different size. This serialization of number relations is a cornerstone of arithmetical ability.

Stage No 4: The Stage of Formal Operations

(Chronological Age 12 years upwards)

Operational thinking proceeds. The adolescent is capable of:

(1) Considering the various ways in which a problem may be solved and the possible forms a variable may assume, eg symbolic *x* of algebra or the best way of plotting a graph. Asked what could account for an abandoned car found halfway between Beaufort West and Hanover, he is able to *generate* or evaluate all the possible solutions.

(2) *Directing purposeful deduction to problems*, scientific and otherwise: He can evaluate hypothetical propositions, discriminating the possible from the impossible, eg 'I have three sisters, Mary, Ellen and myself'.

What is wrong with this?

He is able to work with, and to think through, the impossible as if it were real.

He is able to accept the statement as impossible nonsense, at the same time explaining in rational terms why it is impossible.

(3) *Using abstract rules to solve a whole classification of problems*, eg Application of Archimedes' Principle to a whole classification of appropriate problems.

He is able to combine the separate processes of addition, subtraction, multiplication and division into a more complex algebraic equation and *understands the general principle underlying the process*.

These complex units are termed *combinative structures* and involve the discriminatory ability *to generalize from specific experience*.

It will be noted that Piaget's theory of self-generated, adaptive, problem-solving behaviour, proceeding in harmony with the child's stages of physiological development, is not altogether a new one.

We have seen how in the late 1940s Piaget himself, Jersild and others were stressing the *primary importance of inborn maturation or blossoming points*. Given opportunities for practice and learning it is these inborn maturation points which, within wide individual differences, initiate learning.

Piaget assigns an important role to the infant's motor activity, implying that a normally endowed child who could not use his arms and legs would encounter great difficulty in intellectual growth.

Mussen, Conger & Kagan in *Child Development and Personality* advise caution in generalizing thus. These authors suggest that Piaget's disciples investigate the indispensability of motor activity by studying the cognitive, intellectual growth of thalidomide babies.

Certainly Piaget's principle of primary *self-generating activity and problem-solving* is an important one in planning programmes by which the underprivileged child may overcome his environmental limitations. It constitutes the basic principle determining programming in the Head Start Project sponsored by the United States Office of Education, and designed to raise the educational level of economically and culturally deprived children.

Can enriched training programmes, if applied early, offset inborn cognitive deficiencies? In the opinion of Mussen, Conger & Kagan 'the available data permit cautious optimism'.

In the context of intensive efforts by nursery school teachers, motivated parents, social workers and community workers, together with much individual attention, it is possible to overcome some of the adverse effects of early deprivation.

CHAPTER 13

THE EMOTIONAL EFFECTS
OF ILLNESS UPON CHILDREN

Children enjoy being active. They like to be free to explore the world. They enjoy using their bodies. They like to feel strong.

For the child sickness means entering a strange, frightening, sad and uncomfortable world. No one likes pain, but a child finds it harder to bear than an adult. Usually he does not understand his illness; his time concepts are immature and he fears that the pain will never go away. His confusion and his fears may be increased if he has a high fever and frightening dreams. Fear, tension, and hence (via the Sympathetic Nervous System) biochemical tension-energy, increase his physical symptoms. *Removing him from the comfort, reassurance and love of his parents' presence when he needs them most is a powerful aggravating factor.* He may express his fears and discomfort by becoming irritable, demanding or regressing to babyish overdependence and lack of self-control. He does not know how to reassure himself, and wants somebody else to reassure him.

Hospitalization ('Hospitalism', the classic detrimental effect of hospitalization and other institutionalization on personality development is detailed on pp 46-47)

A hospital is a lonely place, especially for children. Its very cleanliness and efficiency, its lack of casual disorder and comfortable untidiness, deprive it of intimacy and warmth. Gone are all the child's playthings, his precious possessions, his familiar surroundings, his companions, and still in so many cases his parents' comforting presence. The doctors and nurses, although friendly, are extremely busy. Undoubtedly, the most difficult aspect of hospitalization is the uprooting of the child from his secure family life. A stay in hospital can be a frightening and confusing experience for a child. In discussing the Mal-effects of Maternal Deprivation upon Personality Development (p 44) reference was made to Spitz's film 'Grief'. The findings of these individual film records were confirmed and summarized by Robertson (1970), who reported thus on the behaviour of hospitalized children aged 6 months to 4 years:

1. The Initial Protest ('Fight') Phase during which the child, bewildered by his mother's disappearance, cries loudly, pulls at the bars of his cot and throws himself around in desperate frustration.
    This phase may last from hours to days.

2. The Middle Phase of Despair which may be mistaken for 'settling down'. The child gives up hope—he weeps quietly, is apathetic and withdrawn. He retreats to fantasy compensation or depression. He is, in fact, mourning the loss of his mother.

3.   The Final Phase of Denial, when the child may appear more responsive to his environment and may even appear fairly happy—in reality this is the phase of repression of anger, distrust, rejection, guilt and anxiety.*

However, hospitalization *is* sometimes unavoidable, and much can be done to alleviate its unpleasantness and trauma.

Preparation for hospitalization

Parents should be truthful to the child who has to go to hospital. Transporting him to a strange building and, without warning, handing him over to strangers in his time of greatest need can be a terrifying experience. *He is apt to feel betrayed and abandoned by his parents, and to regard all adults, including the hospital staff, as his enemies* against whom he has to defend himself. His resentment, and sense of abandonment by his parents, may cause long-term distrust and doubts of his parents' love for him, thus affecting the precious parent–child relationship. If his parents have at some time made the mistake of threatening illness as a punishment for lack of co-operation, he may even feel that his hospitalization is some sort of punishment—guilt thus increasing his anxiety and tension.

He should be told that he is going to hospital, and why this is necessary, in simple terms that will satisfy his natural concern over what is going to happen to him. He should be told what to expect of ward geography and routine, of nurses, doctors and fellow-patients. He may have to stay in bed all the time, but he is going to hospital so that he can get well quickly.

To lie about the expected length of his stay is an ill-advised effort to console him. If the doctor is sure of the expected length of hospitalization, the child should be told that he will have to stay 'about' that number of days. If the doctor is uncertain, he should be told that his parents honestly do not know how long the treatment will take, but he will go home as soon as the doctor is sure that he is well enough to do so.

He should not, of course, be told of impending hospitalization too long in advance—in the absence of a specific preparation programme a day or two is usually sufficient.

The paediatric department of Charing Cross Hospital, London, places great value on its *play specialists*, whose role includes:

> pre-admission preparation—puppets illustrate what hospital will be like—what the doctors and nurses will do to make Tommy better—He is reassured that his parents will be with him and his brothers and sisters will visit him.

Billy hand-puppet, all soft and cuddly, introduces him to his fellow-patients, nurses, doctors, ward maids and all his new friends.

In teaching nursing students the late Dr Hugh Jolly (1983), described how a play specialist, trained on a unique course in Holland, had, within an hour, prepared a young child for a double leg amputation through telling the story of Johnny puppet, whose legs were so sore that he'd rather get rid of them and buy new, strong toy legs. Then he was able to run and play much better than on his own sore and broken legs.

'I don't know what we would have done without that girl that day!'

---

* Robertson, J. *Young Children in Hospital*. London: Tavistock.

In the film 'To Prepare a Child', produced by the Washington Children's Hospital, Washington DC, USA, participants are children preparing for elective surgery as well as nursery school children who were invited to an amended community outreach programme.

'The *objectives* of a good programme should include:

— assisting the child in the expression of his feelings generated by hospitalization
— increasing the child's knowledge of what is happening to him
— making use of *anticipatory anxiety*
— reducing complications
— enabling the child to return home with a positive feeling towards the hospital and his parents (Kaplan, 1980) . . .'*

The programme

The chid for elective admission is introduced to the programme on a date prior to admission. He is welcomed by the child care worker on duty, who gives him a name tag, while his mother fills in an attendance register. The patient, where possible, is introduced to other patients who are to undergo similar procedures. The child care worker, by means of toy models, demonstrates who doctors and nurses are and shows that mum can be in the ward too. The children are then given a puppet show where procedures such as taking of blood and anaesthesia are emphasized. They are also shown slides and flipcharts of hospital situations and encouraged to dress up in gowns, masks and caps.

'Just because the doctors and nurses wear masks, it doesn't mean they are angry with you—they can't smile with their mouths, so they smile with their eyes instead.'

The children are encouraged to talk to each other. Parents have the opportunity to ask nursing staff and child care workers questions. Siblings are allowed to attend this part of the programme, but only patients and parents are permitted to attend a tour of the wards to which they are to be admitted.

On return from the tour, and before leaving, each patient is given a specially designed colouring-in book of hospital scenes, a syringe, mask and theatre cap to take home. This enables the effectiveness of the programme to be taken into the home . . .

Follow-up

After eventual admission and surgery children are visited post-operatively, wherever possible, by the child-care worker who conducted their particular preparation programme. She also offers *support to the parents at the time of the surgical procedure* as they wait in the specially allocated waiting area adjacent to the theatres. If the design of the theatres permits, parents should accompany their children into

* Kaplan, D. When young children face surgery: The effectiveness of a pre-operative preparation programme for the patient and his family. Unpublished thesis. For further details refer to author.

induction and recovery areas. This allows the child *to go to sleep and wake up* in the presence of loved and familiar faces.

Open visiting hours and rooming-in facilities for mothers also contribute to improved quality of management of hospitalized children. Among the advantages young nurses 'introject' mothering behaviour. Siblings are allowed to visit in some areas. This is an area which requires some consideration, especially for children who spend long periods in hospital.

That pre-operative preparation results in reduction of distress and trauma is a widespread qualitative observation. Among scientific assessment studies is that of Visentainer & Wolfer,* who demonstrated that systematic preparation and support increased patient co-operation and decreased behaviour problems and post-hospital trauma: reduced anxiety, improved communication and total patient care.

Favourable results warrant special efforts to accommodate working parents and those from lower socio-economic groups who do not always enjoy transport facilities.

While one certainly lauds and encourages such preparation programmes, one should also be alert to 'split-off' between *intellectual-level* play-play and *emotional-level* reaction to *reality*, pain, surgical 'invasion', physical restraints and some degree of maternal deprivation. One should blame neither the child nor the parent nor oneself when faced with emotional trauma in spite of preparation programmes. *In the final analysis it is parental presence and support that are the child's greatest comfort and source of security.*

Handling of surgery and other psychologically traumatic procedures

Children, like adults, experience mutilation anxieties and castration fears.

Around 5 years, when parents have tried to assuage impinging death fears by comparison with sleep ('Grandfather has gone to sleep in heaven'), children, like adults, are convinced that they will never awaken from an anaesthetic.

Children should be as unconscious as possible before leaving the ward for the theatre.

One knows there are technical difficulties involved, but one looks forward to the day when the child can be at least lightly anaesthetized in the ward, in his own bed. This would, of course, involve research by anaesthetists into the most suitable anaesthetics to be used. It would also probably involve extra equipment and even special theatre architecture; above all it would involve some imaginative thought; but to those whose duty it is to handle the pathetic and even tragic emotional aftermath of thoughtless routine exposure of the child to the terrifying sight of the theatre, with its dreadful-looking instruments and ghostly white-garbed staff, pinning him down to the table and forcing the mask upon his choking face, no effort to spare him is too great.

Even children who accept anaesthesia bravely, without fuss or protest, often suffer from *internal* suppressed strain and tension, developing a *post-operative trauma* or long-term emotional shock, all too familiar to psychologists. Night terrors; loss of confidence in adults in general; acute, painful over-dependence on parents;

---

* Visentainer & Wolfer. 'Psychological Preparation for Surgical Paediatric Patients. The Effect on Children's and Parents' Stress Responses and Adjustments.' *Paediatrics* **56**(2): 187–202. August 1975.

psychosomatic symptoms such as asthma, urticaria and headaches; fear of the dark, and, above all, fear of falling asleep are common post-operative symptoms, manifesting themselves at varying periods after surgery.

It is indeed the inexperienced or the unimaginative who judge only by external reactions: it is the internalized effect which is strongest and most persistent.

Sodium pentothal injections have, of course, in many cases removed knowledge of the dreaded mask; but there is still the forced separation from mother at this time of crisis and terror, the frightening journey to the theatre, and the painful intravenous injection. *Many influential authorities insist that a mother should remain with her child until he is unconscious.*

Nursing Time 1987 (83: 51, 53-4) reported an opinion survey of members of the British Association of Paediatric Anaesthetists in which 55% of those replying supported parental presence in the anaesthetic room.

In a survey reported by P J Hawthorn (1974) a similar proportion of nurses supported maternal presence.*

In her article 'A Proper Place for Parents' (*Nursing Times* (11–17 May 1988)) Deborah Coulson reports a study of 32 operations in which mothers were allowed to accompany their children into the anaesthetic room, remaining with them throughout induction.

'I wanted to know:

  (i) what strategies parents used to support their children in the anaesthetic room;
 (ii) how the child reacted during the induction of the anaesthesia;
(iii) how the parents behaved during the induction;
 (iv) what feelings parents had about the experience;
  (v) how past experiences of general anaesthetics affected the reactions of parents and children to the procedure;
 (vi) post-operatively, what the child remembered of the experience in the anaesthetic room . . .

> The results indicate that almost all parents who were present with their child during induction of anaesthesia made some effort to comfort him/her, and felt their presence was of benefit to the child. Although some may have been distressed by the procedure, which would be expected when they are watching their own child lose consciousness, the findings suggest that such parents still feel it is helpful to be present.
>
> Along with other researchers who have conducted experimental studies on parental presence in the anaesthetic room, I did not find parents to be disruptive of the procedure.'

A negative factor in providing support and comfort appeared to be requests to parents to assist with physically resistive children. *73,3% of parents believed their children had benefited from their presence.*

Children were significantly more disturbed if they had previously experienced general anaesthetic in hospital.

---

* Hawthorn, P J. *Nurse - I want my mummy*. Royal College of Nursing. London 1974.

Almost all children for whom an appropriate questionnaire was returned remembered some of the events in the anaesthetic room with general accuracy.

Ms Coulsen presents the following recommendations for achieving maximum benefit from parental presence.

1.   Parents should be given guidance as to how they may help. Both parents and children should be prepared in the ward pre-operatively by the anaesthetic and nursing staff. This preparation should include discussion of the parents' own fears of anaesthesia and provision of necessary information and reassurance to overcome these fears.
2.   Where possible the parental role should be that of 'comforter' only, being seen by the child as trying to protect him rather than taking part in the procedure.
3.   Parents should also be given support on leaving the anaesthetic room, since several were found to be distressed (an observation pertaining, of course, to all parents in the ordeal of awaiting the return of a child from surgery—Author).
4.   At this time a nurse is needed to reassure the parent, to give directions back to the ward or to the coffee room, and to provide information on how long it will be before the child returns from the operating theatre, his condition on recovering consciousness, etc.

In conclusion Ms Coulson emphasizes that each parent and each child is an individual with his or her own personality and needs.

Unconscious but nevertheless potent childhood fear associations with surgery have in later years turned many an adult patient to flight, avoiding surgery until it is too late to help him.

For many reasons, both preventive and therapeutic, careful psychological handling of the child in hospital pays rich dividends.

Partial solutions to the trauma of hospitalization and surgery appear to lie in more thoughtful hospital architecture. An interesting innovation emanates from the Amersham Hospital near London.

THEATRE SUITE—AMERSHAM HOSPITAL, LONDON

Anaesthetic in Ward	Preparation Room	Operating Theatre	Recovery Room

The patient is received in Room A—a pleasant ward with coloured walls, floral curtains and taped music. Here mother sits beside her child while he receives his pentothal injection. He is then 'prepped' unconscious in Room B. This takes trained staff approximately five minutes and avoids frightening and humiliating associations. He recovers in Room D, a replica of Room A. Mother is still sitting beside him and, apart from physical discomfort, there is no knowledge of surgery.

Indeed, this simple plan would also be welcomed by adults.

Parental role

Lacking long-term association in the child's mind with pain-relief, safety, security, comfort, with the best intentions, nurses cannot be mother substitutes.

Thus it is a wise policy to encourage parents to participate in the care of their own children in hospital.*

It is true that a child knows that his parents are more likely to be sympathetic and responsive than the doctor or nurse. But he needs responsive sympathy. He wants them to know he is unhappy and he doesn't care what others think. He may make a bid for their support with screams and tears. But for the sake of his mental health, and thus also for his speedy physical recovery, he needs this comfort and tension outlet.

Painful medical treatment, especially surgery, imposes a severe strain on a child. He is still a child, and has the need and the right to act like a child. His crying and distress in the face of his pain and terror should *not* be taken as a signal for his parents' departure, but as a sign of his great need for their love and reassurance.

Most children, through long-term experience, have developed feelings of confidence in their parents, whose very presence is a sign that they approve of what is being done, so that the child more easily accepts that what the nurses and doctors are doing is right and good. Parental presence, wisely handled, may thus constitute an important aid rather than a hindrance to the hospital staff.

A function of the *paediatric social worker* or the senior nurse should be to invite parents to express to her their worries, hostilities, dissatisfactions; to explain to them hospital procedures and the reasons for them, and to outline what to expect of the child's physical and mental reactions to treatments.

That a few parents impart (quite involuntarily) their anxiety and distress is true, but because his parents are so important to the child *the establishment of a positive relationship with parents should be of primary concern to the hospital team.*

Nurses and 'hostess–social workers' can do much to encourage parents to be calm and cheerful, thus giving the child the confidence he needs to win his sickbed battle.

Nurses should try to remember that surgery is a fearful ordeal for parents: an operation may be routine to the nurse, but to each parent a life more precious than his or her own is endangered. Natural logical anxiety may well be complicated by guilt feelings, lest they themselves are in some way to blame for their child's illness or accident. Parenthood, like all strong relationships, is marked by the natural love–hate swing of *ambivalence*. An accident following closely upon a parent's normal hostility swing may well lead to terror lest the child die as a 'punishment' for the parent's hostility. In these circumstances intellectual-level reassurance is a feeble antidote to a mother's feelings of guilt and terror.

The nurse who observes that her intellectual-level reassurances are failing to relieve anxiety should not dismiss the mother as 'just neurotic'. Rather should she try to find time to talk to the mother of the deeper-level conflicts and anxieties of parenthood—stressing the universality of passing anger and guilt and giving the mother opportunity for catharsis.

In showing the mother that she really cares and feels with her—and is prepared to share her anxious hours of waiting—the nurse is giving the deeper-level emotional support inherent in the mental mechanism of *identification*. Even though

* Von Geuren, S G. 'Growth in the Training for the Paediatric Diploma *J*, October 1973. For further details refer to author.

nurse and mother are only two, together they form a supportive group, easing the burden of unhappiness and tension. In this context mother finds it easier herself to identify with similar successful cases.

In many cases the real trauma comes after the operation when the child's appearance might be terrifying to parents. They should be prepared, by nurses or a 'hostess–social worker', for the peculiar pallor, odd breathing, gagging, vomiting, etc, which are common post-operative features. It is the nurse's job *to reassure and support the parents—not to dismiss them*—for their presence is ultimately of great advantage to the patient. Besides which, they too are human beings in distress.

To include and, indeed, welcome the parents is also the finest way of reassuring them that their child is receiving the best possible attention.

The inclusion of parents also serves the important function of convincing some that their emotional responsibilities do not cease when their child is admitted to hospital.

Preserving relationships in the face of hospitalization and painful treatments

Whether they like it or not, in the child's eyes his parents share with the hospital staff responsibility for everything that happens to him. It is his parents who brought him to the hospital and turned him over to the doctors and nurses. If the child is convinced by their behaviour that they *do* share this responsibility willingly and with confidence, he himself will be a more confident and co-operative patient and will recover more quickly.

Of course, parents cannot always be expected to agree with everything done in a hospital, especially in these days when the community is constantly becoming more sophisticated and better informed. Nurses, doctors and hospital officials should be *prepared to discuss these disagreements openly*, although, of course, not in the presence of the child. Sometimes some minor concession to the individual circumstances of the case will improve happiness all round.

If some aspect of treatment is going to *hurt* a child, he should be prepared. The assurance that 'this won't hurt a bit' followed by the jab of a hypodermic needle will neither ease the child's pain nor strengthen his trust in the parent or nurse.

The nurse or doctor who looks so nice and friendly suddenly does something that hurts. In the child's mind the doctor has used his friendliness to deceive and hurt him. Probably telling the child that he is about to be hurt will provide a signal for him to start fighting against it. This is the time for firmness and speed. Prolonged cajoling, coaxing or threats are pure torture for all concerned. What has to be done has to be done sooner or later, and the sooner the better.

The unpleasantness over, the child needs to be comforted and diverted. Remarks such as 'Now, that didn't hurt much', or 'stop crying you big baby', are likely to shame and upset the child further. It is better to dismiss the experience with 'There, that's fine' and to change to more pleasant topics. His mother can take him in her arms and get him interested in a story or game.

It hardly seems necessary to remind nurses that *their job is to heal the sick, not to impose their ideas of discipline and child-rearing upon someone else's child*. In any case, the discomfort, distress, fears and insecurities involved in hospitalization do *not* constitute a situation conducive to the imposition of someone else's disciplinary fads.

Similarly, *this is no time to attempt to 'wean' a child from a customary source of comfort* and security, such as a 'sleep blanket' or a bedtime bottle. A sister may consider a bottle inappropriate to a 3-year-old; she would be wiser to be thankful for the opportunity of providing a component of the 'mother, love, safety, security' formula.

Parental visiting, open wards and sleeping in

One of the worst shocks a child experiences when hospitalized is sudden separation from his parents. It is in extreme situations, such as pain and fear, that children have greatest need of their parents' reassurance, and familiar, comforting presence. Realizing the value of maternal support, the consequent easing of psychosomatic tension, and the preservation of physiological resources, which accompany parental presence, many hospitals have sought ways of amending their routine, so as to allow parents access to their children in times of emotional crisis. Daily visiting, or preferably the 'opening' of wards to mothers before and after surgery, at meal-times, bedtimes, etc, is becoming established practice.

It is true that many children cry after their parents leave, but this is infinitely preferable to the feeling of being unwanted, forgotten and abandoned. Were visits more frequent and informal, parting would not be so sad.

Nurses should not allow their desire for an externally peaceful ward to endanger their patients' long-term mental health. For mental health pivots on the strength and support inherent in mother's presence.

There is certainly a move among the world's paediatric hospitals, great and small, to permit frequent contact with parents. Many have 'opened' their children's wards, waiving official visiting hours.

'OPEN WARDS' AND SLEEP-IN MOTHERS

The Great Ormond Street Hospital for Sick Children has provided sleeping accommodation for mothers living outside London in order that they may be available to their children. Charing Cross Hospital provides simple stretchers which slip under children's beds.

The hardest time to be with a child, and to leave him, is at night. This is when he is most likely to be upset. Hospitals obliged to operate on 'skeleton staff' at night should be especially interested in the Amersham experiment, in which mothers of children under 6 are accommodated with their children in two-bedded wards—with very little structural alteration and considerable reduction in routine nursing and comforting. Wards accommodating children between 6 and 12 are 'open' to parents. The experiment is recorded admirably in the film 'The Two-year-old Goes to Hospital with Mother'.

Paediatricians revisiting England have noted the changed atmosphere in formerly tense, over-quiet or sob-laden wards—now, beside most beds, there is usually a mother, a granny, an auntie, sitting reassuringly knitting, reading or chatting, creating a warm, familiar, comfortable, atmosphere, and, strangely enough, seldom interfering with ward procedures and routine—in fact she often helps by taking upon herself unskilled but important tasks such as feeding, tidying, and reassuring other parents by identifying with them as only a mother can.

When the new Athens Hospital was completed, in order to counteract a staff shortage, mothers were invited to participate in caring for their children as a temporary emergency measure. So successful was this arrangement that the participation of mothers is now encouraged as a matter of policy.

Not all young nurses slip easily into mothering behaviour. The presence of mothers provides role models.

Ward sisters and charge nurses report happier, more confident children, shorter stays and improvement in nursing—especially on the part of young nurses who have introjected patterns of mothering.

The sick child will recover more rapidly if he feels emotionally secure and he is more likely to get this sense of security by having with him someone he knows, who he knows loves him, and will see that he comes to no harm.

Parents, because they know their own individual child in sickness and in health, have much to contribute in judging a child's response to treatment.

It is the wise, experienced paediatrician who opens his examination with the question: 'Now mother, how does Tommy look to *you* today?' Post-hospital psychological trauma and persistent personality maladjustment resultant upon long-term hospitalization have already been discussed. Suffice it here to reiterate that insecurities and fears, which haunt long after hospitalization, are often the result of obeying sincere but ill-advised recommendations by hospital staff to 'keep away, because he's always upset when you have been'.

Visiting a child lets him know that his parents are thinking of him even when they are away. It shows him that they care that he is not being abandoned or forgotten. It also gives him an opportunity to unburden himself, to confide to a sympathetic and loving ear some of the unpleasant and disturbing things which have happened to him.

Even better, sleeping accommodation should be available.

> 'Lack of "special facilities" is no excuse. A day nursery may serve as a parental night dormitory. Put-up beds may be placed beside or even under children's beds. If you have a floor you have accommodation for mothers. Mothers provide a huge source of efficient and caring nursing potential.'*

A child in pain and terror is a child in crisis. He will bear his ordeal and recover more quickly and completely if reassured by his mother's constant presence and support. To deprive him of this courts the danger of long-term and maladaptive after-effects.

In any case, *a child should know that either or both parents will visit regularly and frequently (certainly at least once a day)*. If humanly possible, the child should be visited at each visiting period. He will feel lonely and depressed if he sees other children with parents and friends when no one visits him.

If it is not always possible for parents to come at each and every frequent visiting time, this should be foreseen and explained to the child. He may be unhappy about it, but not nearly as unhappy as if waiting in vain for his parents' appearance. Once a child is disappointed, he will never again be quite sure that his mother or father will come next visiting time. Instead of awaiting each visit with eager anticipation as he should do, he will instead dread the possibility that he will be alone again. If

* The late Dr Hugh Jolly, formerly Paediatrician-in-Charge, Charing Cross Hospital, London, speaking at 'A Global Look at Children', sponsored by Purity, Cape town, 8 March 1981.

the parents cannot manage a visit, then a relative or close friend should, if possible, substitute.

A visit from his teacher often provides the child with a happy thrill—it shows him that he is not shut off or forgotten by the outside world. It will also help him put himself in the future, looking forward to his return to school when he is well again.

Dr Hugh Jolly was adamant in his belief that *children under 12 should be allowed to visit their siblings in hospital.*

'Infection is spread patient to patient by staff, not by visitors. Apart from emotional involvement and support, parents, siblings and patients themselves serve an important role in health education. Our hospital welcomes visiting groups of children and their teachers who are shown the wards, the playrooms, the laboratories and other interesting projects. Every child in hospital should learn more about himself and his illness. To this end we provide *project books* in which the child is encouraged to keep charts, X-rays, syringes, etc. This activity provides both catharsis and evidence that hospitals are not such bad places and health is important.'

Gifts

Besides being amusing, gifts have a special meaning for the hospitalized child (or adult for that matter). They are tangible evidence that, even in his absence, he is frequently in the thoughts of his family and friends. A gift is also a *part of themselves* which they will leave behind to comfort him when he is once again alone. This is the reason why sick children are often insistent that parents bring a gift. Since it is primarily a token, it need be neither elaborate nor expensive. It is the proof of feeling for him that counts.

When he enters hospital, a child should take with him a few toys or other possessions to make him feel more at home, more secure and less lonely.

Sometimes nothing his parents bring appears to please the child—his dissatisfaction with the gift is a displaced symptom of his dissatisfaction with life in general, of his resentment of being shut in and in pain. Or he may just be homesick or bored. A wise parent or friend, a kind nurse, whose attentions are rebuffed, will realize that nothing personal is intended.

Preserving the unique bond between mother and child

An interesting article in the *Nursing Times* of 22 July 1966 illustrates the growing extent to which the medical and nursing professions are becoming aware of the fundamental nature, and indeed indispensability, of the mother–child relationship in achieving physical recovery and long-term mental health. In his article 'Home and Hospital' Dr J L Burn MD DHy DPh, Lecturer in Public Health, University of Manchester, and Medical Officer of Health for Salford, writes:

'A chance remark of a ward sister, at a children's hospital thirty years ago, taught me to realize the supreme influence of the home on the growth of the body, mind and personality of the child. A little girl suffering from a chronic illness was making no progress despite the efforts of everyone concerned in her care. One day sister surprised me by saying "all she needs is to be back in her own home". I knew that the home was poor and the mother inadequate; by contrast the hospital ward was so hygienic, the food was far better and the skill and care provided by the hospital were infinitely superior. Surely the sister was wrong. But she was proved right; the home factor was decisive. Like a flower opening up to the light, the child blossomed in health with the sunshine of mother-love at home. On the other hand I recall, to my regret, agreeing many years ago to a request from a matron of an infectious diseases hospital to abandon the system of parents visiting their children, because it upset the children so much. They cried copiously when their mothers left. We failed to realize that this was just a natural healthy reaction of the children—to be welcomed, rather than deplored.

One of the great lessons, of the last twenty years, has been the irreversible deterioration which often occurs with very young children to institutionalization of the wrong kind.

When we say to a toddler that "mummy is going away to hospital, and will be back in a few days' time" it seems for ever to the child who needs support, food and comfort from the mother. No wonder that small children, on admission to hospital, want their mummies and are naughty. How often one saw in the diphtheria and scarlet fever wards of long ago the apathetic small children who were good patients; for they had been in hospital a long time, separated from their parents. Inwardly they grieved. They were good but withdrawn, lacking the lovely vitality and spontaneity of children. And so, whenever possible, we should support home-care schemes, bring the health services to the child in the home instead of the other way about.

Johnny, as he lay in a hospital bed was a frail pathetic little boy and a woman registrar took a special interest in him. The two got on famously throughout a long illness, and the doctor became genuinely attached to the little boy, whose mother did not visit as often as she might have done. After discharge from hospital, Johnny came back to "Outpatients" in his mother's arms. The doctor saw him a long way off and rushed to meet him and said, "Oh, Johnny, how nice to see you". For no reason Johnny smacked the doctor's face. She was deeply hurt and only later did she realise that the mother, even a poor and inadequate mother, occupied the whole of Johnny's affections.

Michael, aged 7, was admitted to a children's home on account of neglect by the mother, who punished her children excessively. This boy became the special object of care by an excellent nurse. She took him out on little trips. She felt so sorry for the way he had been treated at home. She became very fond of him. All the more was she disappointed when, at the end of two years' stay, Michael said that all he wanted was to get back to his mother. This was very upsetting, but it must be remembered that there are bonds between mother and her children that are not obvious when we visit the home on some occasions when tempers are lost and the picture is one of bad family life.

In the majority of cases there still remains a unique bond between the child and the mother and it is to the ultimate good of all that this bond should be recognized.'

(See The Dying Child, p 548-9).

Role of hospital social workers and Community Nurses

There are, of course, those parents who, for their own reasons, both conscious and unconscious, are only too ready to 'hand over' their children to the hospital staff, disappearing as soon as possible.

They certainly should not be encouraged in so doing, the resources of the hospital team being mobilized to make them aware of their special parental role and obligations. If necessary, visiting should be facilitated by providing fares, contacting employers concerning the granting of off-time, etc. Realizing the importance of parental visiting, the hospital social worker should purposefully direct her energy towards helping parents to realize and fulfil their obligations.

The importance of better transport to improved outpatient departments, and local day hospitals with periodic intensive short-term hospitalization is finally becoming recognized.

It is certainly of extreme importance to long-term mental health that the mal-effects upon personality development of hospitalism or long-term institution-alization (described in chapter 3), be avoided. Mobilization of community resources and provision of a home-care network are important functions of the Community Nurse.

Convalescence

The last few days of a child's hospitalization are often the worst. He feels fine and cannot understand why he must stay in bed. His energy is returning and he is restless and bored with the routine of his illness. This is no time for the staff to be suddenly less attentive or to ignore him. After all the care and attention he has been receiving, sudden withdrawal is too abrupt for him. A smooth return to normal living demands that we give the child sufficient time to make the adjustment back to independence. If one does not taper off attention gradually, the child is apt to become whining and over-demanding of reassurance that he is still loved and important (*regression*).

A child's irritability during convalescence is further increased by the fact that he still feels weak and tires easily; also he finds it difficult to concentrate on any one thing for long. He can be encouraged to play quietly in bed and as a 'bonus' he could be provided with a 'surprise' in toys or games. These will help stimulate his interest while he is alone, and will also show that he is still being thought about with love. He will gradually learn to get along with less attention, but this does not happen quickly. The 'weaning' process may require to be continued until after the period of convalescence.

Another important cause for that aggression, rudeness or sulkiness marking the convalescence of both children and adults lies in the fact that they are now sufficiently strong and independent to express their resentment and anger at the painful and humiliating procedures to which they have been subjected.

The child is still near his illness. Quite frequently, fearing a recurrence, his anxiety becomes focused on his own body processes. Normal psychosomatic sensations become exaggerated and he develops distressing hypochondriacal symptoms. It is important to avoid or counteract such symptoms before they entrench themselves.

David Levy* found the following factors to be potent in the development of childrens' hypochondriacal interest in their bodies:

1. Exposure to disease, deformity, accidents, death in others; disease emphasis in the social milieu.
2. The child's own memories of those events and his relation to the individuals thus affected.
3. The child's own illness, contacts with physicians, hospital experiences, and type of convalescent care.
4. Utilization of body ailments in avoidance of difficult situations and as a bid for sympathy; 'exploitation of illness, real or imaginary'.
5. Body sensitivities (awareness of variations in body form, insufficiency feelings, compensatory striving).
6. Anxieties about illness, especially in response to ill-advised threats regarding the effects of masturbation.
7. Parents plagued by hypochondriacal fears tend, unconsciously, to project these fears on their children's bodies. Their over-attention to bodily function creates a home atmosphere resembling that pertaining in a hospital. Very soon the child absorbs these painful hypochondriacal anxieties.

Children's fears are accentuated by the loneliness, reduced resistance and confusion of illness.

Common fears of children

The 3-year-old — Animals, darkness
The 4-year-old — Animals, darkness, sirens, elderly persons, cripples, death.
The 5 to 6-year-old — Animals, darkness, sirens, elderly persons, cripples, thunder, that his mother will not be there when he awakens.

Castration fears. By 2 or 3 years the little boy has become intrigued by his penis. He derives considerable pleasure from handling this organ and is naturally fascinated by the way it changes size and shape and moves involuntarily up and down.

However, through detrimental environmental pressures (such as 'It'll fall off if you play with it') or an innately over-strict conscience, the little boy may well come to feel guilty and anxious about these pleasures. He fears he will indeed damage or lose this symbol of male dominance as punishment for his 'forbidden' pleasures or some other misdemeanour.

Psycho-analysts describe this distressing anxiety as 'castration phobia'.

Clearly, stressful physical examination or surgery, especially as pertaining to the genitalia, may well reinforce his castration fears, exposing him to much guilt, terror and distress.

This is certainly emphasized when a beloved, or at least an ambivalently viewed parent is involved, as in the Cleveland RAD (reflex anal dilation) affair. In addition to the trauma of parental separation, pain and humiliation,

* Levy, D M. 'Body Interest in Children with Hypochondriasis.' *Am J Psychiat.* 1932. 295–315. As reported by Kanner in *Child Psychology*.

'Vanessa recalls that she and her sister were woken on one occasion to have their bottoms photographed. "I kept saying, 'Why can't we see Mum?' Loads of my clothes got lost and I had to wear pants made of paper. It was horrible."'

(See also p 298.)

Such a child requires an opportunity for verbalization, interpretation, catharsis and repeated reassurance lest painful guilt and anxiety persist, to permanently affect not only his sexual fulfillment but also his life relationships.

Regressing in illness or stress, the adult male patient will experience similar castration fear and distress in the fact of genital surgery, such as prostatectomy.

Little girls, too, tend to the idea that the penis is an intricate, fascinating and superior piece of equipment of which they have been deprived, perhaps as a punishment—

'Worse still, they often fantasize that they were once provided with a penis, but that their parents have condemned them to femininity by cutting it off. On the other hand, the little girl who really wishes to be like her mother will be proud of the fact that her valuable genital organs are better protected.'*

By 3 to 4 years of age the child has already been conditioned to feelings of 'dirtiness', guilt, anxiety and shame towards organs and products of elimination and hence to sex organs (see p 64).

It is a mistake to think that young children are not embarrassed, shamed and distressed at exposure to public toileting and procedures.

Alice dreaded, cried and fought against her second X-ray session, until it was realized that her resistance stemmed from the removal of her nylon briefs. Reassured that she would be allowed to wear cotton panties, her resistance to the investigation subsided.

The practice of refusing older children in a paediatric ward the privacy of screens during toileting may well impose a long-term traumatic experience.

During Tommy's stay in hospital the puppets, dolls, plasticine, and other creative toys will distract and comfort.

Because toys are tangible, small and accepting, Tommy can use them to express his anger and his hurt.

The play therapist encourages Tommy to obtain catharsis by doing to the dolls what he would like to do to the doctors, nurses, and even Mommy and Daddy for bringing him to the hospital.

The play therapist tells him it is quite in order to do these things to dolls, and even to think abut doing them to grown-ups—this way, nobody will be hurt.

The play therapist, through her friends the puppets, dolls and furry animals, teaches Tommy a lot—in fact, his friend Johnny the puppet shows him how to prepare and use his own insulin syringe. He teaches Mary in the next bed to use her crutch until her leg has mended.

The movement towards bringing the Arts (painting, drawing, puppet-making, music, modelling and drama groups) into hospitals is fast expanding in England. The author attended a congress at the Edgar Wood Centre, City of Manchester

* Portia Holman. *Psychology and Psychological Medicine for Nurses.*

College of Higher Education, in December 1981 where the voluntary services of a wide spectrum of artists were presented. Washable murals, in which both staff and patients participated, decorated the hospital corridors. A large wooden soldier pointed directions, and a fairy queen guarded the door to the operating theatre. Busy gnomes, snakes and ladders and stretch-ball games illustrated movements in the physiotherapy department. Murals with period pictures, old movie-strip pull-outs and zippered pictures of royal weddings decorated the geriatric out-patient department. Taped music soothed the journey to the operating theatre and welcomed patients back into the recovery room.

The contribution of voluntary artists to the National Health Service was indeed impressive, and the author agreed with Professor Neil Kessel, professor of psychiatry in Manchester University, when he said:

> 'Art in hospital is a stimulus—people, when involved, find it stimulating. It is togethering—that is, you can do art together as a group activity, or as a private activity, but alongside other people . . . There is additional benefit in being able to look at art rather than looking at blank walls—a particularly valuable experience if the patients have in any way contributed to the pictures.'

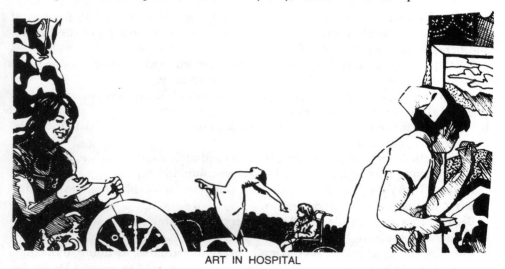

ART IN HOSPITAL

Congress Report cover, 1981.   Edgar Wood Centre, Manchester.

Children often find it easier to communicate their feelings through handling toys, through their drawings, their songs and their drama. Certainly in the magic world of creative make-believe there lies the possibility of vicarious satisfaction—as one saw in the animated face of a paraplegic girl watching the freedom and the grace of creative dance . . .

(For a behaviourist 'unlearning' or 'elimination' technique in overcoming hospital precipitated night fears see p 165.)

Eating patterns and problems

In convalescence some parents and nurses feel duty-bound to coerce patients into a balanced, nutritious diet. To this end they plead, bribe and even threaten.

The youngster becomes angry or anxious, his Sympathetic Nervous System is aroused, his gastric juices inhibited, his peristalsis reversed; the circular muscles of the stomach and throat go into spasm and his food is either regurgitated or spoilt by poor digestion.

Between one and two years, a child often has definite tastes in vegetables, cereals, milk, etc. If he should suddenly turn against one of these vegetables he previously liked, try not to make a fuss of it. If left alone, he will probably come back to it next week or next month. It is important to remember that a child just beginning to get acquainted with a great variety of new foods cannot be expected to adhere to only one kind. It is naturally very irritating to have prepared food just to have it refused, but this is the time to make the child like his food and to make meal-times happy. Associate food with unhappiness, pressure, strong words and unpleasant experiences, and food itself will become something unpleasant to be avoided.

How far can one trust a child's own dietary choice? The most famous experiment in this area is that conducted by Dr Clara Davis of the Chicago Memorial Hospital for Children. As her patients were all suffering from orthopaedic handicaps and one half of them had had tubercolosis or some other bone infection, her theories were put to a very stringent test. The children needed their food to replace damaged body tissue as well as for normal growth. In the 'control' ward the children were strictly supervised as they partook of a conservative balanced diet at regular intervals. In the experimental ward the food was wheeled in from the kitchen on trolleys which contained a large selection of as many foods as possible. Each child chose his own food and no one was urged or obliged to eat.

Results

1. A lessening of food waste and a decrease in kitchen work.

2. The experimental children throve on their new diet. There were very few digestive disturbances, and diarrhoea and constipation were almost negligible—in fact incidence was less than in the 'control' group. Experimental children showed a greater and more consistent weight increase.

Self-choice from a selection, including a reasonable range of natural, unrefined foods, over a period of time resulted in a well-balanced and nutritious diet.

3. At first the children made for the dessert before the soup, but usually settled into a more conservative menu when they became convinced that no pressure would be imposed.

4. Some children did show 'food-jags'. One ate nothing but oranges for 30 hours—appropriately he was known to be suffering from a vitamin C deficiency.

One child with an iron deficiency showed a very marked preference for beetroot and spinach.

However, over a longer period these also showed themselves spontaneously capable of choosing a healthy, well-balanced diet.

One often finds that some children have an artificial craving for *sweets*. This has developed largely because their mothers have boosted the value and enjoyment to be gained from sweets as a means of bribing the child in order to overcome disciplinary problems.

On the other hand, some foods have been given negative value by a mother's insisting that they be eaten before something pleasant. The child is thus given to believe that this food is unpalatable and that something else is nicer. Left alone, children often like foods that adults spurn.

Nutritious snacks

What of the child who craves snacks between meals? If it is a sensible nutritive food, it seems irrelevant when the child eats it. Fruit juice, fruit, biltong, nuts and wholewheat crackers are all healthy foods that are easily digested. Many children have small stomachs and become excessively tired and hungry if they have to wait for big meals. Often they thrive when given small nutritive snacks. It makes little difference when the food is eaten as long as the child eats a reasonable quantity of healthy foods.

Some mothers complain that a child refuses to eat at meal-times but as soon as the meal is over starts demanding snacks. This is nearly always caused by unpleasantness at meal-times. The mother tries to push the child to eat. The child becomes upset, nervous and unhappy. His digestive system is upset and he cannot eat, but as soon as the meal is safely over, he begins to feel hungry. The solution is therefore not to withhold between-meal-time food from him, but rather to make meal-times a pleasant, peaceful and therefore more suitable situation for the intake and digestion of food.

Study of child development has shown us that a satisfying feeding relationship is basic to a loving, outgoing mother–child relationship. From the earliest hours of life pleasant eating experiences are symbolic of mother, love, safety and security. The mother who in later years renders eating unpleasant detracts from the food-symbol and imperils the all-important mother–child relationship.

Unnecessary unpleasantness caused by meal-time moans does not end with childhood. It aggravates the adolescent revolt from home authority.

Adam Block, the author of *American Adolescent Conflict Survey* found that 82% of the boys questioned had fights at home because their mothers insisted that they eat foods they did not like.

It seems such a pity to let meal-times detract from relationships. Worry, bad feeling and irritation can so easily be avoided in remembering that every child is an individual in his own right and appetites are at their best at a table set with laughter and peace.

(Children, like adults, may lose motivation to eat in general depression. They may also withold from eating as a plea for help. (p 90) See also Eating Disorders p 324)

The chronically ill or physically handicapped child

Here parents cannot console themselves that the condition 'will pass in time'. They are faced with a permanent situation within the framework of which they must reconstruct the child's future and, to a large extent, their own. It is natural in these circumstances that they should feel incredulous, even resentful. 'Why', they ask themselves in sorrow and pained frustration, even illogical guilt, 'did this have to happen to *our* child?' They may feel that his whole life is ruined. To see heartbreak and diminishment in a beloved child is worse than to suffer them oneself.

It is the task of the hospital team to convince them, often painfully and with much reiteration, that when such calamities occur many disabled children learn to live comparatively normal lives. What is the best advice we can offer parents facing this problem?

1. We should convince them that the child's disability should be accepted not denied, or hidden or fought by those around him. If the disability is accepted for what it is, neither minimized nor exaggerated, he himself will learn to accept his disability and to live with it. All of us have our limitations; admittedly a paralysed limb is a greater handicap than near-sightedness, but it is none the less only a limitation to activity, not the end of all aspects of normal living.

2. We should help them to see the whole child, and not just his handicap. Let us take, for instance, a boy who has lost an arm in a motor accident. His parents in their grief and illogical feelings of guilt and anxiety for his welfare, may overprotect him, thwarting his every activity until he regresses to loss of confidence and motivation for independence.

Eventually their concept of their son is whittled down to his empty sleeve. They should be shown that, despite his loss of an arm, he has the same emotions, hopes, ambitions, curiosities—the same eagerness for life—as any other boy. It is their duty, and their comfort, to discover and develop the many other aspects of his body and mind.

A kindly, imaginative nurse may well through identification utilize her long-term nursing contact to introduce new *compensation* outlets, which provide alternative, even enriching, fulfillment.

The youngster might, for instance, make as good a debating chairman or magazine editor as he did a rugby captain. Often tests of aptitude and interest can help ascertain and convince him of what he *can* do.

Computers requiring only one simple movement, open up a whole magic world of communication and environmental control. The psychology department of Keele University has even invented a computerised bionic arm!

Telling the child

One cannot hide a chronic illness or a significant handicap from a normally intelligent child. Keeping him in ignorance of the real facts may increase his anxiety. Where a child feels that pleasures are being unreasonably withheld from him, his resentment may imperil the parent–child relationship.

'Why', he asks himself, 'am I in some way different from other children?'
'Am I being punished for something bad I've done?'
'Am I on the verge of dying?'
'Are my parents denying me something because they don't love me?'

The explanation he imagines will, in all probability, be much more fearsome than are the facts. Not knowing the true facts he may rebel, doing just those things which are most dangerous to his condition. Only if he is helped to *understand* it, can a child learn to accept his disability.

There is no need to give the child a full clinical description of his case, but after he is over the first onslaught of his illness and beginning to feel a little better, we can tell him of his condition, not in fearful tones of doom, but simply, directly and even a bit casually. The small child, naturally, cannot grasp very much, but he will learn by experience of living with his illness. The epileptic child, for instance, soon takes his pill-routine for granted.

Arousing self-pity in the child does not help him at all; in fact it can cause serious harm to his personality. A more *constructive approach* is called for. A *diabetic child*, for instance, must be shown that there are other things in life besides forbidden sweets. The child should be helped through the enthusiasm of the parents, nurses and teachers to think more of what life offers him and less about what it denies. He should be helped to discover new interests and abilities through which his physical condition permits him to *compensate*. The case of the diabetic child is a little special, for here the mother figure, formerly associated with the satisfying comfort of pleasurable mouth activity, is forced to withdraw this long-established symbol of her love. Now intellectual-level reasoning is not enough. Mother should go to considerable trouble to substitute acceptable mouth activity, such as sugarless chewing-gum. Above all she should make sure she is giving the child extra attention, spending happy times together, and in other ways demonstrating the constancy of her love and support.

When a chronic illness or an injury strike it is not easy for either the parent or the child to accept the situation—it means a complete emotional readjustment. It sometimes entails complete reorientation of parents' plans for their children and themselves. This is particularly difficult in adolescence when the youngster himself has already formulated many hopes and dreams. He is forced to face life's cruelties before he is ready—in fact while still engulfed in the emotional turmoil of adolescence.

He certainly needs all the companionship, support, ingenuity, strength and serenity his parents, teachers and the medical team can muster. But the greater the hurdle, the greater the reward. Chronic handicap is not the end of life. It is the beginning of a new kind of life—a life which, in its new breadth, may well evoke unexpected talents, philosophy, accomplishments, awareness and fulfillment.

Parents of disabled children should be careful, moreover, not to treat them as asexual: They should ascertain that sex education is appropriate to the disability, which should not be confused with the total person.

Information regarding the importance of the self-image and the warmth, intimacy and fulfillment that come from close bonding should be stressed, and a wide interpretation bestowed upon the whole sphere of sexual activity, together with the alternative sexual satisfaction that a specific handicap may indicate. (See Rehabilitation of the Spinal-cord Injured, pp 508-11.)

There is no greater handicap than to be without love: participation in a warm, loving relationship is a far greater joy than physical perfection. (For self-help support groups, see p 613.)

Support group: Voluntary Council for Handicapped Children, National Children's Bureau, 8 Wakley Street, London EC1 V 70E, Telephone: 01 278 9441.

Helping children cope with serious parental illness

Children are good observers but poor interpreters. For example: 'Grandpa died in the hospital—now dad has to go to the hospital. He's going to die too.' Or 'I got mad at mum when she told me to pick up my toys. Then she got sick. Maybe I made her sick.'

'What should I tell my children?'
How much should I tell them?'
Children need to be told information they can understand.

— Tell them what has happened.
— Explain what will happen next.
— Leave them with feelings of hope that even though you are upset now, there will be better times.
Assure them they will continue to be loved and cared for.
Listen to them—it lets you know what they can handle.
— Answer their questions **simply**.
— Ask them what they think, for example, cancer is.
— Ask them if they are worried about you.
— Correct any misinformation they may have.
Communicate feelings as well as facts.
Some **don'ts**:
— Don't lie (For author's reservation see Chap. 23.)
— Don't trouble them with frightening medical details, financial concerns (except as it will affect them), test results that are not yet in, etc.
— Don't make promises you may not be able to keep. (Say "I think I will be able to . . ." or "I'll try to . . .")
— Don't be afraid to say "I don't know."
— Don't push children to talk.
Some ways to say things:

— "I have a sickness. It is called cancer. The doctor is giving me medicine to help me get well. Sometimes I will feel sick or tired and sometimes I will be just fine. Dad will help me take care of you until I feel better."*

The overriding *fear* of young children *is separation from mother*. If hospitalization is necessary, arrangements should be made for a familiar person to stay with them. *They should be assured that nothing they have done or said or thought could possibly have caused the illness.*

In the case of school-going children, it is probably wise to tell teachers and school counsellors to ensure maximum understanding and help. *Regression in school work, difficulties in friendships and sibling rivalry may all increase.*

Teenagers caught in the emotional disbalance and over-reaction of adolescence may suffer *role reversal*. Just when they are trying to be independent, a parent may need to depend upon them. Some may rebel or regress. Some mature too rapidly.

* *Helping Children Understand—A Guide for a Parent with Cancer.* Prepared by Carol Lindberg of the Minnesota Division, American Cancer Association.

Some take this experience in their stride. Parents should try to communicate understanding, love and acceptance, but still show disapproval of misbehaviour.

Co-operation at this difficult time should be especially rewarded. The support of the extended family and the diversion of friends is important.

'Children's feelings

If you never show how you feel, chances are they won't either. But covering up strong emotions is like sitting on a time bomb. A child can become frightened of his/her own feelings instead of accepting them as O.K.
. . .

- Some children will try to make up for these guilt feelings by being super good and setting unrealistically high standards for themselves. (Reaction Formation)
- Some children will cling to you too much, afraid something will happen if they are not there.
- Some children will withdraw from you, unconsciously trying to become more independent in case something else happens to you or perhaps fearing contamination or that you may die there and then . . .
- Some children will be afraid they'll get cancer too.
- Know that these things will pass with time but let your children know that you understand and accept them as they are.'

Hospitalized parents should make arrangements for their children to:
— visit;
— make phone calls;
— share tape-recorded messages;
— exchange pictures or photographs with each other;
— exchange presents—small remembrances give children a piece of mother to take home;
— explain procedures if children show interest or concern;
— help them prepare for your homecoming.

CHAPTER 14

CHILD ABUSE

(see also Sexual Assault pp 355–9)

At some time, perhaps devastatingly frequently, the nurse will encounter a child who has been severely maltreated usually by one or both of its parents.

Child abuse comprises children being

(1) *beaten violently in temper, in despair or in plain sadistic bullying;*
(2) *emotionally scarred by witnessing physical brutality or long-term violent arguments between parents or other adults;*
(3) *left by themselves for long periods, sometimes days on end, lonely, frightened and at physical risk—often neglected to the point of dangerous malnutrition,* or even beyond, to death.

In the United Kingdom it is estimated that every day a child dies as the result of parental abuse.

Each year 400 babies, under 12 months of age, suffer irreparable brain damage at the hands of their elders. One thousand are physically injured.

The problem of child abuse continues to grow. The increase has been largely in types of abuse other than physical injury (ie sexual and emotional abuse, neglect, and failure to thrive). There was a 115% increase in children reported for these types of abuse since 1985. The most dramatic increase has been in the number of sexually abused children placed on the NSPCC registers. In 1986 some 527 children were registered as having been sexually abused, a 137% increase over the 1985 figure.

The majority of the abused children, as in previous years, were physically injured. Figure 1 shows how the reported physical injury rate to children has increased over the past five years.

The NSPCC's register research is the largest continuous study of child abuse being carried out in this country. The research is based on the information on the children placed on NSPCC child abuse registers. These registers are maintained on behalf of local Area Review Committees. The geographical areas covered by them include over 9% of the children living in England and Wales. This paper looks at 2 137 children placed on these registers during 1986.

Among these children, the number of them who were fatally or seriously injured fell from 99 in 1985 to 87 in 1986. They represented 9% of the physically injured children, a drop from the 11% in 1985 but still slightly above the 1984 figure. 1986 also saw the first registered death from abuse other than physical injury.

The following etiological analysis tells something about the types of people and situations precipitating abuse.

Rate of Physically Injured Children per Thousand by Year

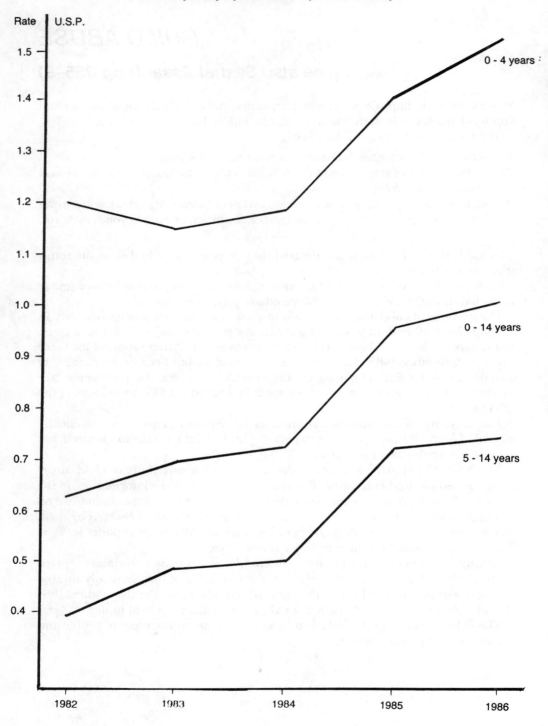

Family Composition

Type of abuse	General	Physical injury	Sexual	Emotional	Neglect
Victim living with both parents	Less than 50%		Just as likely to be living with father as father substitute		
Natural mother + father substitute	27%				
Natural mother	23%				More often

Rate of Physically injured Children per Thousand by Year

Suspected Perpetrators*

Recorded: more than 90%				Unrecorded: less than 10%
Type of abuse	General	Physical injury	Sexual	Emotional
Natural father	31%		31%	15%
Natural mother	32%		1%	More than 50%
Father substitute/ stepfather/ cohabitee (not casual boyfriend)		18%	26%	4%
Siblings/other relatives/ neighbour/ casual boyfriend		6%	35%	7%
Child living with natural father		60%	55%	
Child living with natural mother		36%		2 x as likely as when with father/father substitute
Child living with mother substitute		26%		
Child living with father substitute		61%	69%	
Parent/parent substitute not living with child (on visit to or from custodial parent)		3%	9%	

* Creighton, Susan J. These statistics are derived from the National Society for the Prevention of Cruelty to Children Research Briefing No 8, 1988.

- Precipitating Factors

Factors ranked in order of stress precipitation

Type of abuse	General	Physical injury	Sexual	Emotional	Neglect	Failure to thrive
Marital problems		most often	most often, most severe	most often most severe		
Inability to respond to maturational needs of child					most often most severe	most often most severe
Unrealistic expectations of child		most severe				
Unemployment	Second most frequent stress factor but not among most severe					

Reports of child deaths during 1985 (taken from the *Guardian* newspaper) and reported by Corby* shows that:

There were eight cases reported in the *Guardian* in 1985 where children were abused by their parents or care-takers while social services department, social workers or those from voluntary agencies were involved. In six of these cases the children died.

> Jasmine Beckford (Brent SSD)
> Samantha Waldram (Nottinghamshire SSD)
> Tyra Hendry (Lambeth SSD)
> Heidi Koseda NSPCC Hillingdon)
> Jane Oliewicz (Leeds SSD)
> Charlene Salt (Oldham SSD)
> Bethan and Nicholas Clemmet (S Glamorgan SSD)
> Gemma Hartwell (Birmingham SSD)

Another such case was reported in January 1986, that of Andrew Riley (on the child abuse register of Cheshire SSD) who was murdered by his mother.

Clearly social workers tread a worrisome tightrope between the trauma of family breakdown and the phenomenally persistent losses of maternal deprivation on the one hand, and, on the other, the client's physical safety.

Fatal cases where social workers were not involved include:

The Kerry Babies inquiry—an inquiry into the deaths of two new-born babies in Tralee, County Kerry, Eire.

Louise Brown—new-born Down's Syndrome baby who was allegedly abducted, but whose father was later tried and convicted of her murder.

Christoper Stock—a Liverpool child who was murdered by his stepfather.

Michael Brophy - a 6-year-old child alleged to have been ill-treated by his parents and to have suffered eye damage as a result. His father committed suicide during the trial.

---

* Corby, B. *Working with Child Abuse - Social Work Practice and the Child Abuse System* (Open University Press, Milton Keynes 1987).

In addition there were reports on a wide range of child murders/accidental deaths, three of which pointed to the possibility of some neglect by public authorities.

Natasha and Michael Hurst, aged 11 and 13, who, along with their mother, died in their home as a result of central heating fumes. Originally it had been thought that they had died of hypothermia.

The deaths of *children from a junior school in Stoke Poges* while on a school trip to Land's End.

Adrian Wright, a 6-year-old boy, who drowned in the lido at Hyde Park while on an outing with day centre workers from Southwark SSD.

Several other child deaths—all murders—received widespread press coverage, among the most widely publicized being the murder of a 10-month-old baby who was so hungry he was forced to eat his soiled nappy, and whose parents have been gaoled for causing his 'horrifying and agonizing death'. The father, a 38-year-old security guard, was gaoled for 10 years for deliberate neglect of baby Dean, and his common-law wife for seven years.

Both parents stood emotionless as the judge, Mr Justice Owen, said in the Old Bailey: 'This was a horrifying case and the sentence expresses the horror of society. In the final analysis, you as parents must take the main blame. The agony of this small boy is almost too much to contemplate. To appreciate the enormity of what happened to him, it's necessary to have in mind the words of the ambulanceman who took him away and said he had never seen such a horrifying sight in his career.'

The cause of death was severe malnutrition. Dean's body was wasted and he was half the weight he should have been. When officials arrived to take the child's body away, they found a squalid, filthy room reeking of urine and faeces.

But the couple spent money on food and drink and cigarettes and even the family dog was better fed than Dean.*

Clearly this is only a very small sample of the total number of child deaths and incidents of mistreatment which took place in 1985.

TABLE A.1
Child deaths in suspicious circumstances
Cat E980–989. Injury undetermined whether accidentally or purposefully inflicted

Age	1975	1976	1977	1978	1979	1980	1981	1982	1983	1984
Under 1	9	10	2	11	17	13	25	23	16	11
1—4	12	11	11	3	21	12	24	15	19	22
5—9	12	5	1	5	6	6	15	9	6	5
10—14	10	9	16	16	20	12	27	15	6	8
15—19	62	56	59	64	64	67	140	81	81	72
Total	105	91	89	99	128	110	231	143	128	118

* Argus Foreign Correspondent. June 1988

TABLE A.2
Child deaths as a result of inflicted violence
Cat E960–969. Homicide and injury purposefully inflicted by other persons

Age	1975	1976	1977	1978	1979	1980	1981	1982	1983	1984
Under 1	33	36	18	29	28	13	10	13	15	9
1–4	30	26	33	38	28	17	6	19	22	23
5–9	12	11	13	14	14	10	10	11	3	9
10–14	11	12	14	11	14	7	4	12	5	9
15–19	45	41	35	47	42	37	10	44	34	25
Total	131	126	113	139	126	84	40	99	79	75

The child who has been violently beaten or otherwise injured by his parents

Julie, thin, naked and covered in filth, was cowering in a corner like a small, terrified animal. In hospital they discovered that, at some time, almost every bone in her frail body had been broken. She had been ill-treated and beaten every day of her young life.

'Julie lived in a comfortable, middle-class "chintzy" home behind the blooming roses and pin-tucked velvet curtains of better-off suburbia, where neighbours tend to pride themselves upon "minding their own business and not getting themselves involved in other people's affairs".'

Julie lived in such a home for three years before a neighbour, having been told by mother that Julie was 'away on holiday with her grandparents', saw the child, quite by chance, staring wan, pale and obviously terrified, from behind a closed curtain. After much misgiving, and against her husband's wishes, the neighbour had finally taken it upon herself to report the case to the NSPCC. Indeed, it is this apathy or unwillingness to become 'involved', which often leads to a distressing 'snowballing' of child abuse.

At first, confronted by the NSPCC inspector, (predecessor to the social worker) the mother denied that she had ever had a child. Eventually, cornered, she admitted, that he could find her 'in a bedroom at the top of the stairs'.

On investigation it was found that the mother, in spite of being devoutly and puritanically religious, had become pregnant prior to her marriage. She loved her husband and he loved her.

Nevertheless the child had been conceived 'in sin', and she was living, daily proof of that sin. So she had to be punished, in a perverted effort to expunge the mother's guilt.

Clearly the mother was a deeply disturbed woman who was *projecting* her own feelings of guilt on the child, to the point of considering Julie 'unclean', unacceptable and thus unworthy to exist.

Confronted for an explanation, the father, a successful business executive, 'denied' his knowledge of the situation. Judged charitably, one may assume that he loved his wife so much that he was unable to face the horror of her wrongdoing (*'denial mechanism'*).

'Each day when I came home there was just a little more; I hardly noticed. Whereas you see all at once the result of three years', *he rationalized*.

Both parents were charged and eventually fined £30 each.

The child was placed, on a semi-permenent basis, in 'approved single care' under the supervision of a social worker.

Resolution

The resolution of such cases is no easy matter. The child needs her parents, and it would be permanently emotionally destructive to her personality growth were she to remember her mother-figure only in such rejecting and cruel circumstances. A positive maternal role model is important for future identification.

Like virtually all other children, Julie needs her *mother-figure, irrespective of the way she has been treated* by her. This is typical of the child role within the mother–child relationship in both human and sub-human situations. (See Harlow's monkeys, p 43 and 'Johnny', p 280-1.) It is for this reason that specialized welfare services attempt to reach the *deeper emotional precipitating factors* existing in parents. Attempts to heal the mother–child relationship are intrinsic to rehabilitation. This is also the reason why official organizations tend to avoid normal court procedure.

'We obviously don't fiddle about if a child is on the point of death', said a legal spokesman at the British NSPCC headquarters, 'but sometimes, although we have an open and shut case, we might not see a prosecution as being of benefit to the family as a whole'. Court appearance may impede the resolution of long-term family relationships; yet court procedure is sometimes the only way to force unwilling parents to accept psychiatric treatment.

Sometimes children are used as rejection compensation weapons of revenge or as aggression displacement outlets

Billy's teacher noticed that he had been quieter and more withdrawn than usual. Eventually she realized he was severely hurt and in considerable pain. In fact, Billy could hardly walk and his trousers were stuck to his body by congealed blood. His buttocks were covered by lacerations and indentations of the flesh. Untended, these raw wounds had festered and were weeping through the seat of his jeans.

It emerged that Billy had been beaten by his father with a belt—including the belt buckle. There were signs of similar, older injuries.

The father claimed that it was 'his right' to chastise and correct his child, who, he declared, was 'lazy' at school and could do better.

Billy's little sister was clearly well-cared-for, happy and outgoing.

Investigation revealed a deeply disturbed parental relationship.

The father claimed that his son 'has his mother's stupid brains and looks just like her. He is her favourite—she neglects both the little sister and me.'

It became apparent that the father was 'getting at' the mother through her favourite and beloved child. He was deriving obvious pleasure from his aggressive displacement upon the child. His *'rationalization'* to the effect that Billy 'deserved' such chastisement removed his feelings of guilt, and thus any self-control which he may have exerted.

The mother, on her part, was too frightened to defend her son and in fact had a deep need for the sexual attentions of her husband.

Some children are mishandled or neglected due to the inherent intellectual inadequacies of their mentally sub-normal parent:

Persons with IQ range approximately 60-85, and ultimate Mental Age range between 8 years 6 months and 13 years, relative to normal MA 16 (see p 144), appear, on the surface, sufficiently 'normal' to mislead family and community workers as to their ability to cope with the responsibilities of child-rearing. In reality, they lack the ability to exert normal self-control and to achieve insight into more abstract human situations. Classically they do not possess the time concepts, staying-power and ability to place themselves in the future which are necessary for the achievement of reliable family planning. They have large families for which they are frequently unable to provide the fundamentals of food and living conditions. In the face of their children's demands, unable to cope with the situation, they resort to that physical aggression which is the normal frustration outlet of the intellectually sub-normal. Classically, they are unable to accept that the inadequacies of their children are natural to their appropriate developmental stage. They insist that natural developmental inadequacies require punishment and their over-reaction is classically uncontrollably violent. Such parents will always require close supervision and control in their handling of their children.

Children neglected deliberately or through ignorance

Also very typically, the children of intellectually sub-normal parents constitute a significant proportion of this unfortunate classification of child abuse. Lacking time concepts such parents are likely to forget to feed their children, or do so inappropriately and inadequately. A vicious circle is set up. The persistent crying of a hungry baby is sometimes enough to trigger off an uncontrolled physical outburst in an already mentally defective or disturbed parent. Unable to hold in mind several complementary tasks, they omit to perform essential routine physical care.

A mildly handicapped mother IQ ±70, and thus with an ultimate Mental Age of approximately 11 years, may well forget to test the temperature of the bath, causing very severe burning by forcing her child into scalding water.

Mentally ill parents may appear to commit purposeful child-abuse

Alan was 9 months old and weighed less than his birthweight. He had been fed sporadically and inadequately, and was brought to the hospital in a coma, almost on the point of death from malnutrition.

Mother was found to be in a state of withdrawn lethargy, without motivation or appropriate emotional reaction. Psychiatric examination revealed her to be distinctly mentally ill, in fact, in a depressed phase of schizophrenia. Had neighbours insisted on remaining 'uninvolved' Alan may well have died, and his mother may have advanced into a state of psychotic illness from which it would have been difficult to extricate her. Her grief and guilt on returning to reality would have further complicated her rehabilitation.

It is, of course, true that many cases of child-abuse result from *uninhibited sadism* on the part of one parent and spineless over-dependence by the other. A sane, balanced approach on the part of those professionals who have to deal with the child's tragic predicament is indeed difficult to achieve—but does constitute the cornerstone on which meaningful, comprehensive treatment is founded.

The British system of NSPCC workers fulfilled an important role, frequently not so effectively performed by social workers who enjoy less official status and are frequently 'off duty' when the abuse occurs.

An official operating with specific legal authority is in a stronger position to deal with those adults who are capable of brutality. In the words on one such inspector:

'Men who beat children are cowards. I have never yet had one who directed physical violence at *me*.

Of course alcohol and drug-taking, clouding the reality situation and the ability to exert self-control, constitute an important precipitant of brutality and neglect.

Poverty and crowded conditions do increase the tension situation, precipitating frustration and temper outbursts which are *displaced* upon children. Certainly children living in bad social conditions are more at risk than others.

Exposure to danger factors is sometimes involuntarily increased by the **necessity for both parents to work**, hours of duty sometimes 'overlapping'.

Yet to some extent protecting the child living in overcrowded and poverty-stricken conditions is the fact that cramped and economically deprived situations do render privacy almost impossible. Everybody knows everybody else's business, people are more friendly and their lives are involuntarily interwoven. The news of child abuse thus reaches official quarters more easily.

The child from a middle or upper socio-economic group, whose home is relatively isolated, enjoying greater privacy, has to suffer much longer before his plight is detected and reported.

In the words of Rev Arthur Morton, Director of the NSPCC:

> 'Constantly we ask ourselves how many more children are suffering today because those who could help are reluctant to get involved.'

Danger signs[1]

According to United States statistics 15–20% of injuries in children under 4 years old are due to abuse. Apparently professionals are not picking up nearly enough cases in casualty departments. One way to detect such cases is to note any deviation from the norm in <u>parents' and children's behaviour.</u>

Professor Ounsted of Park Hospital, Oxford, maintains that some children evoke abusive reactions in their parents—'the child sends out signals.' These include children suffering from *organic cerebral impairment or dysfunction.* They tend to be screaming babies, restless and hyperkinetic, who frustrate their parents until they 'are beside themselves.' Feeding problems and other sources of unresolved and persistent crying are also provocative in tired, immature or *isolated* parents.

Child abuse is not confined to infants. Frequently it consists of a pattern. <u>Attempting to solve human and discipline problems by physical attack easily slips into uncontrolled personal and social violence.</u>

Latest statistics in the U.S.A. show

(i) one-third of abused children to be between 12 and 17 years of age
(ii) 50% of abuse cases started out as 'discipline'.

---

* Hare, Isadora, 1978. Further details from author.

The following are typical pointers suggesting child abuse and warranting further attention by community and social services:

'A baby crying for hours on end; a toddler seemingly overprone to tumbles and bruises; a child sick-looking and undernourished; a suspicion that all isn't well. Nothing is lost in investigating, or reporting your doubts to the NSPCC. Much might be gained—a child helped, its happiness, maybe even its life.'

Typical injuries are:

weals and bruises, especially to the neck and head
broken bones
burns and cuts
dislodged vertebrae and shoulders from violent shaking (these injuries often result in permanent visual disturbance, mental defect and cerebral palsy, scarring and deformities).

The child's behaviour varies:

(i) inability or refusal to communicate, verbally or non-verbally, or to relate to persons in the environment;
(ii) an expression of 'frozen watchfulness', depression, withdrawal;
(iii) refusal to eat;
(iv) almost desperate clinging to staff, and, at times, to parents.

These are typical signs.

The inexperienced may negate a diagnosis of abuse when they observe such children's need for their parents. But Bowlby* comments, 'the attachment of children to parents who by all ordinary standards are very bad is a never ceasing source of wonder to those who seek to help them'.

Of Irwin's† 67 cases, 29 were first-born. Siblings had been abused in 12 of the remaining families. Children had already been officially removed from 7 of the families. One of the hazards of removing children from their families is the parents' motivation to embark on a further pregnancy while still under treatment; this in order to prove their competency for the parental role.

In addition, removal results in increased anger and hostility towards their children, the hospital staff and society as a whole.

Some authorities believe that nurses, being more confident in physical diagnosis and its implications are more prepared to take necessary and decisive action than social workers whose concern may focus on parental psychodynamics and future cooperation.

Is child abuse an increasing phenomenon?

Child abuse is a syndrome as old as mankind.

Perhaps to some extent the strains, stresses, both financial and environmental, of our highly pressurized, small unit society, squashed into confined living-space, are important factors. Probably ever-increasing academic demands, irrespective of the intelligence of either parent or child, result in frustration and anxiety, in *over-idealization* and inappropriate pressure to achieve the unobtainable.

* Bowlby J. *Maternal Care and Maternal Health.* Geneva: WHO 1951.

† Irwin, Claire. Senior Psychiatrist. Establishment of a Child Abuse Unit in a Children's Hospital. 1975. Refer to author for further information.

Very possibly it is our enlightened attitude which sees the sadistic and destructive evil of parental beating for the emotionally and physically devastating experience which, in truth, it is.

Of course, some parents who have been brought up at the end of a cane or leather belt have an unconscious need to *displace*, or 'take out', their aggression in such treatment of their own children. At last they have the chance of directly expressing that hostility which has been festering in them ever since they themselves were thus mishandled. They *rationalize*: 'I was brought up that way, and I am none the worse for it. Now it is his turn to learn the hard way.'

This pattern of physical abuse has been passed down (*introjected*) from one generation to another, and it is to the credit of our society, whatever its shortcomings, that this behaviour is seen as humiliating, destructive and brutal.

Child abuse may mean different things to different people and societies. In Victorian society, and in those groups which believe (or at least *rationalize*) the Biblical caution 'spare the rod and spoil the child', there is an acceptance of parental justification for severe beating. In fact such aggression, sometimes concealed in coldly inflicted official punishment, is still the established pattern in certain socially valued schools, juvenile judicial systems, as well as certain institutional establishments.

United States child abuse authority Isadora Hare maintains that dependence on discipline by corporal punishment easily slips into abuse. Legitimized patterns of solving problems by physical attack are soon 'introjected'. She quotes studies to show that 30% of abuse cases start out as discipline.

> 'Child abuse is not confined to infants. Latest (1978) statistics show one-third of abused children to be between 12 and 17 years of age.'

Presentation and etiology

A pioneer and standard work is that of C H Kempe, F N Silverman, B F Steele, W Droegemueller and H K Silver 'The Battered Child Syndrome' 1962 *Journal of the American Medical Assoc vol 181 pp 17–24. This article is currently reprinted in Child Abuse and Neglect* (1985) vol 9 pp 143–54, considers child abuse to be an emotional rather than a class phenomenon.

This landmark article presented important clinical material in association with innovative radiological findings—it also popularized the term 'battered child syndrome'.

Kempe's findings included:

1. Physical ill-treatment of young children is a *far more frequent phenomenon* than previously assumed.
2. *Psychological* rather than environmental stressors (such as poverty, overcrowding and educational deprivation) are predominant precipitators of child abuse:
    (i) parents who have themselves been deprived and mistreated in childhood were unlikely to possess the emotional make-up necessary for adequate parenting of their own children;
    (ii) these parents tended towards unrealistic, excessive expectations of their children →

This pattern of

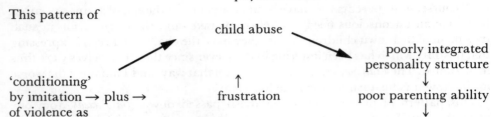

repeats, strengthens and persists <u>unless positive and effective intervention and positive reconditioning takes place</u>.

Kempe recommends:

1. protect the child by:
    removal from parents
    admission to hospital, with or without parents
2. focus treatment on parents by:

    (i) psychotherapy, mainly individual
    (ii) if successful, reunite with parents at home (if indicated, under professional supervision)
    (iii) follow-up social work
    (iv) failure—continued separation of living arrangements.

Response to treatment: Kempe claimed

    80% success rate
    20% unsuccessful due to factors such as severely disturbed or psychotic parents

Further work by Kempe and his associates confirm their basic principle that:
Extraneous factors such as stress and poverty remain secondary to the predominance of parents' own childhood experiences. Child abuse, they claim, is thus a *'classless phenomenon'*. Kempe's treatment programmes are thus concerned with <u>emotional aspects</u>.

Individual psychotherapy is complemented by

group therapy
behavioural therapy } for parents
family therapy

crisis hotlines
crisis nurseries/day centres } for children
play therapy

The important role of physical contact

It is important to impress upon parents that

> although *hurtful* physical contact is *harmful* and *destructive, warm* loving physical contact is *essential* to relationships, to conformity (pp 48-52), to mental health, and to eventual loving sexuality.

So kids, like grown-ups, need plenty of kissing and cuddling.

Preventive community work emphasizes techniques for *prediction of abuse potential* from birth and the neonatal period. Kempe and his workers claim 75% accuracy.

In the late 1960s and early 1970s research focused on the undoubted long-term and irreversible effects on personality of maternal deprivation (see Levy, Bowlby, Goldfarb pp 42-50). Since then other studies have broadened the etiology of child abuse.

Gil presented findings on a nation-wide U.S.A. study of 1 380 cases of child abuse between 1967 and 1968.

Findings

1. Most subjects were from financially deprived backgrounds.
2. Only half the fathers had been employed throughout the year.
3. Almost one-third of the children lived in homes without a father or father substitute.
4. More than one-third were in receipt of public assistance relief.
5. Parents were not as young as in the previous studies.
6. Only 14% of mothers/7% of fathers were reported to have been themselves abused as children.
7. More than half the incidents were not considered serious.

Conclusion

> 'Thus by looking at a broad sample of child abuse, Gil widened the parameters of the subject, and pointed to <u>major structural changes in society as a means of tackling child abuse.</u>'*†

Pelton, in his survey of child abuse, concluded that, contrary to Kempe's theory of classlessness, child abuse and neglect are strongly related to poverty in terms of prevalence and severity of consequences. Again, these views do not refute the psychologically focused explanations of child abuse, but they do emphasize other factors more strongly, and have different implications for official responses to the problem.‡

* Corby, B. *Working with Child Abuse—Social Work Practice and the Child Abuse System* (Open University Press, Milton Keynes 1987).

† Gil, D. *Violence against Children: Physical Abuse in the USA* (Harvard University Press 1970): 'Unravelling Child Abuse' *American Journal of Orthopsychiatry* (1975) vol 45 no 3 pp 346–56.

‡ Pelton, L H 'Child Abuse and Neglect—the Myth of Classlessness' *American Journal of Orthopsychiatry* (1978) vol 48 no 4 pp 608-17).

Developments in Great Britain

The NSPCC had been, in intent anyway, much influenced by Kempe. Now there were amendments. The society substituted qualified social workers for psycho-therapists, their main techniques involving ego-supportive case work. Case work and facilities appeared largely procedural and administrative rather than based on planned methods facilities and specialized training.

An exceptional British facility adhering closely to the work of Kempe is the Park Hospital in Oxford which provides:

> joint residential facilities for parents and child;
> psychtherapeutic counselling;
> group work;
> play facilities and play therapy.

The unit mobilized community-based resources, especially monitoring of maternity wards for 'at risk' parents.

Report on the Maria Colwell Inquiry (a child who died violently in spite of warnings by relations to police and social workers)

The report in this case:

1. highlighted the need for professional co-ordination and communication;
2. alerted social service authorities to the problem of physical child abuse and the extent of public indignation pertaining thereto.

As a result, the Department of Health and Social Security established the existent framework for the:

detection
investigation } of child abuse
processing

Cornerstones of their framework are:

1. Area Review Committees (ARC)
        Composition: higher levels of staff of relevant health and welfare agencies
            Function: to make and implement policy decisions.
2. Case Conference Systems
        Composition: frontline practitioners from relevant agencies.
            Function: in individual cases—to assess, make decisions.
    Parents present with two main complaints concerning the Case Conference system:

    (a) denial of parental right to attend;
    (b) powerlessness to obtain information.

'I don't think it's very nice sitting there discussing someone's whole future, someone's life, and they've got no say. I just think people have a right to know what's being said about them at case conferences.'*
'I was sitting there and I must have smoked 40 cigarettes in the hour they were in there. I was in a terrible state. The woman social worker came out and said,

* Corby, B. *Working with Child Abuse — Social Work Practice and the Child Abuse System* (Open University Press, Milton Keynes 1987).

"It's all right, you can take Terry home." She said, "Everything's been sorted out." They didn't tell me what had been said or nothing.'*

As expected, the 'Cleveland Affair', the matter of Drs Marietta Higgs and Geoffrey Wyatt, in which diagnoses of sexual abuse were based on the reflex anal dilation (RAD) method, and as a result of which 120 children were diagnosed as abuse victims and, at one stage, 250 were removed from their parents and foster parents, has done little to improve the relationship between professional committees and parents.

Upon the pages of her school exercise book Vanessa projected her trauma:

'They said we were abused when we weren't. They (the social workers) kept saying "Why won't you tell us what is wrong?" I kept telling them "But there is nothing wrong."

They said "Daddy has done something to you." But I said I would know if anyone had done anything to me and no one has done anything to me. I got so fed up with them not believing me that I wouldn't talk to them in the end.

I am mad with Dr Higgs. I want to destroy her because she said our Dad had done something when he never did.'

Vanessa's protest reflects:

(i) the danger of generalizing a diagnosis from one diagnostic feature—it is a poor surgeon who would remove an appendix from an x-ray alone in the absence of clinical symptoms. A diagnosis of child abuse should present evidence from the *case history, generalized case presentation, interviews* with and without parents, *projective techniques and other psychological evidence* as well as *more* extensive *physical trauma.*

Shortcomings in the case study methods presented by Drs Higgs and Wyatt are confirmed by the 32 senior doctors on the British Government's Standing Medical Advisory Committee, who opined:

'It cannot be emphasized too strongly that no physical sign can, at the present time, be regarded as diagnostic of child sexual abuse. The most RAD could indicate is a limited level of suspicion.'

The Cleveland report described the doctors as 'zealots' who were 'well intentioned but inexperienced'.

(ii) the readiness of children to jump to the defence of their parents—in almost any circumstances, even, in some cases, where there is justification for suspicion. Sometimes fear impedes case work. But clearly the parent–child bond is important, deep and not to be trifled with. *Separation may be more traumatic to the child than abuse*—herein lies the professional's dilemma!

Some critics maintain that the case conference is an arena for inter-professional rivalry rather than an effective decision-making body.

3. Chile Abuse Registers

Function: to record the names of children deemed to be 'at risk' of abuse or further abuse.

---

* Corby, B. *Working with Child Abuse — Social Work Practice and the Child Abuse System* (Open University Press, Milton Keynes 1987).

Aim: to ensure that:
(i) previous instances of abuse of the child in question are not overlooked
(ii) every precaution is taken to prevent occurrence.

4.   Child Abuse Manuals (issued by the ARCs) provide agencies with procedural guidelines.

Since 1976 there have been legal restrictions preventing adults, with criminal records for offences against children, from living in a joint household with them.

As the result of the 1980 DHSS circular, the definition of 'child abuse' has been extended to *emotional abuse* and *physical neglect*.

The 1980s have seen mounting interest in *sexual abuse* of children within families. Although this is not officially classified as grounds for registration, it is in practice considered as such in many parts of the UK.

However, relative to Kempe's recommendations, emphasis remains administrative, procedural and managerial rather than therapeutic and preventative.

Establishing therapeutic relationships with parents

Among **Corby's** *25 research cases* (1981–5) some social workers established fruitful relationships with mothers. These reflected a *warm friendly climate* upon which to build and reward amended behaviour patterns.

> 'Mrs McIntosh became like a friend. It's a pity people aren't more understanding of social workers.
>
> Me and Joan have always been like friends. We've never been formal. She's come in, I've made a cup of tea, we've sat and had a laugh or joke. If she did get that (a supervision order) it'd change everything between us because I'd know she was coming and checking up on me. I don't like that.'*

Nevertheless, there was an element of unspoken tension about the role of the social worker as child protector. The study suggested a need:

1.   *to define, repeat and bring into the open the reasons for supervision* —
     'Let us state again our problems with Stevie's injuries, how they happened and what we can do to prevent a repetition.'
2.   *to structure intervention* by setting goals and targets in order to achieve specific parental response.

(See Therapeutic Recommendation p 308.)

Extended families were involved in 8 of Corby's 25 sample cases. In most cases the extended family was asked to, and indeed did:

(i)   provide temporary relief, an opportunity to break the cycle of family stress and recrimination, by providing temporary care for the index client;
(ii) prevent more traumatic and painful separation for all concerned;
(iii) facilitate parental visiting, reducing shame and embarrassment;
(iv) facilitate surveillance of rehabilitation.

Of course, parental preferences and confidentiality must be observed.

---

* Corby, B. *Working with Child Abuse — Social Work Practice and the Child Abuse System* (Open University Press, Milton Keynes 1987).

Relatives as a source of information in data collection

There is ethical objection to obtaining this information without client permission. However, in order to protect a child's safety such investigation is justifiable.

Sometimes it may be necessary to investigate a resident grandparent relationship, which later may be stressing the parent, with resultant 'aggression displacement' upon the index client (see Granny Bashing p 477).

Work with adult male family members

Frequently male adults are not involved in ongoing case work.

1. Social workers appear to feel more comfortable with females within the family constellation.
2. Many men resist meaningful involvement.

Unless they *do* 'contract' to become involved, social case work and, indeed, the nursing process, will be incomplete and ineffectual.

Siblings of abused children

The procedural stance is that *if one child is shown to have been abused, all other children in the family must be reviewed* and, if necessary, examined as a matter of urgency. A non-abused child may fear lest he too be attacked. His sibling rivalry and subsequent ambivalence may result first in satisfaction, then in guilt and aggravated anxiety.

Community support

Corby* has his doubts as to both the availability and the efficacy of community resources.

In only one of his 25 research samples was a community group-support facility used. In contrast, in two cases social workers were obliged to protect parents from community scandal and ostracism.

Common impediments to effective intervention are illustrated by reference to the post-mortem inquiry on 3-year-old Darryn Clarke,† who died as the result of assault by his mother's co-habitee, even after anxious relatives had appealed to the police:

1. Belief that the case was not very urgent because —

    (i) there was no known history of child abuse;
    (ii) the relatives may have been over-reacting.

2. The non-abusing parent was acquiescing and 'covering up' due to fear of rejection or 'punishment'.
3. The events took place over the Christmas holidays.

---

* Corby, B. *Working with Child Abuse — Social Work Practice and the Child Abuse System* (Open University Press, Milton Keynes 1987).

† Corby, B. *Working with Child Abuse — Social Work Practice and the Child Abuse System* (Open University Press, Milton Keynes 1987).

Certainly child abuse, like many other social problems, is a real or potential crisis situation, which cannot be adequately treated nor prevented by '9–5' workers. These personnel are based primarily in interview rooms far from the 'hot' on-the-spot catharsis, guidance, support and often life-saving removal required by the gross, physical and emotional trauma involved. One's chances of entering the client's deeper personal world are better when his entrenched defences are down.

An additional frequent impediment to effective action is the health visitor's/ social worker's reluctance to be honest and decisive. She fears lest firm action may imperil her relationship with her clients. As one father shrewdly observed:

> 'She's frightened of the whole thing! So she's wishy-washy—sometimes she's all smiles and out before she's in.'

When is intervention successful?

The Kempes present the following four criteria for their claimed 80% successes who return home from hospital and foster care and who, to the researchers' knowledge, have never been injured again:

1. 'First, the abusive parent's image of himself must have improved to the point where he has made at least one friend with whom he shares regular and enjoyable experiences, such as bowling.
2. Second, both parents must have found something attractive in their abused child and be able to show it by talking lovingly, hugging or cuddling.
3. Third, both parents must have learned to use lifelines in moments of crisis, so that they telephone their social worker, a friend, a member of Parents Anonymous, or else take their children to a crisis nursery.
4. Fourth, weekend reunions with their child in hospital or foster care must become more and more enjoyable, and increasing responsibility must not have strained the family.

It is premature to return the child home if these criteria have not been met.'*

Recommendations

Apart from Kempe, virtually all researchers present findings to show that many cases of child abuse take place amongst the socially and environmentally deprived.

Among recommendations made by the First Report from the Select Committee on Violence in the Family, Session 1976-7, Violence to Children, vol report, London HMSO, were the following.

1. The Health Education Council should consider giving *preparation for parenthood* a greater priority within its existing resources which have recently been increased.
2. Whatever other cuts are made as a result of recent reviews of expenditure there should be no reduction in the number of places available for the under-five's.

---

* Corby, B. *Working with Child Abuse — Social Work Practice and the Child Abuse System* (Open University Press, Milton Keynes 1987).

3. Social services departments should be well known, accessible and welcoming and should provide an open-door policy for worried parents.

4. Greater co-operation and equal status between professions.

5. Greater use of structured models.

The Nursing Process *(ch 9)*

(*Data collection*: Socio-economic status: the geneogram (p 419); ego strengths and weaknesses (p 225); mores; ambitions, etc. Presentation and history of the child's injuries or other abuse. Other physical features, eg mental handicap, or physical resemblances.

(ii) *Assessment*: the nursing diagnosis (p 225): In terms of deviation from goals (Maslow's Hierarchy of Human Needs p 100). Definition of areas in which index client and family require help in overcoming environmental and personal psycho-social stresses in order to achieve the child's safety and well-being.

(iii) *Planning - the contract*: Definition of the client-professional therapeutic relationship. Setting a mutually acceptable programme in terms of goals, behaviour modification, etc. Because the safety of the child is involved, the role of the nurse/social worker may be more directional, even to the extent of statutory back-up for co-operation, removal, return, etc.

(iv) *Implementation*: Participation in goals, tasks, timing.

(*Evaluation/feedback*: (p 231): How far have family relations and socio-economic conditions improved in the programme towards confidence in resumption of parental responsibility or return of the child?

Illustrative Case

Five-year-old Peter came to school with bruises, welts, and a cigarette burn in the palm of his right hand. His teacher's enquiries were met by his stepfather's verbal abuse and allegations that the injuries had been inflicted at school. Peter no longer came to school. When school attendance officers were turned away from the home, the police called, demanding that the child be medically examined. He did not turn up for his appointment. When removal was threatened, his mother took an overdose of sleeping pills. A statutory order compelled the family to attend a case conference.

Planning

An interim compromise resulted in

(a) social case work

(b) compilation of a mutually agreed social case work contract aimed at communicating to the parents:

    (i) the concern of the professionals

    (ii) conditions required to safeguard the child and to avoid his removal.

The contract

For the following 10 weeks Peter would remain at home as long as:

He was taken to school every day by his mother.
She would hand him over to his teacher, from whom she would collect him after school, thus disproving the accusation that the child's injuries were due to the school's negligence.
Peter would be medically examined every Monday.
He would visit his grandparents every Wednesday and Saturday.
Mother would take Peter for a walk or read him a story every day.
Stepfather would play with him for half an hour every day.
The social worker would have regular and free access to Peter.
Mother and stepfather would call at the social worker's office every second Wednesday.
The situation would be reviewed at the end of the 10 weeks.

Contract compliance—implementation at the end of weeks 1–10

Compliance

It was ascertained that

1. Peter was taken to school every day, being handed over to and collected from his teacher as arranged.
2. He attended his weekly medical examinations—there were no further injuries.
3. The child confirmed walks, stories and play in respect of both parents.
4. He visited his protective grandparents every Wednesday and Saturday.

Non-compliance

1. Stepfather did not once attend the social worker's office.
2. Mother came alone and only twice.
3. She failed to communicate meaningfully—rather did she weep, sidetrack and retreat into silence.
4. On reiterated threat of removal both parents attended an 'evaluation interview.

Evaluation

Compliance was praised and the child's good physical condition noted.
Non-compliance areas were defined.

Parents were confronted with:

(i) the implications of these failures—the limitations of symptom eradication without insight, ventilation and changes in basic emotional and thus relationship dynamics.

'Unless you come to feel differently about Peter and want to react differently towards him, no improvement can last'.

(ii) the options of deeper-level investigation, discussion and problem-solving or reconsideration of removal; if, on the other hand, the parents did co-operate fruitfully, eventual lifting of the statutory order.

Re-planning

Parents agreed to a new contract for the following 12 weeks.

Re-implementation

Mother and stepfather both attended social work interviews and succeeded, with reassurance and support, in ventilating their marital, financial and child care problems—which included the stepfather's alcoholism and the mother's endogenous depression, for which he was referred to Alcoholics Anonymous and she for psychiatric treatment.

Re-evaluation

Parental participation appeared to:

ease stress
improve parent-child relationship
prevent further child abuse.

The statutory order was removed but supervision continues.

Unfortunately not all case work succeeds in its <u>primary object of relationship reconciliation</u>: neighbours reported two emaciated, bruised and terrified children to health visitors who called police to break into the house and take the children to hospital. The case was handed over to a social worker who, on attempting intervention, was verbally abused and shoved towards the door.

The children remained in hospital for two months and were then placed with short-term foster parents. The parents visited them there on three occasions, but after two months ceased visiting altogether. They made no efforts within the two-year period to see them again. The social worker wrote to the parents to encourage contact but eventually no further efforts were made in this direction and the children were placed with long-term foster parents. Social work focus switched to finding suitable substitute parents and encouraging visits from the paternal grandmother who provided a blood relationship and ongoing loving support.

Of Corby's six most seriously abused cases

3 resulted in permanent substitute care;
3 in rehabilitation of parents under supervision orders with no further evidence of abuse.

To what extent is the professional justified in taking risks in order to keep the family together?

In 18 of Corby's 25 cases the children remained free of further abuse incidents. In 3 serious cases, further serious abuse occurred while under social work supervision, leading to firmer response within legal provisions.

It should be remembered that although comprehensively researched, Corby's was a small sample.

Prognostic factors appear to include:

1.   assessment of parental personality
2.   co-operativeness of parents

3.   previous history of child abuse
4.   availability of police and medical evidence
5.   seriousness of injury
6.   age and thus potential vulnerability of child
7.   degree of suspicion surrounding the cause of the injury/neglect
8.   socio-economic status.

'The abused child needs help himself: he needs assistance in improving his self-concept, in loosening his inhibitions and in learning to enjoy life. He needs help in expressing and acknowledging his feelings about assault, neglect and separation from his parents. It may be necessary for him to live adaptively and to negotiate healthily in a family with parents who have numerous emotional problems themselves. In as much as the parents usually cannot give this help, it must come from someone outside the family.'

Hospital case procedure (based on the work of Claire Irwin MB ChB DPM)

Child abuse units are attached to hospital paediatric departments. Their goals are:

  (i) to provide safety for the child;
 (ii) to involve the family in a long-term rehabilitation programme designed to return the child to his home;
(iii) to educate hospital staff of all disciplines to develop an awareness, that they may recognize the syndrome; and
(iv) to research the psychopathology and management of the problem.

At the outset it is necessary

  (i) to record the history of at least two generations of the family (see also geneogram p 419); abuse behaviour patterns are introjected (p 107) from one generation to the next;
 (ii) to hold lengthy interviews in order to get to know the parents;
(iii) to create an opportunity for the staff to discuss their own attitudes and feelings toward the problem;
(iv) to conduct regular team, parent and child case conferences in order to assess progress and 'contract' treatment procedures.

While a suspected abused child is admitted to the ward, a member of the psychiatric unit interviews parents or relatives.

Although ultimately each family is interviewed by a psychiatrist, initial information is obtained by any member of the unit. Care is taken to conduct the interview 'along non-accusatory, non-persecutory lines', in order to 'establish a working relationship with hostile, guilty parents. To extract a confession is not the intention.'

'The parents are told that our hospital is concerned with small children who sustain injuries, and that it is routine for these children to be admitted to the ward for investigation and treatment. It is also routine for the parents to be seen in the Child and Family Unit, and time is available for discussion, for home visits and for the establishment of rapport with the family. . . . Legal action is not taken unless parents are unco-operative and it is unsafe for the child to be allowed home. Such action hinders a therapeutic alliance and every attempt is made to avoid it.

The mother is requested to visit the ward daily, so that she can care for her own baby under the watchful eye of the nursing staff. The relationship between mother and child is observed, and a member of the psychiatric unit sees the mother daily to establish a warm, trusting relationship in which the emphasis is on *her* needs. If necessary, fathers are seen after working hours or during home visits.'*

(Special problems of sexual abuse are discussed on p 355.)

Dr Irwin stresses that surveillance of the parent-child relationship during visiting hours only is no substitute for the above programme and may give rise to false impressions.

'Steps are taken to ensure that the mother spends enough time at home to fulfil her household duties and to give time to her other children. Arrangements are made for the supervision of these children while the mother is at hospital. Thus, the abused baby is not exposed to the effects of maternal deprivation, a hazard incurred during the hospitalization of small children.

After a full skeletal and haematological survey, the child is kept in hospital until the paediatric and psychiatric teams are satisfied of its *health*, the *diagnosis* and the *safety of discharge*. Six to nine months' hospitalization may be necessary before it is finally decided whether the child should be returned to his home or whether he should temporarily be in an institution or in foster-care. If the child returns to his home, our *intensive home care programme* is instituted. Daily home visiting, gradually reduced over the months and years, continuity of care by the psychiatric unit and community agency and a 24-hour call system, all help ensure that crises are managed. If necessary, the child may be re-admitted to hospital. . . .

Institutions are poor substitutes for a family, and suitable foster-homes are at a premium. If a child has to be removed, all attempts must be made to establish an ongoing therapeutic relationship with the parents, with the goal of the possible ultimate safe return of the child to its home.'*

British hospitals are developing specialized Mother and Baby units where both sleep in together. Mother is 'mothered', and physical treatments are complemented by group identification, protection, guidance and support.

Pathology of Abuse

Associated factors, both medical and psychosocial, are found to aggravate and precipitate child abuse.

1. *Medical problems*, such as obstetric difficulties during pregnancy and labour, prematurity, congenital defects, minor physical illness during early weeks of life, feeding problems and failure to thrive, are factors. This observation is

---

* The establishment of A Child Abuse Unit in A Children's Hospital', by Claire Irwin, MB, BCH, DPM, Senior Psychiatrist. Any correspondence will be forwarded by the author.

cohesive with that stressed on p 397 of this book, to the effect that the <u>mother–child relationship is frequently complicated by involuntary associa-</u> <u>tion of the child, in the mother's mind, with a traumatic pregnancy and</u> <u>confinement.</u> Thus the necessity for *increased attention to mothers' physical and emotional experiences in childbirth, and during the puerperium, is endorsed.*

2.   *Psychosocial problems,* such as marital disharmony, inability to respond to maturational needs, unrealistic expectations of the child. Unemployment. Some children resemble, and are thus associated with, a disliked spouse or relative.

3.   *Psychopathology* prevailing in this sample is similar to that described in other literature. The majority of abusers evidenced mild or moderate psychopathic traits. Ten abusers were classified as 'severe' psychopaths.

4.   *Many abusers have themselves been subjected to physical and emotional abuse as children,* appearing to unconsciously 'introject' this behaviour pattern unto themselves, or, in their turn, unconsciously 'displacing' their hostility on their helpless children. (See Mental or Adjustment Mechanisms, chapter 5.)

5.   While *unplanned pregnancy,* even within the framework of marriage, clearly constitutes a dangerous predisposing factor in child abuse, *some pregnancies* appear to result from the parent's motivation to 'find a human being who will make up for my own emotional deprivation'.

   When the immature child is unable to fulfil this great love-need of the mother, the latter, fearing a repetition of that rejection which she had suffered as a child, becomes hostile towards her own baby.

6.   Sometimes adjustment to the *sex of the child* has not occurred.

7.   *Emotional immaturity* is a keystone to psychopathology in child abuse. Abusers are not adult parents in a psychological sense. They are unable to control their angry feelings. Concerned primarily with their own needs, they have unrealistic expectations of their children. They are *incapable of frustration tolerance.*

   The abuser has <u>few ego strengths</u> and thus encounters difficulty in coping with even minor crises. A 24-hour supportive service should be available to provide crisis intervention in such precipitating instances as minor illness in parent or child or the visit of a critical friend or relative.

Response to treatment

   Saving children is not enough; we must ask ourselves why we are saving them. Will they lead unhappy lives as a result of the physical and emotional sequelae of abuse? Will they grow up into adults who will breed yet another generation of abusers? The <u>abused child is the index patient, but the symptoms are merely a</u> <u>reflection of a wider disturbance and disorganization within his family and the</u> <u>community at large.</u>

   Statistics to date tend to be somewhat discouraging. A study conducted in the U.S.A. in 1973 maintains that one-half of abused children returned to their families will ultimately die of abuse. However, details of therapy available to such families are unknown.

Within the context of the very comprehensive and detailed therapy provided by Irwin's unit, or in combination with welfare agencies and private practitioners, of the 67 cases studied

1 child died before therapy could be instituted;
1 child died after the unit was established;
18 children had to be placed in foster care or institutions;
9 children and their families have moved, leaving no address;
36 families 'are receiving on-going counselling or psychotherapy, plus regular home visiting' by nurses or social workers.

Recommendations

Irwin maintains that the most hopeful response is to the policy 'mother the mother'. In order to save the child both physically and emotionally the full force of family and community medicine must be implemented. Better screening facilities must be provided at ante- and postnatal clinics, well-baby clinics, nursery and primary schools. There must be suitably trained staff to assist parents where children are 'at risk' for physical or psychosocial reasons. This includes round-the-clock supportive services.

Self-help groups have been successful.

Parents Anonymous is a self-help group of abusing parents who meet regularly and exchange telephone numbers. They are available to one another in time of crisis. They all feel they could lose control when disciplining their children.

London contact

Parents Anonymous for Distressed Parents: 01 263 5672
NSPCC 24-hour Child Protection Phone-in Service: 01 404 444

In case of injury the child should be taken to a hospital casualty department with the request that the family be screened for child abuse.

If the child is thought to be in danger of imminent physical injury the police should be called.

STOP PRESS In its annual report (1989-90) the National Society for the Prevention of Cruelty to Children draws attention to an increasing number of children being sexually, physically and emotionally abused in bizarre ceremonies often involving "satanic rites". NSPCC's director, Jim Harding reports that, of 66 teams of reported cases where children directly experienced ritualistic abuse, and another 14 cases where such abuse was suspected. Up to 20 boys and girls were forced to take alcohol or drugs and watch adults perform sexual acts. They themselves were sexually abused or subjected to other physical violence. Threats were used to control them and to force them to recruit other victims to people's houses or ceremonies in the open.

CHAPTER 15

ADOLESCENCE

Note: This chapter should be read in conjunction with Erikson's Maturational Crisis Theory (see pp 245-253) which latter outlines the positive growth force of adolescence.

The keynote of adolescence is *transition* between childhood and adulthood, involving great changes in every sphere of the individual's life—physical, intellectual, emotional and social.

The primary school years from ages 6 to 12 have been called the Latency Period during which physical growth continues at a fairly steady pace; intellectual growth is closely tied to environmental realities, and the pupil devotes much of his reasoning and understanding to the routines of learning. Emotionally the child in the Latency Period tends to be relatively phlegmatic. This is the 'golden age' of learning and physical skills.

Although sexually curious, he does not appear, on the surface anyway, to be as intensely interested in sexual matters as he was previously, or will be during adolescence.

The Latency Period has been described as Nature's 'breathing space' before the 'rebirth' of adolescence.

The period of relative calm ends with the onset of puberty. In hot climates girls tend to show signs of physical development from about 11 years of age, and boys from about 12 or 13.

As the pituitary gland (the 'orchestrator') stimulates growth, the youngster experiences marked changes in every sphere of development.

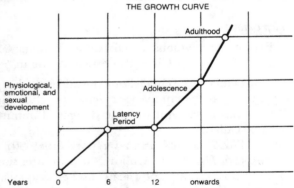

THE GROWTH CURVE

These changes are complex, rapid and unpredictable. Old feelings of security and stability are swept away, and the child and parent are together tossed upon the stormy sea of adolescence.

Adolescence: the 'Oedipus revisited' (refer to p 57)

Hormonal changes contribute to the upsurge of sexual and aggressive unconscious (Id) processes. Fulfillment of libidinal (sex drive) energy now becomes a reality. Sexual desires and phantasies in respect of the opposite-sex parent resurface, plunging the adolescent into Erikson's conflicting developmental crisis situation (chapter 11). Each sex uses the opposite-sex parent as a model for developing heterosexual phantasies with resultant guilt and anxiety for so doing.

The adolescent wants to escape from home into independence and heterosexual fulfilment, but still needs parental support and protection. He may escape into ego-defence mechanisms (chapter 4) such as 'denial' or 'flight' into religious ascetism, or 'sublimation' in political or intellectual outlets.

The classic normal *homosexual phase* of early adolescence may provide welcome respite from the stress engendered by the 'Oedipus revisited'. In that it directs love attachment outside the individual and his family, this phase also prepares for transition to heterosexual relationships.

Many of the adolescent's difficulties are due to the fact that his physical, emotional and social development are themselves uneven and out of step with each other.

Owing to rapid physical growth the adolescent may be gawky, gangling and awkward, overweight and clumsy, at just that period when he or she is becoming self-conscious and over-sensitive about physical appearances. His self-concept is endangered by his fear of physical non-conformity and anxiety lest his body be rejected by those near to him. Corporal punishment may well be interpreted as rejection of his adolescent body.

Physical-emotional development

Unevenness of development results in alternating spurts of physical energy and lassitude. The adolescent loves to partake of, and shine in, active sport, but he also loves 'just hanging around'. This is but one of those conflicts which are the keynote and the source of greatest strain in this period.

Glandular reactions and emotions are closely associated. Any period of *glandular imbalance*, to which the body has not yet adjusted, is marked by *emotional disbalance*—as is seen in the puerperal 'post-natal blues'; at certain times in the menstrual cycle; in the course of the menopause and in adolescence.

In adolescence glandular disbalance is reflected in *strong conflicting emotions*. The adolescent loves intensely and hates intensely. His emotive swing alternates illogically from feelings of exhilaration to depression. He is swayed between the wish for complete independence and persistent need of parental protection.

Characteristic *intensity* of adolescent emotion increases the stress inherent in ambivalence. All of which emotional imbalance certainly disturbs the youngster's sense of proportion, especially in late adolescence. Adolescence thus constitutes a particularly difficult phase for entrance into a stressful occupation such as nursing or exposure to the separation from parental and community support and life-threatening circumstances inherent in army life.

Social development

The process of socialization

As a baby he receives his love within the close mother–child relationship. Although altered, parent attachments persist.

EMERGING FEATURES OF SOCIAL DEVELOPMENT

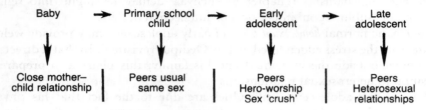

Baby →	Primary school child →	Early adolescent →	Late adolescent
Close mother–child relationship	Peers usual same sex	Peers Hero-worship Sex 'crush'	Peers Heterosexual relationships

As a primary school child his sources of love, satisfaction and security extend to peers, usually of his (or her) own sex.

In early adolescence he finds love-inspiration and outlet in an older man (or woman) relative, teacher, nurse or in the hero-worship of a member of his (or her) own-sex peer group. This is known as the homosexual 'crush' stage—and is normally only a developmental stage, having positive value in externalizing love.

In late adolescence the search begins to reach out for love in a member of the opposite sex (but fulfillment is thwarted by the demands of our society), resulting in further conflict, anxiety and frustration.

Further conflict lies in his spasmodic need to be alone. On the other hand, he wants to be part of 'the group', *identifying* with his peer group in an effort to find protection from the unknown, and from a frightening sense of being 'different'. He thus adheres closely to the clothes, mannerisms and standards of his group, whether this group be a socially approved organization such as the Boy Scouts or a socially disapproved group such as a violent gang.

Against 'the group' he will rebel very little; the normal rebellion of adolescence is reserved for parents and work superiors. These, the adolescent believes, have old-fashioned, unreasonable 'square' standards, which are to be resisted at all costs.

Sensible parents realize they cannot help assuming the responsibilities of parenthood, responsibilities which imply the application of limits which adolescents will resent, yet value as an escape from their own unacceptable emotional drives.

While the adolescent is 'caught up' in his own developmental and emotional entanglements, his parents are also enduring a period of disturbing readjustment. On the one hand they have the desire to help their child grow up successfully; on the other hand they have an understandable fear of losing for ever their relationship with him.

A friendly, relatively uninvolved, adivser, such as a youth counsellor, psychologist, family doctor, church minister, teacher or nurse, can play an important 'middle-man' role in helping adolescents and their parents understand, tolerate and thus find compassion for each other.

The adolescent's ego defence mechanisms are threatened and exposed by his transitional crisis. One sees clearly the different layers at which individuals operate:

Layer No 1—At Work: The person who confronts one in the work situation.

Layer No 2—Among Friends: In his peer group.

Inner World: The Inner World which even the adolescent's parents do not know:

a new world of hopes, ambitions, fantasies and fears ... especially of non-acceptance within the social group and by a marriage partner.

Early Adolescence (12 to 16)

For example:

'Not belonging to any group; there is a feeling of not fitting in anywhere: being neither an adult nor a child. I feel indignation because my opinion is never accepted at home, or by elders anywhere. Too young to know what I was talking about—"you will know better when you get older", they said.'

'When one gets home one makes for the pantry first and gets something to eat, and then you go for your book and shut yourself up with these two—it is a wonderful form of escape.'

Late Adolescence (16 onwards)

'My interest in sport has declined—especially since I have had a steady girl friend.'

'Feeling my parents were unjust in their attitude towards me, not understanding me correctly.'

'I was very concerned over religion—I tried practically every available church: deeply conscious of social problems and intensely interested in them.'

'I felt I as abnormal and that nobody else does these same dreadful things or has the same dreadful thoughts; nobody else has any sex temptation; nobody else has any strange or queer ideas—it would have been a great consolation had I known that most people suffer from these same problems.'

'The relationship with parents is smoothing out now, particularly with mother. No longer class her advice as nagging nor flare up at any occasional remark.'

In our society education has been extended, marriage delayed, and the period of dependence and subjugation to parental authority elongated beyond the point where nature has decreed that young men and women are ready to live independent and sexually fulfiled lives. This period of extended adolescence, beyond natural maturity, has given rise to increased parent–child conflict, unfulfilled physiological needs and a powerful motivation to rebel against the society which has frustrated adolescent goal-attainment.

What constitutes adolescent goal-attainment?

We have seen that by the end of adolescence the young person is expected to:

(a)   come to terms with his glandular disbalance and accompanying physiological changes. His emotional reactions are intense and in conflict. He is caught between his motivation to grow up, and his motivation to stay within the protective care of his parents;

(b)   develop heterosexual interests;

(c)   learn to wean himself from home supervision;

(d)   make new emotional adjustments;

(e)   gain economic independence;

(f)   achieve social poise, confidence and techniques of social acceptance;

(g)   learn how to use his leisure time fruitfully;

(h) evolve a new personally satisfying philosophy: a healthy self-concept and
strong personal identity in family and community.

In fact the main job of the adolescent is to stop being one.

The often unrealistic academic demands set by our society frustrate and
humiliate that 40% (below IQ 98) of all racial groups who are apparently designed
by nature for skilled and unskilled manual (rather than 'white collar' managerial
or professional) work.

Adolescent values

Douvan & Kaye, (1981) conducting a survey of 1 925 girls, chronological ages
11 to 18, at the University of Michigan, posed the following question:

'What would you like to change about yourself if you could—your looks, your
personality or your life?'

Fifty-nine per cent mentioned some aspect of their *physical appearance*, whereas
only 4% mentioned a desire for greater ability.

Jersild in his *Psychology of Adolescence* (1963), emphasizes the important role of
physical characteristics in the adolescent's self-evaluation. The commonest
complaint among girls and boys concerned facial defects, principally acne.

Boys aimed at identifying themselves with masculinity and a large, rugged
physique. Girls wanted to be small and delicate in build, deeply desiring 'a good
figure'.

The adolescent who sees himself as deviating from these cultural stereotypes is
likely to suffer an *impaired self-concept*, becoming anxious about his ability to attract
members of the opposite sex and to achieve all-important social acceptance. In this
important context one appreciates, in chronic cases, justification for cosmetic
plastic surgery or hormonal therapy.

Boys who mature late are anxious about their deviant status, stress often leading
to various forms of antisocial or displeasing compensation mechanisms. They tend
to show off, be arrogant and defiant or sexually over-assertive. Some take 'Flight'
into social withdrawal or drugs.

Rejection for anyone is a most painful, diminishing and sometimes long-term
shattering experience. It is a source of terror for the teenager who fears no one will
ever choose him for a love-mate.

Aggravated by the insecurities, conflicts, self-blame and oversensitivity of
adolescence, the suffering imposed by rejection by a loved figure may permanently
distort self-esteem and damage personality development.

'There is no rejection greater, however, than in love. This is the stuff both of
nightmares and grand opera. Not always is it love for a paramour figure. It can be
because loved ones like parents reject you or your man (Romeos and Juliets) or
loved ones like children reject their parents (King Lears). But the classic fear that
haunts us all is that we will be rejected by the one who holds our heart.

In his autobiography *Confessions of An Actor*, Laurence Olivier wrote that when he
heard his then wife Vivien Leigh saying that she didn't love him any more ". . . it
came like a small bolt from the blue, like a drop of water, I almost thought my ears
deceived me. . . . I felt as it I had been condemned to death."

Coupled with envy, rejection is the cause of wars, the prime motive for murder, the most common catalyst for suicide.'*

The way one meets, and copes with, rejection will depend on the innate, environmental and social factors which have formed one's personality, as well as on the support one receives.

Cultural attitudes of emerging adolescent sexuality.

Mussen Conger & Kagan (1981) emphasize the wide variety of cultural attitudes pertaining towards adolescent sexualtity.

Dakota Indians do not expect children to be interested in sexual behaviour until they have reached puberty, and are capable of reproduction. Among the Melanesian cultures of New Guinea, on the other hand, sex play among pre-adolescents is taken lightly.

A culture's attitude towards sexuality will depend, in part, on whether that culture views sex primarily as a source of pleasure or as reserved for reproduction. The Marquesans stress the pleasure value of sex and are permissive in sexual behaviour in children. Among the Ila-speaking people of Africa, childhood is regarded as a time of preparation for adult life and mature sexual functions. At harvest time each girl is given a house to which she takes the boy of her choice, and there they play as man and wife. It is reported that there are no virgins amongst these people after the age of 10 years.

Astutely, Mussen, Conger & Kagan contrast adolescence in Western culture:

'We have typically spent a great many years teaching the individual to inhibit sexual responses in order to prepare him for a life when he will be expected to make these responses. We have taught him to respond to sex with anxiety when he was a child, and then demanded that he not respond anxiously after he is married.'

The 'new morality' among Western adolescents

The new Western adolescent generation appears to be escaping from bonds of anxiety and guilt, albeit frequently more often in word than in deed.

If one asks 'middle' and 'upper' class youth whether they think there is a 'new morality' regarding sex, the answer definitely appears to be in the affirmative. In a survey of 550 adolescents aged 13 to 20, 75% stated that they had developed 'a new sexual morality'. They do not believe this change to be a lowering of morals: 82% of the sample viewed their moral standards as 'no lower than our parents'. One adolescent summed up the opinion thus: 'Adults are just plain phoneys about sex.'

Clearly the 'new morality' appears to involve a desire for greater happiness and honesty concerning sex. The magazine *Look* in its article 'The Open Generation', published in 1966, reported that 80% of their survey sample felt that a pregnant girl should not marry if she did not love the boy.

Thirty-seven per cent of both boys and girls approved prescription of oral

---

* McGlone, Heather. 'Focus' *The Argus* 23 October 1986.

contraceptives in student health centres. Sixty-six per cent of the adolescent sample expressed the view that sexual intercourse before marriage is anticipated by their contemporaries. Forty-five per cent of the total sample (34% of the girls) agreed that it is 'all right for a boy and girl who are in love to live together'.

Clearly these youngsters placed a greater emphasis on the sincerity of their personal relationship than on the arbitrary judgment of social standards.

In word or in deed?

In view of the changing sex values expressed by adolescents, one might expect these changed values to be reflected in dramatically changed sexual behaviour. Paradoxically, available evidence suggests that the really significant difference in the incidence of pre-marital intercourse does not lie between today's mothers and their daughters, but vis-à-vis both generations and those born before 1900.

	1900	1910	1950's	1980's
Adolescent petting	66%	81%	94%	95%
Pre-marital intercourse before CA 25 years	14%	30%	40%	78%

According to available data, Kinsey, Pomeroy, Martin & Gebhard in *Sexual Behaviour in the Human Females*, report that about 94% of today's mothers engaged in petting as adolescents. In contrast the incidence for their grandmothers varied from 66% for those born before 1900 to 81% for those born in the first decade of the century. These data suggest that the so-called 'sexual revolution' was actually initiated by today's parents and grandparents.

Of females born before 1900 only 8% reported premarital intercourse before age 20, and only 14% before age 25. In contrast, of today's parents and grandparents, 31% reported premarital intercourse before age 20 and 35% before age 25. Clearly it is the attitude of frankness and reduced guilt, rather than frequency, which distinguishes today's adolescents from their parents and grandparents.

'Teenagers involved in the Youthscan national survey will be 18 years old this week.* The 15 000 youngsters have been scrutinized at birth and at the ages of 5, 10 and 16. Their health, development, hobbies, attitudes and diet will be re-examined within the next year. Professor Neville Butler, director of Youthscan, said: "Our next survey will look at how they cope with the prospects of employment or unemployment. Most complain that no one listens to them. If they have low self-esteem and feel disillusioned now, how will they cope with bringing up their own children?"'

Caught in the fertile soil of glandular, and, hence emotional disbalance—the conflict between a 'childish' wish for safety and an intense need for 'adult' self-determination—the adolescent is vulnerable to **stress precipitators**:

* *The Times*, London. Leader page 5 April 1988.

1. The need to find, and define, himself as an individual, with a unique personality, function and honourable place in society—an *identity of his own*:
   'Who am I?'
   'What will I be?'
   'Who will honour and love me?'
2. Parental and school *discipline that is strict and diminishing*, resulting in frustration and anger.
3. *Excessive demands in academic, sporting or other activities* highly regarded by the significant adults in his life.
   or
   parents who are *too busy or themselves too stressed* to provide guidelines or involved, caring support.
4. Lack of *financial security, presentable living conditions*, clothes and reasonable status symbols important to the vulnerable self-esteem of a youngster.
5. Confusion in areas of *sexual acceptance*, success and *identity*.
6. Fear of *army conscription*, removal from loved ones, harsh discipline, combat dangers.
7. *Absence of demonstrated appreciation* of effort and success or, in fact, lack of exposure to situations which may provide *success experiences*.
8. *Pressure from peers* to indulge in alcohol, drugs, fast cars, etc.
9. *Heterosexual transition*: for difficulties in achieving sexual identity see The Sexual Identity Crisis pp 337-40.

In response to these pressures the adolescent may seek tension relief in the unconscious selection of *destructive defence mechanisms* (chapter 5) such as the *'fight'* reaction (p 105):

> physical aggression, bullying: cruelty to animals: passive, recalcitrant resistance, sulking;
> verbal abuse and disproportionate argumentativeness

or the *'flight'* (p 104) reaction:
   social withdrawal to the point of 'unattainable' isolation
or
phantasy escape into an increasingly unattainable and self-destructive dream world;
   actual *running away* from home and school into a self-destructive hobo existence;
   escape into the alcohol and drug 'culture'.

Stress signals

Insomnia	truancy
acne	alcohol, drugs and other substances
headaches	experimentation and dependence
general aches and pains	irritability
altered eating habits—especially	anger
'overeating' and anorexia	depression
rebelliousness	thieving

These behaviours constitute the youngster's efforts to communicate his needs.

Positive Reactions to Adolescent Stress Signals:

'Significant' people especially parents, teachers and nurses should ensure that their 'antennae are up' to receive youngsters' sometimes obtuse 'messages'. Like all relationship-based communication, this is a *two-way process*.

Youngsters are thinking:
'Nobody cares.'
'I've no-one to turn to'
'I couldn't tell my parents *that*.'
Parents are thinking:
'What have I done wrong?'
'What can I do?'

The first priority is to avoid total communication breakdown. Sometimes it is better to 'confront' in a direct but *not authoritarian* atmosphere.

Sometimes an opportunity may be found in *mutual activity* by asking opinions; telling significant stories of one's own youth. In fact, the very act of taking off specific *time* to share mutual and intimate activities on a *one-to-one basis* such as a fishing trip, a hike, a beer at the local pub; a shopping expedition, shared cooking, dressmaking or a trip to the beach . . . all these activities provide valuable and tension-free situations in which to establish that trust relationship and general friendliness so often forgotten in the 'rat race'. The creation of a friendly atmosphere provides the most constructive situation for discussing misunderstandings, conflicts; for providing guidance.

See Berne's Adult–Older Child: Adult–Adult communication patterns p 179 et seq; *Handling Stress* p 32.

Drug use among adolescents—See Chapter 17, Substance Abuse

Eating disorders predominant in adolescence

People's food needs vary with individual metabolism and activity lifestyles.

Loss of appetite

In times of stress, in keeping with Nature's mobilization of physiological resources for the 'fight/flight' reaction (pp 104-105), some people's digestive processes 'dry up' and they experience appetite inhibition:
'I just can't eat—I'm too nervous.'

Obsessive compulsive eating

For others, the more stressed and unhappy they become, the more they are forced by their inner needs to comfort themselves with food, that most primeval mother-associated satisfaction.

From one's earliest hours food and mouth satisfaction have become associated with mother, love, safety and security. Hence the need, in times of stress and unhappiness, to regress. (p 32-5)

Excessive regression to mouth comfort indicates underlying personal, social or work stresses requiring identification, confrontation and solution, perhaps in psychotherapy.

Anorexia nervosa

Anorexia nervosa consists of loss of appetite and refusal to eat even unto the point of life-threatening emaciation.

This self-inflicted physical wasting resultant upon psychiatric illness was first described in 1868 as a disease striking upper-class families in which hunger is not a socio-economic problem. The patient, usually a young, highly motivated woman of perfectionist personality, begins to isolate herself, in many cases working obsessively. She begins to diet strenuously, setting a pattern of increasing stringency which she appears unable to break. The thinner she gets and the greater the attention focused upon her wasting body, the more her dieting crescendos . . . and so does her hunger and preoccupation with food, until the *hunger←→eating conflict becomes so strong that anxiety and resultant tension energy possess her whole being*. Lack of essential food factors contributes to cessation of menstruation and libido. Some orthodox psychoanalysts believe that physical wasting and reduced sexual desire provide escape from sexual conflict and guilt feelings.

Because the seat of satiety is intimately connected neurologically with the hypothalamus, denial of satiety satisfaction may well predispose the subject to gross emotional disturbance—even to the point of apparent hallucination where the youngster 'sees' her shape as quite different from what it really is. She may stare at her emaciated reflection in the mirror, but insists that she sees a fat image.

As starving proceeds the skin becomes dry, rough and grey and teeth loosen and fall out. Some patients 'break out' into obsessive eating jags which they counteract by forced vomiting. This condition termed Bulimia is dangerous to kidney function and may become involuntarily compulsive.

Deprivation of protein reduces efficiency of frontal lobe intellectualization learning functions, and spatial concepts rendering the patient vulnerable to "brainwashing" and perceptual distortion.

Etiology

1. *Biological factors*

New research by Dr Philip Gold, American National Institute for Mental Health, observes that many anorexics secrete abnormal level of vasopressin, a hormone helping to regulate the body's fluid balance:

> 'Altered levels of vasopressin can affect learning in laboratory animals, and Dr Gold hypothesises that they may also influence an individual's perception of hunger and contribute to the extreme obsession with dieting that is the hallmark of anorexia.'

This is one of several biological factors known to be present in anorexia nervosa. Hormonal balance may well constitute a sustaining rather than a causatory factor.

2. *Poor self-image leading to obsessive dieting*

Anorexia nervosa attacks approximately 1 in every 100 dieters, usually women of innately plump or squat build convinced that dieting will make them sylph-like and therefore lovable.

The perfectionist-type patient exposed to environmental pressures such as parent disapproval of 'fatness', and the harping necessity for slimness conditioned by the media, is particularly at risk. So is the aspirant ballerina!

Clearly the insecure youngster who feels generally inferior and poor in self-concept will be most vulnerable to this type of disapproval and pressure. Sometimes mothers, themselves of ample proportions, who have always been frustrated in their attempts to achieve a sylph-like shape, try to compensate for this status symbol by pressurizing their daughters to diet. A girl seeking to please an unaffectionate or demanding mother may introject false standards and an impossible self-image. Conversely a youngster may refuse to eat in order to "spite" a nagging food-pushing mother.

3. *Common psychodynamic theories* in the etiology of eating illness are based on underlying conflict:

(i) Of a sexual nature: Caught in ambivalence between: new adolescent sexual awakening and the desire for fulfillment   *vs* fear and guilt feeling

↓

'denial' (p 115) of the wish for sexual fulfillment

↓

'reaction formation' (p 118)—the adjustive technique of offsetting a very strong, unconscious guilt-laden drive or urge by doing the opposite in one's conscious behaviour

↓

assuming the unattractiveness of the extremely thin in order to camouflage femininity or even assume masculine characteristics, thus safeguarding oneself from "sinful" or fearsome sex activity.

(ii) Another school of thought believes the etiology of anorexia nervosa to be associated with an underlying desire for gluttony or excessive, obsessive eating in an effort to 'take in' love as a 'compensation' (p 112) for feelings of rejection and deprivation. The adolescent, feeling guilty and anxious lest she be even further rejected due to obesity, embarks with varying levels of intention on chain reactions of self starvation.

(a)   indulgence *vs* fear of rejection
↓
establishes patterns of food refusal
↓
digestive disturbances
↓
pathologically reduced food intake
↓
cerebral perceptual disorders in which she actually "sees" her body shape as distorted—though emaciated she sees her body as obese; or

"Self Portrait" of a slim twenty-year old anorexic

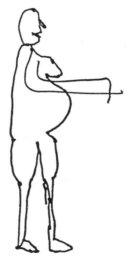

(drawn by an anorexic patient known to the author)

(b)   develops patterns of *bulimia* in which eating jags, to the point of engorgement, are followed by the insertion of the finger in the throat in order to induce vomiting. This pattern may lead to various chronic digestive disturbances and acute kidney conditions.

Psychoanalysts believe that disturbed eating behaviour represents a desire to return to infantile dependency (to "regress") in response to acute emotional deprivation.

4.   There may be *inverted, angry, passive 'fight'* (pp 104-105), an element of the 'hunger strike', in the etiology of anorexia. The patient who feels hurt, rejected, diminished and victimized, personally, socially or by illness, is able to inflict feelings of concern, or at least guilt, upon those 'indifferent' people or circumstances at whose mercy she feels herself to be. In actual fact, eating refusal is a masked plea for involvement, support and affection. Soon the biochemical reactions of anorexia set in and enmesh her, until the illness is established.

Treatment

Because this condition may proceed to serious illness and death, hospitalization is usually indicated. Forced tube-feeding is outdated, having been replaced by intensive psychiatric treatment. "Forced Feeding" has given way to methods based on:

(i) persuasion within involved staff relationships,
(ii) psychotherapy,
(iii) behaviour modification; privileges "open wards", shopping vouchers, use of telephone etc, when food is eaten,
(iv) relaxation therapy,
(v) family therapy, etc.
(vi) Modified insulin treatment (10–20 units), given half an hour before meals, has the effect of stimulating the appetite and is an effective aid in the treatment of anorexia nervosa.

Reference

Welburne J, Purgold J. *The Eating Sickness: Anorexia, Bulimia and the Myth of Suicide by Slimming.* Harvester Press, 1984.

The special implications of adolescence in the nurse herself

The student nurse is herself usually a late adolescent. In addition to the turmoil and conflict of adolescence she is required to adjust to the emotional shocks, physical strain, and tensions of a highly responsible and highly personalized adult profession. In the midst of her own sexual turmoils, embarrassment and anxieties, she is required to make highly personalized daily contact with all ages and types of the opposite sex.

She is under pressure from study and examinations. She is having to accept unquestioningly and continually that very adult discipline under which she is rebelling at home. In many ways the authority of her superiors is an extension of that authority from which nature is forcing her to rebel.

These pressures may, in terms of Erikson's life-crises, result in the recurrence and precipitation of unresolved and vestigial developmental tasks and conflicts. Flare-up reactions to parents and authority; social aggression or withdrawal, are common. Problems of sexual acceptance and identity, with consequent indiscriminate and unwise sexual experience may present. Generalized anxiety, reaction-formation in obsessiveness and psychosomatic tension symptoms may indicate the need for professional help. Some are 'introjections' of patients' symptoms.

If she understands the cause of her tensions, that they are common to all student nurses—past, present and to come—and that most will soon resolve themselves, then these very tensions will become easier to bear. The mechanisms of adjustment through *identification* and *introjection*, which we have discussed in a previous chapter, will help her cope with these temporary disturbances and tensions. (See pp 106-109.)

In the senior nurse, understanding of the adolescent difficulties of her juniors will help achieve tolerance of their shortcomings, and with insight should come ability to ease their anxieties, guilt-feelings and tensions.

The teenage patient

To the adolescent patient, caught in his headlong dash for independence and freedom, divorced from the strengthening influence of his 'gang', torn by the intense conflicting emotional upheavals of his endocrinological disbalance, moody, uncompromising and painfully self-conscious about his sexual development, hospitalization is a traumatic experience. Vulnerability to castration fears persists.

Owing to the development of his sex organs he is experiencing strong new emotions which are the source of conflicting pleasure and anxiety; excitement and guilt; pride and shame. If during this period he is robbed of his privacy and exposed to frequent examination, surgery and post-operative procedures, his embarrassment, humiliation, resentment, guilt and anxiety are unbounded. It is less traumatic to perform operations such as the bringing down of undescended testes and the repair of hypospadias well before the onset of adolescence, preferably before the child goes to school.

Since Western society causes the adolescent to postpone for several years the fulfilment of his sexual urges, he turns increasingly to 'masturbation' or, in modern terminology, relief in self-stimulation. Although this is a normal activity, usually shed in maturity, social and religious taboos are liable to attach to it unnecessary, but none the less crippling, feelings of guilt and anxiety.

We know that in the stress of illness people are liable to *regress* to earlier forms of satisfaction. The nurse should not be shocked by adults who, accustomed to regular sexual outlets, *regress* to sexual self-arousal during convalescence.

The adolescent is resentful of the disciplined dullness of hospital life; he is anxious about his physical condition and about his place in society when he returns to the 'gang'.

Placed in an adult ward, the teenager may well become lonely and isolated. Surrounded by older patients who are filled with anxiety, obsessed with ill health, rendered morbid by incurable disease, he may well *identify* with their anxiety depression and hopelessness.

Exposure to death of his fellow patients will almost certainly constitute a terrifying and depressing experience. So marked is *identification* with the dying patient that the youngster may well develop similar phantom symptoms aggravating his terrifying fear of death (necrophobia).

Clearly the unique problems of the adolescent patient, and the most compassionate way of dealing with these problems, warrant special study and amended ward routine.

Because most hospitals allow persons over 13 years to visit, the teenager is somewhat luckier than younger patients. The visits of classmates and friends do a great deal to relieve the monotony of hospital regime, and to brighten the outlook of the teenage patient. These young visitors, coming to the hospital without gloom or anxiety about the patient's condition, bring news of people and events in which he is keenly interested and which may help to *motivate* him back to health. (See the Dying Adolescent, p 551.)

SEXUALLY ORIENTATED PROBLEMS: INFERTILITY; SEXUAL IDENTITY; SEXUALLY TRANSMITTED DISEASES; SEXUAL ABUSE

INFERTILITY

'And when Rachel saw that she bare Jacob no children, Rachel envied her sister; and said unto Jacob, Give me children or else I die.
And Jacob's anger was kindled against Rachel: and he said, Am I in God's stead, who hath withheld from thee the fruit of the womb?'

Genesis 30: 1,2.

When couples cannot share in the triumphs and delights of childbearing, when their seed is cut off from the chain of life, there is grave disappointment, bitterness and diminishment. Muslim women may face social rejection and divorce if their marriage is without issue.

Although up to 20% of couples cannot conceive without medical help, the very word 'infertile' carries a stigma, lowering the woman's self-esteem and dealing a blow to the male ego.

Treatment for the problem places strains on sexual, personal and family relationships, while the woman has to face months, if not years, of investigations that can include experiences ranging from comic to those causing utter despair.

Members of Infertility Self-help Support Groups in sharing their disappointments, failures and successes, help others to cope with theirs. Among members' comments are:

'There are major emotional and psychological effects to be faced: you feel subhuman, not a proper woman.'

'Wives have to contend with thoughtless or callous remarks from family and friends. 'We're compiling a list of hurtful comments!'

'Unlike the regular exchange of news between women on ante- and post-natal matters, there are no cosy chats about infertility tests. Patients should be warned about the embarrassment of post-coital tests, the pain of tubular surgery and sometimes the costs of the *in vitro* fertilisation programmes. But the hope offered with new treatments, in particular the IVF, make it worthwhile and patients are immensely grateful to have an opportunity to participate.'

One of the group's objectives is the fostering of communication between patients and hospital staff.

'After the implant, it is most important to lie absolutely still for two hours . . . then along comes a porter who decides to run a Grand Prix, with you on the trolley, from theater to the ward . . . and I've had young nurses who tried to force me to get up when I've got there.'

Doctors, including gynaecologists, are not interested in your problem until 'you've tried for two to three years.' The next step is usually prescription of a fertility drug: any further investigation has to be earned.

'Group members may well benefit greatly through sharing experiences.

'A year ago I would not have been able to talk to anyone as I am talking to you.'

Pre-menstrual syndrome (PMS)

Until recently, the gynaecological establishment tended to tell women their pre-menstrual problems were psychological, and had no physiological basis. These 'experts' were predominantly males who, of course, had never menstruated. Their condescending attitude has at last been replaced by acceptance of the fact that the *pre-menstrual syndrome* is psycho-hormonal in nature—emphatically, it is *not* 'all in your mind'.

Medical researcher Dr Katharine Dalton and her co-worker Dr Raymond Green describe the PMS as swelling and tenderness of the breasts, a bloated feeling, acne, lethargy, tension, anxiety, depression and heightened irritability. Dr Dalton quotes Queen Victoria as presenting with typical monthly 'personality change'.

> 'Once a month, Queen Victoria would become unaccountably enraged at Prince Albert, screaming accusations and hurling across the room any objects that came to hand. If the Royal Consort tried to reason with her, she would only shriek more loudly and vituperatively.'

Etiology

Most experts suspect an imbalance in female hormones, specifically oestrogen and progesterone.

Drs Y Samuel Yen and Robert Reid of the University of California suggest that women susceptible to PMS suffer a defect in the hormonal 'messages' put out by the pituitary gland and the associated hypothalamus. The so-called hypothalamic-pituitary axis, being the body's master control centre for hormones, plays an important role in associated emotional fluctuation.

Therapy

The most popular treatment is by prescription of natural hormone progesterone and mild cases often respond to diuretics, which, by promoting excretion of water, relieve the typical bloated feeling.

Psychotherapy, relaxation techniques and emotional support are important therapeutic adjunctives.

Presentation

Table 1. Symptoms of premenstrual syndrome*

(a) Somatic symptoms	Psychological symptoms
Feeling 'bloated'	Irritability
Feeling of weight increase	Aggression
Breast pain/tenderness	Tension
Swelling of ankles	Anxiety
Skin disorders	Depression
Headache	Lethargy
Pelvic pain	Insomnia
Change in bowel habit	Change in appetite
	Crying
	Change in libido
	Thirst
	Loss of concentration
	Poor co-ordination/clumsiness/accidents

Table 2. Reported consequences of premenstrual syndrome*

Incidence of psychiatric admissions	Absence from work
Suicides	Poorer performance at work
Alcohol abuse	Epileptic fits
Child abuse	Asthma
Accidents	Cardiac failure
Accidents to children	Varicose veins
Examination failures	Rheumatoid arthritis
Marital disharmony	Glaucoma
Crime	Hospital admissions in general (eg, for appendicitis)

Not all women suffer from PMS and there is a large variation in those who do. Experts estimate that 20-30% suffer symptoms sufficiently severe to warrant treatment, and perhaps as many as 5% are so seriously affected that work function decreases in the pre-menstrual week.

'The majority of women experience some change prior to the onset of periods, but it is probably true to say that about 40% of women appear to get significant premenstrual syndrome at some time in their life. Some of these tolerate the symptoms, others request therapy.'

It is beholden on those fortunate women who do not suffer significantly to understand and support those who do.

It is equally beholden upon sufferers to attempt insight into the etiology of their impaired self and social functioning, to enlighten their colleagues as to the involuntary and impersonal basis of any difficult behaviour and, possessing self-insight, to attempt increased self-care and self-control at these times.

* O'Brien PMS. Premenstrual Syndrome. Part 1. *Psychiatry and Clinical Psychology in Practice.* A Medical News Group publication. Vol 1 no 4. August 1986

Dysmenorrhea

Is dysmenorrhea responsible for the disruption of important activities such as work, school or social activities? The following research suggests a positive answer:

Dysmenorrhea, or painful menstruation, affects between 25% and 75% of women (Coppen & Kessel, 1963; Klein & Litt, 1981; Weideger, 1976). It is considered to be a leading cause of school absenteeism among adolescent girls (Klein & Litt, 1981) and the greatest cause of lost work hours among women (Novak, Jones, Jones, 1975). Based upon Kistner's (1979) estimate of 140 million work hours lost annually due to dysmenorrhea, Sobczyk (1980) calculated that an average of 2 or more work days is lost per female employee per month. Others have suggested that menstrual cramps cost the US 600 million lost work hours and $2 billion annually (Dawood, 1984; 'Monthly Downtime' 1984).

However, *empirical data do not seem to support these estimates*. While 20-40% of adolescent girls in various studies blamed dysmenorrhea for missing school occasionally, only 3-14% reported missing school every month or every other month (Andersch & Milsom, 1982; Heald, Masland, Somers & Gallagher, 1957; Klein & Litt, 1981; Widholm, 1979).

Findings that (i) dysmenorrhea primarily affects women under the age of 25 (Sobczyk, 1980), (ii) absenteeism occurs primarily among the relatively small proportion of women with severe dysmenorrhea (Klein & Litt, 1981) suggest that dysmenorrhea may not have the economic impact suggested by Dawood (1984) and Kistner (1979).

In their study 'The Impact of Dysmenorrhea on Daily Activities' Valerie A Gruber and Beth G Wildman of Kent State University[*] set out *to investigate the discrepancy between research findings as opposed to empirical observation.*

Their subjects were 293 women between 17-24 years recruited from full- and part-time introductory psychology classes at a Midwestern university.

Procedure

All subjects completed questionnaires, concerned with menstrual experiences and daily activities, at two testing times five weeks apart. During both testing sessions, subjects were given the Menstrual Symptom Questionnaire—Revised (MSQ-R; Chesney & Tasto, 1975; Stephenson, Denney, & Aberger, 1983; Wildman & White, in press), a questionnaire about their daily activities, (Activities Questionnaire) questions about remedies and coping methods used, and questions concerning perceived consequences of missing scheduled activities.

Findings

Pain severity:

'Bothersome or worse'	:	70,8%—7,8% reported 'severe' or 'excruciating pain
'Mild discomfort'	:	23,4%
'No pain or discomfort'	:	5,8%

68,0% reported using prescription pain relievers.

* This paper was presented at a Poster Session at the 94th American Psychological Association Convention, Washington DC, August 1986

Although 60,7% of the sample reported spending extra time resting during their menstrual periods, the majority of women did *not* report disruptions in their daily activities due to menstrual discomfort.

33% reported missing one or more of the following activities on the day before, or on the first two days of, menstruation:

    classes   :   12,6%
    homework   :   14,7%
    social activities :   16,5%
    routine tasks   :   17,2%

(less than 1% of employed women missed *work* due to dysmenorrhea)

Predictors of activities missed

Amount of pain

The relationship between the amount of pain experienced and activities missed was positive:

    'Severe and excruciating pain' — $1/2$ missed activities
    'moderate pain'   — $1/3$ missed activities
    'mild discomfort'   — $1/6$ missed activities

SEXUAL IDENTITY

As research into the delineation between men and women proceeds, we are constantly becoming more aware of the merging of sexual characteristics.

Recent research conducted by Ounsted & Taylor* stresses what they call the 'plasticity' of the sexes, maintaining that distinctions between men and women are by no means fixed. Each sex bears some glandular potential of the other. Environmental pressures may stimulate and change endocrinological and personality balance.

The hereditary equipment of males and females differs only in the Y chromosome, which they maintain acts merely as a *developmental decelerator*. Their analogy is that the girl-child skips quickly, blithely, perhaps somewhat carelessly, up the staircase of life.

She may even sometimes skip a step.

She maintains her lead throughout life, reaches adolescence about twenty months before her male 'competitor', and begins to shrivel to old age five years before he does.

In fact, it may be his prolonged exposure to periods of vulnerability, such as in childhood, in adolescence and in ageing, which predispose him to a higher death-rate before old age.

The boy-child derives his greater physical strength and claimed higher level of intellectual flexibility, even his added physical appendages, by virtue of his slower, surer and more thorough progress up the developmental spiral. During his more leisurely and thorough climb he has frequently stopped to absorb, organize and digest each developmental innovation.

---

* Christopher Ounsted & D C Taylor. *Gender Differences—their Ontogeny and Significance.* Churchill-Livingstone. 1972

Given a basically common reservoir of hereditary factors, both sexes bear the ability to modify physical and mental features in response to environmental demands, stresses and rewards.

Among many lower-life examples, that of the 'voidie' fish impressively illustrates sexual flexibility.

The male voidie, aggressive, large, with well-developed sexual features, effectively leads and protects a 'harem' of females ranged in descending order of strength and aggressiveness from a large, dominant but definitely female first wife, to an essentially weak, retiring passive and very feminine last or youngest wife.

If the male leader deserts his harem or perishes, the first and most aggressive wife begins to lose her female characteristics and becomes a physiological male.

In this role she—now 'he'—takes the place of, and in fact *becomes*, the male of the family, effectively Fighting off enemies, where necessary taking to effective 'Flight' and fathering his young.

However, if *during* this process of sex-change 'he' is attacked by a larger, stronger and more proficient male fish, being no believer in 'Woman's Lib', the temporary inter-sex fish reverts to her female role and rushes off to the safety of the harem. The oyster also alternates. He starts off as a male, becomes a female, and may return to male status.

Every kind of human sexual intergradation has been found from males with undeveloped masculine genitalia to males with all degrees of female genital development; from females with undeveloped or incomplete female organs to those with well-developed male organs. Between the two are many gradations of sexuality.

GENDER IDENTITY DISORDERS

The hermaphrodite

Professor Hugh Hampton Young of Johns Hopkins University has published a treatise on twenty indisputable cases of true hermaphroditism in which the same individuals had within them both ovaries and testes, a situation not uncommon in the lower animals, such as the tapeworm, the snail and the Drosophila fruit fly.

The true overt human hermaphrodite, who possesses organs and characteristics of both sexes, is extremely rare. Such cases show a physiological defect of the sex organs which renders normal sexual relations impossible, which condition is usually due to *pathological* genetic inheritance. The true hermaphrodite possesses organs and characteristics of both sexes.

Trans-sexualism

This condition is distinguished from homosexuality in that the client's main distress lies in his *own inappropriate body and feelings*, rather than in his fixated interest in the same sex. The client's <u>outer physical</u> make-up indicates his or her own <u>sex</u>.

His or her own <u>inner world</u> of feelings, attitudes and self-concept indicate <u>gender</u>. And the two do not match. If they did, sexual motivation would be directed towards the opposite sex.

It is as if the soul of the male is trapped in the shell of the female and vice versa. This is the reason for *transvestism* or pleasure in dressing in the manner of the 'opposite' sex.

The etiology of inconsistency between external sexual characteristics and inner gender is uncertain. Among probable causes are

(i)   imbalance of foetal hormones—in animal experiments if a pregnant mother takes certain barbiturates, antibiotics or psycho-active drugs, there may occur distortion of gender identity,

(ii) viral infection leading to improper programming of gender-role signals in the developing brain, causing confusion in the child's response.

Sex chromosomes are not the sole key to sex differentiation.

The recognition of such cases and the decision to embark on surgical treatment—the only effective treatment so far established—is of course a very specialized process.

Usually, the treatment consists of drastic surgery comprising mastectomy, hysterectomy and phalloplastics.

Those authorities who report a high rate of post-surgical success claim the following prognostic criteria:

1.   Normal and above Intelligence Quotient—in order to weather the trauma of surgery and readjustment, sustained insight and mental flexibility are essential.

2.   Long-term personality presentation should be sound, featuring:

a good work record,
stable relationships,
a history of religious and moral integrity,
an accepting family and strong social support.

The ideal age for surgery is around 21 years.

Appropriate motives in client's own words:

"Relief from mental suffering"
"To be myself"
"So people will treat me as I am"
"I will be able to be truthful"
"To love and enjoy my life"
"To marry and have children. (By adoption of course.)"*

It is difficult for a normal woman to accept the desire on the part of another to destroy the deepest and most precious evidence of womanhood.

Nurses are often worried by their own feelings of embarrassment, awkwardness and disapproval. Group discussion to provide

(i)   ventilation of problems and feelings,

(ii) guidance in addressing patients,

* Dr R Hempill, Lecture: Psychological and Surgical Implications in Transexualism, August 1988. Further details available from the author.

(iii) advice in handling compensatory over-aggressiveness in the patient of male gender, and submissive helplessness in those of female gender, is reported to be helpful.

It is helpful to try to identify with the poignant feelings of the transexual.

I'm not a woman—that's the whole point. I'm a man inside myself. 'I'm a man and as a man it's a horror for me to have breasts, bearing constant reminder that Nature made a dreadful mistake in putting me together. I have to get rid of all the woman in me, and surgery is the only way.'

The sexual identity crisis (see also Erikson, chapter 11 pp 246-8)

Many people do not understand Nature's <u>graduating continuum</u> between the rare conditions of complete 'maleness' and, at the other extreme, complete 'femaleness' and the <u>many interweaving patterns</u> between the two; together with the changing personality components of sexual identity throughout the life process. Indeed in later years differences between the sexes narrow.

Adolescents especially may become unnecessarily anxious about developmentally normal, and environmentally provoked, interludes of homosexual interest and perhaps activity. Counselling designed to work through these experiences, to guide and reassure, may prevent considerable anxious soul-searching and suffering.

Homosexuality

Homosexuality is that form of sexual behaviour which swerves individuals away from heterosexual relations, inclining them towards relations with, or interest in, their own sex.

Etiology is probably both

(i) constitutional due to endocrinological and perhaps chromosomal irregularity

(ii) environmental

The homosexual of basically normal appearance and physiology

There are two kinds of such homosexuals. The active plays the part of the male; the passive plays the part of the female. Thus the active male homosexual, although he prefers the company of males, may be outwardly no different from other men, and may even be more 'masculine' than the average man. Similarly the 'passive' female homosexual who plays the female role in relations with other women, is often extremely feminine in her behaviour. It is the passive male who acts like a female and the active female who often looks and acts as a man.

Terman & Miles formulate a frequently observed phenomenon to the effect that both men and women tend to become more 'feminine' as they grow older—men especially move nearer women in their sexual interests, behaviour, etc.

In his report on *Sexual Behaviour in the Human Male*, Kinsey claimed that at least 13% of the Unites States male population are classifiable as 'predominantly homosexual'. Clearly not all these homosexuals are overt hermaphrodites. Many, especially the 'active' male and the 'passive' female, are appropriately male and female in appearance. <u>Features of diagnostic syndromes presented on page 339 may be present in various combinations.</u>

Environmental Etiology

Certainly environmental factors can provoke homosexual interest and activity patterns.

Typical environmental and psychogenic factors are frequently related to:

1. *The one-sex boarding-school, hostel, military academy, etc*: Normal socio-sexual development proceeds from

> the mother–child relationship
> complemented by the
> Peer relationship—same-sex relationship ('crush' stage)—
> to the heterosexual relationship.

Each stage constitutes an important 'stepping stone' on the path to that sacrifice, tolerance and outgoing-love essential for maintaining satisfying, long-term relationships. The presence of the opposite sex stimulates heterosexual interests.

Deprived of the opposite sex, boarding-school pupils may well fixate at the same-sex 'crush' stage, turning to their own sex for love, warmth, approval and excitement. Once this pattern is established it may prove difficult to 'move on' to heterosexual behaviour, especially in the context of residential life in predominantly one-sex professions.

Indeed, Kinsey points to a high correlation between wealth, social status and homosexuality. Boarding-schools, military academies, college hostels, etc tend to be the prerogative of wealthier families. Regression to same-sex interest and activity sometimes occurs through 'necessity', as in long-term imprisonment.

2. *A poor or hostile relationship with the 'same sex' parent*: A youngster who resents his father's loud, abusive language, financial selfishness, bullying and aggressive behaviour towards his mother may dissociate himself from his father's male role, *identifying* instead with his loved mother figure:

'If that's how men are, I'd rather be like my mother!'

Clearly strong, positive identification with her mother is important for the establishment of a girl's sound sexual self-concept.

3. *Loss of the mother-figure leading to fixation on another older woman.*

4. *An instilled impression that heterosexual relationships are sinful, immoral, 'dirty' and bad: a history of sexual abuse*

5. *In women, a fear of pregnancy.*

6. *Personal unattractiveness to the opposite sex.*

7. *Admiration for another girl with the beauty, accomplishments or social status she lacks, and consequent vicarious satisfaction.*

These etiological factors combine to distinguish most homosexuality not as an innate deviation but rather as a choice related to the individual's developmental history. <u>If during transitional stages people are "seduced" or habituated to homosexual satisfactions, they may become "fixated" therein.</u>

DIAGNOSTIC FEATURES are consistently present since

For Females:

A. Strongly and persistently stated desire to be a boy, or insistence that she is a boy (not merely a desire for any perceived cultural advantages from being a boy).

B. Persistent repudiation of female anatomic structures, as manifested by at least one of the following repeated assertions:

(1) that she will grow up to become a man (not merely in role)
(2) that she is biologically unable to become pregnant
(3) that she will not develop breasts
(4) that she has no vagina
(5) that she has, or will grow, a penis

C. Onset of the disturbance before puberty.

For Males:

A. Strongly and persistently stated desire to be a girl, or insistence that he is a girl.

B. Either (1) or (2):

(1) Persistent repudiation of male anatomic structures, as manifested by at least one of the following repeated assertions:
    (a) that he will grow up to become a woman (not merely in role)
    (b) that his penis or testes are disgusting or will disappear
    (c) that it would be better not to have a penis or testes

(2) Preoccupation with female stereotypical activities as manifested by a preference for either cross-dressing or simulating female attire, or by a compelling desire to participate in the games and pastimes of girls.

C. Onset of the disturbance before puberty.

Dreams and masturbatory phantasies according to inner gender rather than outer sex are an important diagnostic factor.

Treatment

Should homosexuality be treated, or is it a natural phenomenon, the satisfaction of which is the individual's own private business? The answer must depend upon the individual's own adjustment.

Therapeutic indications

1. People of heterosexual identity, because of environmental or life-change circumstances, may also undergo sexual identity crises. An important role for therapeutic help lies in areas of unestablished sexual preference where the client is confused, guilt-laden and anxious, even terrified, about his sexual identity. Faced with the possibility of 'differentness', rejection by loved ones, and, perhaps above

all, rejection by his own inner self-concept, he may encounter great difficulty in sorting out his sexual identity.

2. Where the main factor is of environmental, psychogenic etiology, intensive psychotherapy and environmental manipulation are indicated, should the client feel the need for it.

3. Where true homosexuality is established, the client may profit from help in making his or her transition to full participation in the homosexual culture, free of vestigial guilt feelings, anxieties and impaired self esteem — free to start life anew. His "significant people" may also require psycho-therapeutic help in amending atitudes and relationships.

SEXUALLY TRANSMITTED DISEASES

Sex always was, and will continue to be, a basic instinct. No attempt to control disease by curbing this instinct is likely to succeed. The answer must lie in some other approach.

This is an area of medicine to which there clings an attitude of blameworthiness and culpability soon introjected by the client. The client's self-image is impaired by shame; his or her guilt is in-turned and treatment may be avoided. So intimately does medical literature link promiscuity with sexually transmitted diseases, that one begins to suspect that microbes and viruses are capable of reading marriage certificates!

Are psychiatrically disturbed people more prone to sexually transmitted diseases?

Pedder & Goldman, using a questionnaire in a series of new patients attending consecutively at a venereal disease clinic in London, found that 30% of 219 patients were probably 'psychiatric cases'. This figure approximates that found in general practice and in a medical out-patient setting.

Mayou, interviewing 100 first attenders at a venereal clinic in London, found 'a considerable amount of psycho-social morbidity' and rated 20% as 'psychiatric cases'.

There was no specific psychiatric pattern, but a rather mixed neurotic symptomology. While the majority reported anxiety about their possible illness, in a quarter of cases anxiety appeared to be long-standing and related to chronic social and psychological difficulties.

Of course the more sex partners — the more chance of contracting STD. But it can happen to anyone — even an unlucky virgin!

The truly promiscuous male has difficulty in forming lasting relationships with women, of whom he may well be fundamentally afraid. His need may be to dominate and humiliate the woman and to him copulation may be a means of achieving this. If ever he does fall in love, he may well become impotent. The above type of true promiscuity should not be confused with bouts of periodic promiscuity which may occur in otherwise non-promiscuous persons, eg when they are away from home.*

The following sexual problems appear to be specifically associated with venereal disease clinics:

(i) *Unsatisfactory sexual relations with the spouse.* If the primary sex partner acquires an infection as a result of an extra-marital episode, and transmits this infection to the spouse, he may well develop feelings of guilt, anxiety, aggression, Fight or Flight in the marriage relationship.

Clearly, if underlying psycho-sexual problems are not dealt with, the whole process is likely to be repeated. Sex therapy may well be indicated where:

(ii) *A pregnancy may have resulted in transient loss of attraction.*

(iii) *Restriction of sexual intercourse may have been advised for medical reasons.*

(iv) *A genital condition may cause pain or discomfort* in intercourse and thus remove the partner's desire for sex relations—this is especially true of urethritis.

(v) There may be *underlying emotional impediments derived from subtle conflicts* and challenges in the mating relationship, eg an impaired sexual self-concept and consequent fear of failure leading to an unconscious clinging to symptoms as an excuse to avoid intercourse.

(vi) The *need for dominance in the male and submission to a powerful male partner in the female*, with resultant inability to fulfil these roles.

Venero-phobia

The patient complains of symptoms which, after a full investigation, cannot be explained on any physical basis. The persistence and accuracy of these symptoms and the distress they cause illustrate the manner in which *a phobia may become so strong as to be experienced as a delusion.* Patients may attend several hospitals, demanding further tests, insisting that their belief may eventually be verified.

Underlying psycho-sexual etiology of venero-phobia

So great is the emotional trauma associated with a previous sexually transmitted disease that the patient cannot accept that he has been cured. His strong guilt feelings and consequent generalized anxiety, lead to

(a) obsessional avoidance neuroses, or

(b) rationalized frigidity and impaired sexual function.

---

* King, Nicol & Rodin. 'Veneral Diseases—1964-1980'

Faced with deep-seated conflict between

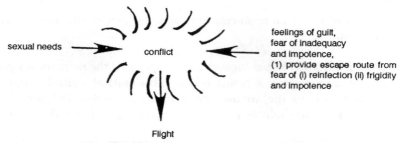

sexual needs → conflict ← feelings of guilt,
fear of inadequacy
and impotence,
(1) provide escape route from
fear of (i) reinfection (ii) frigidity
and impotence

Flight

the patient may unconsciously avoid confrontation by *'Flight' into the protection of disease*. At the same time, the delusion of his disease safeguards him from the fear of frigidity and impotence.

Further etiology of the frigidity and pseudo-impotence consequent upon the treatment of sexually transmitted disease may lie in:

(i) constitutional depression, or
(ii) paranoic schizophrenia,

the patient's impotence presenting as a *typical delusion that his body has been attacked by an evil, bad or punitive 'agent'*.

The World Health Organization and other international authorities appear to agree that sexually transmitted diseases are on the increase. The USA is virtually the only country with notification regulations both for doctors and laboratory reporting. Returns from STD clinics in the United Kingdom show over half a million new cases each year.

Specific psychological components of STD and their treatment.

In chapter 2, we read how the mother–child relationship becomes the nucleus of the socialization process.

Through association of the *removal of hunger pain* and *a general feeling of physiological well-being with the mother figure*, the configuration of *mother love, safety and security is established*.

Then, as the child develops and experiences the *reward of her love and praise*, this becomes an important stimulus-goal-satisfaction sequence in the establishment of *those sacrifices necessary for a socially acceptable behaviour pattern*.

The *loving approval* which she bestows upon him when he has subjected himself to the physiologically uncomfortable process of specific defecation *reinforces positive toileting habits*.

When this all-important mother figure expresses *disgust at the misplaced products of elimination, he soon develops the idea that the products of bowel and bladder are dirty, disgusting and 'forbidden'*.

Owing to the *close anatomical association between organs of elimination and sex organs, strict toilet training*, so typical of our Western culture, soon conveys the *message that the closely located sex organs are also dirty*, nasty, untouchable, and disgusting to the all-important mother figure.

These negative associations are often reinforced by social and religious taboos.

So closely are the sex organs associated with shame, guilt and stress that even normal sexual activity within marriage is often rendered distasteful and 'shameful' in our Western culture. Sometimes specific sex therapy is required to teach people to become 'comfortable' with their bodies—to touch and be touched—to give and receive pleasure.

When the sex organs, as a result of 'forbidden', promiscuous (or even acceptable) intercourse, have become *diseased, 'dirty' or untouchable, feelings of 'sin' and shame predominate*. The desire to avoid exposure of 'guilt laden' sex organs, especially in public clinics where environmental privacy is questionable and 'cross-questions' by officials rife, is certainly understandable.

It is important that the *community worker* is equipped with mental health education and insight into the process of

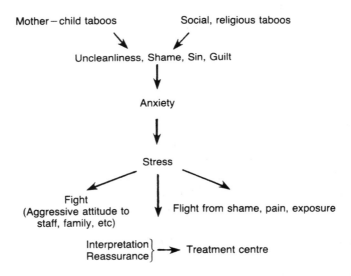

Naturally, local social attitudes, specifically *traditional sex taboos*, may aggravate the stress → Flight–Fight reaction. It is important that the community worker be sufficiently enlightened in local moral traditions to reach the client at an emotional level appropriate to his long-term mores.

Clearly the *administration of the treatment centre* is of importance, irrespective of the socio-economic group for which it caters. Both building structure and atmosphere should convey the strong reassurance of *privacy* and *confidentiality, respect and compassion*.

Considering the treatment of sexually transmitted diseases within the context of the 'nursing process', the following plan evolves:

1. *Data Collection*: The client's view of his problem within the context of his social and family relationships.
2. *Assessment—The Nursing Diagnosis*: Does he think STD is *always* associated with promiscuity and 'immorality'? Does he anticipate painful treatment as a

'punishment' for his 'sins'? Does he feel guilty and anxious? How does he feel his wife, extended family and peer group would react if they found out? Is he optimistic about the power of medicine to cure him? Are his doubts about attendance valid or do they constitute rationalizations? Is his reaction to his illness appropriate to normal group expectancy?

Assessment should take cognizance not only of conscious attitudes but also of those lying at deeper levels:

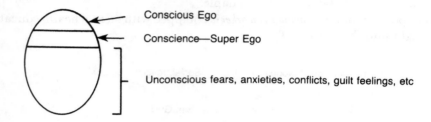

3. Planning and Implementation

Discussion of the goals of physical and social treatment with the client. It is important to ask his permission concerning any liaison work envisaged.

Medical pitfalls and prognosis are of importance, as well as details of appointments, liaison with employers concerning time off work (if desired) etc.

Discussion with the client about his expectations of his wife's response should she be invited to participate in the treatment programme . . . interpretation, catharsis, reassurance.

It is important to *separate the clinical realities* of physical diagnosis, treatment programme and the prognosis from *internalized moral judgements*, guilt feelings, fears of punishing pain, etc.

One must expect, at conscious or unconscious levels, feelings of *anger and hostility* towards the partner who has subjected his or her lover to the pain, humiliation, anxiety and violation of a sexually transmitted disease.

Some sexually transmitted diseases such as herpes genitalia are *treatable but not curable*.

Will the woman *ever find another lover* if he knows her condition?

Will she ever be able to *relate confidently and pleasurably* to this or another partner?

Will her *child-bearing* be affected?

Will her *attitude to sex* become fearful, hostile, bitter?

Will she *pass on these negative feelings* to her children?

Can herpes cause cervical cancer? A positive, although not necessarily causatory, relationship does exist. Six monthly pap smears are indicated. But remember that cancer phobia is almost as bad as the real thing! (p 520)

How crippling are the partner's *guilt feelings*—is he covering up by hostility or "flight" abandonment?

Physical and emotional pain, and the suffering they impose, may demand in-depth *counselling or psychotherapy* for both partners who are inextricably bound in their predicament.

Somehow they must find a "modus vivendi".

Establishment of Positive, Healthy and Responsible Sex Attitudes

It is important to separate, in the client's mind

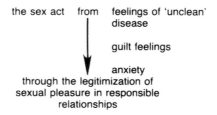

A punitive, anxiety-provoking attitude on the part of clinic staff may result in such strong feelings of guilt and self-disgust that the client may seek 'protection' in compulsive, obsessive neuroses (see p 58) and isolation.

It is important to avoid

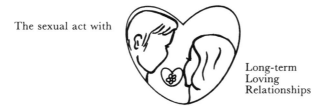

Rehabilitation should rather attempt to connect

The sexual act with

Long-term
Loving
Relationships

4.   *Evaluation* of physical and emotional progress: Physical recovery, restoration of self-worth; healthy, positive attitude towards love, sex and marriage.

At a Sexually Transmitted Disease Convention (1982) the author requested delegates to complete a simple questionnaire rating importance of treatment–avoidance factors:

'Please number these stumbling blocks in treatment compliance in order of importance as you see them:

	I*	II
1. Distance	☐	☐
2. Expense	☐	☐
3. Penalization for time off work, etc	☐	☐
4. Pain	☐	☐
5. Ignorance of etiology, treatment, prognosis	☐	☐
6. Tribal or cultural fears concerning sexual practice and illness	☐	☐
7. Personal shame (a) exposure of sexual organs (b) feelings of anxiety concerning sexual irregularities	☐	☐
8. Anxiety regarding a lack of privacy and confidentiality	☐	☐

* Column I   Your personal feelings
Column II Your perception of your patient's feelings.'

It is interesting to note the strong emphasis on

ignorance of the nature of extensive complications and on the other hand favourable prognosis within the context of timeous treatment.

Incidence of first choice

'Ignorance' constitutes by far the most conspicuous causatory factory precipitating treatment failure at 80%, followed by

shame, guilt, anxiety—16%
penalties relating to loss of pay and fear of loss of job—16%
social and personal fears—12%
pain—10%
expense—10%
others—10%

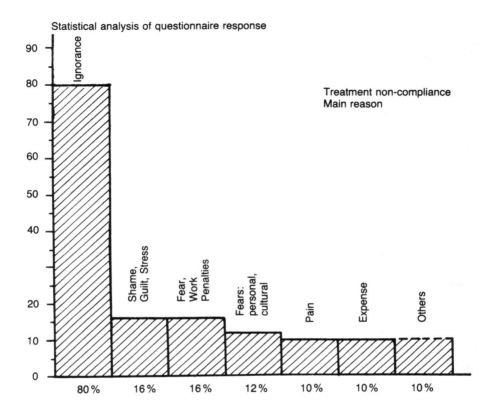

Statistical analysis of questionnaire response

Treatment non-compliance
Main reason

Very clearly the general feeling of nurses responding to this ad hoc questionnaire rated ignorance, shame, fear, (personal and social) and possible employer difficulties as being more important than the more obvious 'stumbling blocks' of pain and finance.

Doctors, on the other hand, gave more importance to pain and expense.

AIDS—the modern plague

At least in the Middle Ages the Black Death came, ravaged, and went. Victims died or were only temporarily contaminated and outcast. Now they are under permanent sentence of death, forever untouchable, feared, despised, stigmatized and isolated.

And all the while their ranks grow. The number of AIDS sufferers in the UK is doubling every eight months.*

* Miller D, Weber J, and Green J. *The Management of AIDS Patients*. MacMillan Press, London. 1986

The effects of diagnosis

First reaction to the terrible news will certainly throw the patient into 'crisis'. (Chapter 24, especially pp 563-7).

1. IMPACT PHASE

In the beginning he may be numbed, stunned. He may 'deny' or be filled with anger or wild grief. In such crisis the personality is laid bare.

At diagnosis his 'support system'—lover, close friend, family—should be mobilized. However, in AIDS diagnosis *confidentiality is imperative*—the patient may fear his lover will blame or desert him. Fearing contamination, his lover may leave him to suffer and die alone.

Not all homosexuals have stable, loving partners. The homosexual 'community' is composed of many sub-groups. The patient who has not been part of an established social circle, who has irregular employment or a 'difficult', 'unpleasing' personality, may have no enduring relationships or friendships. His family may be ignorant or rejecting of his sexual preferences. His illness highlights his loneliness and his isolation. Professionals must step into his lonely, frightening void.

Because of the intolerance and rejection surrounding homosexuality, and the isolation which follows diagnosis, most patients are defensively secretive. Others, in the shock of diagnosis, may lose their protective inhibitions, seeking catharsis in telling too many people of their plight, thus further endangering their social and occupational lives.

In clear structuring of their diagnostic model, staff will find security, support and increased efficiency. Models will vary but, in the experience of St Mary's (Paddington) team, *in initial intervention no prognosis nor statistics are given.*

  (i) In the first place, no one can predict the individual course of the disease;
 (ii) in the second, there is no purpose in removing hope and reinforcing terror.

> The patient's counsellor is introduced.
> Ventilation and catharsis are encouraged.
> Information and constructive suggestions are submitted
> *(Consistency, regularity,* and *good liaison* are cornerstones of successful counselling).
> *Support groups* are identified and the *hospital relationships offered as a lifeline.*
> The patient should not be allowed to leave the hospital in shocked isolation.
> He is usually admitted for further investigation and counselling.

2. POST DIAGNOSTIC TURMOIL—THE RECOIL PHASE (pp 525–9): The

patient now realizes the terrible realities of his predicament. David Miller, clinical psychologist at St Mary's Hospital, London, in his masterly presentation 'Psychology AIDS, ARC and PGL', gives the following moving account of the effects of diagnosis:

> 'A diagnosis of AIDS has profound implications for the patient. The prediction of death that most make in conjunction with diagnosis, the chilling realization that no cure yet exists and that friends and others are dying of AIDS, and the widely unsympathetic response of the public to affected homosexuals, generates a sense of entrapment for most patients, especially in the first few months following the news. Some of those affected have described

AIDS, ARC or PGL as a prison from which there is no escape. Understandably, many have talked of experiencing a "revolution" in their life since they became aware of their condition. Accordingly, the effect of diagnosis is felt in many important ways.'

Table 7.1 Some emotional implications of AIDS and PGL diagnosis

Shock:

of diagnosis and possible death; uncertainty

Anxiety:

uncertain prognosis and course of illness (the disintegration of death—Author)
effects of medication and treatment
status of lover, and lover's ability to cope
reactions of others (family, friends, lover, colleagues, employer, etc)
loss of cognitive, physical, social and occupational abilities
risk of infection from and to others

Depression:

helpless to changed circumstances
virus in control of life
reduced quality of life in all spheres
gloomy, possibly painful, uncomfortable and disfiguring, future
self-blame and recriminations for past 'indiscretions'
reduced social and sexual acceptability; isolation

Anger:

over past high-risk life style and activities
over inability to overcome the virus
over new and involuntary life style restrictions

Guilt:

being homosexual
'confirmed' unacceptability of homosexuality via illness

Obsessions:

relentless searching for explanations
relentless searching for new diagnostic evidence on his own body
inevitability of decline and death
faddism over health and diets

Especially those patients who have never really accepted their homosexuality may believe, at conscious or unconscious levels, that their terrible predicament is a punishment for their 'sin'. Self-reproach, guilt and fear mount to aggravate their distress. Counselling and psychotherapy are important sources of reassurance and support.

For management of three particularly painful aspects of serious and life-threatening illness with special reference to AIDS, see

Anxiety (p 32)

Depression (Care of the Dying and the Bereaved pp 534 et seq: Emotional
Effects of Illness p 479)

Obsessions (pp 120 et seq)

Clearly it is within his relationships with his loved ones, support groups and
professionals that the patient can best be supported and comforted.

Subsequent management includes

contact *with lover and family* in technicalities of testing and infection control

emotional ventilation and support

interpretation of the patient's needs

problem solving: problem breakdown

possible solutions

goals and timetable

Does the client's emotional attitude affect the course of the disease?

Jack Gorman, associate professor of clinical psychiatry at Columbia University
College of Physicians and Surgeons in New York City is currently researching 450
people infected with the AIDS virus.

He is not sure of the effects on prognosis, but he does opine:

"We certainly want to encourage people to remain optimistic and cheerful, but
we don't really know if it makes a difference or not, and that's what we're trying to
see."

Others believe that while a positive attitude cannot eliminate the virus, it can
reduce stress, which is thought to inhibit the body's immune system.

Judith Wiker, a Chicago holistic therapist who counsels people with AIDS or
AIDS-related problems, believes "there is a certain kind of person that is a survivor
with AIDS.

"That kind of personality is one that starts living in the moment, a person that
is letting go of their past feelings and fears . . . and they're letting go of future
projections about death."

Managing the suicidal patient

Understandably, the AIDS patient may see his only solution in suicide. The
most provocative professional stance is not to take his threat seriously, implying
indifference or challenge. Thus *talk of self-destruction should be treated with the greatest
concern* (chapter 25).

Because the patient's predicament is so terrible, his prognosis so hopeless, his
threat confronts the professional with her own ethical dilemma. To guide and
support the professional as well as the patient, St Mary's Hospital has constructed
the following format for dealing with the many suicide threats presented by AIDS
patients:

Intention for self-harm is routinely but sensitively probed.

Where a patient indicates his desire to take his own life, he is told that to
'determine his own death is his right as long as others are not implicated'.

Where the professional judges the suicide risk to be increased by reactive or
endogenous depression or other psychiatric disorders:

(i) the patient is told that all reasonable measures will be taken to prevent
its occurring;

(ii) emergency psychiatric referral is indicated and, where appropriate, psychiatric hospitalization and medication are instituted.

Miller believes that, with a minimum of planning and encouragement, the *quality of patient life can be significantly enhanced*, even where patients have only a short time left to live.

Typical psycho-emotional problems in the post-diagnostic 'turmoil phase'

According to Dilley et al,* the most typical psychological problems presented by AIDS sufferers result from:

(i) real or imagined *isolation* following diagnosis. (A cat or dog, being immune to the disease and unafraid of infection, may well provide loving and tactile comfort . . . Author)

(ii) *uncertainty* about the future;

(iii) *sadness* at the loss of health
income
employability
future relationships
(impending separations in death . . . Author)

(iv) *fears* for the fate of his *lover*—that he has infected his lover, that his lover will abandon him.

The patient *feels contaminated, unclean and untouchable*. His hope and self-esteem are shattered. These feelings may be aggravated by constant examination and experimentation. The patient comes to resent, and resist, what he sees as his *'guinea-pig' role*.

Jenner et al† believe that AIDS patients should be cared for in *single rooms* within a specialized complex. Among other advantages this arrangement

(i) protects them from the curious and rejecting

(ii) prevents negative identification by the sero-positive with diagnosed AIDS patients, for *the former live in hope that they will not develop the disease*.

To counteract feelings of isolation, visiting hours should be flexible and a mobile telephone available.

The role of the nurse vis-à-vis her patient, his lover, his family

The nurse may need help in becoming really accepting of homosexuality. By reviewing her own sexual development and that of her friends she may become aware of developmental changes, environmental influences and the many gradations of sexuality (pp 337–40).

Miller is clearly not a disciple of facing the patient with the reality and imminence of his death.

'Both patient and lover may derive strength from shared hope of recovery; the nurse must avoid destroying this hope even if, in her view, it is unrealistic. She may help modify the hope as part of a team approach—for example, focus

* Dilley J W, Ochitill H N, Perl M and Volberding P A. (1985) 'Findings in psychiatric consultations with patients with acquired immune deficiency syndrome' *Am J Psychiat* 142(1), 82

† Jenner E, Levi A and Houghton D. *Nursing—The Management of AIDS Patients*. MacMillan Press, London 1986

attention on the recovery from the present opportunistic infection rather than the long-term outlook.'*

(Communicating with the terminally ill: see pp 546-8; for the nurse's role in the imminence of death, see pp 551-3.)

'The nurse must not feel that it is a failure on her part if . . . depression shows little sign of lifting. It has been our experience that few AIDS sufferers reach a state of verbalized acceptance of death.'†

The lover/partner faces a multiple burden

1. From the time of his partner's diagnosis, AIDS dominates, encloses, restricts and takes over his life at both emotional and physical levels.
2. He fears (and, indeed, sometimes knows) he has contracted the virus or the disease. He watches the path of disintegration and suffering he himself may, or must, tread.
3. He is socially shunned.
4. His sex life is shattered.
5. His employability, and thus his financial status, are threatened or destroyed.
6. He must assume a constellation of new roles:

full-time domestic
         nurse
         counsellor
patient caretaker, comforter, support and companion, even unto death
go-between in negotiations between patient, hospital and family—by which latter he may be battered, insulted, blamed, rejected and hurt.

Despite their intimate, longstanding and loving relationship, which may be as meaningful as any heterosexual marriage, and in which the partners regard themselves next-of-kin, the lover may be treated as a contemptible outsider by hospital staff and family. His hurt and anger may be *displaced* in misunderstood aggression. *The nurse requires sensitivity to both patient and lover.* She may, with the patient's permission, increase mutual trust by informing, comforting and supporting both at the same time, and by inviting the partner to share in nursing care. Certainly, like the patient, the partner needs counselling and support, especially in his grief and bereavement (pp 553-5).

7. As the patient's illness proceeds he may suffer cerebral damage, personality change and impaired self- and home care skills—even to the point of constituting a danger to himself and his lover.

To all of these pressures the partner must surely react with ambivalence, hostility, guilt, anger and distress. *Some lovers cannot tolerate their burden*, taking to 'flight' or begging release—which the counsellor must 'grant' by giving 'permission to go', thus dispelling conflict and guilt.

In the difficult and heart-rending decisions of this terrible personal and social illness the nurse should not advise—*rather she should sit quietly, conveying acceptance and*

---

* Miller D, Weber J and Green J. *The Management of AIDS Patients*. MacMillan Press, London 1986
† Miller D, Weber J and Green J. *The Management of AIDS Patients*. MacMillan Press, London 1986

reassurance. Her role is that of a "sounding board" for the intense emotions and difficult decisions which burden the participants. It is important not to impose upon the partner a level of involvement he is unwilling or unable to attain.

The family

To family and friends *AIDS may confirm the 'sin'* homosexuality embodies and the punishment it deserves.

Fear of contamination and infection may be so unbearable the family become hostile and resentful, displace aggression, or 'take flight'.

To the parental family their son's illness may constitute many-faceted *shock and grief*: because many homosexuals continue to conduct their lives in separate avenues, even unto death, their son may have excluded them from an important part of his life.

> Now they learn he is a homosexual.
> He has AIDS.
> He is dying.

In her role towards the patient's family the nurse should allow them to ventilate their

> shock
> sorrow
> anger
> guilt lest they have in some way caused the painful predicament in which their son/brother finds himself

If the patient is bisexual there may be a *rejected, hurt, angry wife* who will almost certainly displace her anger on the patient and his lover.

The *nurse will certainly require support* in her efforts to reconcile and defuse this potentially explosive interplay of hurt emotions. If, through insight, sensitivity, tact and a big slice of luck, she is able to arouse initial sympathy and support, she will extend the breadth of her patient's resources and thus his affection and comfort. In this area at least the lot of the heterosexual woman patient and the haemophiliac is eased.

SPECIAL EMOTIONAL INVOLVEMENTS IN NURSING AIDS

(1) It is important that the nurse feels really comfortable with homosexual patients and their partners

  (i) in the intimate and sometimes involuntarily disconcerting details of their lives;
 (ii) in their tortuous swings between hope and despair.

(2) She also needs to feel comfortable with death. In facing another's death she needs to come to terms with her own mortality and that of her loved ones. *To identify constantly with the dying can be a very distressing way of life*. This is the stressful price she pays for high-dependency nursing in terminal illness.

(3) In addition, she is continually exposing herself to risk of infection by a lethal virus on a long and broad basis. Although the risk of infection by inoculation of patient blood and exposure to excretions is very small indeed, there is *constant need for minute care*—on her part as well as that of her *colleagues, on whom she depends both*

technically and emotionally. The result of a mistake anywhere along the line could be disastrous. Here is a situation particularly evocative of *painful obsessional neurosis*.

4. *Cumulative stress* is assuredly aggravated by skimpy staffing.

5. The nurse has a *separate life outside the hospital*. She (or he) is someone's daughter (or son), wife (or husband), mother (or father). She is haunted by fear, overt or covert, logical or illogical, that she may infect her loved ones.

They, under pressure from the media, friends and their own natural fears, exert constant pressure that she change her work. She may even fear they may desert her, should she continue to expose herself to even a remote chance of contracting and spreading this dreaded disease.

The <u>NURSING/CARING TEAM SUPPORT GROUP</u> should be capable of identifying with, and providing catharsis and support for, nurses' acute and recurring problems. It should

    (i) meet regularly, at least every fortnight;

    (ii) be free from professional hierarchy;

    (iii) be led by a facilitator well trained in group dynamics (p 170);

    (iv) for intellectual level reassurance, be well supplied with latest research and other information (eg *Morbidity and Mortality Weekly Report, Communicable Disease Report*).

<u>Obstacles</u> to be catered for include:

  (i) nurses' commitment to 24-hour team care;

  (ii) their need to 'escape' when off duty.

These lead to poor and irregular group attendance.

It is thus beholden upon nurse management to provide opportunities for group meetings during duty hours by appropriate staff rotation and within the context of intact financial benefits.

The author pays tribute to David Miller and his associates from whose book "The Management of AIDS Patients" she learned so much, not only of technical skills, but also of companion, caring and true humanity. If she quotes him often it is because she could find no better source by which to help, guide and remind her nurse-readers.

<u>Workshops</u>

AIDS Workshop: David Miller, St Mary's Hospital, Praed Street, Paddington, London W2

Life, Death and Transition: E Kubler-Ross, Shanti Niyala (England), PO Box 212, London NW8

CRUSE Counselling Workshops and Support Groups: C Spence, Lifestory Counselling Centre, 178 Lancaster Road, London W11

Addresses for high-risk self-help support groups:

Body Positive: A resource and support organization for those who are HTLV III sero-positive. Address: Body Positive, BM Aids, London WC1N 3XX

The Terence Higgins Trust: A registered charity providing face-to-face and telephone counselling, support groups and 'buddy' services for those with AIDS, and an information service for those with AIDS-related worries. Address: Terence Higgins Trust, BM Aids, London WC1N 3XX. Telephone Help Line: 01-278 8745 (8.00–10.00 pm, Mon–Fri)

London Gay Switchboard: A telephone advisory, counselling and referral service for gay people and for those with health-related concerns, run completely by gay people. Telephone: 01-837 7324 (24 hours daily, year-round)

Haemophilia Society: Information, research and advisory service for haemophiliacs and their families. Address: PO Box 9, 16 Trinity Street, London SE1 1DE. Telephone: 01-407 1010

Health Education Council: 78 Oxford Street, London WC1A 1AH. Telephone: 01-631 0930

SEXUAL ASSAULT/CHILD ABUSE

Sexual 'interference', where children are sexually manipulated, occur most frequently at the hands of *older relatives and male friends* (usually middle-aged) of the family, who use an innocent entreé into the home as a means of exploiting young children. It is very easy for 'Uncle John' to peep into a little girl's bedroom to say 'Good night', undress her and initiate what is usually forced sex play. Shy and over-obedient children, afraid to assert themselves, especially with adults, are more at risk. Because the family do not wish to create an embarrassing situation, they usually 'cover up', and avoid asking the offender to their home again, which is probably the most sensible thing to do under the circumstances.

In guarding children from sexual abuse, the crux of the matter is the establishment of *optimum self-protection, while at the same time refraining from instilling fear of, and disgust at,* sexual relations, and of men in general.

A child rendered fearful of sex may become permanently inhibited and withdrawn, spoiling those adult sexual relationships which should be the source of love and warmth, and that ultimate sexual friendship which is the core of marriage.

Nevertheless some precautions are necessary, and will be most effective and least frightening within the context of a warm, understanding, affectionate and easily approachable parent–child relationship in which all sorts of life-experiences, emotions and challenges are freely and spontaneously discussed.

Awesome clinical, biologically orientated interviews are not conducive to the informal discussion of every conceivable subject. In sex education we still have a long way to go. Many parents will still balk at actual verbalization of the simplest explanation of sexual intercourse, and the physiological functions of menstruation: If parents are embarrassed to talk about such natural functions, how much less enlightening will be their discussion of sexual deviation!

It is necessary to be specific about what is meant by 'interference', lest the child generalize feelings of disapproval and fear to all aspects of healthy sex.

Where the *father is the abuser*, the incestuous relationship may be complicated by:

Straight terror, anger and fear of no escape from the powerful father figure upon which the child is dependent.

Ambivalence—the 'love swing' leads to feelings of guilt and distress and disloyalty towards the mother. These emotions may in turn lead to 'cover up' mechanisms such as 'denial' and 'flight'.

Electra attachment to the father figure (p 57)—where this attachment is intense and unresolved, the girl's satisfaction, conscious or unconscious, in the relationship conflicts with feelings of betrayal and guilt towards the mother figure upon whom she is heavily dependent.

Oedipal attachment—in homosexual paternal abuse the boy's Oedipal aggression flames into hate and fear towards the father and guilt feelings towards his beloved mother figure.

Permanent damage to the child's own eventual lover and parental roles.

Some mothers, frightened lest their husbands resort to further abuse or desertion, protect them even at the expense of their children's mental health.

Recognizing the need for a 24-hours service where adults and children may seek protection, anonymous support, catharsis and guidance without fear of repercussion, Child Protection Line phone-in service was established (01 404 4447). This service operates on the assumptions that

1.   The child is telling the truth.
2.   The child's needs are at the focus of intervention, superseding those of other family members.

During the first seven months of its existence this service has received over 2 000 calls, of which 400 involved physical violence. The service, provided by two professional counsellors, is conducted by the National Society for the Prevention of Cruelty to Children.

(The Cleveland Inquiry and Dr Higgs' anal dilation technique is referred to on p 305.)

Precautions

Young children under 6 years of age can only be protected physically. By the time a child is about 7, it is possible to be more explicit about undesirable situations in a commonsense, non-frightening way.

At this stage children will have learnt from their parents' reactions that some strangers are acceptable, friendly and reliable, while with others one should exercise a certain caution. They should be told in simple direct terms:

1.   Don't talk to strangers—there are people who appear very friendly but who are not. In fact, they are somewhat 'sick' in the head, trying to use children's bodies as if they were adults, in a way which could be hurtful and unpleasant.
2.   Stay in groups—avoid isolated and secluded places such as lifts, stairwells, underground garages and construction sites.
        On a bus or train sit near other passengers or the bus driver.
        If someone you do not fancy pesters you or is insistent on speaking to you, giving you sweets or taking you to a quiet place, tell a conductor, a policeman, a passer-by—but don't go with him, even if you feel sorry for him.
        Pretend the nearest occupied house is your own.

According to police statistics, youngsters in their *mid-teens are at greatest risk.*

In the natural hostility and rebellion of adolescence, seeking more physical freedom, they expose themselves to more dangers. Adolescents who have grown up with a knowledge of deviants, the necessity for self-protection, and a reasonable degree of discretion regarding with whom they should mix, and whom they should avoid, are certainly better protected that those who are suddenly—too often traumatically—enlightened! Girls should be warned against 'petting' with boyfriends in lonely places. They should also be well aware that drugs and alcohol lower a person's discretion and sense of control.

It is just as important to warn a boy of the danger of abuse by an older man. Expensive meals, visits to his house or 'pad', quiet beaches and drives in the country, provide opportunities for sexually oriented contact. Sometimes a young 'recruiting' agent lures a youngster into groups where homosexual patterns are established, and intense group pressures strangulate a return to heterosexual interests.

What should one do when abuse has actually occurred?

It is most important to *avoid feelings of guilt, self-distaste, 'dirtiness'*, and the idea that one is *for ever 'blemished'*. Above all, the integrity of the victim's self-esteem is of primary importance. One should reassure a victim that no serious or permanent damage has occurred.

While it may be more public-spirited to lay a criminal charge, physical examination, police questioning, formal statements, court cases (albeit *in camera*) will all overemphasize the incident, and increase the victim's feelings of fear, guilt and impaired self-image. The sooner the whole matter is forgotten the better.

A remark such as: 'The silly old fool should have his head examined. There's no permanent damage done; just keep away from lonely crackpots in future' is a healthier reaction than the tearing of hair, court cases, vengefulness, etc.

The child or young person should, of course, be praised for having brought his experience to his parents, assured of their understanding and support, and reassured by their sensible reaction.

Just as each child's personality, and the extent of physical and mental injury, vary, so does each individual case differ in both presentation and prognosis.

Where injury is painful, requiring traumatic procedures, and the child has a sensitive personality, nightmares, sleeplessness, inability to separate from parents, fear of the opposite sex, preoccupation with cleanliness, and other anxiety obsessions may indicate deeper-level anxieties, feelings of guilt, dirtiness and 'sinfulness'. Difficulty in freeing oneself from an isolated incident, and withdrawal from the joyful things, the good relationships in life, may well herald the need for individual psychotherapy. It may also be necessary to reassure against fear of pregnancy and sexually transmitted disease.

When, due to deep and persistently painful and destructive emotional trauma, it becomes necessary to reach, release and relieve the sequelae of sexual abuse, the psychotherapist must tread carefully in order:

(a) to give the child tools at his or her own developmental level, including projective techniques such as miniature toys, family dolls, picture-story cards with which to *expose, express and handle deep feelings* of aggression, fear, shame, guilt and anger (see chapter 3 and Projection p 122).

(b) not to project her own interpretations and mores but rather to release the child's experiences and feelings.

The keynote of therapy is always relief from guilt and anxiety, restoration of self-esteem and provision of new, more constructive behaviour models.

The same is true of formal judicial investigations when, in the course of justice, children are required to undergo painful and frightening clinical examinations and to relive traumatic experiences for officers of the law. In court they must face the feared accused and the cross-examination of his lawyers.

In order to reduce the trauma of so doing the NSPCC has secured an amendment to the Criminal Law Amendment Bill of 1885.

In a letter to The Times, London (14 March 1988) Alan Gilmour, Director of the National Society for the Prevention of Cruelty to Children, writes:

> 'We support the points made by Esther Rantzen,* particularly on the admissibility of <u>video-taped recordings</u> and the need for *skilled child-care "interpreters"* through whom defence lawyers can examine a young witness during the recording.
>
> American experience suggests that many perpetrators admit their guilt when shown video-recordings which will be used in evidence: *the child is spared the necessity of appearing in court.* Of course, the status of these recordings will need to be regulated in law, but this need not be an insurmountable barrier.
>
> Children seldom lie about sexual abuse, but in the often lengthy run-up to a trial they may come *under pressure to change their evidence.* It is far better that an interview with a child should be video-recorded *while the incident is still fresh in a child's mind* and that such a recording should be admissible as evidence.
>
> We fervently hope that such provision will be introduced during the later stages of the Bill's passage.'

'Hot' on-the-spot ventilation, before guilt feelings, anxiety and defence mechanisms solidify, is also <u>more effective</u> than delayed therapeutic intervention. However, replying to the controversy, Greg Knight MP insisted in the House of Commons:

> 'It would be wrong to deny the accused the right to insist that the child appear in court to be cross-examined.'

Dr Robin Moffat, senior Forensic Medical Examiner, London Metropolitan Police, warns that built-in preconceptions may slant both the victim's evidence and the interviewer's interpretation.

> 'Over 75% of child victims are in the same family as, or are related to, the alleged abuser. Interviewers are often met with a denial by the victims because they are under threat from a parent, or the child feels intensely guilty about what has happened.'†

It should also be acknowledged that, to some children, who are strongly attached to their parents, or for whom the 'love' swing of ambivalence is strong, the <u>prospect of family break-up, or imprisonment of the offender on their evidence, is more traumatic than the abuse itself.</u>

Therein lies the child-carer's dilemma!

---

* Chairman of Child Line (phone-in service)

† Letters to the Editor, *The Times*, London, 14 March 1988

And what of the paedophile whose apparent preference is for sex with children?

1. Because most paedophiles begin with phantasy before they embark on actual molestation, there is a time lag which allays suspicion and diverts prevention.
2. A 'regressed' paedophile usually seeks adult sexual relationships but, when stressed or rejected, he regresses to relationships with children.
3. A 'fixated' paedophile is more difficult to help. Due perhaps to parental rejection, unattractiveness, rebuffs in adult overtures, he permanently seeks compensation in sexual exploitation of defenceless children who will not taunt his sexual inadequacies.

Rape

Much of what has been said about the prevention and handling of sexual abuse in general applies to rape specifically for, despite our living in a 'permissive' society, the *violation* of one's person, one's emotions, one's self-respect, the very temple of one's being, in the form of enforced intercourse, is certainly a *most traumatic experience*. Some women even *feel guilty to have survived* so humiliating and indeed devastating an experience. Rape *smashes apart all the love associations* built up throughout one's life in the sex act, which is thereby transformed from the ultimate dream of joy to the most degrading and painful of experiences. Feelings of violation, humiliation, anger, dirtiness and sorrow almost always outmeasure the physical damage.

It is customary to speak of women being raped, but this also applies, in the homosexual act, to men.

Underlying a woman's 'shame' is the *unconscious fear that rape really is impossible* and that she may, even at an unconscious level, have acquiesced in the most intimate of relationships with a repugnant stranger. It is these feelings of *guilt and shattered self-worth* that usually impose their heaviest burden upon the victim.

If a woman lays a charge, she is exposed to the impersonal, perhaps even rough, handling of a district surgeon, cross-questioning by the police and efforts on the part of defence lawyers to 'break' her story in order to reveal her as a culpable, willing party to repugnant intercourse. Experience has shown that even a verdict of proven rape casts a shadow of suspicion or distaste upon the victim. Thus the trauma and shame are emphasized and aggravated. It is little wonder that many genuine rapes remain unreported, and even hidden from professional help.

The advice to report a rape must depend on individual circumstances, including the victim's age, the stage of her oestrous cycle and thus the likelihood of pregnancy.

If a charge of rape is to succeed it must be reported to the first responsible person whom the victim meets after the attack.

Exclaimed one victim: 'The humiliation was unbearable, as is the judgemental attitude of doctors.'

A 'Rape Crisis' specialist psychiatrist criticizes legal procedures thus:

'The victim is thrust unwillingly into a fragmented system with many pitfalls and hardships, involving being passed from police to district surgeon, then home, and perhaps psychiatric help, a train of events contributing to her trauma.

A major trend has been to centralize facilities by setting up *'sexual trauma units'* within hospitals, precisely because of the need of the sexually traumatized.

The rape victim in then in a setting to undergo the necessary processing where not only expertise is available but protection and support are also forthcoming. She is spared the difficult and draining task of seeking out help.

The police statement, the medical examination, treatment and psychother-apeutic support all take place in the same room with the same skilled staff. Crisis-intervention is initiated immediately, and helps to mitigate the trauma of the investigation.

Of greatest importance is the continuity of follow-up care, especially with regard to medical and psychological needs.'

This does not, however, protect the complainant from the emotional *trauma* of cross-examination and attempts to discredit her by defence lawyers.

The most important aspect of post-rape rehabilitation is the *ability to convince the victim, at both the intellectual and the emotional level that she is not blameworthy, 'soiled' or in any way diminished. Rape is not the end of the world, and life still holds great joy and fulfilment.* For every demented, violent sexual deviant there are thousands of warm, loving, considerate and appreciative lovers and husbands.

The following are amongst significant causes of rape:

1. Frustration against women generally, due to some insecurity or inability to relate to them.
2. Defence against strong homosexual tendencies.
3. Reaction to strong heterosexual impulses, although this is rare.
4. Isolation and sexual deprivation in institutions (gaols, army, mental hospitals, etc.) resulting in homosexual rape, especially amongst men.
5. The tradition of coercive sexuality, in which men, to a large extent, still see themselves as the dominant sex, and regard women as objects.
6. Psycho-pathological tendencies, giving rise to child rapists and rapists such as Jack the Ripper.
7. Mental retardation and consequent reduced self-control, and impaired insight and foresight.

Wife-battering

Why do women stay?

'May you never be tried with what you can get used to.' Old Jewish proverb.

Janine Turner, herself a former battered wife, author of *Behind Closed Doors* (Thorsons) and founder of Lifeline, maintains that

(i) A young, inexperienced woman may know no other relationship.
(ii) The man may displace his guilt (p 121), *blaming her* for causing his outbursts, for 'deserving' to be beaten, to be sexually hurt, until her whole self-concept is an apology. "The way you nag makes me beat you up."
(iii) Although she does not love the violence, she may love the man; so she

(a)   begins by rationalizing—drink, financial worries, 'the in-laws', all provide 'excuses';

(b)   nurses the false hope that she'll be able to change him.

(iv) She fears the unknown, she doesn't want to leave 'everything'—her children, her home.

> 'So the boundaries of normality stretch and her pattern of acceptance solidifies . . . abuse becomes the norm.'

Indeed, this pattern of 'conditioned' (p 156) acceptance may become so entrenched that, if she does free herself, a battered wife may step into another violent relationship.

Other factors preventing 'breaking free' are:
lack of job qualifications to support a growing family
an innately passive dependent personality.

In some relationships one should be aware of a strong element of masochism/sadism, with an underlying satisfaction in this kind of intense emotional—physical experience

Can the man change?

> 'If he becomes frightened of himself—what he is doing to others and to himself—then he may seek help in overcoming his childish outbursts ['fight' mechanism] in the face of frustration.'

(Inter alia, pp 26, 104-105).

Breaking the pattern: women breaking free:

> Stop hiding and making excuses.
> Talk to as many knowledgeable 'concerned' people as you can—health visitors, doctors, family, solicitors.
> Find all the help available: whom to go to, where to turn.
> Then, make a plan!
> 'They said I'd never be able to drive a car/earn money/break away—so I did!'

Warning 'Plan to leave when the shelters are not so full—avoid public holidays, especially Christmas.'

Self-help support group

> Janine Turner
> Lifeline
> P O Box 251
> Marlborough
> Wilts SN8 1EA
> Telephone: 079-373 286

(From 'After Nine' BBC. TVAM, 13 April 1988.)

EROTOPHOBIA—THE FEAR OF MAKING LOVE

Experiences such as

1.   actual physical pain due to, for example,
        an adherent hymen
        anatomical disparity
        infection
        obstetric suturing
2.   imposition of guilt feelings and fear of punishment
3.   horror stories about sexual diseases
4.   sexual abuse

may lead to persistent obsessional terror or other destructive imprints. Such imprints constitute stimuli to

fear, anger, shame, panic
biochemical tension energy designed for 'fight or flight'
overactivity channeled to the muscles of the walls of the vagina, further impeding intercourse

Vaginismus,
ie involuntary spasmodic closing of the vaginal entrance preventing penile penetration.

In the woman	*In the man*
pain,	conviction that the woman is voluntarily blocking, shutting him out,
fear,	
frustration,	physical discomfort,
anger,	emotional hurt,
loss of self-concept,	anger,
avoidance,	frustration,
distress.	aggression,
	forcing partner to participate in that which she dreads,
	losing interest and abandoning partner.

Some possible solutions

communication between partners
better options in achieving a fulfilling relationship
marriage guidance
professional psychotherapy
sex therapy and counselling

Countering the effects of sexual abuse

Suggestions for complementary self-help

(Although these suggestions are directed towards sexual abuse, they may well be amended to achieve catharsis and therapeutic displacement in other traumatic areas.)

1. Write an Anger Letter to your abuser, venting all the anger you never allowed yourself to feel. Write as if you are experiencing the abuse today. Give HIM the guilt, the degradation. You need never show this letter to anyone.
2. Remember and talk about your experiences. Although painful, they are now nothing more than memories. Draw them out, then let them go.*

Contraception—the psychology of non-compliance

Very few people choose not to have children because they are concerned about overpopulation. Finances, health, readiness, fear of the responsibilities of child-raising and the simple fact of not wanting children, all motivate contraception. Why then do so many unwanted pregnancies occur?

Psycho-social mechanisms

No doubt, psycho-social mechanisms, both conscious and unconscious, affect contraception compliance, among which the following are of import to the nurse:

1. In purposefully denying herself the satisfaction and self-enhancement of procreation and, in some religious contexts, preventing divinely ordained life, a woman undergoes considerable *psychological conflict* at both conscious and unconscious levels. Deeply ingrained cultural values are defied by the woman who prevents pregnancy, with consequent painful ambivalence, guilt and anxiety.
   Guilt reinforces the socio-religious belief that sexual pleasure without procreation is especially sinful. Hence the acceptance of pregnancy as punishment for extramarital lovemaking. 'I must expect to suffer for what I did.'
2. *Denial*:
   (a) that pregnancy can occur: 'It just didn't seem possible—we only did it once
   (b) that statistics apply. We all believe 'accidents' happen only to other people.
   (c) that contraception works: 'I don't see how a little pill like that would have helped.'
   (d) personal responsibility: 'It was up to him to protect me.'
3. *Loneliness*: 'I was so lonely, I couldn't say "no" in case he left me.'
4. *Love*: 'I didn't want to spoil his pleasure. I love him.'
5. *Embarrassment*:
   Deeply ingrained feelings of shame lead to avoidance of admitting to ignorance, and of exposing the genitalia (inter alia pp 67-8) in medical examination. The intimacy of the sex act is very different from 'cold-blooded' clinical exposure.

---

* Lifeline self-help support group for victims of domestic violence: abridged from *Sufferers of Sexual Abuse*. PO Box 251, Marlborough, Wilts SN8 1EA

6. *Gamesmanship*:

    (a) In terms of Berne's 'Game Playing' (p 178ff) the non-use of contraception may constitute a weapon:

        (i) to a forced marriage or continuation of a waning relationship;
        (ii) for punishment of over-protective or 'restrictive' parents; to prove independence or to escape from home.

    (b) In some cultures men are convinced that removal of fear of pregnancy will encourage female infidelity. There is also belief that pregnant women 'won't get into trouble by sleeping around.'

    (c) Insistence on a large family in order to provide an income and protection in old age. This applies particularly to some third world states where state pensions are very small and land requires much labour.

7. *Masochism*: Fulfilment of an unconscious need for suffering and self-debasement: 'Look what he made me go through.'

8. *Sexual identity conflicts*: Self-esteem and social recognition through proof of desirability and procreativity:
    'This proves I'm a real woman.'
    'Now they can't say nobody wanted me.'

9. *Eroticism and immature irresponsibility*:
    'To hell with it—sexual pleasure comes first.'
    There is almost a gambler's pleasure in tempting fate. The greater the risk, the greater the fun.
    'He dared me to make love then and there.'

10. *Crisis and pressure* may provoke uncharacteristic behaviour.
    'Death was all around us. It was now or never . . . and we needed to comfort each other.'
    'If he were killed, at least something of him would go on living.' (This type of motivation usually does lead to unregretted acceptance.)

11. *Grief and loss*:
    pregnancy provides a replacement 'object' to replace a new life for an old: to overcome the finality of death. Where death is especially guilt-laden, as in the case of accidents, the need to compensate in a new life may be overwhelming and the pregnancy welcomed.

12. *Fear and anxiety pertaining to physical risks* as a consequence of the 'pill', eg:
    cancer
    weight increase
    superfluous hair growth
    prevention of later desired pregnancy

13. *Immaturity or mental retardation* may prevent risk evaluation, judgement and responsibility.

14. *Availability of abortion*—which also allows for preliminary manipulation and 'game-playing'.

15. *Iatrogenesis*—socio-cultural ambivalence, religious or ethical conflicts and anxiety.
    Disapproval or lack of concern *within the professional* herself may result in half-hearted, inaccurate advice and failure to motivate compliance.

'I don't want to encourage promiscuity.'

'They mentioned the pill, but really didn't tell me much.'

'Just another burden in the hopelessness of life: Oh well, so what—everything is hopeless anyhow.'

The nurse's role in counselling

Personnel working in family planning clinics who have negative feelings about contraception, sexuality, or the clients themselves, may transmit these feelings and attitudes to their clients, and thus influence their contraceptive behaviour.

Nurses need to remain aware of the goals of their work in family planning—to provide individuals with the knowledge, self-confidence, and tools to control their own fertility according to their own desires and beliefs, not those of the nurse.

For **counselling** in both group and individual counselling sessions a twofold approach is advisable.

At the intellectual level, topics profitably discussed include:

> *a cost-benefit analysis*: as pertaining to finances, housing, socio-economic demands and responsibilities; the contrasting cost of contraception failure; *contraceptive method choice*: exploring the individual advantages and disadvantages of methods available.
>
> In the final analysis, only the individual can decide which method is preferable to her and her partner. Only when they *both accept*, identify with, and above all *choose* the method for themselves, can any correct, consistent and long-term usage be expected.
>
> In so personal a matter authoritarian prescription is doomed to failure.

The nurse should attempt to develop *sensitivity* to intellectual-level *cover-up of deeper, emotional level avoidance and rejection mechanisms*. Meaningful communication requires opportunity for personal discussion, catharsis, acceptance, reassurance for one or both partners.

If emotional aspects are to be discussed in a *group situation*, it is wise to introduce emotionally fraught areas via impersonal hypothetical cases, inviting confrontation, discussion and group suggestions.

There should be an invitation for follow-up personalized discussion.

When contraception fails, resulting in unwanted pregnancy, it is common that the affected parties transfer, 'take out' or *'displace'* (p 121) their guilt, anger, resentment upon each other and the clinic staff. The latter should be able to accept this emotional catharsis at an impersonal level, reacting with support and reassurance rather than reciprocatory umbrage. (For self-help support groups, see p 613.)

References:
Sandberg E C, Jacobs R T. 'Psychology of the Misuse and Rejection of Contraception' *American Journal of Obstetrics and Gynaecology*. 1971; **110**: 227-42.
Gillmore-Kahn, Oakley, Hatcher. *Nurses in Family Planning*. New York: Irvin Publishers, 1982.

CHAPTER 17

SUBSTANCE ABUSE
INCLUDING ALCOHOLISM

'Boils and abscesses plague the skin; gnawing pains rack the body. Nerves snap; vicious twitching develops. Imaginary and fantastic fears blight the mind and sometimes complete insanity results. Often times, too, death comes— much too early in life. . . . Such is the torment of being a drug addict; such is the plague of being one of the walking dead.'

—US Supreme Court, 1962

Drug use among adolescents

Motivation behind adolescent drug-taking and other socialization problems

1. Today's adolescents are raised in a 'drug culture' in which a wide variety of medically-sanctioned drugs have surrounded them since birth. Pills to sleep, pills not to sleep; pills to calm anxiety, pills to stimulate; pills to alleviate pain; to suppress appetite, to stimulate appetite; to have babies, not to have babies. From earliest years they have been conditioned to attempts to alleviate pain, stress, etc by drugs.

2. Aware of the anxiety, horror, and generally dramatic effect engendered in adults by their drug-taking, it is reasonable that some adolescents may well be utilizing this emotionally fraught activity in order to express their natural rebellion against adult authority, and even to focus attention on their emotional needs. (The Games People Play, p 178ff.)

3. Adolescent drug-taking may well constitute a means of rejecting the values of an adult society which youngsters often find impersonal, heartless and material-istic. In their search for a meaning to life, a set of values, a way of restoring individualism, personal dignity, beauty and creativity, they are purposefully renouncing the 'rewards' of the way of life pertaining in the organized, materialistic 'rat race'.

4. Clearly to the educationally alert, ambitious youngsters who are emerging from underprivileged groups, the world which favours certain socially, financially and racially privileged groups, serves to frustrate, depress and anger them. To this group, emerging from a society in transition and frustration, drugs provide a means of temporary escape and oblivion. Failure to bridge the gap between intellectual understanding and emotional acceptance is reflected in the intelligent adolescent's recourse to drugs when, in his heart of hearts, he knows this behaviour-pattern must prove inevitably fruitless and destructive.

5. Contemporary academic demands which constitute unrealistic and impossi-ble goals for the lower 40% of any population's intellectual distribution, result,

366

inevitably, in failure, rejection, depression and anxiety, from which the innately non-academic youngster may well seek escape or flight in drug bravado or oblivion.

The diagram on page 145 shows that placement within

(i) IQ range 105–110, ie the top 25% of the population, is considered prognostic of success to academic matriculation level;

(ii) IQ range 115 upwards, ie the top 15% of the population, is considered prognostic of success at University degree level.

It is thus apparent that the bulk of the population seeks unrealistic goals.

6. Research sponsored by the New York State Council for Drug Addiction defines the most important factor distinguishing the user from the non-user to be peer group pressure which accounts for more than 50% of the total risk. Effective means of re-orientating peer group leadership and values and strengthening individual resistance is at the heart of drug prevention.

To insist that cannabis 'is no worse than alcohol' is no advertisement for cannabis! A main danger relates to progression to more dangerous drugs.

Many eminent authorities believe that cannabis can cause permanent brain damage. In a paper presented to the 12th International Congress on Therapeutics, Professor Gabriel G Nahas, on behalf of a Columbia University research team, described how tetrahydrocannabinol, the active constituent of cannabis, can penetrate the interior of the cellular protoplasm to damage the structure of 'life formula' deoxyribonucleic acid (DNA).

He said this effect could be produced by smoking hashish three times a week over a period of two years. It would appear that the cells of cannabis addicts no longer renew themselves at a normal rhythm, which phenomenon is loosely similar to the effect of exposure to radioactivity. Severage of a chromosome link had been observed in all 32 subjects.

Professor Nahas claims that lowering of cellular immunity level opens the door to diseases of metabolism and cancer. On the other hand, a pharmaceutical 'cannabis' derivative is unique in its ability to counteract the distressing effects of chemotherapy, probably by distorting perception.

DRUG DEPENDENCE

In law an 'addict' is defined as someone who has become so dependent on a drug that he has an 'overpowering desire' to continue its use.

Interviewer: Why did you try heroin again, if you got sick from it the first time?

Addict 1: Cause I liked, you know, like the high.

Interviewer: You said you got sick?

Addict 1: I got sick, but I got loaded. Got bombed . . . You get sick at the stomach, you know, but when you're loaded, you just don't care [You] just sit there nodding. [If you] feel sick, you just go, come back, and nod some more.

Addict 2: Well, I know one broad in particular. She begged me to give her . . . a shot, and she got deathly sick. And that was the last time she used it.

Interviewer: Did she say anything about it?

Addict 2: She said, if that's the way it is, she didn't want anything to do with it.

—W E McAuliffe. *A second look at first effects.* J. Drug Issues, 1975.

Presentation and etiology

The effect of drug-taking is to disturb cerebral functioning, over-stimulating and distorting the perceptual functions of the occipital, parietal and temporal cortex, as well as the hypothalamus, the seat of the emotion. At the same time the inhibitory function of the frontal lobe is depressed, reducing anxiety and causing a feeling of well-being.

Thus, in the short-term, drugs may impart an over-reactive 'high', trouble-free 'floating' feeling, providing temporary escape from:

(i) *Feelings of inadequacy in the intellectually limited* upon whom there are, in our society, stressful pressures for unattainable academic and social goals;

(ii) *Conflicts within the familial and school situations* where the adolescent revolt is aggravated by authoritarian parental and school situations; over-protection or withdrawal of involvement in favour of the parents' own social and career-oriented demands. Poor relationships within the home lead to exaggerated and painful ambivalence, guilt and anxiety, from which the young person may seek to escape;

(iii) *Difficulties in establishing a healthy self-concept and strong feeling of personal identity* in family, job and community. Rural youngsters moving to cities are particularly vulnerable in this respect;

(iv) *Innate personality disorders* such as crippling depression, anxiety and aggression; the painfully stressed obsessive-compulsive personality; the troubled paranoid personality and the extroverted, easily influenced hysterical personality; the passively dependent asthenic personality; the psychopathic personality who, being unable to postpone the satisfaction of his immediate needs for the sake of long-term, more worthwhile material and social rewards, is particularly vulnerable to any temporary self-gratifying behaviour.

These 'at risk' people find in drug use an artificially relaxed or self-aggrandizing state in which problems are solved and their suffering, albeit temporarily, is assuaged.

Pretty soon a *vicious circle* of 'high' relief, followed by a return to painful, unbearable reality and further attempts to escape in escalated drug-taking, is established.

As the body chemistry adjusts to each drug-dosage level, *an increased intake is required to achieve a 'high'*. The desperate need for drug relief increases. Only within the greedy tentacles of the *drug sub-culture* does the dependent find acceptance, sympathy, support and contacts for his crucial drug supply.

It is important for anyone dealing with drug dependants to realize the powerful and comforting bonds—and, indeed, the strangulating hold—of that tight drug-dependent group.

'Recent increases in the drug problem should be viewed against the wider socio-economic, cultural and political events in Great Britain. Economic growth, rising living standards and relatively full employment of the 1960s and early 1970s have given way to recession and economic stagnation. Unemployment has risen sharply, more so among the young, the unskilled and minority groups. Many inner-city areas have experienced steady deterioration in housing conditions, transport and other services.

Over the same period, the youth cultures of the late 60s and early 70s have disintegrated, loosening informal constraints which helped define what drug use was acceptable to particular groups and what was not. Optimism has been replaced by cynicism, despair and anger, particularly among the young, unemployed working class and minority groups. Ageing "hippies" have few options left.

Such a sketch of Britain sliding deeper into gloom is neither complete nor "balanced". Nor is it a sufficient explanation of problem drug use. The rapid expansion of non-medical drug use in the 1960s occurred at a time of boom.

But it does provide part of the background against which some groups and individuals start or continue to use drugs.'*

In poorer people drug addiction is more closely correlated with socio-economic problems and sub-cultural norms. Over-population, alcoholism, parental absorption in the problems of survival rather than child-raising, lack of middle class goals and motivations and 'hand-to-mouth' survival rather than long-term life-structure, all combine to diminish individual worth and responsibility. An escape to identification with self-destructive gang-norms, including drug-taking, both as a Flight mechanism and as a contributor to the 'big man' image, is reinforced.

However, within the *middle class stratum* there is more personalized adolescent revolt, search for personal identity and escape from excessive familial pressures.

As his dependence increases, so his environment and life pattern constrict to satisfaction of his drug needs. His whole life revolves around his painful efforts to fight his craving: the financial and other intricacies involved in obtaining a 'fix'; his mechanisms for avoiding the 'interference' of family and teachers; the love–hate, and sometimes the power demands of his sub-culture peer group; and coping with the anti-social and sometimes criminal behaviour inherent in their norm-pattern.

Drugs and the pattern of use

Cannabis

Cannabis is the drug most commonly used for non-medical purposes in Britain. Use increased dramatically during the early 1970s, may have stabilized in the mid-70s and has since steadily increased. Eight out of ten drug seizures and convictions involve cannabis, usually small amounts. Since the 60s cannabis use has diffused across all classes, though it is most common in the under-40s.

Cannabis ('ganja') is deeply embedded in the culture of certain black communities—to a lesser extent among Asians and to a greater extent among Africans and West Indians. But as communities assimilate they take on the general pattern of drug use in Britain.

Cocaine (coke)

During the 1960s cocaine use was largely on prescription as a therapeutic substitute for weaning heroin dependants from that drug. When treatment for this addiction was transferred to special drug dependence clinics 'prescribed' cocaine use dipped.

During the mid-1970s cocaine gained popularity, especially where there was style, champagne and money. But its use, usually on an intermittent basis, spread to all classes, by whom it is usually sniffed rather than smoked free-base.

'Cocaine sells for £55–£70 per gram (typically 30–70% pure). A couple of casual users might consume a quarter gram in an evening. Regular users with

---

* Hartnell, Richard. Drug Indicators 1980. Recent Trends in Drug Use in Britain. Institute for the Study of Drug Dependence.

sufficient resources might use one or two grams a day. Since 1983, prices have fallen while Customs seizures have markedly increased.'*

Although this suggests increased supply, cocaine is not a favourite drug amongst British adolescents. It is more popular in London and the South. ('Crack' is cocaine converted for smoking.)

Amphetamines

'Amphetamines are stimulants capable of giving a "lift" lasting three to four hours. Feelings of exhilaration, confidence and alertness and the temporary elimination of fatique are what the user looks for, but these are "paid for" by after-effects including hunger, fatique, and sometimes depression.

Frequent repetition to maintain the "high" can result in irritability, anxiety and paranoid feelings. In extreme cases these can develop into a psychotic episode. At such times the overwrought user can be a danger to himself and others.

The attractions of amphetamines make psychological dependence a problem. Amphetamines can be injected, eaten, or smoked, but are most commonly sniffed or "snorted" up the nose and absorbed into the bloodstream via nasal membranes.

These drugs were once widely prescribed for the treatment of obesity and depression, accounting for two and a half per cent of all NHS prescriptions in 1961.'[†]

These stimulants, once popular for medical purposes, are rarely prescribed today. Nevertheless, after cannabis, amphetamine is the most popular drug used by adolescents. Although more of a working-class drug, amphetamine is used across various social groups.

'Amphetamine is common in some colleges, studios, construction sites, and in the music business. In some of these groups it is used as an aid to maintaining long periods of concentration or physical work; in others purely as a recreational drug. A minority of individuals are compulsive users. . . .

Amphetamine sulphate powder 20 to 40% pure, retails at around £10-£12 per gram, similar to the price ten years ago. A compulsive user might get through several grams a day, while a casual user with no substantial tolerance to the drug's effects could take several weeks to consume half a gram.'[‡]

When combined with opiates and used in other multi-drug combinations (barbiturates and stimulants), amphetamines are injected.

LSD

This drug has lost 'its mystique and is now used less as a self-conscious instrument of "mind-expansion" than as simply a "fun" drug, a trend associated with the dissolution of the 60s "counter-culture" movement.

Although used more casually than in the 60s, LSD is supplied, and therefore probably used, in units of lower than average strength. Today a single, usually weak, dose of LSD costs around £2–£3.'[§]

---

* Ibid.

† Shapiro, Harry. *Focus on Amphetamines*. ISDD.

‡ ISDD publication *Drug Use in Britain*.

§ Ibid.

Barbiturates and tranquillizers

Although caution in prescription has reduced availability, 'barbs' remain a problem among multi-drug users. Sources are prescriptions, legal and 'diverted' pharmacy thefts. In London use of these drugs is largely restricted to 'chaotic' multiple drug use in the city centre where they are sometimes replaced by tranquillizers.

Solvents

Sniffing of glue, Tipp-Ex, Spray 'n Cook, now switched in some areas to butane gas.

Use of solvents appears to concentrate, 'fad', and then fade in certain schools, gangs and areas. However, a minority of maladjusted, environmentally and socially stressed youngsters become heavily involved in search of coping or escape mechanisms.

Synthetic opiates

'Diverted' from the legitimate medical market, these include cough mixtures, pain killers, laxatives containing codeine, diconal and methadone.

Both solvents and synthetic opiates are used as substitutes for heroin and as drugs of choice, especially by the young and inexperienced.

Abuse presentation

In order to be drug-effective these preparations must be taken in such large doses as to cause serious organic side-effects, such as neurotransmitter disorders, dangerous respiratory spasms, kidney failure and liver disease. It is the frightening suffering of these side-effects that usually brings the drug-dependent youngster for treatment.

> 'Younger drug users appear to be using cannabis, solvents, amphetamines, pills such as Valium, and alcohol. Apart from alcohol, these are inexpensive and unlikely to lead to convictions for drug offences, though the consequences of use may still be disturbing. In the past five years a minority have started to use heroin. In areas such as Wirral or Glasgow, this is a substantial minority.'*

Heroin *is one of a group of drugs (the 'opiates')* derived from the opium poppy with generally similar effects, notably the ability to reduce pain and anxiety. As well as being prescribed as pain-killers, opiates are used medically to treat coughs and diarrhoea. Opium is the dried 'milk' of the opium poppy. It contains *morphine* and *codeine*, both effective pain-killers, and *from morphine it is not difficult to produce heroin* which in pure form is white fluffy powder with twice the potency of morphine.

Since 1970 the number of people using opiates regularly has risen, probably at least ten-fold. Most of the increase has occurred since 1978. The primary drug involved is illicitly imported heroin. This increase may now be slowing down.

Since heroin addiction first presented a 'problem' in the 1960s the number of known addicts has increased dramatically. At first excessive heroin prescriptions by a small number of doctors was virtually the exclusive source.

---

* Ibid.

In 1968 prescription for addicts was restricted to licensed doctors at special dependency clinics and psychiatric units. Then drug importers from South-East Asia took over, but a series of bad harvests and successful police seizures limited supplies and prices rose steadily until the fall of the Shah of Iran. Then the first major increase in heroin supply was associated with the influx of Iranian refugees. Since 1981 Pakistan and Afghanistan have become the primary (albeit illegal) suppliers.

The current price of illicitly imported heroin in London is £80-£100 per gram (typically 30 to 60% pure) in gram quantities. Prices are highest in Scotland.

Opiate addiction clinics have significantly reduced their heroin prescriptions, substituting methadone. But illicitly imported heroin has become much more available.

Pattern of use

Intermittent recreational use of heroin (sniffed and smoked rather than injected) has become widespread.

1960s: heroin use was mostly an adolescent/early adult phenomenon
1970s until 1980/1: addicts were more likely to be in their mid- to late twenties and
      thirties
1981 onwards: much younger people have become increasingly involved. The
      proportion of female addicts has increased to 30%. While addiction has
      contributed to increase in London, other large urban districts, such as
      Merseyside, Manchester, Edinburgh and Glasgow, are seeing increased
      availability and use.

      The pattern of use

1. has become ghetto-like in its distribution in depressed areas with the difference that in the UK heroin addiction is still mostly restricted to the white British or Irish population—though the situation in some black or ethnic groups does seem to be changing as supplies become more available;
2. has also expanded to children of the middle and upper classes.
3. A much smaller proportion of the total addict population is in treatment than 15 years ago (from 50% heavy opiate users to 25% or less). This implies that the number of people in the UK who used opiates regularly at some stage during 1985 was in the order of at least 60 000 and perhaps as high as 80 000.* It does appear that the increase of new heroin users in London may have levelled off, perhaps due to in some degree to increased liaison between drug prevention authorities.

During 1986 HM Customs and Excise seized illegal drugs with a total street value of £85 million. Seizures of cannabis, cocaine and amphetamines were all more than in 1985, although heroin figures were down.

Amphetamines showed the most dramatic *increase*—37 kilograms compared with 26 kilograms in 1985—a 42% rise. Cocaine—up from 79 kilograms to 94 kilograms—showed a 20% increase and cannabis—22,607 kilograms, compared with 20,905 kilograms in 1985—was 8% up.†

---

* Ibid.
† HM Customs and Excise news release, 8 January 1987.

Deep concealments in freight and drugs carried inside the body—what is called 'stuffing' or 'swallowing'—cause concern. There was a huge increase in stuffing and swallowing cases in 1986. Sixty four internal concealments in total were detected in 1985 but the next year there were 135 involving heroin, 33 involving cocaine and 20 involving cannabis. Thirteen per cent of the total amount of heroin and 11% of the total quantity of cocaine detected was being smuggled internally during 1986.

> 'These couriers cause serious problems at the London airports because, after they are detected—and there have been as many as eight detections on one flight—the resources employed to cope with them are enormous. Furthermore, officers dealing with this type of smuggler are exposed to a serious health risk.'*

Abuse presentation

The initial experience of heroin is not always pleasant. Especially after injecting there can be nausea and vomiting alongside or instead of pleasurable feelings. These unpleasant reactions fade with repeated use.

When injected into a vein all the heroin is usually injected into the bloodstream at one go. This can intensify the initial effects into an almost immediate, short-lived burst of extremely pleasurable feelings, often described as a 'rush'. Other ways of taking heroin give less intense feelings, though after smoking the effects are also practically immediate.

Rather than blocking the sensation of *pain*, heroin and other opiates make pain *more tolerable by reducing the sufferer's emotional reactions to it*, so although still felt, the pain seems to matter less. More generally opiates cushion the user from the psychological impact of not just pain but also hunger, discomfort, fear and anxiety. This relief from suffering is also experienced by many people as a positive feeling of well-being, contentment and happiness—a sense of being 'wrapped up in cotton wool'.

Even at doses sufficient to produce these feelings, the user is still capable of functioning adequately—he can, if necessary, think, talk and act coherently. At higher doses sedation takes over and the user becomes drowsy. Excessive doses produce stupor and coma, and possible death from respiratory failure. Diarrhoea may make the contraceptive pill ineffective.

The consequence of injecting opiates and of a drug-using lifestyle can be serious. Among regular injectors there is commonly physical damage or *infection* associated with poor hygiene and the injection of adulterants. These include hepatitis, AIDS (through the sharing of needles), inflammation and obstruction of veins (which may lead to superficial veins being 'used up' as the user searches for healthy veins to inject), *heart disease, lung disorder* (as adulterants clog blood vessels in the lungs).

Whether they inject or not, opiate addicts suffer from a high incidence of *lung disease* (especially pneumonia) caused by repeated drug-induced respiratory depression and decreased resistance to infection. *Reduced appetite* and *apathy* can contribute to disease caused by poor nutrition, *self-neglect* and bad housing. Repeated heroin sniffing may cause *nasal damage*.†

* Ibid.
† ISDD Information Service. *Heroin in Britain.*

Table 3.2 New drug addicts notified to the Home Office during the year by type of drug to which addiction was reported(1)

United Kingdom

Type of drug	1976	1977	1978	1979	1980	1981	1982	1983	1984	1985	1986
									Number of persons		
Heroin	607	613	859	1,110	1,151	1,660	2,117	3,559	4,926	5,930	4,855
Methadone	308	328	321	345	349	431	473	633	686	669	659
Dipipanone	131	233	280	320	351	473	627	539	309	223	116
Cocaine	111	139	142	126	147	174	214	345	471	490	520
Morphine	316	411	411	385	351	355	356	363	357	326	343
Pethidine	33	44	46	47	33	45	20	32	31	34	33
Dextromoramide	32	50	66	66	53	59	68	111	112	104	97
Levorphanol	1	2	1	2	–	2	–	1	1	3	–
Hydrocodone	–	–	–	–	–	–	–	–	1	1	–
Oxycodone	–	–	–	–	–	–	1	–	1	1	2
Phenazocine	1	1	2	2	3	2	3	4	3	3	2
Piritramide	–	–	–	–	–	–	–	–	–	–	–
Hydromorphone	1	1	–	–	–	–	–	–	–	–	–
Opium	–	–	1	2	–	–	2	–	2	14	23
All notifiable drugs	984	1,106	1,347	1,597	1,600	2,248	2,793	4,186	5,415	6,409	5,325

(1) As an addict can be reported as addicted to more than one notifiable drug the figures for individual drugs cannot be added together to produce totals.

Notifications are sent to the Home Office by doctors who are legally obliged to supply certain details of their patients who they know or suspect to be addicted. Excepting notifications from prison doctors, the number of addicts notified reflects the *demand* for medical treatment.

Are 'new' addicts getting younger?

Cumulative percentage of UK addicts notified for the first time aged under 21, 21–29, or 30+.

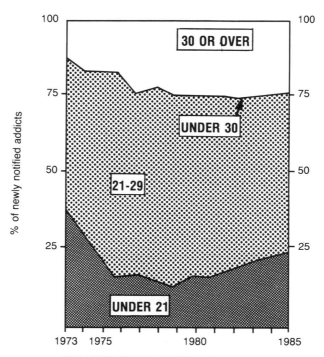

THE NEW YOUNG ADDICTS. Throughout the '70s and '80s newly notified addicts have been mainly in their teens or twenties. Though rising since 1979, the proportion of under-21 year olds is still less than in the early '70s, but the numbers are far larger — over 1 500 in 1985 compared to 310 in 1978.

These statistics were supplied by the Institute for the Study of Drug Dependence Information Service, for whose kind assistance the author is grateful.

Half the addicts notified in 1984 were under the age of 25 years. 'Only a minority of addicts are notified . . . anywhere between a quarter and a tenth according to different estimates.' This implies that there were probably 50 000 to 80 000 addicts in Britain in 1985.

Signs and symptoms of drug abuse:

Distortions of the pupils: dilation of pupils and reddened eyes are usually associated with cannabis and pinpoint pupils with heroin.

Excessive sleeping, voracious appetite, vomiting.
Staggering and stumbling; breathing difficulty.

The *psychological* signs of drug abuse vary with each individual, but the following may be 'suspicious'.

Evasiveness about friends.
Staying away from home without explanation.
Strong mood-swings—rush of enthusiasm, interest in sport, schoolwork, etc, followed by withdrawn lethargy.
Over-excitability and disproportionate laughing and crying.
Bad temper.
Low threshold for frustration, resulting in aggressive over-reaction.
Zombi-like suggestibility to criminal activities, reinforced by need for money to satisfy growing drug dependence.

In contrast with the relatively rapid metabolism of alcohol, the physiological effects of drug abuse are more persistent. The detrimental effects of drugs are 'sneaky'. The victim may consider himself 'cold turkey', but in actual fact the metabolism is slow and the effects long-lasting. Tests reveal *cannabis* in the urine for as long as a week after admission.

By the time the client reaches hospital he is usually in a state of

Sympathetic Nervous System over-arousal, resulting in hot and cold rigors, sweating, tremors, blackouts, spasms, exaggerated startle reflex, high–low temperature swings, diarrhoea.

Especially in advanced cases, he presents with

abnormally high PHL and other cerebral chemical disturbances, with resultant epilepsy

and, in the case of the heroin addict, nausea and vomiting.

Psychologically he presents with acute confusional states and psychotic features such as paranoia with hallucination, acute restlessness and mania alternating with withdrawn depression.

Immediate—and indeed often life-saving—in-patient treatment, is organic in emphasis, involving

rehydration and the therapeutic administration of "bridging" barbiturates of increasing weakness designed to wean the patient from his gross dependence.

This 'cold turkey' process, involving physical withdrawal and painful confrontation with reality conflict, guilt, anxiety, diminishment and the other personal burdens the patient has been seeking to avoid, causes very significant physical and emotional suffering.

Fear of withdrawal effects can be a strong inducement to continue drug usage. This is *physical dependence*. However, even after overcoming the physical agony of 'cold turkey' many addicts return to drugs. This demonstrates the strength of *psychological dependence* upon:

(i)   the mental effects of the drugs;
(ii) the tight drug culture where relationships develop and revolve around the structured routine of buying, dealing in and using shared drugs. Here he finds unconditional acceptance.

Thus, to stand a chance of staying drug-free the <u>user may have to sacrifice his peer relationships and reconstruct his whole social life</u>. He must thus be very strongly convinced that the rewards of staying drug-free are greater than his present drug-laden satisfactions. He must learn to say "NO"!

Treatment trends

In response to the first wave of young heroin addicts in the 60s the government set up a network of specialized *hospital treatment centres*. But the specialist centres have been unable to absorb the much larger waves of 'new' addicts (many will have been addicted for several years before being notified) in the 80s, most of whom have turned to GPs for treatment.

Initially many hospital centres prescribed addicts the drug they wanted—heroin. But in the mid-70s the balance tipped from attracting addicts into treatment and prescribing drugs that would keep them there, towards *prescribing regimes that denied them the legal means to continue their heroin-injecting lifestyles*, and then sought to move them relatively quickly to total abstinence from opiates.

This they attempted to do by weaning patients from heroin, the drug of their choice, to the *bridge of less damaging methadone*, first by injection and then by mouth.

Some observers suggest *'consumer resistance'* to these regimes is why most addicts seeking treatment now go for first to GPs, and why many more do not seek medical help of any kind. In addition, clinics are now in *competition with a well-organized market* that did not exist in the 60s.

Those *fighting drug addiction* now come out on all fronts by

1. attracting new patients into treatment
2. confronting patients' addiction
3. destroying the illicit market—heroin is a class A offence where the maximum sentence for trafficking is life imprisonment plus fine; for possession, seven years plus fine
4. preventing the spread of AIDS
5. co-ordinating research at national and international levels
6. education.

Treatment procedures

Drug users may receive *help from voluntary sector* day centres, advice, counselling and social work services specializing in drug problems. Such centres may take the major role in supporting and rehabilitating their clients, or may refer them to *clinics* or one of the *residential rehabilitation houses*, where drug dependants who have ceased drug use stay for up to 18 months to reconstruct their personal and social lives.

Nursing functions in the Acute Phase

   (i)   *support* free from judgemental censure;
  (ii)   Astute nursing *observation*, not only of vital processes, medication, etc but also of the patient's personal behaviour;
 (iii)   Provision of a *learning experience*. The nurse should have available enough information about the etiology, presentation and implications of drug-dependence to provide a learning situation within that 'hot' stage of the dry-out experience, when the patient is more accessible to motivation for rehabilitation.

A particularly difficult aspect of the *relationship between the nurse and her drug-addicted or alcoholic patient* lies in the achievement of a *balance* between

> *empathy*, that emotional-level 'feeling with' which can only come through an ability to 'identify' and communicate with the patient in his suffering, problems, and weaknesses,

and her ability to
> *remain in alert, and unsentimental, control of the situation.*

Especially as they emerge from the acute phase of physical illness, drug-dependents and alcoholics find themselves in distressing and anxiety-provoking *conflict* between

> *a desire for freedom* from painful physiological symptoms and ego-diminishing dependence on a clearly 'sick' group in which they encounter humiliation, power-struggles, and continual submission to the financial, emotional and personal struggle for drug supplies,

as opposed to

> their exprience of escape, power and 'high' sensory gratification *obtainable from drug 'trips'* in the sub-culture peer group where, alone, they feel confident and accepted.

Within this painful conflict situation the 'dried out' dependant may be overcome by the urgent need for 'a fix'. Desperate, he becomes impressively manipulative, resorting to pleading, bargaining, weeping, and arousing guilt-laden pity within the inexperienced—and indeed sometimes experienced—nurse.

In fact, within the context of acute 'dry out' treatment, as well as the more long-term therapeutic group situation, the nurse herself will certainly need the guidance and support of her colleagues on both an individual and team basis.

Specialized residential group therapy involving a combination of

> confrontation and support
> encounter therapy

is indicated.

John Strang and his staff at the Maudsley clinic in south London report thus on 31 patients accepted for treatment:

After the initial handing-over period *an agreement is negotiated* with addicts that they will start to reduce and/or switch from injectables within a few months. Dr Strang was 'surprised' that reaching agreement with most had been an easy, two-way process, with the planned schedule often coming from the patients themselves. But he admits that only time will tell whether the co-operation holds up when the contracts 'come to the crunch'.

There is concern that existing treatment and rehabilitation services are inappropriate for women and those with child-care responsibilities, most having been developed to cater for the young, rootless and possibly homeless men that typified the early 70s drug scene.

There, group members are taught to recognize within themselves and each other conflict, anxiety, stress and resultant adjustive mechanisms such as flight, denial, withdrawal, aggression, displacement. The keynote of successful therapy consists in communcation of loving concern; the promotion through group and individual therapy and environmental manipulation of emotional security, self-expression and recognition of realistic goal achievement.

New goals and motivation fulfilment patterns are worked out, implemented and evaluated. Thus the facilitator and group members provide a learning experience for the achievement of more acceptable social skills and personal satisfaction. But care must be taken with *more introverted personalities*, who can be so inhibited and insecure in group cathartic situations that their rehabilitative programmes must include significant individual therapy.

The role of the nurse in post-acute rehabilitation

While it is essential that she identifies with the pain, humiliation, guilt and anxiety of her patients, especially in their struggle between motivation for:

freedom from:		blissful escape on
(i) physiological suffering		a drug 'high' from
(ii) dependence on the	vs	(i) the agony of withdrawal
destructive, all-absorbing		(ii) reality
drug culture		confrontation

the nurse must manage to keep her distance. Her role is neither that of a puppet to be manipulated nor an authority symbol to be challenged.

This latter role will soon arouse and cause to be transferred to the staff the defiant or smouldering aggression of that adolescent rebellion which has probably been a causatory factor in drug dependence. *Rather, she is the warm, supportive 'umpire' in the patient's own inner battle.*

Participation in the therapeutic group requires a *high level of tolerance in order to cope with patients' intense feelings* as they alternate between rejection, dependence and aggression. In fact, so great are the demands upon the therapeutic nurse that she can function productively, and at peace with herself, only within *her own group-support team system.*

The team, through discussing and reliving their own personal and professional experiences and feelings, afford each other catharsis, insight, guidance, support and an opportunity to analyse, understand and handle their own projections, introjections and emotional responses to the larger therapeutic situation. Thus they are equipped to handle, and feel comfortable within, their own feelings— aggression, dependency needs, depression and job satisfaction. Without insight into her own feelings and reactions, the nurse will become so solidified that she will be unable to participate profitably in the dynamics of the therapeutic situation.

Prognosis

Prolonged use of drugs can cause:
1. lung and kidney damage and serious respiratory problems;
2. damage to the reproductive cells, which may influence future generations;
3. suppression of hormones concerned with normal sexual functions thus increasing infertility;
4. long-term behaviour disturbances and permanently impaired brain functioning;
5. premature brain cell deterioration and thus premature aging.

Therapeutic planning depends on the patient's accessibility to new values, goals and the attainment of them through the acquisition of new living skills.

The prognosis is dependent upon reliable *treatment screening* designed to bring together for intensive personal and group therapy *those who are capable of commitment to a changed lifestyle.*

This will depend upon factors such as the individual's innate personality structure: pre-dependency history, intelligence, familial and social support systems and, above all, the possibility of participating in programmes designed to achieve dynamic change.

Impediments such as brain damage and advanced organic defects resultant upon the biochemical mal-effects of drug and alcohol addiction, innate personality defects such as a dependent asthenic personality, psychopathology, an innate tendency towards withdrawn depression, general intellectual and emotional rigidity, and thus inability to achieve an ideational, dynamic and motivated change in behaviour pattern, certainly detract from a positive prognosis.

Advice to parents and community workers

1. Recognize your own panic, anger, fear and distress, but do not let them get the better of you. It is important to avoid over-reaction.

2. Show confidence in the youngster—also show your love and your willingness to help, but *do not*

> over-react,
> shout, and
> preach or moralize.

Alienation will threaten the very relationship that is the most important rehabilitative lever.

3. Specialized professional counselling should provide

 (i)   knowledge of the facts of drug abuse;
 (ii) a neutral, calm approach;
(iii) catharsis and support;
(iv) positive group identification;
 (v) parent counselling.

With increasing spread of drug problems, especially among young people, *volunteer services based on parent concern* have become more of a feature. These

(a)   act as self-help support groups for parents
(b)   run advice services for drug users.

To prepare these and other groups for dealing with drug problems, training resources are required.

Drugline drug advisory centre

9a Brockley XSE4 692 4975
28 Ballina St SE23: 01 291 2341
Lambeth 01 677 9541

Drugs, Advice and Information—The Blenheim Project 01 960 5599

Drug Concern (Barnet)

Woodlands Ho, Colindale Hospital 01 200 9525
The policy of most social agencies who work with young people is to remain objective—to point out the health hazards of addiction and the possibility of permanent brain and other physical damage.

Most like to talk to the family even when there is the merest suspicion that the child is experimenting. Families whose children would seem in any way involved in the drug scene should seek help at once.

Education for prevention

The upsurge in use has stimulated *educational initiatives* including videos and teaching packs for use with young people in schools, youth training and other youth-work settings. One favoured objective is to give youngsters the *social skills to refuse drug offers* from their peers. This approach recognizes that <u>friends of the same age are the usual source of drugs for young people</u>.

> "I have learned that drug abusers prefer to use drugs in the company of other people. For this reason, they are always looking for others to convert to their 'way of thinking'.
>
> This is the dilemma of many teenagers: on one hand, they *know* that drugs are dangerous; on the other, they don't want to be rejected or dismissed as a 'straight' by their peer group.
>
> So what do you do if your friends offer you drugs? Just say 'no'. It's as simple as that. If you have already thought about the drug issue, you will have a clear idea of the consequences involved and will probably find it much easier to say 'no'. Tell your friends what you have learnt about drugs: if enough of *them* say 'no', you'll soon find that you are in the majority and others will follow your lead."[*]

An effective way of backing-up the parental role in fighting the 'big man' image of peer group drug-identification lies in *early contra-indoctrination*.

---

[*] Searll Adele: 'It can't happen to me'. The mother of an ex-addict tells her story. Further details from author.

A novel approach, sponsored by Mrs Nancy Reagan, wife of the former President of the United States, is a comic book entitled *The New Ten Titans* (published by DC Comics Incorporated and underwritten by the Keebler Company). *The comic provides young readers with the opportunity of identifying with anti-drug hero models* in exciting emotional experiences. The story portrays teenage heroes such as 'Cyborg', a slick, smart half-man, half-robot who spreads the word about the damage drugs can do to children. There is also a character called 'Speedy', the baffling Bowman who acknowledges he was once a child heroin addict, who was saved by the kindness of a super hero.

> 'I'm Anna Jurez and I am 12 years old. I've taken pot, hash, oil, dilaudid, cocaine, downers, and qyaaludes. I've been taking them for three years. My brother Juam, he was the one who started me using drugs. Now look at him —he's dead'

Says Mrs Reagan:

> 'Don't let anyone tell you that you can't be a hero. You can, and you are about to learn how. Picture yourself in battle. In fact, it is one of the most important battles our nation has ever fought.'

'Super heroes', whose adventures rival those of Superman or Buck Rogers, spread a consistent message: 'Stay off drugs!' The comic is being distributed free at 35 000 United States' schools and is aimed at children as young as 10.

Alcoholism

When the social habit of drinking escalates into alcoholism its complications affect the entire community.

Uncontrolled drinking disrupts all spheres of human functions:

At work → impaired motor co-ordination
         disturbed human relations
         disrupted teamwork
         inefficiency, reduced productivity, industrial accidents
         job loss and unemployment

in the motor car → road accidents, death and maiming
in the family → loss of self-control, arguments, fights, abuse, assault, unwanted pregnancy, foetal alcohol syndrome and mental defect.
in the community → drain on welfare resources

An especially disruptive aspect of alcoholism is its 'spin-off' into unhealthy role models. Some children must attempt to assume parental roles. Others either reject, or 'introject' (p 107) the mother or father role. 'Introjectors' take the same path to self-destruction.

A cycle of alcohol abuse from generation to generation is established. It has been estimated that 40–60% of children of alcoholics become abusers themselves. Here is Liza Minnelli's story:

> '"My whole family had it. My sister beat it when she was 15. My brother has had trouble, but he's all right now. I was the strong one. It took longer to catch up with me."

She was 38 years old and reeling from an exhaustive diet of drugs and booze. She was haunted by the spectre of her mother Judy Garland, killed by a drug overdose at the age of 47.

Her mother and father, director Vincent Minnelli, were divorced when she was five. She spent her formative years caring for a younger half-brother and half-sister and a mother who staggered between hysterical highs and crushing lows.

Liza started on Valium for a back problem. Then a sleeping pill, then a diet pill. She punctuated drugs with hard liquor.

"I didn't think I was addicted." she said.

She was into her third marriage and had two miscarriages. The marriage to sculptor Mark Gero was hanging in the balance. He too was hitting the bottle and "travelling in the fast lane".

In 1984 Liza began missing performances on Broadway and showbusiness braced itself for a disastrous rerun of the Judy Garland story.

She said she lied about her drug taking because she didn't want anyone to know she was imperfect. "I was constantly fooling myself."

Her sister Lorna Luft finally confronted Liza with the truth and she followed other stars like Elizabeth Taylor into the Betty Ford Clinic.

The real battle started when she came out and resumed her career. Now at champagne parties she drinks Coke.

'Yes I have had a drink but I went out and got help straight away. I felt terrible and I went and said "I'm scared." You think you can handle it but you can't. It is much smarter than you are. It's cunning, it's tricky, its baffling, it's tough."

She says she now knows what her mother went through.'*

Frequently alcohol addiction links with drug addiction. Self-control and insight are grossly impaired. Accidents and violence and the need for money to buy more soon bring the abuser into conflict with the law and into jail.

Alcoholics find that only alcohol can make them feel self-confident and at ease with other people; often want 'just one more' at the end of a party; look forward to drinking occasions and think about them a lot; get drunk when they had not planned to; try to control their drinking by changing types of liquor, going on the wagon, or taking pledges; sneak drinks; lie about their drinking; hide bottles; drink at work; drink alone; have blackouts (that is, cannot remember the next day what they said or did the night before); drink in the morning, to relieve severe hangovers, guilt feelings and fears; fail to eat and become malnourished; get cirrhosis of the liver; shake violently, hallucinate, or have convulsions when withdrawn from liquor.

'Alcoholics Anonymous' considers an affirmative answer to four or more of the following questions indicative of a significant drinking problem:

	Yes	No
1. Have you ever decided to stop drinking for a week or so, but only lasted for a couple of days?	( )	( )
2. Do you wish people would mind their own business about your drinking—stop telling you what to do?	( )	( )

---

* Gordon, George 'No More Lying from Liza'. 1986.

3. Have you ever switched from one kind of drink to another in the hope that this would keep you from getting drunk? .... ( ) ( )
4. Have you had a drink in the morning during the past year? ... ( ) ( )
5. Do you envy people who can drink without getting into trouble? .... ( ) ( )
6. Have you had problems connected with drinking during the past year?   ( ) ( )
7. Has drinking caused trouble at home?.................................. ( ) ( )
8. Do you ever try to get 'extra' drinks at a party because you do not get enough? .... ( ) ( )
9. Do you tell yourself you can stop drinking any time you want to, even thou you keep getting drunk when you don't mean to?.. ( ) ( )
10. Have you missed days of work because of drinking? .... ( ) ( )
11. Do you have 'blackouts'?... ( ) ( )
12. Have you ever felt that your life would be better if you did not drink? .... ( ) ( )

There is little doubt that body tissue—especially in the liver and Central Nervous System—is, within the context of long-term intake, *permanently damaged* by alcohol. This damage presents in *Delirium Tremens*, marked by involuntary shaking movements, hallucinations and *impaired* memory, self-control and judgement. Alcoholism is recognized as a major health problem. In the USA it is ranked as the third greatest killer after heart disease and cancer. And the network of suffering spreading out from the alcoholic himself reaches the home, the job, the road. . . .

Etiology

Who is particularly at risk for alcoholism?

As in the case of drug addiction, alcoholism provides a 'Flight' escape mechanism in the face of pressure, anxiety, stress and generalized fears and feelings of inadequacy.

Persons least able to withstand stress or who are directed most easily into destructive adjustment mechanisms are those suffering from:

   (i) A childhood deprived of mother love, safety and security; those positive experiences necessary for the development of confident self-assertion;
  (ii) Personality disorders reflecting over-dependence, acute anxiety, psycho-pathology, depression and other disorders predisposing towards drug abuse;
 (iii) Low intelligence;
  (iv) A loosely structured environmental and familial support system, lacking constructive role-identification, where 'anything goes'.

Also especially vulnerable to mal-effects of alcohol are people with an innately slow metabolic rate for alcohol, resulting in a build-up of biochemical vulnerability. However, such etiology is rare and may be used as a conscious or unconscious 'rationalization'.

A particularly dangerous combination is the 'escape route' afforded by mixing alcohol with:

> sedatives and tranquillizers which, being psychotropic drugs, 'double up' on hypnotic effects in the Cenral Nervous System;
>
> amphetamines and stimulants, which combination is not only biochemically more potent but also provides a strongly euphoric aura upon which it is particularly easy for a vulnerable personality to become 'hooked'.

The effects and withdrawal effects of the alcohol–amphetamine combination are particularly long-lasting, often resulting in marked debilitation.

The therapeutic role of the nurse

In hospital 'dry out' therapy the nursing role is similar to that pertaining in drug dependence, as is her *supportive, observational* and *educational role*. Likewise she should be able to *balance empathy and supportive involvement with a certain 'distance' and ability to withstand 'feeling sorry'* for the patient. She should remain watchful lest she be manipulated by him to obtain money, alcohol, etc.

Alcohol-dependent clients are often older than those suffering from drug dependence, and their drinking habits are more subtle, more deceptive.

For long periods they are 'protected' from diagnosis (and thus from help) by social mores which accept social drinking and nights 'out on the tiles'.

The gradual accumulation of alcohol, and its biochemical mal-effects, results in a heavy build-up of alcohol in the metabolic system, and hence in additional retardation of therapeutic effects.

Prognosis:

The more long-term and insidious the alcohol build-up,

(i) the more the cerebral organic involvement, and hence retardation of mental processes, especially as pertaining to ability to 'shift' or change, particularly within the context of advanced age;

(ii) the more difficult it is to inspire, and achieve, motivation necessary for enduring the discomfort, even the suffering, involved in the 'drying out' process;

(iii) the greater the difficulty in involving the older client in

> the intellectually oriented emphasis, and free-flow intercommunication,
>
> the acceptance of criticism,
>
> the pressure for building new behaviour patterns, inherent in therapy.

All these factors combine to render treatment of alcoholism, especially in older people, a slow, frequently impeded and not always successful process.

Alcoholics Anonymous believes that only through *a spiritual awakening* within the context of warm, critical yet supportive, group work is it possible for an alcoholic to recondition his behaviour pattern towards a more satisfying and constructive way of life.

AA support group work:

'Because AA meetings are held every day and night of the week, AA *groups* offer continuing supportive contact to help the alcoholic maintain recovery. And in addition to offering almost unlimited time to the alcoholic, AA offices and groups can make available a wide variety of AA publications.

By far the best way to refer an alcoholic to AA is to *take* him or her to an AA office or meeting. Establishing direct telephone contact between the alcoholic and AA while the client is with you can also be effective.'

CHAPTER 18

THE FAMILY

STRUCTURE, DYNAMICS, FUNCTIONS
BREAKDOWN: PREVENTION, DIVORCE, CUSTODY
REHABILITATION

The *family* is a kinship group which provides for the raising of children, and for certain other needs varying from society to society. In some very simple societies the family educates, heals and fulfils religious goals. In more sophisticated societies, outside agencies assume specialized functions. Like all social institutions, the family is a system of interrelated

    norms—conventional, expected behaviour,

and

    values or social controls, (p 234)

fulfilling a set of purposes.

Functions of the family*

1. *Marriage* in our society is the approved pattern for establishing a family. Marriage and family are found in all societies, having evolved from the need for stable and defined relationships for raising children and assigning the work essential to survival. For founding members (parents) marriage provides the physical and emotional satisfactions inherent in the security of a long-term relationship.

2. *Reproduction:* In all societies children are produced and raised by families, of which at least one member is socially designated as responsible for the child's survival and nurture. From this familial function there develops the concept of 'legitimacy'.

3. *Regulation* of sexual activity: Irresponsible and unstructured sexual function, endangering 'bonding', has never been tolerated for long in any society.

4. *Socialization:* Because the first few years of a child's life are spent almost entirely within the family, it is from this institution that he introjects (p 107) long-term perspectives, values and norms. As we have seen in considering personality development, it is within the intimate and loving atmosphere of parental, especially maternal relationships, that the child learns to make the sacrifices inherent in socialization (p 48 et seq). Although in adolescence there is temporary rebellion against familial norms, in general children introject and retain more of their parents' values than they may realize.

5. *Provision of healthy role models:*

    The admired father figure motivates his son's positive identification with a strong, protective, sexually vigorous male figure.

---

* Horton & Horton. *Introductory Sociology Learning Systems* Ontario: Irwin-Dorsey Ltd.

The admired mother promotes in her daughter positive identification with a warm, nurturing, sexually loving woman figure.

When role models are poor, they are either ineffectual or resented; avoided or negated. Thus is repeated the cycle of ineffectual life adjustment. Owing to the intensity of familial relations, rejection of family norms may lead to conflicting loyalties, anxiety, guilt and prolonged stress.

6.   *Status ascription:*

Parental family patterns, norms and values tend to perpetuate. Because poor parents provide limited opportunities and expectation, their children are exposed to neither motivation nor ambition. Children of higher-status families are exposed to both opportunity and motivation.

7.   *Affectional function:*

Hopefully meeting members' need for affection, love, intimacy and emotional involvement, the family is society's basic 'care unit'.

The family provides the natural haven for comfort, recovery and rehabilitation of both physical and emotional hurt.

Its safe structure accepts catharsis in the expression of ambivalence, disappointment, anger, loss, anxiety and frustration in reaction to the world's harsh demands. Home is the place for 'letting one's hair down'.

Demonstrations of 'reaching out' in loving and caring help family members achieve, accept, contain, support and make constructive use of strong emotional needs.

8.   Introjection of a code of religious and socio-political ethics, values and beliefs, spreading out from the family's introjected tolerance of each other, compassion, sense of justice, respect for the rights of others, to the community, the nation and Mankind.

Thus the family spreads its ethical heritage.

The family is a dynamic unit—experiencing, adapting, changing. Ties are amended by 'letting go' of authority and dependence to allow experiences of outside love, mating and parenting. The life of the family unit, like that of the individual is subject to Erikson's concept of life-change through the resolution of developmental conflicts and crises (chapter 11).

Applying Erikson's model to the family, nuclear parents are faced with the resolution of conflicting:

 (i) individuality vs closeness and sexual fulfilment → to meet the needs of both founding partners (p 249) → Love and Basic Trust

(ii) having achieved *autonomy* the unit is able to assert *initiative*
      personal goals vs sacrifice of attention—focus involved in accommodating new, helpless and dependent member → self-actualization and community status

(iii) parental authority–child dependence vs leadership, decision sharing, acceptance of children's experimentation, interests and value expansion into peer group and community

(iv) leisure and freedom vs the discipline imposed by industry → financial security and status → socially accepted, achieving and happy children

(v) self-absorption vs generativity; adolescents move towards peer group, self-decision, career absorption; parents move towards career fulfilment and authority, responsibility for their own ageing parents, civic and other group responsibilities and satisfactions

(vi) integrity of family unit vs feelings of personal, physical diminishment:
the 'empty nest' syndrome,
vicarious achievement in children's independence, career and other achievements,
personal genetic perpetuation in grandchildren, return to husband–wife one-to-one intimacy and mutual satisfaction,
own peer mutual interests and civic groups

(vii) family functions completed:
security and intimacy of shared life vs despair of aloneness
loss of spouse
adjustment to reduced physical and emotional resources → comfort in religion, wisdom, philosophy, contact with children and grandchildren → peer group and community interests and companionship.

While confirming the need to 'let go' of one's children that they may be free to go forth into their own careers, personal and familial relationships, the experience of the past few generations, in which the nuclear family pattern has been reinforced, is emphasizing the traumatic financial and isolatory experiences of reduced family cohesion. Throughout the Western world sociologists and psychiatrists are reconsidering their emphasis on the pre-eminence of independent living. There has been peril in young people's search for substitute families in peer 'communal living' groups. These latter are often either unstable and emotionally demanding, or manipulated and exploited by the mentally ill or unscrupulous.

Very painfully, divorce statistics, drug dependence, suicide escalation, lonely and abandoned old age, have reinstated the life-long value of the family—Nature's basic, natural, blood-unit—and the conviction that 'No man is an island'.

Types of family structure

There is wide deviation in the manner in which societies aim to achieve the important goal of appointing some male as responsible for each child.

While all marriage patterns insist on mating outside the nuclear family (to exclude incest and its dangerous genetic and emotional results), some insist on *endogamy* within the extended family, clan, village, tribe, race, religion, etc.

This is Kutum, the traditional marriage pattern of many Indians. *Exogamy*, the norm in Western countries, requires that marriages take place outside some prohibited degree of relationship.

Classification

The *nuclear* or *conjugal* family consists of one married couple and their children. Fulfilment and durability of all family functions are dependent upon the survival and romantic attachment of the two marriage partners.

This is the predominant family pattern in most Western societies.

The *consanguine* family is based upon blood rather than marriage relationships. The family consists of blood relatives, together with their mates and children. A man's responsibilities and primary emotional bonds lie within the family in which he is raised, rather than that into which he married. Permanent, indissoluble blood relationships, and the flexibility of responsibility flowing therefrom, pertain in Zulu, Xhosa and Muslim families and, to a diminishing extent, in Indian families. Some features persist in Jewish families. Usually consanguinal families are patrilineal, authority lying with senior male members.

Responsibility extends to a dead brother's family, but not to his divorced family.

Historically, most societies evolve from *polygamy* or plurality of wives. However where males are particularly threatened by environmental hazards, as pertains in the hunting perils encountered by Greenland Eskimoes, polyandry, allowing several husbands to one wife, is the accepted pattern.

Monogamy (one wife to one husband) has now become the legally enforced custom of most Western Societies.

Nuclear Family	Consanguinous Family
Advantages:	*Advantages:*
Self-decision, especially in love relationships, career choice, mobility, privacy	Security and protection within the flexible, 'umbrella' relationships of the extended family, a chain of successive standards, traditions and cultural supports
Disadvantages:	*Disadvantages:*
Being dependent on one precarious, 'romantic' relationship the family *lacks:* (i) transmission of folklore, standards, traditions, close relationship with grandparents, (ii) the 'safety net' of emotional security, protection and succour extending not only to children but also to the frail and the old, (iii) pooled work and financial resources.	*Reduced:* (i) personal freedom, (ii) educational and vocational choice, (iii) opportunity for travel and development. Family roles are 'predestined', (iv) status of women, who are usually diminished to a subservient role, sometimes within the restrictive structure of polygamy; many are bound by 'displacement' traditions, suffering forced marriage, and, in many third world countries, mutilating female circumcision.

The New family

Pregnancy heralds the end of the honeymoon

Love in the attic; the amorous blending of two individuals into a self-contained oneness must yield:
at best:

to the mortgaged, self-contained, two bedded flat, or 'semi'. Pizza and Coke at the corner must be balanced against prams, cribs, 'sitters', educational endowment policies. Albeit temporarily, soiled nappies and yelling hunger invade the love-nest.

at worst:

the circling stork casts panic-stricken shadows of unsupported rooflessness, devastated income and isolation.

CHANGED ROLES

Fundamental to stressors of pregnancy are the changed roles facing the new family's founding members.

Long before the baby's birth, especially when she feels life:

(i) The mother's participation in the marriage changes.
    The baby's presence intrudes upon her sleep, her social life, her career and financial contribution, her thoughts, her hopes, her dreams.

(ii) The physical discomforts of pregnancy bring feelings of heaviness, nausea, lethargy, depression, anxiety. Hormonal changes stimulate fears; thoughts and dreams of procreation and motherhood *from which the father is largely excluded.*

These psycho-physiological changes in Eriksonian terms (p 245ff), upset the marriage equilibrium necessitating resolution of the crisis caused thereby.

The wife must attempt to face, resolve and integrate into her *new wife–mother role* the following stressors:

resolution and abandonment of the pampered, indulged and idealized wife–child role,

attenuation or sacrifice of her career: the stimulation, ego-satisfaction and haven of independence this has afforded her,

acceptance of home-based chores,

threat to her figure and personal appearance.

All these 'sacrifices' she must balance against the unknown and sometimes unrealistic dreams of the maternal role.

Father's role crisis may be precipitated by the following stressors:

Abandonment of the idealized boy–hero, central lover role in favour of a more restrained, sometimes secondary place in his wife's thoughts and care.

Dominance of the breadwinner role over that of lover. Possible assumption of sexual abstinence in the last months of pregnancy, and the initial post-natal period.

At this time psychoanalysts believe *paternal jealousy of the infant usurper, especially a boy rival,* for mother's loving attention, reaches a peak. According to the Oedipal Theory (p 57) anger, jealousy, guilt and anxiety conflict with the paternal role, especially when father sees his 'rival' on the maternal breast, invading, in an especially tangible manner, paternal territory.

'Will my wife ever love me passionately again?'

'What if the baby dies as punishment for my jealousy?'

Father is required to find a *way of combining the husband–father role* in assuming responsibility, in providing physical and financial safety.

His new role should be balanced by his satisfaction in the dependence, status and love he receives from the genealogical line he has founded.

In attempting to resolve the ambivalence, conflict, anger, guilt and anxiety inherent in their developmental conflict, both parents, in Eriksonian terms, utilize the mental mechanisms of *Identification* and *Introjection* (pp 106-109) finally achieving the peace and fulfilment of parental homeostasis (pp 245, 388). Women who have observed their own mothers' joy and satisfaction in the combined role of wife, mother, homemaker, will more easily identify therewith, introjecting similar behaviour patterns and satisfactions. Those who have observed the successful and satisfying extension of the maternal role, to one of career participation, may well introject skills for compromise and amendment. Negatively, where new founding members have:

(i) suffered from environmental exposure to rejecting, resented or confused parental roles,

(ii) been exposed, in their own formative years, to parental influences caught in the conflict of class, socio-economic and cultural changes, lacking familiar traditional guide-lines and success models,

they may encounter confusion, failure, disappointment and ego impairment in their own unstructured parental role.

Yasmin looked down on her mother's 'primitive' and 'embarrassing' beliefs and behaviour. Yet she never felt accepted and confident among her middle class sophisticated elegant school peers. She followed mothercraft books assiduously but lacked faith and peace of mind, until a respected Hindu woman doctor pointed out the positive traditions of their mutual culture.

The intense experiences of pregnancy and childbirth:

negatively, in their distaste, panic and even horror, positively, in their excitement, anticipation, intense involvement and achievement,

do much to set the pattern of familial roles.

Socio-Economic 'class' and culture are important determinants of attitudes towards love-making, extra-marital intercourse, sexual fulfilment and hence, obstetrics.

Despite the 'sexual revolution', there persists in Western culture, partly through pressurized *toilet training and insistence on perfect cleanliness*, the impression (conscious or unconscious) that faeces, organs of elimination and hence, by association, the closely associated sex organs are 'disgusting', unacceptable, shameful and therefore guilt-laden. (Diagram p 343.)

Reinforced by *cultural and religious taboos*, feelings of guilt and shame may be strongly attached to the sex act and the whole obstetrical area. Indeed, throughout the Judeo-Christian world, and in the case of extra marital intercourse, amongst Muslim women, there persists the stricture that sexual activity is for procreation rather than 'forbidden' pleasure. Ingrained negative attitudes may persist in spite of the licence of marriage.

Among Hindu women there is, according to the custom of Kutum, dependence on a family structure in which relationships stem from a common grandfather and his sons.

The family is much involved in important decisions including marital choice and relationships. In fact marriage primarily involves families rather than individuals.

Some African men are still emotionally tied to the concept of circumcision as a necessity for initiated manhood—and, totally destructively, there still persists among the simplest traditionalists, insistence of the mutilating practice of female circumcision. Where individuals flout family-based traditions they may, in crises, present with such guilt and stress as to impede familial function and relationships, and even, via the arousal of the Sympathetic Nervous System, the normal physiology of labour.

Here the techniques, catharsis, reassurance and positive group identification of ante-natal preparation aim to break the destructive tension cycle.

Obstetric arrangements

Upper and middle class women are often delivered in private hospitals by doctors of their choice and, increasingly, by methods selected and insisted upon as a result of ante-natal preparation, education and information, eg
Grantly Dick Read's method of achieving 'natural' childbirth by breathing and relaxation techniques and active participation: *Leboyer's* 'gentler' methods of reducing trauma of loud sound, bright lights, precipitous cutting of the umbilical cord; his technique of underwater delivery and, above all, family participation. *Jolly* and other followers emphasize the importance of close, unimpeded maternal, and indeed paternal, bonding flowing from father's supportive presence at birth.

For the woman who avails herself of formal and informal birth information, there is a choice of methods involving various body positions devised to minimize pain, enhance descent and delivery of the baby. She claims the right to replace the passive, recipient role with one of active participation.

One wonders whether reluctance to include the mother as an active partner is unconsciously motivated by the obstetrical team's need to project an image of magic power, rather than of understood efficiency and mutual accomplishment.

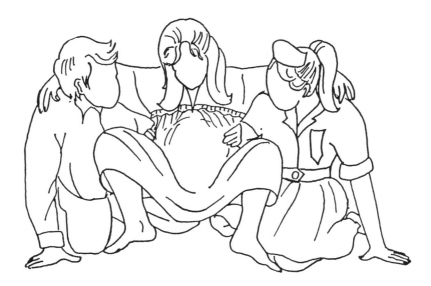

The "crouching" position of active labour enforces mothers controlling participation, and the supportive roles of father and professional team.

'Active labour and the adoption of a natural, upright or crouching birth
position is the safest, most enjoyable, most economical and sensible way for
the majority of women to give birth. There is no disruption of the normal
physiology of labour, no interference with the hormonal balance, post-natal
depression is rare and problems with breast-feeding and mothering are less
likely.'*

Some patients and practitioners favour a modern version of the old birth stool.

Janet and Arthur *Balaskas* and Dr Yehudi *Gordon* in England, and Dr Michel
Odent in France, aim to 'restore the balance between women's instinctive ability to
give birth, the skills of birth attendants and the safety of modern technology.† It has
taken a long time since the 1930s when *Russell* and others demonstrated
radiographically that the cross-sectional surface area of the birth canal may
increase by as much as 30% when a woman changes from the supine to the
squatting position. One wonders why. Is there some truth to the opinion that the
obstetric team feels more powerful, more 'in control' when standing authoritatively
over their supine, restricted patient?

'Lower working class' women are usually obliged to conform with whatever facilities
local state hospitals or midwives provide.

Immigrant women especially those from Africa, Middle Eastern cultures and the
Caribbean may, by introjecting maternal patterns, be attended by 'traditional'
midwives or senior 'family women' rather than those provided by the National
Health Service. This happens in spite of a conflicting desire for westernized
facilities. This is a pity. There are many ways of adjusting the home or hospital to
cater for more informal physically supportive birth customs.

Antenatal preparation

A. In the First Stage—As pertaining to the uterine muscles

Uterine muscles consist of:

(i)   the closely packed circular muscles of the lower segment;
(ii) the wider spaced circular transverse and longitudinal muscles comprising the
       upper segment

HYPOTHALAMIC—OXYTOCIN—PAIN CYCLE

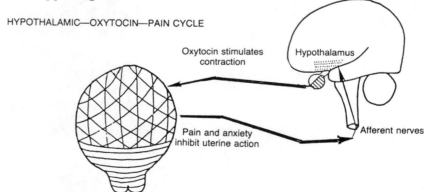

---

* G Hofmeyr and E Sonnendecker: The place of 'active birth' in present-day obstetric practice, 1985.
Further details obtainable from author.

† The International Centre for Active Birth, manifesto undated.

Preparation aims at assisting the patient to participate actively in breaking the vicious circle of

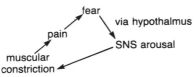

B. In the Second Stage—As pertaining to the cervical muscles

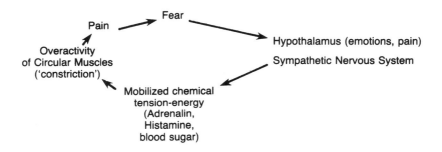

Fear-stimulated over-activity of the involuntary circular cervical muscles causes counter contractions to interfere with, and even to strangulate, freedom of movement in the voluntary longitudinal muscles.

Thus fear-stimulated over-activity distresses, disorganizes, prolongs labour; increases pain and fatigue, and renders unlikely that purposeful, active participation in the second stage which is essential for the conclusion of a successful and fulfilling delivery.

It is important that, from the outset, the word *contraction* be substituted for *pain*. The word 'pain' is in itself a stimulus for painful interpretation of what may otherwise be felt as strong sensation.

Important ways of counteracting this 'vicious circle' of fear, SNS tension-energy, and pain include:

(1) forestalling the fear–pain link by education, emotional-level reassurance; 'sensation' rather than 'pain' interpretation conditioning, and a positive attitude towards childbirth. Familiarity with common technical terms such as dilation, first and second stage, amniotic sac, counteract tension triggers, and include mother as an active member of the team.

Obviously this involves fairly long-term antenatal preparation within the context of an amiable, trusting relationship.

(2) Adopting breathing and muscular techniques permitting *overall relaxation* (thus including relaxation of the involuntary circular muscles) at contraction-peak, when tension over-activity and muscle conflict would otherwise have caused pain. Breathe deeply. Hold on for contraction peak. Exhale slowly letting all your body flop forward.

(3) A soft tennis ball, held in the palm of the hand, compressed in inhalation, slowly released in exhalation, helps 'condition' the mind to work in unison with the contracting uterus.

It is not easy to achieve voluntary relaxation, especially in the enormous experience of childbirth. Repetitive rehearsal involving 'suggestion' and 'auto-suggestion', to the point of self-hypnotism, may well prove helpful. Hypnotism is a trance-like state produced in a co-operative subject. This trance-like state reduces the inhibitory power of the conscience, enabling the hypnotist to reach into subconscious, and even perhaps unconscious strata. Here 'suggestion' may result in deeper-level relaxation, and conviction that pain perception will be reduced, or interpreted as strong sensation rather than suffering.

Nobody expects the midwife to be a professional hypnotist, but soothing music, repetitive humming, rhythmic inhalation and exhalation, associated with the soothing, pleasantly monotonous voice of the instructress may well condition the mind to deeper-level relaxation (p 32).

Especially in the case of first births, it is necessary to remove, or at least to alleviate, the greatest of human fears—that of the unknown. Repeatedly in the classes, it should be pointed out that *childbirth is just another physiological expulsive mechanism*, comparable with other familiar expulsive mechanisms unassociated with pain, such as the stretching sensations, the pressure, the elimination and the relief of defaecation.

Antenatal preparation is designed

(i) to give essential information,
(ii) to establish between midwife or hospital team, and patient, that long-term relationship of friendship, confidence and trust which is essential for emotional-level reassurance and fear alleviation.

Within a close, intimate and permissive relationship, deeper level emotions emerge, often prompted by the cathartic revelations of other group members. Remarks such as:

'My aunt died in childbirth—they say she bled to death' may trigger opportunity for valuable insight and reassurance. Common feelings revealed in communication with sympathetic professionals are:

Feelings of vulnerability, especially if it is a first pregnancy.

Feelings of ambivalence, even if the pregnancy was planned and desired.

Feelings of being trapped; that life will never be the same again.

Mood swings, ranging from euphoria to depression to cow-like serenity.

Sudden, irrational fears of having an abnormal child or of dying in childbirth.

Unmarried women may have special worries, eg little support from family, or friends or financial difficulties. These result in feelings of apprehension and loneliness and isolation and disturbing stress.

Nurses need to be aware of these normal feelings which require special sensitivity.

Beischer, Mackay, Bailliere and Tindall present the following table (28.1, p 225 2nd British Edition 'Obstetrics and the Newborn')

TABLE 28.1
STRESS AND ANXIETIES IN PREGNANCY

Past Medical History
- Infertility
- Termination of pregnancy
- Obstetrical problems in pregnancy
- Significant family history
- Genetic/inherited problems

Social
- Feelings of inadequacy
- Single parent. Present partner not the father of the child
- Dependent or sick relatives
- Poor supporting family network
- Marital dysfunction (eg infidelity)
- Interpersonal conflicts
- Problems related to finance, housing, career
- Drug addiction

Current Medical
- Pregnancy unplanned/not wanted
- Obstetrical complication (minor/major disorders)
- Medical/surgical complication(s)
- Separations from family (eg in hospital)

Rational/Irrational Fears
- Normality of reproductive organs
- Normality of baby (malformed, too large, dead)
- Loss of figure, attractiveness
- Labour, delivery (pain)
- Haemorrhage, dying
- General ability to cope

In hospital delivery, it is important to achieve continuity or 'carry-over' from the antenatal class to the obstetrical unit. If possible, the nursing roster should be arranged so that midwives or physiotherapists conducting antenatal classes will be on duty in the obstetric unit when their group of mothers is due for confinement.

It is important to include in the course at least one visit to the hospital, so that mothers may have an opportunity of meeting the staff and of becoming familiar with the hospital situation.

In order to promote compromise between domiciliary and hospital delivery, the obstetrical unit should be as homelike as possible. Admission followed by relegation to bed sets the stage for association with illness, the mother lying stiff and tense in bed, awaiting pain. An informal lounge, homely decoration and taped music, provide a peaceful, pleasant, natural setting for the first hours of labour. Long lonely hours spent in the bleak sterility of a formal labour or grim, instrument-decorated delivery room are unlikely to promote confidence and happy anticipation. Both parents are often helped by taking with them tapes of the instructress' voice in explanation, reassurance and as relaxation reminder cues, all to the background of familiar soothing music.

Why is it so important to alleviate the terror, the horror, the passive, helplessness *and pain of childbirth?* The mother who has had a painful or terrifying delivery may, through association, consciously or unconsciously, *blame and resent her baby* for having 'subjected' her to this ordeal. This illogical but strong negative association constitutes a burdensome start to motherhood and, impedes bonding.

Even more frequent are mother's *feelings of blame and hostility towards father*, whose impregnation she feels to be directly responsible for her painful and horrifying ordeal. Determined that she will not again allow herself to undergo childbirth, she rejects her husband's sexual advances, imperilling home and marriage.

The advantages and purpose of antenatal preparation

Antenatal classes are supplementary to, and in no way a substitute for, good physical supervision. They should not claim to replace supervision nor to interfere with obstetrical handling. Taught simply, and conducted by the obstetrical team which is actually to attend the patient in labour, they may perform important functions in:

(1) Allaying fear and thus preventing the establishment of the vicious cycle of fear and psychosomatic tension.

(2) Presenting the possibility of making childbearing an enjoyable and fulfilling experience.

(3) Affording an opportunity for establishing that long-term relationship between obstetrical team and patient which may reach her fears, anxieties, hopes and dreads at deeper emotional levels than is possible in casual, fleeting ordinary clinical contacts. It is often only in the context of such a long-term relationship that the patient is able to reveal the superstitions, old wives' tales, and other anxieties to whcih she is victim.

(4) Providing the reassurance of *group-identification*, helping mother forget herself, finding comfort in the successful experiences of her classmates. It is comforting to know that others share the same misgivings and anxieties, ultimately to learn from classmates who have already had their babies that most of one's own fears are groundless. Return visits with baby or letters are thus recommended.

(5) Reducing pain and shortening labour.

(6) Avoiding unnecessary anaesthesia, drugs, post-anaesthetic hangover and anoxia in the baby.

(7) Replacing nine months of fearsome dread and unhappiness by nine months of relaxed and joyful anticipation. To the expectant mother the antenatal class can give high morale, companionship, pose and serenity, the right attitude to pregnancy, childbirth and motherhood.

Obstacles to successful antenatal preparation

While maintaining a confident and optimistic attitude towards her antenatal programme, the midwife or physiotherapist should be warned of several obstacles, of which the most important are:

1. The difference between *intellectual* and *emotional acceptance*. In the general nursing course, the difficulty involved in bridging the gap between understanding and feeling is emphasized (see pp 66ff). With the best will in the world, the woman who has been exposed during *her life-history to strong fear or guilt associations* appertaining to the whole process of sex and childbirth may encounter real difficulty, in spite of intellectual insight, in overcoming her unconsciously motivated fears. In such cases, the *midwife should invite personalized discussions* in which mother is encouraged to think or 'associate' back to her earliest memories pertaining to sex information, childbirth, etc. *Linking back*, she may reach deeper levels of consciousness where she may be helped to locate, recognize and reveal traumatic experiences. Opportunity for *catharsis*, and reiterated *reassurance* by the midwife, who has by now achieved some measure of long-term relationship, should help achieve emotional-level relief (p 64 et seq). Should a mother remain unrelieved of her fears, agitated, and unduly tense, it may well prove wise to refer her for psychiatric help.

2. Especially frustrating is the *apathy, disinterest* and *resignation* to pain manifested by some mothers and their families. Sometimes an older 'traditional' relative may *displace* her own resentment, hostility or fear experienced in childbirth:

'I went through the suffering, now it's *your* turn.'

3. In poorer communities, bus-fares and working hours constitute strong obstacles to participation in the antenatal programme. In such cases the good offices of the *Community Nurse* or hospital social worker should be solicited in making an interpretative home visit to the mother's family, or in making appropriate financial or work arrangements.

4. The real apathy and even resentment felt towards childbirth by mothers already burdened by too many children. One can hardly expect the mother with seven children, and food for two, to anticipate with excitement the wonder of childbirth, when this merely imposes another mouth demanding attention and food.

Clearly, rewarding childbirth and a good mother–child relationship are largely dependent on reliable family planning.

In spite of these difficulties, the successful and enthusiastic midwife and physiotherapist will soon form that nucleus of 'converted' mothers, who will spread abroad the good tiding that childbirth can be a joyful, creative experience, instead of a disorganizing, emotionally traumatic nightmare.

Psychological involvement in labour

Labour, like most other strong human experiences and relationships, arouses *ambivalence*—those mixed feelings, that swing of the pendulum between wanting and not wanting, loving and hating, which are often manifest in the obstetrical unit. Provoked by intense discomfort in labour, or anxious about her new responsibility, the mother may declare that she does not want the baby; that she is angry with her husband for having placed her in this position. She may fear she is about to give birth to something 'bad' or deformed. These natural feelings should be accepted: it is a stupid or insensitive midwife who would reproach mother at this stage, or indeed afterwards, arousing feelings of guilt and anxiety.

Hypersensitivity and personalization in labour

In the gross arousal of labour and the hormonal disbalance of the lying-in period the mother is hypersensitive, tending to apply overheard irrelevant remarks (and obstetric complications) to herself. She may become deeply emotionally upset by a short retort or an unkind word. The staff, remembering this, should not react personally to her exaggerated reactions and displaced aggression.

Midwifery procedures, concentrating as they do upon areas of deep emotional significance, *expose and 'rip away' the patient's deeply engrained defences* against her shame and guilt. Thus she may react very strongly, at an emotional level, *experiencing procedures as a humiliating assault upon her person*. Indeed, some patients insist that the embarrassment and humiliation they experience in procedures such as enemata, shaving, douching, etc constitute the most traumatic and dreaded aspects of the whole process of childbirth.

The impersonal and clinical atmosphere of the obstetrical unit is very different from the passionate abandon of the sex act. Politeness, courtesy and good manners are therefore essential in good midwifery.

While many such procedures are indispensable, every effort should be made to safeguard the patient's privacy through the use of screens, dressing towels to ensure minimal exposure, allowing the patient to do as much for herself as possible, polite dignified address, etc.

It is during labour that mother's <u>familiarity with a simplified explanation of the</u> <u>mechanisms of labour</u>, and with common <u>technical terms</u>, becomes especially valuable, reducing her fear of the unknown, alleviating tension and including her as an active, organized participant of the obstetrical team.

Left at the mercy of grim stories told by other patients, she is liable <u>to introject</u> <u>fear</u>, to panic, and in so doing become entangled in the vicious circle of fear, psychosomatic tension, pain and more fear. Large indiscriminate labour rooms are thus a technical disadvantage in the conduct of satisfactory natural childbirth. On the other hand, *the patient should not be left alone*, to become frightened by her own thoughts. Alone there is nothing to distract her, no one to advise. Neither is there any relationship upon which to lean for reassurance and support in the context of the strange, enormous sensations of childbirth. The mother needs support and guidance in carrying out the instructions received in the antenatal group.

Constant reassurance, encouragement and inclusion of the mother in procedures, and in the *progress of her labour, are essential* if she is to remain co-operative. The more intelligent mother, especially, is made to feel resentful and unhappy if treated as an interfering schoolgirl. A high-handed attitude on the part of the obstetrical team, will certainly reduce her active co-operation.

A helpful procedure in rounding off antenatal preparation consists in asking each mother to write back to the group an account of her experiences, sensations. <u>If the</u> <u>father is not available an alternative 'birth companion' should be provided</u> <u>throughout labour and delivery</u>, perhaps the patient's own mother.

It is a mistaken interpretation of the new approach to childbirth to exclude the *use of those pain-relieving drugs which help relaxation* and do not cloud the ability to participate in the first stage and to appreciate the fulfilling climax of the second stage. Thus no mother should be made to feel guilty, or a failure, if a drug such as Pethidine is asked for and administered.

Pain

Unfortunately not all labours go smoothly, and many are marked by painful complications. At this point I would appeal to the midwife to reread the section on Pain (p 480 et seq). Tactile comfort and identification are stressed.

Insight into regression to generalized pain helps mother 'isolate out' and localize acute sensation to specific areas. Concentration on a 'stretched vagina' is easier to handle than generalized swamping pain.

There is strong support for *epidural anaesthesia* for pain relief, or, where women are likely to experience significant pain, prevention. Many obstetricians believe, on the following grounds, that this form of analgesia should be available by patient choice:

1. It prevents pain-stimulated inference with first-stage muscle work.
2. The strangulating constriction of fear-induced over-activity of the circular cervical muscles is avoided.
3. It being impossible to cut off sensation completely, the mother still feels pressure as a guide to contractions, and thus the necessity to bear down. She is thus able to participate actively in the birth process.
4. Freedom from exhausting pain
    (i) is more conducive to joyful participation in the moment of birth than resentment and exhaustion;
    (ii) preserves parental and mother–child relationships.

There being no virtue in suffering, and creation bringing its own unique satisfaction, one can find no psychological fault in this argument.

Participation by fathers

It is becoming common practice to invite fathers to attend appropriate antenatal classes and to be present in the delivery room. Among advantages thereunto pertaining are

1. Interpreting to father the physical and emotional changes his wife is experiencing in pregnancy—this with a view to eliciting his interest, sympathy, tolerance and feeling of *actively sharing* in the development and eventual creation of the new life in which he is an essential, although often neglected, partner.

The father does not automatically share the mother's strong creative drive and nursing satisfaction.

His routine is disturbed, he is called upon to make sacrifices, and he may feel that his pre-eminent position in his wife's thoughts is being usurped by this new rival for her love and attention. (p 57)

2. Showing father how his presence during labour and delivery enables him to

(a) remind mother how to breathe, move and relax as labour progresses, and sensations become so strong that it is not always easy to carry out instructions on her own. The all fours, standing or crouching positions of active labour reinforce father's supportive and team roles; (Diagram p 393)

(b) massage the cranial-sacral parasympathetic nervous system, stimulating the secretion of soothing antihistamine, thus counteracting the disorganizing Fight–Flight tension-energy cycle initiated by fear stimulation of the sympathetic nervous system;

(c) isolate out localized strong sensation from swamping, overall pain.

Father's presence in labour and delivery rooms provides

(i) the support of a long-term relationship in which the mother has learnt to find safety, comfort and strength;

(ii) enrichment of this relationship by together triumphing over pain to achieve the miracle of creativity;

(iii) an opportunity to participate in the actual birth of his child, thus identifying with creation and sharing the most fundamental bonding experience.

To quote Prince Charles when he faced the press as he emerged from sharing Princess Diana's first delivery 'I'm emotionally exhausted. That sixteen hours was a very adult experience.'

Bonding—The mother–child relationship in the lying-in period

About fifty years ago Dr Truby King of New Zealand and his grimly starched Plunket nurses took to the four corners of the newly scientifically bemused world a doctrine of baby-care based on coldly scientific scales, clocks, schedules and fanatical antisepsis. Heaven forbid that a mother should spontaneously pick up, hug, kiss and rock her baby! What infections, what selfish, criminal self-indulgences and irresponsibilities would result!

From this cold, unnatural handling there resulted emotional and physiological tensions in mother and baby—the inhibition of her milk supply, and disturbance

of her peace of mind, 'feeding problems', protracted crying and general lack of
spontaneous contentment in her baby.

In contrast studies by Spitz, Levy, Bowlby, Harlow, Rheingold, and others, have
resulted in a 'swing-back' to the best aspects of natural 'baby in the cradle beside
mother' midwifery (see pp 43-50).

As a result of modern experiments with babies and animals there has been a
'swing-back' to the realization that Nature's plan of keeping mother and baby close
to each other, both environmentally and emotionally, is the least traumatic and
most desirable way of bridging the gap between parasitic and independent
existence.

Bonding begins inter-utero, the mother responding to her child's movements with
protectiveness, fascination and increasing anticipation. From this symbiotic
relationship grow feelings of closeness, warmth and involvement which may well
trigger off those endocrinological developments which prepare the woman for
motherhood, both psychologically and physiologically. To quote Dr Hugh Jolly,

> 'Our birth rooms at Charing Cross are certainly cosier and less clinical places
> than the labour wards I have seen in some other places. When father is not
> available, our obstetricians record who is to be mother's "labour companion".
> Bearing in mind that she must *not* be alone, if nobody is suitable from her
> immediate circle we will provide somebody. While still on the umbilical cord
> (thank God for making it long enough) the baby is placed on mother's tummy.
> We advise her to turn on her side "en face", *so baby and mother can look into each
> other's eyes*. Among other studies, the Cleveland Technical Investigation has
> shown that, in these circumstances, the *baby focuses his eyes on his mother's face for
> the first hour of life, as Nature designed it.*'

Thus they find joy and contentment in each other.

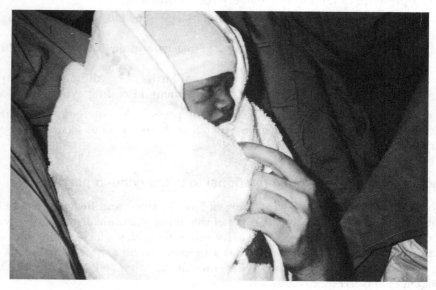

David, the authors' first grandchild, <u>wide-eyed</u>, meets mum's entranced gaze, 10 minutes after Caesarian
delivery, at the Royal Free (15.11.89).

We are becoming increasingly convinced that one should not announce the sex of a baby as soon as it is born. When a mother has been hoping for a boy, or vice versa, her first reaction on hearing that her child is of the other sex may be one of disappointment, and a degree of involuntary rejection, guilt and distressing, disorganizing anxiety may be experienced. It is wise to avoid this unwelcome intrusion into the triumph and joy of birth, substituting joyful congratulation and the immediate placement of the baby on the mother's breast. By the time she has herself discovered the baby's sex, bonding will already have commenced unhindered; and whether she has been blessed with a boy or girl will probably have become immaterial.

> 'Our obstetric unit likes to leave the family alone together to get to know each other—this is an inflexible rule at Charing Cross.'

A reflection of the unique and lifelong importance of the birth experience lies in an African custom of enquiring about one's origin: One does not ask 'Where were you born?' but rather 'Where is your umbilical cord buried?'

Every man has a right to the dignity and security embodied in his roots. His self-image is enhanced by the conviction that somewhere in this world is the spot whence he emanates, whence he takes life, whence he goes forth and whereunto he has a right to return, to live, and to die amongst his fellows.

No doubt, caught in traditional conflict, some immigrants may suffer from feelings of disturbed identity and isolation when unable to comply with this deeply rooted tradition.

Imagining the effect of such 'rootlessness' in the face of strong, time-long tradition, one realizes again the need for attempting to cater in our highly specialized, technical and quick-turnover hospitals for those traditions that time and custom have rendered so important.

We have read in chapter 2 how the neonate develops from a mass of generalized feelings and responses to a specific integrated personality, and how closely this process is dependent upon the mother–child relationship.

When frightened or frustrated the baby cries and panics with his *whole* tensed-up body. When happy, he relaxes and smiles with his *whole* warm cuddly self. When *hungry* his *whole* being is racked with pain. (Crying—see p 38-9.)

Soon after birth he becomes aware of his instinctive needs, and experiences pleasure and gratification, when they are satisfied. His physical needs centre on sleep and food, and the *soothing feeling of physical and emotional well-being which results from mother's removal of hunger pain through feeding.* If, at the same time, through holding, stroking, fondling and nursing, she stimulates his *parasympathetic nervous system*, with consequent outpouring of *soothing antihistamine*, she establishes a close, physiologically based mother–child bond.

Touch is a need rather than an indulgence. It is the main medium of human bonding. It becomes part of our ritual, our play, our care.

Formula for the establishment of a satisfying mother–child relationship

(i) Removal of hunger pain
(ii) Fondling stimulation of parasympathetic nervous system → soothing antihistamine → physiological well-being
(iii) Mouth activity

} mother love, safety and security

This formula constitutes the basis for that close, primitive, deeply engrained mother–child relationship which will spread out to influence the baby's human relations as a whole. For *the mother–child relationship is the pattern upon which all other relationships are modelled.*

Deprivation of touch experience is a serious obstacle to that mother–child bonding fundamental to mental health. There is much evidence that deprivation of body touch, contact and movement are important contributors to a number of emotional disturbances including reactive depression, anxiety, withdrawal, hyperactivity, sexual aberration, violence, etc. Because children in intensive care are particularly vulnerable to touch deprivation, David Todres, of the Massachusetts General Hospital a paediatrician, anaesthetist, neonatologist and director of the hospital's ICU is insistent that:

> 'The parent looks past the machine and sees the baby. Because there's a need for bonding, I try to get the parent to hold the hand of the baby in the incubator. . . .'

Rooming-in

For obvious reasons, successful demand feeding is more easily organized in the context of 'rooming-in'. The mother, too, is usually greatly helped by 'rooming-in' of one form or another. The baby's presence is comforting and elevates childbearing above mere illness, giving it purpose and dignity.

The advantages of rooming-in

1. Seeing her baby sleeping peacefully beside her, the mother is not disturbed about his well-being. Closeness, warmth, freedom from anxiety, liberate maternal feelings and enhance emotional unity of mother and child.

2. It affords her the opportunity to enjoy her baby unharried by domestic and family responsibilities.

3. Continual presence of the baby, contentment, demand feeding and thus increased handling of the breasts, stimulate lactation.

4. It affords more freedom from infection than does the general nursery.

5. Watching and participating in the handling of the baby, the inexperienced mother becomes accustomed to correct mothercraft procedures, and also to her baby's own individual habits, while still within the secure and protected environment of the hospital.

6. It affords the father an opportunity to share these important familial experiences. Some units provide double-bedded rooms for family intimacy.

7. The baby's presence is an effective antidote to the post-natal blues as has already been referred to.

Of course, some overworked, tired mothers welcome the rest afforded by the lying-in period and do not wish to be continually 'disturbed' by the presence of the baby. Such mothers are probably not spacing their confinements, and would be well advised to attend a birth-control clinic in order to avoid the recurrence of an unwelcome pregnancy. Others may, of course, need rest in recovering from a difficult delivery. In such cases a compromise form of partial rooming-in should be devised. Perhaps the baby can spend days with his mother and nights in a central nursery. One imaginative United States architect has designed an ingenious scheme whereby four units of two-bedded wards are grouped around a central, common eight-bedded nursery. The babies lie in drawer-like cribs in which they may be drawn at mother's will into the maternal ward.

The *famous Sheffield Experiment* conducted by the Sheffield Royal Infirmary demonstrated that demand-fed 'rooming-in' babies ('experimental' babies) were more contented, slept better, regained birth weight more quickly and showed fewer feeding problems than those in the more strictly scheduled 'control' group. In addition, mothers in the experimental group showed better lactation, more strongly developed maternal instinct, greater pleasure in their children and less susceptibility to the post-natal blues.

The obstetric unit at Charing Cross Hospital is convinced of the advantages of placing the *baby in bed beside his mother* rather than in an adjoining crib. This allows for the complete union of mother and child as Nature intended:

> 'Careful follow-up and national research have convinced our unit that this is a perfectly safe practice, provided the mother has not had a sedative, and is not under the influence of alcohol or other drugs.'

Breast-feeding versus artificial feeding

Most mothers enjoy the pleasurable physical sensation and emotional satisfaction which they experience in breast-feeding. Certainly there can be no tactile satisfaction and warm interflow as close and intimate as that between the mother and the child at her breast. For the child, the *breast-feed bond establishes a love–comfort association with a warm, human contact, as opposed to a cold, impersonal bottle-object.* This association augurs well for lifelong ability to seek, develop, and value warm human relationships.

A compromise for the mother unable to breast-feed might well lie in holding the baby to her bare breast while bottle-feeding, thus enabling him to fondle the breast, maintain close contact, and receive (both orally and by touch) the soothing rhythm of the familiar maternal heartbeat.

Regrettably the Western world has taken a long time to move away from Truby King's restrictive pattern of physical and psychological mother–baby separation. Paradoxically it is middle-class women who have taken the initiative in returning to breast-feeding as a natural and important mother–baby bond.

Pressurized by the strong conditioning of the mass media, unaware of the potentially fatal effects of misusing formulae, and desperately wanting the Western 'best' for their babies, many women especially in transitional and immigrant cultures—have turned to artificial feeding. They stint on other basic needs, believing that money buys the 'best'.

Anthropologist and childbirth counsellor, Sheila Kitzinger, believes the choice between breast- and bottle-feeding is not only an individual one: it has become a 'political issue' for women in developing countries desirous of introjecting the role model patterns of Western women.

Some mothers definitely resent breast-feeding. The reason for this resentment may be fairly obvious, such as insecurity in the marriage relationship and fear that their husbands may no longer find them desirable should their breasts begin to sag. Even surface fears are real, tension-fraught, distressing, and therefore worthy of respect. Some experience discomfort as the uterus contracts.

Other avoidance associations are embedded in deeper levels of preconscious or unconscious emotional functioning. The mother may sense father's jealousy of the resented son–rival hungrily possessing her breast, and symbolizing this usurpation by his hungry possession of her breasts.

A normally jealous elder sister, cast out at feeding time, may always associate breast-feeding with her mental picture of the hated sibling–rival possessing mother's body in the intimate feeding relationship. These unconscious negative breast-feeding associations involve resentment, guilt, tension and a recourse to avoidance–escape.

These associations are long-term, deep-seated and powerful: certainly the midwife, in her short, relatively fleeting relationship with the mother, will not remove them. Her *pressure will only arouse guilt feelings and anxiety which, resulting in physiological disturbance of the mammary glands, will defeat its purpose*, leaving mother miserable, guilt-laden and tense.

Well-managed artificial feeding is preferable to unhappy, tense, resented breat-feeding.

Provided that:

(i) feeds are self-regulated,
(ii) they are conducted in a leisurely manner by mother herself to her accompaniment of cuddling, nursing, etc.
(iii) the teat hole permits sufficient sucking activity (it should not allow more than twenty drops a minute when the bottle is inverted),

artificial feeding need not impede healthy personality development. Well-conducted artificial feeding is certainly preferable to pressure exerted on mother to breast-feed if, through a lifetime of 'shame' or resentment-associations, logical or illogical, she has come to regard breast-feeding with distaste and disgust.

Fortunately today's young women are more natural and uninhibited than their own mothers, most finding delight in spontaneous breast-feeding.

Caesarian section—psychological involvement and bonding

What must it feel like to have a baby *and* an operation? It is unrealistic to expect 'Caesarian women' magically to transform themselves into 'good' and caring mothers in a context of post-operative trauma, both physical and mental.

In the case of a 'hot' Caesarian delivery, an epidural may take too long to work, necessitating general anaesthesia. Mother and baby having had no contact for many hours, bonding is imperilled. In 'cold' surgery preference is moving to *epidural anaesthesia which has many advantages*. The mother is able to see her child while he is still on the cord, as if he were vaginally delivered. Routine use of a screen separating mother from the birth-scene is certainly being questioned.

As soon as possible thereafter, she should be able to touch and stroke him, and look into his eyes; one would hope that one arm would be free, but if this is not possible the father should hold the baby to her face.

So now even a Caesarian birth can be a family-centred occasion. The baby is usually handed to the parents while the doctor sews up the incision. When the operation is over, all three can be moved together to the recovery room so that they may spend this all-important hour in the intimate privacy of family bonding.

This is a good time for the mother to commence breast-feeding.

It is becoming common practice for the anaesthetist to give the mother a little extra epidural anaesthetic so that she may bond comfortably with her baby during this first hour. If this precious time is spoilt by pain she may unconsciously blame the baby for her discomfort, and as a result develop negative feelings towards him.

Fortunately the practice of placing all Caesarian babies in incubators for the first day of their lives is becoming less frequent. But where this *is* necessary, the incubator should accompany the mother into the recovery room, and also into her ward, so that both mother and child may benefit from 'rooming-in'.

Post-natal psychological implications of the Caesarian section

The new 'Caesarian mother' may be *angry with herself*. She may resent her own body for being too small, too unco-operative, to allow her to give birth normally. She may think she did something wrong; she may feel guilty that she has deprived her child, and herself, of a normal birth. For the rest of her life she may feel, whenever anything goes wrong: 'If only I hadn't given up so soon. If only I had done my exercises' etc.

She may feel inferior and frustrated when she listens to friends repeating their beautiful experience of vaginal delivery. She needs to discuss and be reassured about these feelings before they escalate and become engrained.

'Rooming-in' and father's presence and reassurance will help counteract normal post-natal depression aggravated by post-surgical trauma.

Engaging the services of a sympathetic paediatrician in advance will assure the baby's health and the mother's confidence, while at the same time removing the necessity for routine placement in an incubator.

Breast-feeding is particularly important post-Caesar. Not only does the colostrum help break down mucus, but successful breast-feeding will help to counteract any unfavourable psychological effects of Caesarian section while at the same time strengthening the bonding process.

Father's role in the Caesarian section

The father sits or stands at the head of the delivery table, beside the mother's head, where he can reassure and support her.

A new parent, he has every right to participate in this special moment in the family's life. He may stand up and watch as much, or as little, of the operation as he likes—he may even take snapshots if he wishes.

Mother is shown the baby on the cord, and he is taken to her face while still unwashed. Then the delivery room nurse attends to the baby in view of both parents. She wraps baby in a blanket and gives him to the father, who then cuddles the child close and takes it to the mother.

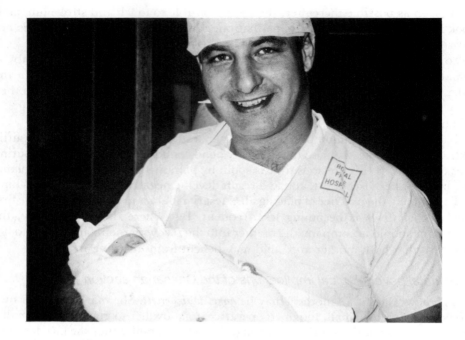

The presence of the father may make the difference between a successful surgical procedure (from a medical point of view), and a joyful, meaningful occasion for the parents and their baby. A problem does arise if father becomes so interested in the operation he forgets the mother!

Post-natal blues

Basic to mother's emotional state after delivery is her *hormonal disbalance*. Pregnancy is marked by growing *intensity of glandular activity* (and thus *emotional over-reaction*), probably culminating in the onset of labour. After delivery, there is abrupt cessation of the endocrinological build-up of pregnancy. This sudden endocrinological anticlimax brings a feeling of depression 'emptiness' and unmotivated lethargy.

A few days later, with the onset of the intense activity of the mammary glands, *hormonal disbalance* again leads to that distinct depression and irritability known as *post-natal blues*. *Depression* and *inability to cope* increase as the day wears on, the patient longing to escape into sleep. There is continual longing for fluids and fattening foods; diffuse pain and marked irritability. Mental confusion in time and space makes the mother frightened of herself and her baby whom she may come to resent. Ambivalence, guilt, disappointment and general misery may, in severe cases, lead to suicide. In distinct cases hormonal treatment, usually by progesterone is indicated.

References: 'Bonding with Your Caesarian or Premature Baby' *Odyssey*, March/April 1980; Bonny Donovan *The Caesarian Birth Experience*. Beacon Press: Boston, p 562, 1978.

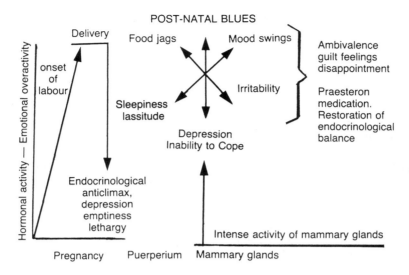

POST-NATAL BLUES

It is certainly the unwise nurse, or misguided husband, who reacts personally, who 'take umbrage', who 'reacts back' in the face of that involuntary lability (mood swings) which classically, accompanies endocrinological change and which will disappear with the return of normal endocrinological balance.

Depression or anxiety, aggravated by personal and environmental factors and endocrine changes, may underline a wide range of symptoms such as anorexia, vomiting, palpitations and urinary frequency, all of which require individual counselling. (Extreme care should be taken not to mistake puerperal psychosis for 'post-natal blues'. Puerperal psychosis, p 411).

Sibling rivalry

Because the midwife shares intimately in a most important family experience, because she deals with a family excited, stimulated and rendered impressionable by a great event, hers is the opportunity to promote good human relations in many spheres. She can influence mother to be warm, loving, demonstrative and easy-going, so that the child she has helped to bring into the world will grow up in warmth, security, contentment and that love which frees him from the necessity to hate.

One person to whom the baby's arrival may bring insecurity, hate, aggression, guilt-feelings and permanent personality maladjustment is the elder sibling, who is now undergoing perhaps the most difficult of human adjustments—that of learning to share love. In the excitement surrounding the birth of the baby, the elder sibling is often cast to one side. From being the focus of love and attention, his position is often usurped by this newcomver who demands, and receives, affection, love, presents and attention which were formerly his. Naturally, his feelings towards this rival, whom he feels has usurped the all-important mother love, are *ambivalent*. His feelings toward the baby, and, indeed, towards his mother, swing between love and distressing, guilt-laden hate.

During his 'love periods' he feels guilty and anxious about his 'hate' periods.

If he is punished for his aggression, cast out during feeding time, or in other ways rejected, his festering hate will come out in aggression, or, more serious, be suppressed, causing powerful subconscious guilt-tension, anxiety and painful neuroses.

In several important ways, the midwife can help to alleviate this damaging experience:

1. She should explain to mother and relatives the strength of the elder child's primitive needs, loves and hates. Every elder sibling is a potential Cain.

2. Now, while the baby is still a bundle of sleepy peacefulness, safe in his cradle, is the time to show the elder child love, warmth and extra attention.

Visiting relatives and friends should be asked to bring a small present for the elder child, rather than a large one for the baby. They should be asked to give him that love and attention to which he is accustomed.

3. Obstetric units should not exclude sibling visits.

Dr Hugh Jolly, Paediatrician-in-Charge, Charing Cross Hospital Psychiatric Unit, London, was insistent that the growing practice of inviting young siblings to visit their mothers in obstetric units should be routine. 'Scientific research has shown that infection spreads through staff contact, not through sibling contact.'

Almost universally the elder sibling feels *'Mum has got herself another baby because she thinks I am not good enough'*. This conviction is certainly reinforced, 'to hazardous proportions', by exclusion from this emotionally charged family experience. The Charing Cross unit prepares mother for sibling visits by advising her to feed the baby before the visit, thus keeping both arms free to welcome and caress the elder child. She should not demand that he meet and welcome the new arrival, but allow him to discover the baby himself, when he is ready to do so—a development which may in fact occur only at subsequent visits.

If daily visiting is impossible, she should telephone him, or send home with father a small gift or note as a token of the fact that she is well, safe and still loves him.

4. Some children, especially girls, are comforted by presentation with their own 'baby' doll, 'trousseau', baby bath, etc.

5. It is often a good idea to have the elder child out of the house when the baby is brought home. With baby settled, mother will be free to give to the elder her usual loving attention, when he arrives home.

6. At feeding time, the elder child should be encouraged to snuggle close to mother.

The mother who resents these physical demands may be reminded that all too soon, when her children grow up, she will crave such attention.

In his excellent book *Baby and Child Care*, Dr Benjamin Spock presents an astute illustration of a baby, crying and nursing a minor hurt inflicted by the elder sibling. Mother, realizing that 'the aggressor needs reassurance rather than punishment', is restraining the elder in a hug.

Remarks such as 'Heaven will punish you for hurting your little sister' are especially dangerous (p 63 et seq). It is important that the aggressive sibling does not learn to push his hate into 'the unconscious' where it will cause festering, long-term guilt and anxiety. Rather should he be encouraged to express his hate verbally, at a level where, through *catharsis* and *reassurance*, he may be helped to know that his feelings are understood and accepted—that he is still his mother's important and loved first-born.

'You don't have to hate the new baby. You are my especially loved big boy.'

Puerperal psychosis

Behind almost every case of infanticide and maternal suicide lurks a sad, and often reprehensible tale of failure to observe, understand and emphasize the presence of puerperal psychosis.

The patient suffering from puerperal psychosis is mentally ill, and for her own protection, that of her baby, and society as a whole, she should be treated as such. Properly treated, usually by drug therapy, the acute stage of this condition should pass within a few weeks. However, if taken lightly, puerperal psychosis may lead to far-reaching tragedy in mother's self-destruction, her destruction of her precious baby or the killing of innocent persons about whom she has paranoic (persecutory) *delusions or hallucinations:* 'If I don't kill her first, she will kill my baby!'

In contrast with the 'slowing down' of post-natal depression, the psychotic patient, early in her illness, presents as *over-active, interfering, suspicious, tense and agitated. Insomnia* features strongly as do persistent *ruminative 'circular' disconnected thoughts.* Later she retreats into her own fantasy world where *delusions* (false, impossible beliefs) and hallucinations (unreal sensory perceptions) destructive to her baby and herself, abound.

> 'Isobel, a 24-year-old mother, noticed a small pimple the size of a pinhead on her daughter's face when she was two days old. Isobel was in tears when she asked:
>
> "Could it be a misplaced testes? Do you think Julie has spina bifida? Nobody tells the truth here, everyone is in conspiracy against me. They all say it's nothing, but it is something, I can see it." '*

She talks of self-destruction, of destroying the baby, of killing people attacking her child. These symptoms should not be cast to one side nor their verbalization stifled. Utilizing her long-term contact with the patient, the midwife should rather *seek to enter into her fantasy world.* By encouraging the patient to talk, the midwife may discern those painful and terrifying delusions and hallucinations which underlie the patient's withdrawn, suspicious, aggressive or otherwise inappropriate behaviour. The midwife should not be lulled into false security by the fact that the patient's symptoms are not always present: classically, they come and go. It is the nurse's duty to observe carefully, record and draw the attention of the doctor to any such abnormal behaviour in her patient.

Etiology and handling

The etiology of puerperal psychosis appears to be twofold:

1. That which is due to a temporary *toxic condition.* The patient who is carefully observed, protected from herself, and biochemically treated with antibiotics, tranquillizers and other drugs, will probably emerge none the worse within about three weeks.

2. A *latent form of schizophrenia* which, like diabetes, can be precipitated by the biochemical and endocrinological changes of pregnancy, childbirth and lactation. Promising research indicates that schizophrenia is due to impaired secretion of an unknown endocrine essentially for metabolism and other biochemical processes. Stelazine, and similar drugs, appear to help control endocrine disturbance. It is

---

* Dalton, K. *Depression after Childbirth.* Oxford University Press. 1980.

important that the patient and her family realize that medication is not a form of drug addiction. Rather does it consist in the artificial application of *a biochemical which the body lacks*. In all probability such a patient requires long-term supervision and adjustment of her body chemistry. Serious psychogenic conflict, fears or environmental stresses may increase the possibility of puerperal psychosis.

The type of schizophrenia encountered in puerperal psychosis is, apparently, of a relatively serious and long-term nature. The mother may require in-patient, followed by out-patient, treatment over a long period.*

It is my earnest hope that no reader of this book will ever find herself in the tragic circumstances of having, through negligence or poor observation, misinterpreted puerperal psychosis as the post-natal blues. Such a mistake may well be responsible for a long string of preventable tragedies.

Parents in bereavement (Stillbirth, Miscarriage, Adoption)

One should never forget that bonding begins in utero.

'There is a vital need for the mother and father of the child who is born dead to see and handle their baby in a natural way. They need each other's support in sensitive sorrowing. This is still their beloved child. A birth without a baby is an empty birth. If the baby is whisked away there is no feeling of accomplishment—no memories. Even if the child is malformed, nothing is so frightening as an imagined monster. Using carefully draped towels one can show first the normal face, and then the deformity. (This principle is also true in the case of abnormal living children, whose mothers should be given the opportunity of getting to know and love them, primarily as their baby, and then as children who need special care.)'

Whatever the circumstances, the midwife should, as usual, remark 'It is a lovely baby', thus relieving feelings of emptiness, depression and guilt by the conviction that the parents have, after all, been able to produce something beautiful and worthwhile. It is often consoling to provide parents with a sensitive photograph of their dead baby.

'There is enormous pain within bereaved parents, and we try to dilute this by providing a place for father and mother to sleep together in the hospital. We also ask mother's permission to tell other mothers what has happened, that they may sympathize, rather than ask curious questions. I have seen permanent grief, anxiety, and marital turmoil resulting from callous, unwise or insensitive handling of stillbirth, e g "I'm sorry you can't see her—we've put your baby in the incinerator"!'

Stillborn babies, like other dead children, are worthy of a funeral, of being mourned. From grief and mourning there may emerge reborn hope, readiness to handle another pregnancy or at least that personal dignity which comes of having, at one time produced a thing of beauty.

Interested persons are invited to write to the Still Birth Association, c/o Charing Cross Hospital Obstetric Unit, London, for their leaflet designed to comfort and guide bereaved parents.

Because the mother intending adoption is about to face bereavement, she too should be encouraged to hold, nurse and grieve over her child. If so doing influences her to alter her decision, that is her prerogative.

---

* Dr Hugh Jolly, late Paediatrician-in-Charge, Charing Cross Hospital, London.

A 'mothering' photo of the baby will at least provide a reminder of the gift of life bestowed upon her and her child.

The unmarried mother

Surely it must go without saying that the unmarried mother should be invited to join the antenatal class. Because she may feel socially rejected, it may be necessary for the midwife to make a point of inviting the unmarried mother into the group. The terms on which she joins the group are, of course, her own decision. The extent to which she identifies with the group will depend on the tact of the midwife. Her training both in general and obstetric nursing, should have impressed upon the midwife the fact that each of us plods our way through life, spurred on by a medley of motivations, both social and antisocial, accepted and rejected. All of us are driven by basic motivations for love, hate, anger, the need for acceptance, honour, importance, sexual satisfaction: the manner in which these drives are frustrated or satisfied by the environment is often beyond the control of the individual. We are all ships tossed on the sea of life, and to none of us is it granted to choose the weather!

The midwife should be the last person to sit in judgement. Indeed, it often falls to her to reassure the unmarried mother, to remove that additional guilt and anxiety to which she is subjected, and which may, through over-stimulation of the sympathetic nervous system, prolong and complicate her labour.

The natural mother, married or unmarried, having borne her child, has been prepared by nature for the sacred function of mothering: her endocrines stimulated, her protective instincts aroused, she has something special to offer her child—that acceptance and the unquestioning love which she alone can give!

If widows and divorcees can make a good job of child-raising why not the unmarried mother?

Teenage pregnancy

Daniel Callahan hits the nail on the head:

'One of the main difficulties of being a teenager is sex, at once a great discovery, a great mess, a great pleasure, a great frustration and an all round great muddle.'

Because the nurse is very often the person to inform the youngster that she is pregnant, she is the first person upon whom her client has opportunity to unburden her predicament. It is important to realize that:

(i) most pregnant unmarried youngsters have little self-esteem,
(ii) are in the crisis conflict of lifelong decision-making long before nature intended.

Adolescent pregnancy is a problem of children having children. Indeed the adolescent is not only emotionally, but physically handicapped by her immaturity.

Charles Low, US Department of Health Education and Welfare* presents research to show that:

1.   The babies of young teenage mothers are two to three times more likely to die during the first year of life.
2.   Low birth weights are twice as high among teenagers.

* '11 Million Teenagers'. The Alan Guttmacher Institute, 1976.

3.   Maternal deaths are 60% higher among teenagers.

Her *age*, together with her present *educational level*, must play a role in any teenager's choice, bearing in mind that twice as many teenage mothers drop out of school in relation to their peers. In the United States teenage pregnancy is the most common cause of school drop-out.

Very few return to school to complete their education, with the result that teenage mothers face a high risk of unemployment and corresponding poverty.

The nurse's role should be one of counselling, not advising. The aim is to allow the youngster *to discover for herself the option best suited to her own individual circumstances*. Indeed, it is she, and not the nurse, who must live her life out. Among her options are:

Fostering
Impediments: probably from fear of bonding with the child, and consequent pain of separation, foster mother volunteers are scarce and professional 'approval' rare.
Abortion
Ideally termination of pregnancy should occur before 13 weeks, but can be carried out successfully up to 24 weeks. After 24 weeks, incidence of complications increases dramatically. Abortion being such an emotive issue, both on religious and humanitarian grounds, the mother should be encouraged to clarify her own values.

Because Christian, Judiac, Islamic and Hindu religions frown upon termination of new life, the youngster may be more deeply affected thereby than she realizes. This solution may result in *painful and long-term guilt feelings*. Because the pain and stress caused by guilt may burden personal emotions and subsequent relationships, it may be advisable to refer the teenager who has taken this option for interpretative and supportive psychotherapy or counselling.

Adoption

Unlike many adoptive relationships, the natural mother–child relationship does not involve stressful competition with *over-idealized fantasy mother* and child *figures*. Participants love and accept each other because they *are* one of the other and Nature is contrary, sometimes denying the blood-mother further pregnancies.

In some cases the adopted *child's hereditary attributes*, especially his intelligence and psychoneurological personality structure, *are not truly acceptable to his adoptive family*.

An image of unacceptable 'badness' identified with the blood-mother is certainly detrimental to a healthy self-concept. 'I must be rotten like my real mother.'

It is not easy for the *adopting mother*, who feels herself a failure relative to the successfully procreative biological mother, to enhance the latter's image. Her *ambivalence towards the child's birth-mother* results in a conflict between gratitude and anger, and *renders the adopter vulnerable to phantasies* both of high expectations and the assumption of a 'rescuer' role. She seeks *to assuage her guilt-feelings* at having 'stolen' the child by phantasizing that she has rescued him from a terrible fate at the mercy of 'bad stock'.

Now that phantasy of 'bad stock' becomes so frightening that she develops anxiety phantasies about poor intelligence, inherited disease, 'bad seed', criminal tendencies, etc.

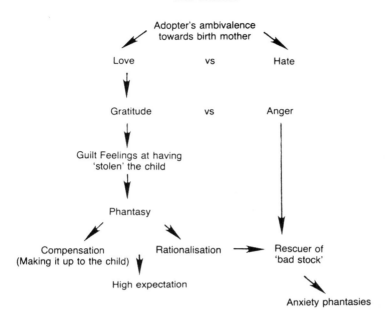

In order to avoid distressing phantasy, many authorities recommend that the adopting mother has access to very thorough, detailed and personalized information about the biological parents and their backgrounds.

Weider (*Psychoanalytic Quarterly* 1977 A, B; 1978), and others, cast doubt on the current theory of informing adoptees at the time of their first questions of origin, which usually present about CA 2 years. At this developmental stage phantasy is not clearly demarcated from reality, and the child takes literally the idea that *he was given away, or even thrown away*, by a non-caring mother. People only give away things they do not want and do not care about. The child expresses his sense of loss, anxiety and guilt by regressing to cleanliness obsessions, nightmares, separation anxiety, etc.

He *dare not offend nor displease his adoptive mother* who may also 'give him away'. He sees his real mother as bad, naughty and unloving—an image the boy may later 'project' upon wife and mother figures, and the girl may 'introject', to the detriment of her own self-image: 'Am I also bad and unloving?'

It may thus be wiser to postpone the idea of the 'chosen baby', sacrificed by the loving biological mother, to a later developmental stage, around six or seven years, where reality becomes more reliably separated from phantasy. Some children, in their anxiety or sorrow, *reject an interpretation of adoption*, requiring loving reassurance and later reapproachment. However handled, the adoptee is *nearly always strongly motivated to seek out the natural mother*, either for reassurance of her acceptability, or to establish blood bonds. Many reputable adoption agencies now provide necessary information.

Especially in adolescence, as the necessity for faith in committed relationships emerges; at pregnancy, when problems of genetics and procreation arise; when adoptees' own children seek their blood relatives, and in middle age when the adoptee craves opportunity for a 'last look' at the blood mother, there is strong motivation to seek roots.*

Insight into the special contribution of the natural mother lies behind British legislation to the effect that no steps in the direction of adoption may be taken until the mother and her family have had time to adjust to the situation and, in many cases, to make plans to accommodate it.

Most young teenage mothers

(i) are dependent on their parents,
(ii) feel they have already let their parents down.

Because *parents may*

(i) genuinely feel adoption to be the best solution for their grandchildren,
(ii) at a conscious or unconscious level, wish to distance themselves from the embarrassment and disappointment of an 'illegitimate' grandchild,

they exert unjustifiable pressure on the confused youngster. Sometimes *parents* attempt to cut the 'Gordian' by *themselves adopting the baby*, a course of action often fraught with dangers of later conflict and identity crises.

Being a single parent

No midwife should presume to dissuade the mother who wishes to keep her baby. Each case rests on its merits. Just as there exist successful adoptions, so there exist many happy, successful well-adjusted children living with their mothers outside wedlock. Most of these never reach welfare agencies.

The unmarried mother can be reassured through *identification* with great and respected historical figures, religious leaders, artists and playwrights, who are known to have been born out of wedlock. There are many who doubt the authenticity of Pharaoh's daughter's report to the effect that she found Moses floating down the Nile in a crib of reeds. Is it not written of Hagar's son Ismail 'Arise, lift up the lad, and hold him in thine hand—for I will make him a great nation . . . and God was with the lad'!

Despite changing community attitudes and the alleviation of many difficulties formerly involved in keeping mother and child together, *problems do remain*. It is essential that the nurse point out these problems, as well as sources of amelioration and support.

The most important criteria for being a successful single parent appear to lie in the physical, mental, psychological and financial support afforded by parents, grandparents and other relatives. Unless this is forthcoming the girl is indeed hard pressed to cope with the financial, personal and social demands of 24-hour child care concurrent to earning a living. To rely on paternal maintenance is unrealistic.

For those who seek the solace and reward from their baby's love, it is important to point out that *motherhood is primarily a giving, not a receiving role*.

The contribution of *community facilities* is of course also vital. Details are available from the National Council for the Unmarried Mother and her Child.

* Kestenberg JA. *Psychoanalytic Study of the Adoptive Child.*

Social isolation of the single mother

Considerable maturity is required in order to cope with reduced marriage prospects, and the social isolation involved in constantly staying at home to mind the baby.

Resentment, jealousy and feelings of having 'lost out' may be displaced upon the child even to the extent of abuse.

The arranged or 'shotgun' marriage

Esther Sapire, 1985* reports a study showing that 60% of 'forced' or 'shotgun' marriages end in divorce within five years. This may be due to the fact that few such relationships are well established, the couple hardly knowing each other.

Indeed 20% of pregnancies in her study occurred within six months of first intercourse.

A bottom line fact is the man's willingness to marry at the expense of his own ambitions and emotions. And many are far too young for a permanent relationship. Irrespective of good intentions, a girl of 14 and a boy of 16 caught in their own adolescent conflicts, have little chance of achieving the sacrifices, understanding, self-control basic to successful marriage.

The teenaged father is himself usually so confused that he is incapable of deciding whether to marry, to leave school, to find a job, etc (see Contraception, The Psychology of Non-Compliance, pp 363-366).

The new family—when things go well

Largely because they are dealt with in other sections of this text, positive aspects of emotional closeness, support, the joys of shared dreams and achievements from young adulthood into old age, are not, in this section, fully expounded.

What rewards await the family that 'sticks it out', walking forward together in the highly pressurized, violence-strewn 'rat race' towards the twenty-first century?

Among the family's long-term goal satisfaction one may list:

Reliable love, safety and self-esteem, not only in the formative, appealing days of infancy and childhood, but also through the illnesses and stresses of adulthood, and the helpless, unappealing diminishments, confusion and dependence of old age;

> Acceptance and supportive tolerance during the conflicts and insecurities of adolescence;
> Reliable group-inclusion in times of crisis and grief, joy and fun—protection from terrifying isolation;
> When things go wrong a safety-net, reliant not on the induced caring or dutiful charity of outsiders, but bound by the exclusivity of the primaeval blood-knot;
> Shared responsibility to relieve burdens of guilt and anxiety, and when the individual fails, a bolster to his self-esteem within the concerted pride of family.
> Only within the genetic family chain can the individual overcome failure, disappointment and the personal disintegration of death, to achieve biological immortality.

* Sapire, Esther: Teenagers Need Sex Knowledge: Executive Health. September 1985. Further details from author.

Family pathology

The functions of the family are intense, long-term, ambivalent, complicated and stressful, calling for maturity, ability to compromise, sacrifice and communicate; flexibility, a sense of humour, common interests and goals, good manners, a fair slice of luck and other factors too many to list.

No wonder, somewhere along the line, family cohesion is threatened and the help of professionals indicated.

Among the most serious etiological stresses are:

> breakdown in communication,
> intrusion and excessive need of the extended family,
> over-investment in children, career or social activities,
> financial stresses and inconsistent ambitions,
> schism and skewing in family relations in which parental relationships are so solidified by hate, anger, lack of communication or indifference that members are aligned in malevolent opposing camps.
> *psychiatric illness*:
> neuroses
> psychosomatic illness per se, introjected, and used as a manipulative tool
> psychoses
> especially reactive depression (p 591)
> personality disorders
> intellectual subnormality

These psychiatric conditions exert such long-term and heavy demands upon tolerance, patience, personal integrity, self-esteem and effective parenting that undermining of family structure and function is virtually inevitable. Socialization is imperilled, sexual identity threatened and the fulfilment of nurturing roles seriously impeded. The healthy spouse is forced into 'role reversal' and pressurized until unable to provide children of the marriage with material essentials, protection, guidance and healthy, self-fulfilment roles.

Lieberman (1979)* conceives the useful *geneogram*—a diagram summarizing and illustrating family structure and dynamics, including vital details of various generations:

> important life events, eg births, deaths, divorces, illnesses,
> family roles,
> emotional bonds and stressors,
> significant persons and their links with focal relationships.

Mary, the index client, is asked to tell the professional about her relationship with her parents.

'My mother, aged 40, and father, aged 45, divorced after a turbulent relationship, but both are strongly attached to me.'

---

* Lieberman S. *Transgenerational Family Therapy*. London: Croom Helm, 1979.

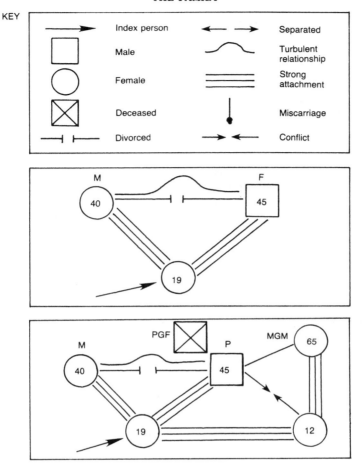

'I have a sister Joan, aged 12, who does not get on with our father, but is strongly attached to our 65-year-old widowed maternal grandmother.'
'I am very fond of Joan' and so forth, to embrace, summarize and illustrate a wide family network.

Familial disruption presents in

(i) family constellations torn by strife,
(ii) 'empty shell marriages', in which meaningful communication has broken down, and parties are joined by mutual hate or severed by mutual indifference, but the unit is held together by external structures such as religious requirements, social mores and financial considerations,
(iii) divorce.

Social research rates alcoholism, chronological and emotional immaturity, sexual problems, infidelity and 'incompatibility' high on the list of causative factors. Yet they all appear peripheral to the fact that *attitudes to divorce are related to political and social trends*. Until late in the eighteenth century, the wife was considered, in law, to be merely part of her husband's property. It was not until early in the nineteenth century that English common-law rights were extended to married women, conferring upon them the status of a 'person' in law and thus capable of entering into contracts, initiating legal proceedings, etc.

Only late in the nineteenth century was the married woman considered worthy of the assumption of custodial rights—ie of ability to assume responsibility for the care of the children of her marriage. Naturally, as soon as her right to apply for dissolution of marriage and to assume responsibilty for the everyday care of her children was acknowledged, divorce statistics began to rise.

Investigating the US divorce-rate for the period 1920–80 Morton & Glick (1976)* illustrated the correlation between changed religious, political and social attitudes, and the dramatic increase in divorce statistics.

There was a notable drop in divorce incidence during the depression of the 1930s when human resources were almost entirely devoted to survival.

No doubt the sharp rise after World War II reflected the difficulty in adjusting to the demands and rights of the returning father–husband figure.

The 1950s witnessed the post-war 'baby boom' and a temporary drop in divorce figures.

These were the years of the great American romantic dream. The marriage age dropped to around 18 years, and women accepted, and sought, security, love, status and fulfilment in the home, the kitchen and the nursery.

But towards the end of the decade the dream began to tarnish.

Women began to ask themselves 'Is this all there is to my life?'.

The early 1960s saw a marked increase in psychiatric problems, especially alcohol abuse and depression, and a renewed recourse to divorce. The mid-1960s and the 1970s witnessed the

> decline, or at least decreased personal importance, or religious and social disapproval;
> increasing influence of the women's movements which questioned fulfilment in exclusive domesticity, and demanded equal pay for equal work outside the home;
> wide adoption of alternate lifestyles less dependent on life-long marital obligations,

all of which are, no doubt, contributing to marital instability and a continued rise in divorce statistics.

Indeed, women's demands for equal rights at home and on the labour market may well be giving rise to ambivalence, conflict, anxiety, stress and thus decreased effectiveness in homemaking and mothering roles.

In response to changes in the female role, men appear to be examining their own feelings and are even finding some satisfaction in the assumption of a more active family and parental role, a phenomenon vividly presented in the film *Kramer vs Kramer*.

Whether such role-changes are actually contributing to contentment and fulfilment would appear questionable; but they are certainly forcing society to provide the means of preventing divorce, and where family breakdown is inevitable, a structure in which the trauma of relationship disintegration may be reduced and mental health preserved in all parties involved.

* Morton, A J & Glick, P S 'Marital instability in America: Past and Present'. *In: Divorce and Separation: Context, Causes & Consequences*. New York Basic Books 1279.

Measures designed to avoid divorce

Lawyers are not marriage guidance counsellors. Yet especially in 'middle' and 'upper' socio-economic groups, they are often the first line of appeal when marriages 'go wrong'. Sometimes the very fact of having consulted a lawyer provides a type of 'shock treatment', bringing parties to their senses. Through the good offices of the legal profession they seek that communication which their pride, their confused emotions and, frequently, the interference of others, has placed out of reach. The protagonistic interactions of their lawyers provide the parties with aggressive representation of their needs, and a relatively 'safe' tool of indirect, aggressive catharsis.

Indeed, most conscientious and sensitive solicitors do attempt to ascertain that the marriage is truly irreconcilable before proceeding to negotiate the best divorce terms for their client. But to impose upon legal representatives the role of marriage guidance counsellors is clearly inappropriate. Partners in a disturbed marriage should rather seek the professional help of marriage guidance organizations, churches, medical practitioners, registered clinical psychologists, social workers, sex therapists and professional nurse–practitioners most of whom are especially interested and qualified in this area. Indeed, the sensible and well-advised client will seek such sources of professional help at the first sign of marriage breakdown. Certainly, once the marriage reaches the divorce court, there is little hope of saving it. To do so is certainly not the function of the judge, whose role is that of an objective, passive and neutral umpire. His main human interest in the case consists in his responsibility of furthering the best interests of minor children.

What troubled marriage partners may expect from professional workers

1. Opportunity for *catharsis*—sympathetic, non-moralistic concern and acceptance of anger, distress, fear, and guilt feelings. In 'hot' situations the professional's role may well constitute appropriately amended Crisis Intervention (see p 563) in providing the 'relief of talking out' and supportive understanding.

2. *Reassurance* that strong feeling and the expression of primitive emotions—love and hate, anger and aggression, self-interest and resentment are all perfectly legitimate experiences within the intimate and often stressful marriage relationship. They certainly do not, on either side, constitute evidence that relationships are irreconcilable.

3. *Interpretation* of the client's own feelings and behaviour, and the responses which these arouse in the marriage partner, the children and the extended family. 'Role play', affording opportunity to experience and express the emotions of other participants in the family scenario is of value—the 'empty chair' technique provides a particularly effective opportunity for catharsis and reflected 'feedback'. Sometimes one counsellor works individually and in confrontation groups with all family members. In emotionally explosive situations it may be wiser to defuse the situation by allotting separate counsellors for identification and support.

    The therapist should be prepared to accept *displacement* of the client's anger, frustration, and guilt feelings in that transference reaction which is often the first intermediary step towards direct communication.

4. Re-opening of that *channel of communication* between husband and wife which so
    often becomes cluttered and bogged down by everyday tensions, frustrations
    and that search for identity which commonly make the marriage relationship
    stressful. Zaihoch, an eminent Israeli *sex therapist*, is on record as saying 'My
    main function often seems to consist in relaying of messages from husband and
    wife which should be directly spoken between themselves'.

    Indeed, many marriage partners, owing to childhood and adolescent
    backgrounds of secrecy, 'respectable' silence, social and religious taboos, lack
    specific anatomical and physiological vocabularies. They thus experience real
    difficulty in communicating basic sexual facts such as love-making tech-
    niques.

5. Help in achieving that *insight*, and enhanced *motivation*, for preserving the
    marriage, from which there may emanate a self-motivated plan for marriage
    rehabilitation.

    Maybe there is validity in a somewhat cynical recommendation that, as a
    last resort, the marriage counsellor should emphasize the *financial burdens and
    material inconveniences* of running two homes.

Women should recognize the frequent necessity for going out into the 'rat-race'
of the working world; of subservience to employers, and often younger, more
specialized colleagues; the psychophysical burdens of working during the
menopause, and the difficulties encountered by most women—certainly by older
women—in achieving social rehabilitation, especially a new life partner. The
definition of these very real disadvantages of divorce may well motivate people to
work for better understanding and more fulfilling relationships.

Of course, some relationships are so empty, so lacking in common goals and
enjoyment, so actively displeasing to both partners, that rehabilitation is
impossible and indeed unwise. *Although most children insist, for many years, on their desire
to keep the home together, in the long run few would wish to carry the life-long burden of
compensating parents for a 'life of sacrifice'.* The pain of divorce may well be justified by
the freedom to forge ahead, free from guilt, to make their own lives.

In such cases it is clearly the duty of the marriage counsellor to advise his/her
clients as to the best way of dissolving the marriage, protecting their legal rights and
achieving personal rehabilitation. Now individual support, group identification
and motivation for a new start, work satisfaction and other post-divorce
rehabilitation facilities come into operation.

Marriage counselling service: Divorce Conciliation and Advisory Service. Phone:
(01) 730 2422.

What about the children

Most authorities agree that, no matter how wisely divorce is handled, the
fragmentation of one's life pattern, relationship-constellation and physical environment
causes an 'inner separation' which may lead to deformation of the 'inner life'. Social
attitudes are distorted. Emotions lose proportion. Conflict, guilt, anxiety and
resultant biochemical tension-energy seek relief in unbearably demanding
behaviour or withdrawal and the single person's greatest enemy—isolation!

If this is true of adults, how much more so of children, whose world is still largely
restricted to home and family, upon which they are so physically and emotionally
dependent? Especially in our Western nuclear family, bereft of the support, comfort

and status-identification of the extended family, the child is particularly defenceless in the face of disintegration of his family unit. He is especially vulnerable if his appearance or behaviour presentation resembles that of the 'deserting' or 'resented' parent.

Defusing the trauma

The most important underlying principle in protecting the child's mental health is reassurance that, *in spite of the split between his parents, they will both stand by him, support him, comfort him, strengthen him.* He must believe that his own particular position in the family constellation is stable, unaltered and rock-strong.

If he is anything but an infant, he has probably long *anticipated and dreaded* confirmation of his ultimate fear that his world is about to tumble around him. Parental explanation should be simple, reassuring and designed to counteract underlying fears:

> 'Mommy and Daddy find we are unable to continue living together. *We have decided that we will get along much better, and be better friends, if we do not live in the same house. So we are getting divorced. You must understand this makes no difference to the way we feel about you. You are still our beloved child, the centre of our lives. You still have a mother and a father, who live to keep you safe, happy and give you the good things in life. For your happiness we shall both always continue to work and pull together.*'

One cannot over-emphasize the necessity for preserving the child's good image of both his parents: If one parent disappears from his life, he will feel deserted, resentful, guilty and anxious.

> 'What have I done to send my Daddy away?'
> 'If my father cannot be relied on to stand by me—if he has deserted us, and all we ever get from him is a monthly cheque and a Christmas card, *how can I ever trust another man to love and care for me?*'

Alternatively, children seeking escape, or compensation, may *over-idealize* or phantasize absent parents, with whom the reality parent is unable to compete. In addition they risk the traumatization of disillusionment. *Lacking an admired role-model to emulate and please*, the child encounters difficulty in achieving behaviour patterns of self-discipline and conformity.

Deserting or diminished parents disturb role-model identification; a father who derogates the mother's image runs the risk of destroying a girl's self-concept, imperilling healthy identification with wifely and maternal roles.

'If wives and mothers are so rotten, I never want to be one.'

A mother who 'runs down' the father may prevent her son from identifying with the strong, reliable male figure. Spurning the male role, he may identify with the beloved mother, running the risk, especially in adolescence, of a sex-identity crisis.

It is thus most important that parents avoid the temptation to derogate the former partner whom they believe to be at fault.

It should be unnecessary to remind parents to *avoid using children as bargaining pawns* in the resolution of their own anger, hate, hurt or jealousy. ('If you go on seeing that woman I will not let you take the children on Sundays!') *Children who are instilled with hate, anger, and resentment against either parent or step-parent*, are not only exposed to painful emotional conflict, guilt and anxiety but, with increased maturity, may well come to 'see through' their parents' hate-displacement mechanism. Thus security and healthy role-model identification are further undermined.

A more subtle complication of self-consolation during the divorce transition is a *tendency to use a child as a sop to the parent's own guilt-feelings*. Thus a mother who has divorced in order to marry her lover may seek to assuage her guilt feelings towards her former partner by encouraging, at a conscious or unconscious level, her daughter to assume her own former role by taking premature and inappropriate responsibility for her father's needs.

The most satisfactory, fruitful and healthy child-care plan in the face of divorce emanates from *meaningful parental communication* in order that those living and educational *arrangements which are least disruptive* and most conducive to the child's happiness and welfare be evolved.

Naturally the *wishes of older children should be taken into consideration*. Only those living arrangements which are *mutually satisfactory* and have evolved from the parties concerned *themselves* can ultimately become consistently effective and congenial. Needless to say, it is impossible, in the light of inevitable changes, evolutions and adjustments, to construct rigid procedures. Hence those plans which are most *adaptable, flexible* and *informal* are the most successful. Once parents become bogged down with insistent delimitation of days, hours, conditions and places of access, and rigid holiday stipulations, the battle is on!

At this point parents may constructively seek the *relative neutrality, and unimpassioned communication offered by expert opinion*. It is imperative that clinical psychologists, church ministers, social workers, nurse–practitioners and others whose opinion may be sought in these delicate negotiations have an opportunity to identify with the feelings, aspirations, difficulties, needs and adjustments technique patterns of *both* the parents and their children. Sometimes parental feelings are so antagonistic that initially each requires his or her own partisan professional in order to work out, and express, individual needs and emotions before more direct communication is possible. It is essential that such professionals achieve a delicate balance between identification with their clients on the one hand and the needs of the whole family constellation on the other.

The most frequent 'trap' into which professionals fall is *involvement in the 'see-saw' bargaining of custody and access details* which will, in any case, usually resolve themselves once the raw hurt and anger emanating from marriage breakdown subsides. Even broken marriages may fulfil masochistic-sadistic needs. It is the task of the professional worker to help achieve an acceptance of marriage breakdown without blame or remorse. Then one works to substitute between the parents a new, less intense, working relationship.

Even if negotiations for an amicable resolution of child-rearing plans fail, it is the obligation of the professional worker to gear the rehabilitation process towards *healing relationships*, rather than to become involved in the legalities of the divorce.

Another frequent pitfall of the professional worker consists in acceptance of verbalized hate and desperation which may really hide *strong bonds of dependency, masochism and sadism*. Husbands use wrangling over legal rights to hurt; women lay charges of physical abuse—and hang around for more. Outraged professional workers become involved in a network of intrigue which is really marital game-playing rather than a real wish for divorce. It is time for the exasperated professional worker to stand back and reassess underlying dynamics.

The involvement of the professional worker is particularly disturbing when *one partner, still being strongly attached and emotionally dependent* on the other, does not want the divorce, but clings tenaciously to the marriage, attempting to use the children to hold it together. Her 'denial' of her husband's real wish to terminate the marriage leads to endless rationalization of his rejection: He is the victim of a cunning adultress, is mentally ill, etc.

Where the initiating partner has already formed a new love-attachment the role of the 'rejected' partner, usually a woman who will experience considerable difficulty in building a new love-relationship, is a particularly sad one. One can hardly expect her to approach a divorce settlement with any degree of equanimity or sweet reason. She may well require the catharsis, support, insight and guidance inherent in individual psychotherapy or counselling, in order to achieve new feeling and behaviour patterns. Reassuring identification of group therapy and support of the extended family are also important.

Within the context of reasonably successful professional counselling, the legalities of the 'Agreement of Consent' should constitute a mere formality. Without a reasonably mature attitude, negotiations leading to the 'consent paper' become entangled in destructive 'game-playing' which has little to do with the welfare of the children. Rather are the parents playing 'Child to Child' (see Berne, p 178).

Financial arrangements do, of course, often constitute a serious stumbling-block to the conclusion of a mutually acceptable divorce.

Most court orders are now based on maintenance for children, rather than alimony for wives, it being held that no man can reasonably be expected to maintain for the rest of her life an able-bodied woman who is capable of providing for herself. Of course, special consideration applies, after long-standing marriage, to the older woman who should beware time limits on maintenance settlements.

The physical disintegration of the home (loss of social status and simultaneous deprivation of toys, books, clothes, motor car and other tangible tokens of love, comfort and security) does certainly constitute an important aspect of the loss encountered by children of divorce. It is little wonder that such things may become bargaining tools in the hands of hurt, angry, or 'rejected' parents. The importance to children of *tangible symbols of their former secure lives* should not be spurned by those seeking to reduce the pain and deprivation of familial disintegration. The financially favoured parent should certainly be discouraged from depriving his children in order to 'punish' his former spouse. It is, of course, important to reassure children that, irrespective of their ability to provide material pleasures and social status, both parents still love them constantly and strongly.

In order to ascertain that a child's material and educational needs will continue to be met irrespective of a parent's insolvency or death, some lawyers insist on an insurance policy to cover such contingencies.

When parents, preferably in consultation with older children, have arrived at mutually satisfactory, or at least tolerable, consensus as to living arrangements, periods with the non-custodial parent, maintenance, etc, the terms on which the marriage is to be dissolved are formulated by the parties' legal representatives into an Agreement of Consent. This document sets out agreed provisions pertaining to

> custody and access,
> maintenance,
> proprietary rights—the division of the assets of the marriage, and
> legal costs of the divorce.

The Agreement assists the judge in compiling his *Custody Order*, a Court Order structured in accordance with the two legal principles of

custody and
guardianship.

When the divorce is granted the contents of the Agreement of Consent and the Custody Order become Orders of the Court, contravention of which constitutes a criminal offence.

Custody

'Custody is that portion of parental power which pertains to the personal life of the child. Spouses who live together share custody, which then seldom attracts judicial attention. But where the consortium is terminated, whether through separation or divorce, custody is entrusted to that parent whom, in the opinion of the Court, is most capable of providing for the nurture and upbringing of the minor children. In this is included all that makes up the ordinary, daily life of the child—shelter, nourishment, and the training of the "mind". . . .

A custodian parent has, therefore, the right to regulate the life of the child, determining with whom he should or should not associate, how he should be educated, what religious training he should receive, and how his health should be cared for.'

If, as is customary in the absence of definite evidence to the contrary, the mother is entrusted with the custody of her child, 'the child passes into the home of the mother, and there it must find all that is necessary to its growth in mind and body'.

Except in very unusual cases of proven and specific situations such as a history of gross, uncontrolled violence or serious, permanent mental disorder, the court gives the other spouse the right of 'reasonable' access to the child, specifying weekends, portions of school holidays, etc.

The Courts have become increasingly insistent upon considering the 'best interests of the child' rather than parental moral blameworthiness. In so doing they have acknowledged the importance of emotional attachment, and the strength thereof, in motivating patterns of conformity. Healthy mental development may well be independent of moral factors. The Court may thus decide that it would be in the interests of the child to remain with a loved mother-figure irrespective of adultery or financial limitations—while at the same time making a maintenance order consistent with the father's financial means.

At the same time, in granting 'reasonable access' to the non-custodial parent, the Court takes cognizance of the child's need for two strong parental relationships.

It is the spirit of compromise—not the letter of the law—that ultimately prevails—and that spirit is most happily and profitably characterized by *communication, flexibility* and *informality*.

What are the traumatic effects of divorce which professionals try to prevent?

Wallerstein & Kelly* (1974, 1975, 1976, 1977) and Kelly & Wallerstein (1976,

---

* Wallerstein, J S & Kelly, J E. 'The Effects of Parental Divorce. The Adolescent Experience'. *In: The Child*

1977) examined reactions of children at different development stages, in the initial stage of divorce, one year later and five years later.

The following table, compiled and presented by Mrs Jennifer Zuck, a registered clinical psychologist, at the Forensic Psychiatry Conference on 16 January 1983, summarizes the findings in this longitudinal study:

1. Pre-school ($2\frac{1}{2}$–6 years)

The children
  were frightened, confused,
  blamed themselves,
  had an intense need for contact with adults,
  had fears of being sent away.

This particular developmental period being characterized by egocentric reasoning, children would say—'Daddy left because of me'. The children saw themselves as responsible, tending towards guilt and anxiety.

2. Early latency (7–8 years)

A stage characterized by ability to express feelings:

  expression of feelings of loss, sadness, depression,
  feelings of rejection and abandonment,
  feelings of anger towards mother for 'sending father away',
  desire to effect reconciliation between parents.

Attempts to deal with guilt and anxiety often involved guilt 'displacement' on parents, eg 'Daddy left home because he was bad'.

3. Later latency (9–12 years)

Children adopted a more realistic approach to divorce and displayed:

  ability to express anger at parents' behaviour,
  divided loyalties and pity,
  feelings of loneliness and rejection,
  feelings of embarrassment at parents' behaviour.

Children rarely felt responsible for their parents' divorce.

4. Adolescence (13–18 years)

In this developmental stage children were seen to be most openly upset and expressed:

  strong feelings of anger, sadness, embarrassment,
  resentment of parents' relationships,
  fears about their own relationships in sex and marriage.

in his Family; Anthony, E J & Kouterlik, A (eds) vol 3. John Wiley & Son, New York 1974; Wallerstein, J S & Kelly, J E. 'The Effects of Parental Divorce: Experiences of the Pre-school Child.' *Journal of American Academy of Child Psychiatry* 14: 600–616. 1975; Wallerstein, J S & Kelly J E. 'The Effects of Parental Divorce. Experience of the Child in Later Latency.' *American Journal of Orthopsychiatry* **36** (2): 256–269. 1976; Wallerstein, J S & Kelly, J B. 'Divorce Counselling. A community service for families in the midst of divorce.' *American Journal of Orthopsychiatry* **47** (4). 2 February 1977.

These children were able to view their parents objectively, and most were able to disengage themselves from parental conflict within about a year.

Generally, it is evident that divorce, irrespective of the age-level, has severe psychological consequences on children.

'A "children's telephone" is a unique service in Sweden. A child in trouble may phone for help or advice and, if necessary, will be seen by a social worker. In seeking help, the child may choose to remain anonymous. Last year over 50% of the children who used the "children's telephone" service did so because their parents were involved in divorce.'

The *concept of 'joint custody' or 'shared parenting'* is not a new one. Within the context of reasonable maturity and psychological health in both parents, where they are able to operate free from a 'continuing acrimonious battle', joint custody may well constitute a more family-oriented arrangement than disputed one-parent custody.

In any case, *only those decisions and programmes which emanate from parents and children themselves, and which meet with reasonable approval, can hope to succeed.*

Post-divorce disposal *usually rejected* by professionals consist in:

Cutting the Gordian knot of tangled family relations by placement in a *boarding school or other institution:*

Except for extreme cases requiring temporary, emergency 'breathing space' in order to defuse emotional turmoil, *institutionalization serves merely to convince* the child that his parents are voluntarily abandoning him. Deprived of his customary support-system, and the intimacy of familial belonging, his long-term confidence in all-important parent figures is seriously imperilled. He loses not only one parent but both!

Separation of siblings: Separation further fragments children's life-structure and self-concept. Splitting children deprives them of comforting identification and the support of the remnants of their family constellation.

Children instinctively 'see through' a mother's efforts to relieve her painful guilt-feelings by sending her daughter to comfort her abandoned husband, or utilization of parental conflict in order to 'rationalize' sibling preferences. Certainly separation will precipitate and influence the painful and dangerous effects of underlying sibling rivalry, both justified and unjustified.

Separation, no matter how overtly logical, increases a child's isolation, guilt feelings and anxiety, pushing him yet further into the lonely pit of 'differentness'.

Easing the emotional trauma of divorce: Rehabilitation

Divorce is preceded, and indeed followed by, feelings of disappointment, remorse, guilt, failure and rejection—that most painful, diminishing and distorting of emotions from which there may appear to be no redemption.

'The stigma it brings has not changed. Way back, even before Guinevere left Arthur to run off with Lancelot and Hamlet told Ophelia she'd be better off in a nunnery, the first caveman came home to find his best friend had not exactly had to drag his wife off by the hair, and the first prehistoric agony aunt patted him on the shoulder and told him the pain would gradually dull.

> Rachel Roberts was so obsessed with the dream that she would get Rex Harrison back, even years after their marriage was dissolved, that Peter Ustinov said of her: "All her conversation came back to one topic—Rex, Rex, Rex."
>
> She took her life the same day that an article appeared in the paper mentioning a small volume put together by Harrison, dedicated to his sixth wife, Mercia . . . "My beloved wife from whom I have learned the art of living and loving at long last."—*Duo Features*'*

Rehabilitation is designed to return the divorcee to the highest possible level of functional ability. This may require crisis 'here and now' intervention and/or referral for individual psychotherapy (p 609 et seq).

Self-help identification support groups

In spite of the concern and care invested in easing the burdens of divorce, the Salzburg workshop observed:

> 'The emotional process before, during and after a divorce can be very painful. Without sympathetic understanding by others, the person who is being left by a martial partner can become ill and desperate. The idea of self-help groups has recently been introduced for people in divorce situations. In these groups everyone may have an opportunity to discuss his or her problems. In the presence of others who are in the same difficult situation, problems are often more easily resolved and self-confidence established. Mutual encouragement helps people to look towards a new future. The self-help group, with the aid of a trained co-ordinator, is a powerful method of prevention for people who are at medical risk of becoming, for instance, alcoholic or depressed, or developing psychosomatic diseases.'

It was, however, a common experience of delegates that women persevered much longer in groups than men, who soon found new marriage partners. In fact remarriage appeared to be the ultimate goal of many women who stayed with the group.

The *role of the community worker* in assisting post-divorce rehabilitation consists not only in co-ordinating, and referring clients to psychotherapy or self-help groups, but also, where indicated, and with the permission of the client, in *rallying resources* such as the extended family, teachers, friends, personnel officers, etc, to provide emotional support and share in child-care when the mother is forced to seek work.

An important principle in divorce rehabilitation consists *in avoiding that isolation* which constitutes the breeding-ground of loss of proportion and withdrawal from potentially healing relationships. Demotivated by reactive depression (see p 591) and thrown back on her own fragile resources, the divorcee may reach 'breaking point' in which she seeks 'Flight' in alcohol and drugs, or displaces her angry 'Fight' in child abuse.

There is certainly a need to extend parent support groups to *child and adolescent support groups*. (See also p 613.)

---

* McGlone, Heather, 1986.

REHABILITATION OF CHILDREN OF DIVORCED PARENTS

Our Western civilization, bombarded by many social and financial stresses, and denied the support of the extended family, places the child of the disintegrated family at particular risk. On divorce, long-term anger, insecurity and anxiety may precipitate reactive depression, acute feelings of 'differentness', 'protective' neurotic obsessions so strong as to imperil social and educational activities, withdrawal or status-compensatory aggressive behaviour, all of which require intensive and individualized as well as group-oriented professional help.

Participants in the Salzburg workshop* were unanimous in their experience of *Children's inability to accept*, at deeper emotional levels, the reality of their parents' divorce.

Young children faced with 'projective techniques' including family dolls, pictures, etc refused to make a consistent parent-identification choice, either placing the 'hero' figure alternately with each parent, or pushing all the dolls together.

Older children, even when parents remarried, admitted to aggressive feelings towards 'step-parents' and compensatory phantasies of family reunion.

Clearly, there is a basic need to counteract that internal and external fragmentation and 'inner separation' which classically leads to conflict, isolation and impaired mental health.

An important counterforce to this fragmentation consists in the custodial parent's ability to foster, preserve and give opportunity for fulfilment of a strong, supportive and loving relationship with the non-custodial parent.

The child of divorced parents is indeed *much conforted by the feeling that his parents are still friends*. It does much for his personal and social self-image that the former family is sometimes seen together in friendly circumstances.

The Swedish idea of a 'children's telephone service' affording twenty-four-hour professional catharsis, insight, support and guidance is indeed worthy of extension to other communities. There is no therapeutic substitute for *on-the-spot 'hot' confrontation with sources of distress, anxiety and anger*.

It is sometimes necessary, with a client's permission, that the community-worker interpret a child's distress, anxiety, isolation and need for supportive relationships to teachers, extended family members, community and social welfare facilities.

The consensus of international opinion is that the responsibility for family breakdown lies not in increased ease of divorce by consent but rather in emotional immaturity and a lack of insight into the difficulties involved in adjustment to a life-long relationship, unique in its intimacy and demands for compromise, self-effacement and personal sacrifice.

In the hope that intellectual insight into this demanding and unique relationship may improve its stability, delegates at the Salzburg World Federation for Mental Health passed the following resolution:

> 'Be it resolved that governments be approached, through the World Federation for Mental Health, to see that all potential parents receive child-bearing counselling, eg during the last year of compulsory schooling.'

The role of step-parents

'By 1990, predicts the School of Sociology at Johns Hopkins University, more

---

* World Federation for Mental Health, Salzburg 1979: "Divorce, Separation and Custody".

than one in two families in America will be "step-families" or single-parent families.

Already one in five American children live in a "step-family" and 25 m adults are step-parents.'

The School submits the following suggestions for successful 'step-parenting':

'Don't rush things. Don't try to make children call a new parent mom or dad too quickly. It takes time to develop trust; keep some of the old family rituals such as a bedtime story so that the child has something to hang on to.

The non-custodial parent should try to set aside a room or at least a drawer that belongs to the child so that he or she feels at home on visits and not like a visitor; it is important for the child to keep contact with the non-custodial parent and at least to know where the other parent is; contact should be maintained with the grandparents on the non-custodial side; most importantly, the child must have the assurance that the new marriage will not diminish the parent's love for him or her.'*

One might add the opinion that step-parents should, as far as possible, avoid the disciplinarian role. Their role is delicate enough without risking the classic 'cruel' step-parent image. The step-parent cannot afford to become associated with punishment which the child will certainly resent, and 'store away', imperilling that long-term relationship basic to any meaningful incentive for conformity. Punitive associations encourage compensation in over-idealized 'real' parents.

The step-parent would be better advised to concentrate his or her efforts on building a relationship based on fond friendship. From the acorn of 'like' the oak of 'love' may one day grow.

Because of the long-term involvement it entails, the conduct of family-breakdown and pertinent rehabilitative services is particularly appropriate to the **Nursing Process**.

In fact, without a structure the whole multi-faceted process might become distinctly unwieldy.

The professional worker may find structure within the nursing process particularly helpful in the compilation of her *court report:*

1. *Data collection*: will take cognizance of family structure, socio-economic background, physical environment both in the home and the community, extended family and community resources; history and presentation of parent–parent, parent–child and other important relationships from pre-conception attitudes through to present emotional commitments, responsibilities conflicts, etc.

    It is useful for the professional worker to note whether the child resembles his father or his mother and the emotions aroused by such resemblance. The child's developmental and intellectual status, his scholastic potential relative to his attainment—evidence of anxiety in obsessions, sleeplessness, psycho-somatic disorders, vocational goals, life-patterns etc.

    The construction of a Lieberman geneogram (p 419) should prove a useful model of dynamic data.

2. *Nursing diagnosis (assessment):* will take cognizance of familial composition, status, relationships, and behaviour relative to the norm.

---

* Lynne Cornfield, Argus New York Bureau. 1983.

Has the family disintegration really resulted in much deviation from the norm in areas of attachments, conflicts, financial, social and religious status; in their own self-images and the images of the extended family and other concerned persons?

What are the family's needs in transitional support, long-term support?

What are the family's strengths and weaknesses?

Is this family capable of restructure and rehabilitation or is it the opinion of family members and professional workers that everyone will be better off within the context of divorce, restructure and new beginnings?

What, in the light of her knowledge, is the professional worker's opinion as to wisest arrangements for custody, guardianship, etc?

What will be the greatest impediment to family restructure or post-divorce rehabilitation?

3. *Planning:* What is the consensus of family members and professional workers with reference to the family's goals in

  (i) financial, social and personal transition
 (ii) long-term support and rehabilitation?

What is their motivation for rehabilitation?

How can their goals be achieved? Programme timing

What personal and community resources can be harnessed for
    immediate tension defusion?
    long-term support and rehabilitation?

4. *Implementation:* Dissemination of information, guidance, catharsis, support:

  the avoidance of isolation: group support, extended family involvement, church, cultural activities, etc;
  financial adjustments: amended budgeting, part-time work, etc;
  adjustment to work outside the home, child care facilities, specific job training;
  change of place of abode, etc;
  formulated by clients, professional workers, etc.

5. *Evaluation:* in the 'feedback' phase there is evaluation of the effectiveness of individual and group support, family therapy, financial, custodial and other arrangements
      relationship readjustment.
  Are the family expectations being met?
  Separate evaluations will no doubt be required pertaining to
      maternal rehabilitation;
      paternal rehabilitation;
      the children's adjustment.

Is there any agreement between pre-divorced expectations and post-divorce reality? Have hopes for a new and fuller life been realized?

Is experience showing that original goals are inappropriate and will need modification in order to be achieved?

In the case of such long-term and highly emotionally charged processes it might well be necessary to go back several times to reconstitute Planning, Diagnosis, Implementation and Evaluation within the essentially dynamic, changing circumstances of family breakdown and relationship regrouping, restructure and, one hopes, rehabilitation.

CHAPTER 19

THE CLIMACTERIC— THE MIDDLE YEARS

MID-LIFE CRISIS

The Menopause (See also Erikson's life crises, pp 245–253, esp 251–2)

'I am proud of my wrinkles. I earned them!'—Elizabeth Taylor.

The most universal shock of 'middle age' must undoubtedly lie in loss of physical strength, of ease of mobility and of emotional resilience: you thought it would never happen to you, and here it is! Can it be that, through her utterance quoted above, Elizabeth Taylor was seeking protection in Reaction Formation?

The endocrinological-emotional disturbances of adolescence, although painful, do herald the beginning of 'the big years'—adulthood, independence, marriage, family and business or professional fulfilment.

Adolescence is a period of excitement and hope.

In contrast, the *endocrinological-emotional* disbalance of the menopause signals the end of a period of personal, sexual, familial and career fulfilment.

The menopause stretches over varying periods between the 40th and 60th year. Physical symptoms, including circulatory changes and reduction of secretions involved in sex and reproduction, result in 'hot flushes', ie embarrassing and debilitating profuse sweating, and hyperventilation; insomnia; momentary memory loss; listlessness; obesity; and the accentuation of former minor ailments.

On the other hand the vaginal and clitoral lining become thinner and more delicate, increasing sensation.

Depression, anxiety and distress take root. The woman fears that, as her glands 'dry up', she will lose her feminine attractiveness.

'What do middle-aged people worry about?

- Possible or actual deterioration in physical health.
- Worry about what to do when the children leave home, the empty-nest syndrome.
- The fear of becoming dependent, either physically, financially or both, on their children, other relatives or community resources.
- A heightened sense of responsibility for their own parents as they increase in age and possibly decrease in independence.
- Apprehensive feelings about retirement, what to do with all that time, the loss of companionship of fellow workers and impending loss of status and a decreased standard of living.
- Retrenchment in favour of younger people is a very real fear in poor economic times.
- Middle-aged women may fear an unwanted pregnancy.

- Thoughts of dying become more frequent and women especially may begin to think about widowhood.'*

To have reached the end of childbearing years is, to many, a sadness. To have reached this turning point childless may be felt as a tragedy.

Surgery such as hysterectomy or mastectomy constitutes a trauma. Women have been known to develop paranoic aggression towards their surgeons, who, they feel, have 'desexed' them.

To equate reproductive capacity with sexual responsiveness and attractiveness is erroneous and may lead to reduced self-esteem and voluntary isolation.

It is important that the nurse talk to her patient, establish a warm relationship and effective rapport in order to assure that the *whole person* is being treated and not just the wound.

Mutilating surgery such as mastectomy is certainly felt as marking the end of desirability (as it may well do) and thus justifying rejection. Movement towards 'lesser surgery' is indeed encouraging (see p 81).

Menopausal changes herald declining power, old age, loneliness and increasing separation from grown-up children—'the empty nest' syndrome.

Involutional endocrine-linked 'melancholia' or depression may add to the woman's tension, irritability, aggression, suspiciousness, demanding nagging and 'snappiness' in home and work situations.

There is an element of truth in Heather McGlone's comment:

'If only Snow White had shown her stepmother a little love instead of spurning her, and told her she looked so terrific that the man down at the mirror store thought they were sisters, the poor woman might never have sought to compensate for her midlife insecurity by fishing for "you are the fairest of them all" reassurances.†

Various research projects show a correlation between the woman's life history and her ability to adjust to life change. The woman who presents with gross psychological disturbances may well have lived through similar trauma in adolescence and pregnancy.

Research in several countries shows physical type, age at first period and the Pill to have little effect on symptomatology.

In contrast, women who have

— never been married
— never had children
— borne a child when over 40 years of age
— enjoyed a better education and earn a higher income

tend to present with reduced symptomatology.

Especially is this true of women who are able to compensate for the satisfactions

---

* Goddard, Jo (Medical journalist and PRO, Plato Healthcare Promotions). Middle Age Crises—a Self-fulfilling Prophesy? 1986. Original article available through the author.

† McGlone, Heather. 1986. *Helpful reading*: Derek Llewellyn-Jones *'Everywoman'* (Faber); Oxford Medical Publishers: *Hysterectomy. A book to help you deal with the Physical and Emotional Aspects*; *Hysterectomy* Family Doctor Publications, British Medical Association: Hysterectomy.

of youth by accompanying the physiological transitions of the menopause by transitions to new careers, interests, etc.

Frequently occurring when her children are adolescent and endocrinologically "uptight" , emotional instability is two-pronged.

Endocrine supplements (especially oestrogen, except where there is a history of oestrogen dependent carcinoma) and counselling by doctor, social worker, Community Nurse or religious adviser are helpful.

It is important to stress the *universality and transience* of this stage—and to put the woman's mind in the more optimistic future when she will have adjusted to glandular and life changes. As pertaining to her career role, she should be strengthened to resist disparaging remarks about 'her time of life'. Identification with a similarly placed women's group is often reassuring.

Unlike Western culture in which a woman's status, acceptability and self-image are very dependent on her youth and physical attractiveness, other cultures have provided honour and status compensation for women who have achieved their menopause. The Xhosa culture, for instance, bestows upon her the title Ukuphela Kwe Thombo, entitling her to a special place of wisdom and honour. Xhosa women are said to show few adverse menopausal symptoms, even looking forward to their new status.

At this time, when the menopausal woman feels very threatened by the strength and confidence of youth, it is especially *important that the nurse treat her client with respect.*

There is a strong tendency for women to associate male doctors with authoritarian father-figures, thus accepting a passive rather than active, participatory role in their treatment. Examples are hormonal treatment and surgical options.

> 'Such decisions affect their lives—mentally and socially. *They should know what the problems are and make up their own minds.* . . . American women are becoming more aware of this, and participation in their own treatment has already brought about some change.'*

The position should improve further as more female gynaecologists and physicians assume an influential role in medicine.

> 'By the time the menopause is passed, a woman begins to reap the harvest of years gone by. The business or professional woman achieves her promotion; the wife shares her husband's success, the mother enjoys her children and grandchildren.'†

Seeking Help:

One may advise: if you find yourself unable to enjoy the things which always cheered you up—music perhaps, or flowers or a bright day, or if you find you are waking regularly at 3 or 4 o'clock in the morning and cannot get back to sleep again because of gloomy thoughts, do go to see your doctor. In addition to physical help he may also suggest a support group:

* Dr Penny Budock, Assistant Professor of Family Medicine, State University of New York.

† Landau, Miss M E, MD FRCS *Women of Forty.*

Woman's Health Concern
17 Earl's Terrace
Ground floor flat
LONDON W8 6LP
Telephone: 01 602 6669

Marriage Guidance Council
76A New Cavendish Street
LONDON W1
Telephone: 01 580 1087
(Local branches are listed
in telephone directories)

Women's Health Information Centre
52 Featherstone Street
LONDON E1
Telephone: 01 251 6580

West Midlands FPA Clinic
7 York Road
Birmingham
B16 9HX
Telephone: 021 454 0236

Sheffield FPA Clinic
17 North Church Street
Sheffield
Telephone: 0742 21191

Well Woman Clinic
Wood House
Park Clinic
Wythenshawe
Manchester
Telephone: 061 437 4625

FPA Clinics which offer counselling
but not medical treatment:

6 Harlow Road
High Wycombe
Buckinghamshire
Telephone: 0494 26666

Mortimer House
13A Western Road
Hove
Sussex
Telephone: 0273 774075

104 Bold Street
Liverpool
Telephone: 051 709 1938

21 Dudley Road
Tunbridge Wells
Kent
Telephone: 0892 30002

8 Fairfields Road
Basingstoke
Hants
Telephone: 0256 2698

From: Living Through Change—Information for Patients. Compiled and presented by Ciba Laboratories.

The involutional period in men

About ten years later in their lifespan, men too tend to suffer involutional distress. Although symptoms are milder, many do suffer depression and anxiety which render them moody, intolerant, unpredictable and difficult in home and work relationships.

Clinical psychologist Jean Coleman maintains that stress related problems are high on the list of male menopause symptoms:

'By the mid-40s, if a man hasn't got to the top at work he has to adjust to the fact that now he probably never will,

'Another aspect is that the middle-aged man's parents will be elderly or dying. More worryingly, some of his friends may be dying of heart attacks. Suddenly he realises he is not going to go on forever.'

'This realisation is probably the reason why so many men have affairs with much younger women or wish to start a new family late in middle age.'

'They may seek promiscuous associations with young women, seeking thus to convince themselves of their attractiveness and potency.

These disturbances are, of course, aggravated by genital surgery such as prostatectomy with its implied threat of castration (see pp 57ff, 283).

Modern surgical techniques enable the nurse (unless otherwise instructed) to reassure her patient that though prostatectomy may result in reduced fertility, it does not result in reduced potency. If she senses this fear she may well take the initiative in verbalizing reassurance.

Although protastectomy may be followed by 'invisible' retrograde ejaculation, neither erection nor the sensations of orgasm are affected.

However, surgery may injure nerves responsible for erection and orgasm, and where this occurs the patient's self-image and sense of attractiveness and power are certainly imperilled. The nurse is referred to the more detailed discussion of sexual rehabilitation presented in the section on the Spinal-cord-injured Client (see p 508).

Dr Barbara Evans in her book *Life Change* maintains that the number of men who are impotent (for physiological or psychological reasons) doubles between ages 45 and 55, to approximate one-tenth of this population group. This drop in male libido is, she maintains, reflected in 'husband induced' alleged loss of sexual interest in one-tenth of women aged 46–50, this statistic later rising to one-half at a higher age. Authorities endorse that many marriages are strained by the inability of tired or stressed men to meet the sexual demands of their wives.

Dr Evans believes that other people's views and social mores, as much as physical changes, affect how women experience the end of their reproductive years. Clearly, sexual desire and its manner of expression and satisfaction depend on the understanding, communication, flexibility and initiative of both partners.

Dr Zaihoch, founder of the Centre for Sex Counselling Therapy and Education at the Rambam Medical Centre in Haifa:

'Researching 100 couples who attended the centre shows that more middle-aged husbands than wives decided on therapy. In spite of this being regarded as a "permissive" age, people still have conservative attitudes about sex. Stereotyped behaviour of both partners often blocks communication, preventing experimentation and contributing to sexual inadequacy. Every couple has the capacity to enjoy an active sex life till a very advanced age—in fact "till death do them part."

All that is required of many couples with problems is a frank discussion, but often I am the one who has to ask both of them the questions they should be asking each other.'

For alternative and complementary sexual fulfilment see Rehabilitation, p 508.

Late middle age may constitute its own *identity crisis* termed 'retirement shock'. The bank manager had his own strong identity. He knew who he was, and the honour and authority his position brought him. Now he's not sure whether he is a gardener, a kitchen hand or an aspirant to the bowls team. His stress level increases, and will erode his self-esteem unless he works out a solution.

Decisions, right or wrong, become important stress releasors.

Now is the time to identify problems, classify possible solutions through speaking and identifying with others, and draw up plans for the future.

Especially as one grows older, it is important *not to be too harsh upon oneself.* In evaluating one's achievements it is important to *'self-talk'*, positively praising one's physical health, one's faculties and one's achievements.

'Well that's pretty good for an old timer. My experience makes me valuable.' 'I'm going to try something new just for the heck and pleasure of it—and it doesn't matter a damn whether the result is good, bad or indifferent. As long as I get a kick out of it, that's all that matters.

The good news: Dispelling the myth

- 'Quality (as opposed to speed) of intellectual functioning is fairly stable throughout life, unless the person is suffering from a health condition affecting his or her cognitive abilities.
- Physical activity can continue throughout a person's life—the type and degree of intensity may need adjusting, that's all.
- Creativity can flourish at any age.
- Personality does not normally change drastically throughout life.
- Sex drive often continues well into the eighties.
- Age is a poor index of the ability of people to find pleasure in living.
- More educated individuals seem to enjoy better health and seem to adapt more successfully.*
- List of Support Group facilities : available from
  Menopause Clinics
  Camden Lock
  London N7 0BJ

* Bridges W. The Discovery of Middle Age. *Human Behaviour* May 1977.

CHAPTER 20

THE CARE OF THE ELDERLY IN OUR SOCIETY

A Crabbit Old Woman Wrote This*

What do you see, nurse, what do you see
Are you thinking when you look at me—
A crabbit old woman, not very wise,
Uncertain of habit, with far-away eyes,
Who dribbles her food and makes no reply
When you say in a loud voice—'I do wish you'd try'.
Who seems not to notice the things that you do,
And forever is losing a stocking or shoe.
Who unresisting or not, lets you do as you will,
With bathing and feeding, the long day will fill.
Is that what you are thinking, is that what you see.
Then open your eyes, nurse, you're looking at me.
I'll tell you who I am as I sit here so still;
As I do at your bidding, as I eat at your will,
I'm a small child of ten with a father and mother.
Brothers and sisters, who love one another.
A young girl of sixteen with wings on her feet,
Dreaming that soon now a lover she'll meet;
A bride soon at twenty—my heart gives a leap,
Remembering the vows that I promised to keep;
At twenty-five now I have young of my own,
Who need me to build a secure, happy home;
A woman of thirty, my young now grow fast,
Bound to each other with ties that should last;
At forty, my young sons have grown and are gone,
But my man's beside me to see I don't mourn;
At fifty once more babies play round my knee,
Again we know children, my loved one and me.
Dark days are upon me, my husband is dead,
I look at the future, I shudder with dread,
For my young are all rearing young of their own,
And I think of the years and the love that I've known,
I'm an old woman now and nature is cruel—
'Tis her jest to make old age look like a fool.
The body it crumbles, grace and vigour depart,
There is now a stone where I once had a heart;

---

* Found among the personal possessions of a geriatric patient, Newcastle, United Kingdom.

439

But inside this old carcass a young girl still dwells,
And now and again my battered heart swells.
I remember the joys, I remember the pain,
And I'm loving and living life over again.
I think of the years all too few—gone too fast,
And accept the stark fact that nothing can last.
So open your eyes, nurses, open and see
Not a crabbit old woman, look closer—see ME!

'Who Do We See . . .?'*

What do we see, you ask, what do we see?
Yes, we ARE thinking when looking at thee!
We may seem to be hard when we hurry and fuss,
but there's many of you, and too few of us.
We would like far more time to sit by you and talk,
to bath you and feed you and help you to walk;
to hear of your lives and the things you have done;
your childhood, your husband, your daughter, your son.
But time is against us, there's too much to do—
patients too many, and nurses too few.
We grieve when we see you so sad and alone
with nobody near you, no friends of your own;
we feel all your pain, and know of your fear,
that nobody cares now your end is so near.
But nurses are people with feelings as well,
and when we're together you'll often hear tell
of the dearest old Gran in the very end bed,
and the lovely old Dad, and the things that he said
we speak with compassion and love and feel sad,
when we think of your lives and the joy that you've had;
when the time has arrived for you to depart
you leave us behind with an ache in our heart.
When you sleep the long sleep, no more worry or care,
there are other old people, and we must be there.
So please understand if we hurry and fuss—
there are so many of you, and too few of us . . .

Old age is a time of stock taking—and the nett result is often disappointing, disillusioning and depressing. Many hopes, dreams, plans, and relationships have failed to meet life's aspirations and ambitions.

Many elderly know the 'self' they project inwards and outwards to be partly a false one. Frailty and rejection strip naked their ego defences. This is the pay-off; now there are no second chances.

---

* An answer to the poem 'A Crabbit Old Woman Wrote This' written by Elizabeth Hogben, student nurse at Sefton General Hospital, Liverpool, England.

The elderly realize the responses they make no longer work—they fail to improve and control their environment.

The ageing person clings desperately to his ego integrity, his self-esteem, his self-image. In accordance with his personality and life pattern, at conscious or unconscious levels, he may

  (i) regress to <u>learned helplessness</u>, reinforced by the stereotyped picture of the elderly he and his 'significant' people have introjected from their environment;
 (ii) become <u>depressed and suspicious</u> to an extent exceeding that prognosed by his failing physical status;
(iii) in accordance with the current theory of narcissism, <u>displace</u> his frustration, his anger, his rage, his impotence upon others—his attendants, his friends, his family—then accuse them of presenting his own projections. The chief nurse stopped me going home to my family who want me. I am a good, honest woman — You broke my vase in jealousy;
 (iv) attempt to draw <u>strength from his auxiliary 'egos'</u> (his support system), and in so doing he may terrorize, victimize and exhaust his family, his workmates and, later, his attendants. The superintendent told me to defy the foreman.

Recommendations

Contrary to destroying his defensive mechanisms, family and medical staff would do well to *encourage his defiance and anger rather than his submissive regression.* You've got a right to get your anger off your chest — to do it for yourself.

Now is the time for *caution (including imposing inhibitory 'safety rules')* and remonstrations *giving precedence to:*

  (i) positive effort and independence;
 (ii) preservation of dignity, status;
(iii) free access to loved ones, (including animals—who do not see deterioration and fragmenting vigour; who do not anticipate helplessness;)
 (iv) preservation of feelings of usefulness and a meaningful life;
  (v) self-decision and creativity to avoid insidious inactivity;
 (vi) freedom – to motivate
            to get going
            to keep going . . . to take reasonable risks

> 'So open your eyes, nurses, open and see
> Not a crabbit old woman, look closer—see ME!'

Now is the time for 'significant' people to introject Eastern respect and honour for the aged, as reflected in the universal greeting of the Hindu world. For when the Hindu joins his palms and bows his head he makes the greeting:

> 'I revere the spirit of God within you.
> I revere the person within you.'*

* Professor Lynn Gillis. Psychology of the Ageing Process, 27 June 1988. (Details available from Author).

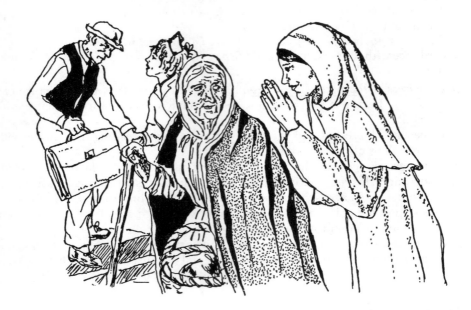

According to Erikson (1963) the final phase of the individual's life-cycle conflict is that of 'ego integrity versus despair'. During this phase he reviews his life and adopts one of two attitudes:

(i)   He may accept and feel good about his life accomplishments. He no longer yearns to have done things differently, and is not plagued by painful regrets. He is thus filled with a sense of integrity, fulfilment and achievement.

(ii) He may view his life with regret, remorse and dissatisfaction, filled with despair and inturned self-blame. He may actually project his discontent and resentment into his interpersonal relationships. It is important that others realize that his feelings are of *self*-disgust rather than contempt for others. His despair may be aggravated by fear of death, and the knowledge that as his life draws to a close it is impossible to change his set of values. He feels he has lived for nothing!

Erikson maintains that preparation for this final phase of one's life should begin in early childhood, for without resolution of previous developmental conflicts, there can be no comforting solution of this final confrontation with personal disintegration.

'An acceptance of physical limitations and reorientation of life style in accordance with these limitations is imperative. The ageing individual then develops a sense of brotherhood with all mankind and is no longer confined to the restrictions of personal conflicts and his vision is directed towards universal strivings and ideals.'

Thus wrote Gail K Luiz Ricciteloi in her prizewinning article: 'The Coming of Age of Mrs H', in which she presented the following Nursing Intervention Plan in the care of an elderly depressed woman:

'The aim of nursing intervention in a psychodynamic unit was to help Mrs H to accept her ageing and consequent changing role; to attempt to resolve residual conflicts; to improve her self-esteem and self-assertiveness; to help her plan for a future that would be more meaningful; to get her to face the prospect of her own death and that of her spouse (a problematic task in the face of depression—author) and to assist her in her efforts to be more independent . . .

In view of the fact that Mrs H received treatment in a heterogenous ward, special care had to be taken by the nurses to see that her individual needs as an ageing person were catered for, while at the same time carefully nurturing a sense of belonging . . .

Life Review

Relating conscious past experiences helped Mrs H to see her life as it really was and to accept it for its worth. Simply *lending an ear to her reminiscing* assisted her in this task. She was also encouraged to write down her memoirs and to make a collage of photographs. The latter was useful in aiding her to accept her changed self-image . . .

Therapeutic efforts had to be directed at supporting her poor sense of identity and building up her sense of self in renewed areas of interest . . .

Another aid to accepting her changing role was the exploration of her talents, abilities and interests. Together with the occupational therapist, a plan was made to help her develop new avenues. She was also informed of and encouraged to use, special community resources available to senior citizens.'*

Psychoneurological changes of the ageing process

Changes are individualized and usually gradual and plateau in pattern.

Modern medicine has prolonged man's life span, but not necessarily his life-efficiency. With age come

decreased efficiency of the heart's pumping action
impaired elasticity of the cerebral blood vessels
impaired quality of DNA resulting in general deterioration of new cell structure

Reduced cerebral blood supply leads to *relative anoxia* and a gradual *deterioration of cerebral tissue and function*. Microscopically, cerebral deterioration is seen in the formation of plaque. *Teeth are lost* and adjustment to new situations, including dentures, is almost unbearable. *Metabolism is not efficient*; old people living alone seldom bother to cook for themselves, and some cannot afford to eat well. Consequent malnutrition and vitamin deficiencies also contribute to gradual but definite deterioration of cerebral function.

Deterioration of sense organs themselves results in impaired information intake.

Impaired visual equipment results in impaired information intake as to the height of

---

* Gail K Luiz Ricciteloi 'The Coming of Age of Mrs H—Nursing Intervention in an elderly depressed woman'—Johnson & Johnson writing competition for the International Year of the Aged, *Curationis* March 1983.

a step, speed of oncoming traffic; incorrectly dialled telephone numbers, mistaken identity and generalized feelings of insecurity, humiliation, anxiety and depression.

Poorly functioning auditory equipment results in incorrect information intake as to prices, times, social arrangements; reduced participation in normal amusement, and general social isolation.

Certainly, within the context of that reality rejection which is so often the lot of the aged, it is natural that erroneous information intake will result in feelings of rejection, suspicion and thus aggressive and displeasing social reactions in the aged.

Impairment of cortical functioning and thus perceptual inaccuracy results in cerebral *misinterpretation* of information intake.

Deterioration of occipital lobe results in occipital *misinterpretation* of what is 'seen'. A flapping curtain may be 'seen' as an attacking robber; rice in his plate is misinterpreted as 'glass' with which a 'hostile' nurse is trying to kill him; flashing lights are seen as 'flashing knives'.

Impairment of temporal lobe functioning results in misinterpretation of auditory stimuli so that casual or friendly conversation may be misinterpreted as 'evil plotting'; an invitation to take a walk as a resented command to do so.

Impaired parietal functioning may misinterpret hot tea as tepid.

Deterioration of the upper motor neurone results in impaired motor processes with resultant loss of bladder and bowel control; palsied, shaky hand movements, difficulties in self-feeding, self-dressing, etc. Left hemisphere problems lead to circulatory blocks and aphasia (inability to match thoughts with words).

Deterioration in the frontal lobe results in reduced flexibility of thought processes which become rigid. Being unable to attain 'mental shift' the old person 'perseverates', repeating over and again 'long-winded' stories and complaints that everyone has heard a thousand times.

'Hold' *abilities*, involving vocabulary, social comprehension, observation of detail and established learning are relatively stable.

There is disproportionate fall-off in *'Don't Hold' psychological processes which are particularly vulnerable to organic impairment*, namely those involving

(i) *fall-off in recent memory*, to the point where a patient, forgetting that his nurse has just served him lunch, may accuse her of starving him;

(ii) *loss of new learning*, so that he finds it impossible to adjust to unfamiliar ward routine, or to the fact that he must take his medicine twice instead of three times a day. New learning is not as efficiently traced on ageing cerebral cells as when they were young and vital. However, the aged are not children. They possess islands of relatively intact old memories and skills, vocabulary and social insights.

The occupational therapist who attempt to teach an old lady a new knitting pattern is indeed imposing a disturbing and overwhelming task. The patient's *spatial concepts* (occipital functioning) are vulnerable, so that in spite of many demonstrations she cannot adjust to changed furniture or new ward layout.

By comparing scores on standardized 'Hold' tests with those on 'Don't Hold' tests, clinical psychologists can calculate, with fair accuracy, the extent of organic impairment. This is known as the Organic Deterioration Index, and is of importance in establishing a patient's

(a) legal status, where it may be necessary to establish that he is incapable of handling his own affairs which are then placed in the hands of the Court of Protection;

(b) organic cerebral loss due to a motor or an industrial accident for the purpose of establishing an insurance claim.

This observation draws attention to the fact that the effects of organic cerebral impairment are similar whether etiology be due to senility, cerebral haemorrhage, tumors, or trauma.

Organic changes in the *tracts connecting the frontal lobe* responsible for inhibition, self-control and foresight *and the hypothalamus* responsible for emotional reactions and motivation may well result in personality changes.

Where the tracts bringing self-control down from the frontal lobe to the hypothalamus are deteriorating the patient may lose his ability to exert self-control, becoming *involuntarily* fractious, childish, demanding, agitated and restless.

Where the tracts 'bringing up' normal emotional involvement and motivation from the hypothalamus are affected, the patient may well become increasingly lacking in drive, depressed and sometimes burdened by overwhelming anxiety and obsessional compulsions.

Complemented by his instinctive feelings of rejection and redundancy; arterioschlerosis and impaired blood supply, cortical impairment results in that suspiciousness, that 'touchiness', those ideas of persecution, in fact that *paranoia* which is a burdensome feature of the ageing process.

Misinterpretation of the reality environment which results from deterioration of sense organs and cortical functioning is *reflected in a type of delusion and hallucination* which presents as similar to paranoic schizophrenia, although the etiology thereof is quite different, as is the prognosis.

The prognosis is one of increasing gradual organic deterioration rather than that return to reality interpretation which one may expect from the younger schizophrenic patient.

These changes are associated with the special anxieties of the elderly.

Anxiety in the elderly

'What do old people worry about? About being alone, not being able to manage for themselves, about ill-health and about having to cope with change. They dread the thought of having to go to hospital or of moving to a new room. Anxiety is in fact, one of the staples of their lives. The main problem for relatives and friends is to recognize it because it may be disguised or appear in different forms. The most obvious are feelings of fear, dread, tension or panic—the same apprehensiveness that everyone will recognize from their own experience. This may be associated with restlessness, agitation, tearfulness and indecision. It may however appear just as "jitteriness", or the person merely complains that he is always fatigued or feels "exhausted" without obvious cause. Anxiety can also be transformed into medical symptoms such as subjective bodily sensations—tense feelings in the abdomen or pains in the chest, sensations of heat, muscular pains, etc. None of these are due to actual physical disease, but the person may think they are and is surprised when his doctor tells him they are merely a sign of psychic stress.'*

Among common psychosomatic symptoms of anxiety in the aged are over-breathing, involuntary swallowing, abdominal discomfort and belching, giddiness, palpitations, a tingling sensation in the fingers and diarrhoea without organic cause.

Medication and the elderly

The type of medication prescribed for this *senile dementia* is usually different from that prescribed for schizophrenia. Prescribing tranquillizers and other medication for the elderly is complicated by their impaired metabolism. Drug retention mounts and accumulative build-up results in over-medication which in turn leads to drowsiness or agitation: *toxicity and confusion are sometimes misinterpreted as senile dementia.*

The elderly are 'touchy' about taking medicine. They resent—and even suspect—the issue of medicine by others. To treat them as children hurts, provokes, diminishes and causes regression. For these reasons, pharmaceutical plans for special individualized daily or weekly packaging to facilitate self-administration are to be encouraged.

Manifestations of cerebral impairment may combine to culminate in general cerebral atrophy with diminution of nerve cells, described as

Irreversible Organic Senile deterioration (Dementia)

A study in England in 1972 found that about 5% of people aged 65 or over and 20% aged 80 or over had some degree of senile dementia.†

Presentation

> intellectual deterioration;
> reduced initiative;
> disorientation for time, place, people, aggravated by removal from familiar environment or bereavement.
> blunting of the emotions—apathy alternating with agitation;
> sleep disturbances; especially night-time restlessness;
> gross memory gaps, the past being confused with the present;
> incoherent and fragmented speech and thought;
> confusion causes misinterpretation, which may appear to result in delusionary behaviour; deterioration in personal hygiene and household order and cleanliness.

Medication:

> phenothiazine and benzochazepine drugs for controlling agitation and sedatives for sleep.

However prognosis is progressive.

---

* Gillis, L S. *Guidelines in Psychiatry.* Juta.

† Age Concern: Elderly people in the United Kingdom: Some basic facts. November 1988.

Reversible Symtomatology

However, *before* irreversible cerebral impairment may be diagnosed the following <u>reversible</u> facilitator ('DIMTOP') components should be eliminated:

D = Drugs—excessive, duplicatory, inappropriate, contradictory;
        alcohol, diuretics (electrolyte balance).
I = Infection—minor or major, especially pneumonia, urinary;
        fever does not always present; faecal impaction.
M = Metabolic—uraemia, hypo- and hyperglycaemia;
        hepatic confusion, dehydration.
T = Trauma—falls→concussion.
O = Oxygen deficit—blocking of blood vessels: arterosclerosis;
        manifests especially at night;
        cardiac impairment;
        reduced oxygen in lungs; hypothermia.
P = Psychological and perceptual—environmental change;
        bereavement, emotional trauma.*

DIMTOP factors should respond to physical investigation, medication, environmental stimulation and manipulation.

Depression in the Elderly

In spite of his reduced mental efficiency the elderly client senses that, in our *specialized, urbanized, small-unit, maximum productivity society*, he is becoming redundant, unwanted, at best impatiently tolerated.

The elderly constitute 15% of the industrial Western population of which group almost half are psychiatrically impaired, most of them by depression.
In the United Kingdom the elderly occupy

40% of outpatient-physician time
30% of inpatient-physician time.

Of these groups, 40% suffer some psychiatric impairment. Depression is twice as common as dementia, which latter affects 20%.

Presentation of depression in the elderly comes in many forms:
Organic cerebral or psychotic illness
Reactive and other depression

Neurotic symptoms
    Psychosomatic ailments with little *overt* sadness.
Depression frequently accompanies conditions such as arteriosclerosis, Alzheimer's and Parkinson's diseases, patients despairing in the realization of their decreasing ability to handle life and to partake in the joys of independence and normal relationship communication.

Potocnik reports a study in which
40% of Parkinson's patients
33% of dementia patients
are depressed.

* L S Gillis. *Guidelines in Psychiatry*. 1977.

Etiology of geriatric depression is multifactorial, individual factor patterns varying at any given time.

Predisposing factors include:

> hereditary factors;
> childhood experiences;
> bereavement and other loss;
> long-term personality structure;
> gender.

Common precipitators of depression are:

> physical illness and its aftermath, e g:
> influenza;
> infectious hepatitis;
> neurological conditions;
> incontinence;
> side-effects of drugs;
> vitamin B12 deficiency→anaemia;
> carcinoma;
> endocrine disturbances—
>> hypothyroidism
>> hyperparathyroidism
>> Cushings.

However, the most important precipitating factor is psychological stress resultant upon a series of 'losses' such as

> status
> income
> health

>> 'In 1980 55% of all elderly people aged 65 and over had a long-standing illness which limited their activities.
>> 36% had hearing difficulties.
>> 12% could not go out of doors and walk down the road on their own.*

> *company and friendship*—especially close familial relationships

>> 'In the United Kingdom 29,2% of pensioners live on their own.
>> 39,8% of old people on their own are aged 75 or over.
>> About 25% of old people in Scotland have no children and 22% have no brothers and sisters.
>> In a 1977 study in England, 30% of the over 75s had never had children and 7,5% had outlived their offspring.'†

> independence
> accommodation
> impending loss of life.

---

* Age Concern, England. Elderly People in the United Kingdom—Some Basic Facts. November 1986.
† Ibid.

These precipitants pressurize coping mechanisms already impaired by inevitable physiological and psychological changes, (pp 443-4). The elderly stagger under the inevitable loss of 'significant people' and the withdrawal of social supports. Their overwhelming psychological reaction may be illustrated by a triangular 'set' depicting the patient's presentation with one, two or all three of the following emotions:

aggression
anxiety
depression.

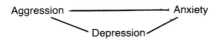

This triangle of emotions interweave, are interchangeable and may mask each other.

Symptomatology

Major depressive episodes present with the following diagnostic criteria:

1. a dysphoric mood, presenting with restlessness and agitation of at least two weeks duration,
2. plus four of the following symptoms presented to a significant degree—

   (a) poor appetite, significant weight loss, or increased appetite or significant weight gain
   (b) insomnia or hypersomnia
   (c) loss of energy or fatigue
   (d) psychomotor agitation or retardation
   (e) loss of interest in usual activities or decrease in sexual drive
   (f) feelings of self-reproach or inappropriate guilt
   (g) diminished ability to think or concentrate
   (h) suicidal ideation

   Minor or milder depression presents as depressive apathy marked by
   loss of former interests,
   social withdrawal,
   hypochondriasis,
   anxiety,
   emotional preoccupation,
   appetite disturbances,
   sleeping difficulties,
   loss of energy,
   irritability.

The *mood* lacks capacity for the enjoyment of life rather than the abject misery of major depression.

Psychogenic pain (real suffering without adequate physical explanation) may present, with the following psychogenic etiology:

Fears of dependence, bereavement, death, conflicts, inability to make decisions, ambivalence and guilt feelings, anxiety→

Autonomic Nervous System tension energy (pp 25-32)→psychosomatic symptoms.

Depression may be reinforced by:

1.   Avoidance behaviour (conscious or unconscious) in response to threats such as hospitalization.
2.   Secondary environmental gain, eg the notice of a normally rejecting family or indifferent staff.

'Denial' conscious or unconscious may impede therapeutic insight.

As evening falls, the elderly often become miserable, wretched and weary. The alcoholic 'sundowner' is a valuable and welcome 'pick-me-up'.

In fact, according to Mrs R Manley, a specialist nurse in the care of the elderly, many establishments for the elderly in the UK are equipped with their own pubs.

Chronic pathological grief reactions present with three classic syndromes, namely

1.   The *unexpected grief syndrome* following the unexpected death of a close relative or 'significant' person, where the sorrow of loss is aggravated by feelings of self-reproach and self-punishment, continued obligation and clinging to the dead.
2.   The *ambivalent grief syndrome* in which hidden hostile feelings towards the dead lead to feelings of guilt, restlessness, anxiety and fears of divine retribution by some terrible punitive happening, such as the person's own death.
3.   *Chronic grief* usually following the ending of a dependent, clinging relationship. In spite of intense mourning and catharsis, this grief persists for an abnormal length of time. (See Grief work pp 556-7.)

Suicide

The frequency of depression, even unto suicide, is high. According to Potocnik, the elderly account for approximately 25% of all suicides. The elderly single male is most 'at risk', followed by the agitated depressive.

The extent to which professionals tend to deny, dismiss and take for granted clients' complaints of sadness, misery and full-blown depression, is revealed by a United Kingdom study showing that:

1.   Most suicides had contacted a doctor within a week before their death.
2.   Most suicides had been known to be suffering from depression for approximately six months.

Treatment of depression in the elderly

On the part of 'significant people':
stimulation of 'ego' integrity through

self-decision
dignity
creativity

even to the extent of bending and reassuring 'safety rules' in order to counteract regression to 'learned helplessness' and loss of motivation to live (pp 441, 459 et seq). At their time of life, many seniors may prefer occasionally to 'take a chance' rather than to suffer repressive diminishment and boredom.

For a specific programme to counteract depression in the ill and elderly, see David Miller's recommendations (p 350).

1. Mobilization of social resources

    (a) family,
         significant persons,

    by means of

         interpretation,
         professional support,
         self-help group participation; (see p 613, chapter 26)
    (b) psychotherapy, individual and in groups, with realization that some personalities have always been 'private' and will understandably reject group participation;
    (c) involvement in social welfare community programmes—
         visitors   occupational therapy, etc.
         social clubs   music, movement, participation
         outings   and relaxation therapy.
         self-help groups   day care centres

2. Grief work
    See pp 556-7.

3. Pets
    Cats and dogs provide unquestioning love, tactile comfort, companionship, safety, motivation for exercise and a purpose in life. The importance of catering for pets in residential facilities is stressed by many authorities.

4. Physical examination

    (a) excluding toxic conditions,
    (b) providing exercise, dietary supplements, etc,
    (c) appropriate medication—

It is important that the elderly be involved in their own individualized medication programmes.
Of importance are:
  verbal communication,

    pamphlets ⎫ explaining drug function,
    videos   ⎬ side-effects,
               ⎭ dosage, etc.

  the provision of innovative packaging:
  calendars—'pop-out' packaging
  illustrated instructions.
  e g:
  with meals

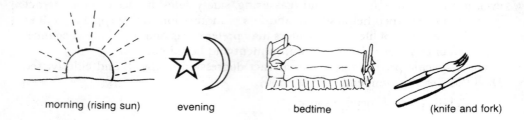

morning (rising sun)   evening   bedtime   (knife and fork)

Prognosis for depression in the elderly

Studies have shown that although there is a natural tendency for depression to get better with improved circumstances, nevertheless

(*a*) the prognosis is less favourable than for younger patients,
(*b*) relapses are extremely likely:
    'Depression in the elderly is eminently treatable, but, because of a high relapse rate, prolonged after-care and maintenance therapy are indicated.'

The Ageing Population

Unlike his counterparts in the East and among certain African people, the Western elderly person is not protected by social mores (community customs or norms) designed for the protection of the aged.

Lack of respect for the elderly, a fall-off in certain religious standards, the widespread belief that he no longer has anything of significance to offer the employer, all lead to an increasingly long period of diminished social influence, financial security, sense of purpose and self-respect.

His own peer group diminishes, and he is no longer able to afford his own home. His self-care, efficiency deteriorates, and he becomes an increasingly unwelcome burden on his family and society. He senses himself to be as a guest who has outstayed his welcome. Soon his family plead inability to provide 'twenty-four hour supervision' and he is institutionalized.

Actually, the aged in Britain are doing well in maintaining their independence. Very small proportions of elderly people live in an institution: 1,2% are permanent residents in hospital and 2% are in residential care. This low figure is a credit to British community services—especially those delivered by District and Community Nurses.

A fall-off in birth rate due to improved standards of contraception, together with a longer life-span, resultant upon improved medicine, is constantly increasing the proportion of elderly people who must be supported by the diminishing proportion of active workers. Widespread reluctance to compromise by accepting the slower output, but increased experience and well-ingrained skills of the ageing, has increased the burden which they reluctantly and involuntarily impose upon society.

'The population of the United Kingdom is 55 767 381 (Census 1981).
9 673 476 people (3 226 298 male and 6 447 178 female) are over pensionable age which is 60 for women and 65 for men.

8 163 241 are aged 65 or over.
3 117 981 are aged 75 or over.
  563 805 are aged 85 or over.
17,3% of the population of the United Kingdom are elderly people.
Between 1981 and 2001, the total number of people of pensionable age will have increased overall by 3,3% having peaked in 1991. The proportion aged 75 and over will, however, steadily increase by 27,6% and those aged 85 and over by 79%.'*

Thus in the UK there are almost 10 million elderly people.

On retirement a woman can expect to live to 80,6 and a man to 77,4. Either from choice or because they cannot find employment, people are retiring earlier. In 1983, in the five years before the basic state retirement age, only 59,5% of men and 50,8% of women were working.

Pensioners in poverty

Basic pensions from July 1986–April 1987 are £38.70 for a single pensioner and £61.95 for a couple. Scale rates for supplementary benefit are £37.90 for a single person and £60.65 for a couple.†

Almost half pensioner households depend for at least 75% of their income on state pensions and benefits.

The proportion of weekly expenditure per person spent on housing, fuel and food is greater in households where the head is aged 65 and over (58%) than it is in those where the head of the household is aged under 65 (43%). Proportionately pensioners spend nearly twice as much as the rest of the population on fuel. The most severe deprivation is experienced by pensioners living alone who are mainly dependent on state pensions. In all, 70,1% of their expenditure goes on housing, fuel and food.

Amongst households with people over 60, 68% have no car, 50% no central heating, 34% no telephone, and 39% have no washing machine.

Living alone

70,4% of men of pensionable age are married, but only 44,2% of women. Widowhood is very common; of the women of 75 or over, 64,2% are widows and of those 85 or over, 72%.‡

Owing to steadily increasing longevity we have reached a situation which is unique. A considerable proportion of the retired have either one or both parents still living. We are the first generation in recorded history with more than one generation in retirement.

The rural multi-generational family has been replaced by the urban nuclear family with the elderly living in separate households without their former roles in family life.

---

* Age Concern, England, with the generous assistance of SAGA Holidays plc. Elderly People in the United Kingdom—Some Basic Facts. November 1986.
† Persons of Pensionable Age: Great Britain Census 1981.
‡ Ibid.

Lack of space is not the only reason for the state of neglect in which many old people are living. Lack of interest and lack of a sense of responsibility on the part of the children and relatives of aged persons are not to be overlooked.

The tendency in modern society is for the elderly to be progressively segregated from the young. This has tended to result in social isolation of the aged with accompanying pathological developments. Welfare organizations have realized that needs in respect of emotional security, social recognition and a sense of worth must be met.

With the change in our life style, older people are beginning to value their independence more and more. Organizations dealing with the aged have found that *by providing certain facilities the aged are able to maintain their independence*, and therewith their self-respect. They are in need of much less intensive care while leading much happier lives. Many elderly people do very well in meeting the change and mastering the new freedom which retirement brings.

They may, however, require some specialized housing and community facilities.

Some Debilitating Difficulties encountered by the Elderly

Incontinence is of four types

STRESS

Urine leakage occurs, without warning, following sudden stress on the bladder, such as coughing, sneezing, laughing or lifting a heavy object.

URGE

This is usually associated with reduced muscle control and is the sudden urge to urinate that is very uncomfortable and cannot be contained.

SENSORY

This type of incontinence usually occurs in older people. The bladder sometimes becomes less sensitive to being stretched and suddenly empties of its own accord.

LOCOMOTOR

This term refers to situations where the person cannot get to the toilet in time because of lact of general mobility caused by old age, stroke, arthritis or some other disease.

For the patient, psychological troubles are often more painful than physical ones. One should always treat the patient — not the bed!
To be negative and depressing only makes things worse.
Negative nursing such as restricting fluids, being dressed in pyjamas by day, removal of carpets, newspapers on the floor and rubber sheets hanging up to dry, destroy the patient's self-image and his motivation to recover or even survive.

There are special incontinence care products specifically designed to cope with the problem. They make life more comfortable for the patient, his family and carers.

Words of praise and encouragement, and the the company of good friends, can be very rewarding in restoring patient confidence.

One should remember that incontinence can sometimes be cured, often improved and always made more tolerable.*

The Psychosocial Aspects of ARTHRITIS in the Elderly†

THE CHRONIC RHEUMATIC DISEASES

BASIC RESPONSES INCLUDE:

- Fear/Anxiety
- Dependency
- Anger
- Loss of gratification

PATIENT MAY GO THROUGH:

- Shock/Denial/Disbelief
- Anger
- Bargaining
- Depression
- Eventual acceptance

PROBLEMS ARISING FROM PHYSICAL DISABILITY

1. Chronic pain
2. Loss of function
3. Deformity

PERSONALITY CHANGES

- Depression
- Rigidity
- Excessive concern with bodily fuction

MAY BE MODIFIED BY:

- Premorbid personality
- Sex
- Degree of socio-economic stability
- Organic Disease (SLE)

OTHER COMMON PROBLEMS

- Secondary gains from sympathy
- Change in family role
- Sexual dysfunction

COPING MECHANISMS:

- Hope
- Covering up
- Lowering of expectations and activities
- Pacing

MANAGEMENT MUST BE AIMED AT:

- Providing patient with a sense of acceptance.
- Providing patient with understanding.

* Smith and Nephew: Incontinence — What is it? How to Cope Better.

† Smith. Peter. Quoted by McDonald Scott WA: Myths in Rheumatology. Details from Author.

Providing patient with some direction to assist with psychological, social, functional, and economic problem solving.

AND INCLUDES:

- A patient-orientated team approach. The nurse is vital in this.
- Counselling (Direct, family group).
- Supportive infrastructure within the community.

The role of the Community District Nurse

A primary role of the community nurse is to protect the elderly from the destructive hospital experience by providing preventive, curative and ameliorative service. Quoting from Dr M Barlow, medical Superintendent:

> 'Hospital is uncomfortable for everyone—how much worse must it be for an old lady half blind, who knows exactly where everything is in her room, who has to go to the toilet 5 times a night and loves her hot water bottle. In hospital she is in a strange atmosphere, she cannot find the toilet so wets the bed (and is heavily castigated by the nursing staff, which upsets her, she cries, has urinary incontinence and promptly wets the bed again), a whole vicious circle [See pp 119-121, 472]
>
> Unfortunately there are times when old people do have to go to a hospital for operations etc but I believe that post-operatively every effort should be made to return the patient back home—or to the halfway house as a matter of urgency. Hospitals have become super-specialized, hyper-efficient institutions and there is very little place for the medical care of the aged in these cold, expensive buildings. Everyone used to die at home. Why cannot we allow the old the privilege of still doing this without the indignities of tubes stuck up every orifice and young brash doctors and nurses only waiting for a bed to be freed.'

It is, of course, the provision of nursing procedures at home which keeps people out of hospital.

> 'The ideal person to seek out the elderly in the community and assess their physical, emotional and social needs is the community nurse (with careful regard to the client's privacy and self-determination—Author). After a complete *assessment*, referral to other appropriate agencies may be made. However, referral does not relieve the community nurse of her overall responsibility towards the elderly person. She must ascertain that the progress of elderly persons is followed up and act as a co-ordinator in their care . . .. The ideal is to help the elderly live an independent, happy and useful life in their own homes, making their own contribution to the community.'

That British Community Nurses are fulfilling their obligations is reflected by the volume of

'Service at Home [1980]
In a year amongst those aged 65 and over:

605 426 are seen by Health Visitors
1 632 881 are visited by Home Nurses
1 732 452 receive NHS chiropody services
765 754 received the services of a home help.'*

Preventive, Promotive and Curative Functions of the Community Nurse

Preventive: Pre-retirement courses designed to counteract and accommodate the physical and psychological changes of ageing.
Nutritional information.
Social clubs—PT, hobby discussion groups, etc.
Familiarity with relevant protective social legislation.
Preventing hypothermia. In 1984, the deaths of 857 people aged 65 or over involved hypothermia according to their death certificates. A 1972 study indicated that 10% of old people are at risk of hypothermia.
Liaison with Occupational Nurses regarding employment opportunities, etc.

Promotive: Home visits, including motivation of family units to become involved in communal care.
Conduct of local clinics on a regular basis, in association with Homes for the Aged, Service Centres, Day Hospitals, etc.
Establishment of social clubs and Day Care Centres.
Liaison with welfare organizations.
Inspection of homes for the elderly in order to evaluate staff training and living conditions.
Organization of paramedical services—ie occupational therapy, chiropody.

Curative: Home nursing—The frail.
The elderly discharged from hospital.
Transport to out-patients clinics.
Specific procedures such as injections, dressings, blood pressure records, urine tests, etc.
Many elderly are concerned about bowel function and incontinence. In this there may be an element of regression to childhood maternal dependence, a bid for approval and security.
Training of nurse-aids.

An elderly person who is treated for pneumonia at home does not become confused. But put that person in hospital, and the unfamiliar environment, combined with poor eyesight and dehydration, can cause confusion.

* Age Concern, England. November 1986.

His distress is aggravated by cot sides which look like prison bars to an elderly person left alone in the darkened room of a hospital for long periods.

Family support: Catharsis and guidance of all family members, including the client herself in order to weather the specific strains involved in supporting and caring for the aged.

Entertainment diversions, including outings, extend survival goals.

Spontaneous approach after bereavement when the Community Nurse will need to utilize and amend the emotional support and assessment, planning and evaluation inherent in crisis intervention (see p 563 et seq; Grief work pp 556-7).

A recent survey in the United Kingdom showed that, within the context of supportive communal services and assistance in arranging accommodation for the aged for two weeks each year, 80% of families were prepared to keep the aged with them.

It is important that no elderly person be deprived of his home and independence for the sake of specific nursing procedures, which may well be conducted in even simple home circumstances.

There is growing criticism of inappropriate utilization of residential care by elderly persons who could have retained their independence in the community. Those residences for the aged which do not favour admission of frail persons as they do not have 'adequate facilities' for their care are said to reflect a fundamental error of planning and design. It is claimed that professionals and support systems do not always seem aware that residential care *should* be for the frail.

Long-term community maintenance services particularly appropriate to the *nursing process* include combating poor nutrition, hypertension, diabetes, leg ulcers, arthritis, poor sight and hearing, dehydration, constipation and resultant feelings of obsessional anxiety and depression.

These long-term, insidious conditions encourage the aged person to regress to childish fears and dependence. The Community Nurse should *utilize nursing procedures and 'rapport' emanating from her ability to provide physical comfort in order to establish meaningful relationships*. Herein lies her most effective antidote to those feelings of depression and isolation which crush motivation to survive.

'I aimed to preserve her dignity and self-respect by arranging my visits to suit her and by being confident and optimistic about her disability. Allowing her to make decisions maintained her sense of self-worth and independence, and giving her the right to choose and informing her of all procedures beforehand, preserved her self-esteem.'*

Impact of surgery—the role of the nurse

'Nurses should realize that the psychological impact of surgery on the elderly can be far-reaching. Firstly, they may feel a *loss of independence and be frustrated by their increased dependence* on others. They often feel useless and unwanted owing to their

* Gersman, Anna. 1986.

inability to perform usual activities. Elderly patients may suffer a *sense of loss after surgery* and must be motivated to resolve possible depression or anxiety.

Secondly, the patient's *emotional and physical environment during rehabilitation is important* to his psychological outlook.

The individual in an institution has little privacy, and relationships with others are reduced. A low range of interests and activities is shown and there is a tendency to be withdrawn and unresponsive. These problems can be solved if the family care for the patient at home where he feels more relaxed. The home environment must be stimulating, with windows to look out of, pictures on the walls, mementoes of past experiences, etc.

Thirdly, *individual behavioural differences must be considered* when evaluating the psychological effects of surgery on the elderly.

One person may respond with so much anxiety and depression that they are immobilized, while another may be upset and concerned about their plight, but be able to make the best of the situation.

Fourthly, *the psychological impact of an operation causes a disruption.* This is always disturbing, but usually temporary. The patient and family must be encouraged to express and discuss their feelings with the help of the professional nurse [who] can often give insight into how strengths, resources and capacities of the family can be forgotten during the crisis period.'*

Unfortunately the health of the aged is not always predictable.

Some service centres liaise with nurses who operate *where healthy aged persons have suddenly become ill* or frail. This is an emergency and sometimes transitory service. It certainly increases the confidence of the independent aged.

Sexual needs of the elderly

Freud believed the two mainsprings of Man's life-force to be:

The Life Instinct, expressed in sexual behaviour,

The Death Instinct, motivating acts of aggression against others or oneself.

Denied satisfaction of their sexual goals, the aged may, at various levels of consciousness:

seek compensation in aggression displaced upon others. (p 121).

abandon the Life Instinct and, in unmotivated depression, seek the final withdrawal of lonely death.

Despite the many diminishing and changing facets of ageing, basic needs remain the same. Need for the close, comforting warmth of intimacy and sexual fulfilment is no exception. Indeed, especially among residents of establishments for the aged, there should be specific approval and provision for the enjoyment of sexuality, as well as information on alternate stimulation of coitus, where this is indicated.

It is important to exclude underlying debilitating factors such as diabetes, neurological or vascular disease and the blunting effects of medication.

* Ibid.

Premature and retarded ejaculation may respond to treatment. Dyspareunia (painful intercourse in women) may be due to atrophic vulvo-vaginitis or lack of lubrication. Oestrogen therapy or change of position may be indicated.

There is often an indication for increased clitoral and other local stimulation.

It is important that the aged should feel free to seek advice about sexual enjoyment.

Dr LJ Abramowitz, a specialist gynaecologist, in his article 'Sexuality in the Ageing' in *Continuing Medical Education* vol 1, no 5 observes:

'It has recently been shown that with ejaculation, testosterone production is stimulated. This may be the physiological basis of the old belief that "if you don't use it you'll lose it!" In the female, too, regular coitus (and oestrogen therapy) help to maintain the vagina as a functioning organ ... patients should be encouraged to think young and keep physically and mentally fit and not to retreat from their environment. This will not only add years to their lives, but will add life to their years.'

Pets and the elderly

Tactile comfort, deeply rooted in its symbolic association with Mother Love, Safety and Security, and the warmth of loving relationships long gone, is especially important to the aged. For those living alone it is important to feel something alive and welcoming in their home.

People laugh at old ladies and their cats, but one is amazed at the intensity of feeling between them. Cats are easier to manage and more tactile than dogs. Research has shown one's blood pressure falls if one strokes a cat.

Another patient has wanted to commit suicide until a stray cat she nursed back to health gave her so much joy she wrote a poem about it. Recent research shows that cat owners are less sociable but more contented than non-owners. Many people do not own a cat for fear of what would become of it if they themselves died. A cat support service—people willing to take in other's cats—to guarantee the pet's future is an idea worthy of costly consideration.

It is of course, very important that, should residential care be necessary, arrangements be made for the client to take her pet with her.

Welfare agencies for the elderly

The aims of most welfare agencies for the elderly are to promote the interests and well-being of the aged, to co-ordinate activities, give guidance and assistance to all organizations interested in the welfare of the aged and to serve as a channel through which the problems, findings and suggestions of member organizations can be conveyed to government and other appropriate authorities.

Training courses and conferences

For matrons and staff of homes, professional and voluntary workers, etc.

Employment schemes

Providing a service to employers and to the elderly seeking employment.

Boarding-out schemes

Finding temporary accommodation and board for a senior person, enabling the family to go away for a holiday, have hospital treatment, etc.

Housing and accommodation

It is becoming prescribed practice *to avoid uprooting the senior citizen* from that domestic and community environment to which he has adjusted in his more flexible years, in which he finds safety, dignity and a sense of personal worth; in which, due to familiarity of spatial arrangements, he is able to function independently within the context of his familiar and long-term peer and social group. Shops, library, clinic, bank, park, community centre are all comfortably familiar.

A compromise consists in economic and sub-economic housing projects designed to cater for the decreasing size, financial resources and physical independence of the family unit.

Danish and Dutch projects for specialized villages, with communal facilities such as cinema and participation theatrical units; participation sports amenities for bowls, croquet, and even yoga; restaurant facilities, hospital unit, etc, are being successfully emulated in Britain and the USA.

It is planned that the retired couple will buy a housing unit, which may later be exchanged for a flat, which latter, when eventually sold, provides for the terminal small-unit hospital care of the frail. Nursing facilities are available throughout.

Other *accommodation alternatives* when original homes become too big, expensive, lonely or isolated are:

Cottages.

Flats, with or without provision of one or two meals a day.

Homes providing comprehensive care.

Important causes for deterioration as clients regress from the relative independence of Category A, to the virtual hospital-patient status of Category C, are *disorientation, social isolation, lack of privacy, impaired mobility and depression*, all of which are associated with environmental dislocation. Research into *optimum accommodation* sufficiently *functional and flexible* for adaptation from physical integrity to frailty (even unto the 'wheelchair stage', and thus suitable for other disables) emanates from the Buildings for Health Services Subcommittee of the Building Research Institute of the CSIR.

Dr E V Macagnano, Senior Research Officer, has designed a double or single bedroom-living room, kitchenette, bathroom unit, fully equipped with adapted apparatus, furniture and open slide doors, 35 sq metres in area. There are no fixed internal walls nor corridors, and the unit, which can be grouped with others round a patio, or quadrangle, is of relatively modest cost.

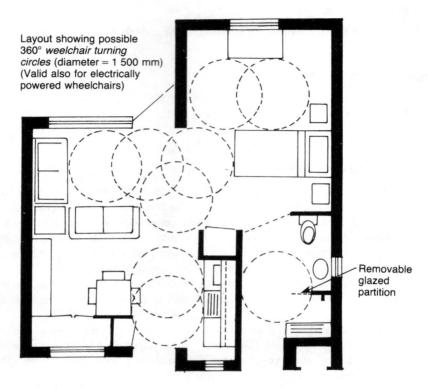

Layout showing possible
360° *weelchair turning
circles* (diameter = 1 500 mm)
(Valid also for electrically
powered wheelchairs)

Removable
glazed
partition

One is frequently distressed by the lack of social facilities and the *loneliness encountered by middle-class senior citizens*. Because their financial needs are not blatantly obvious, their emotional needs are often overlooked.

A growing urban *tendency not to become 'involved' in one's neighbours* results in special painful isolation of the middle-class elderly. Sometimes police, eventually called in by a casual passer-by, find old people who have lain dead in their flats for days, even weeks.

Many do not know of local social, recreational, religious, paramedical and domiciliary services. In Great Britain 35% of pensioners who were entitled to supplementary benefit did not claim.

Casework

Professional social work and community nursing services.

Clubs and service centres

Participation by members in the running of these should be encouraged.

Facilities could include: a workshop and pottery kiln; a shop for the sale of products made by members; food parcels at wholesale prices containing meat, fish, vegetables, home-made cakes and jams, etc; the sale of second hand clothing, furniture, china, etc; occupational, social, drama participation groups; hairdressing at special rates; library; yoga; old-time dancing.

Multi-purpose utilization of some service centres to include day care centre facilities.

Children and families may provide accommodation for their aged, but during the day both husband and wife have to work and the children are at school. Thus the aged have to remain locked up at home, helpless and alone.

The family may choose to drop off their senior citizen at the Day Car Service Centre in the morning and pick her up again in the afternoon.

A day care centre should be designed so the aged are able to rest and sleep if they so desire. This facility entails provision of nursing services.

In Britain some service centres are multifunctional, providing care, creative occupation, recreation and companionship for retarded children, psychiatric patients, the lonely and the aged, many of whom have much to give each other.

Some speak in favour of moving away from segregated and isolated facilities to absorption into those catering for other community activities such as maternal and child welfare clinics, art groups, activity centres for the handicapped. Here the elderly can perform useful functions as part of the general community. Many elderly people crave contact with other age groups.

'Twelve old people—Jack, Bill, Mary, and nine other women and men—sat in a circle. One was in a wheelchair and several leaned on canes or walkers.

The children were on the floor inside the circle: Beth, Nicole, Benny, and five more. They were laughing and talking with the old people and singing nonsense rhymes.

It was "contact time" at the Community Programmes Centre of Long Island, an unusual daycare centre that, under one roof, serves children from infancy through pre-school age, and also the elderly.

Every morning for an hour a group of children visit the old people, touching, hugging, singing and painting funny faces.

"Just being with them," says the centre's director, "so that children can grow up with matter-of-fact awareness of ageing and disability, an understanding that life is a process, that people come in all shapes and sizes."

Jack wanted to see Beth's doll, but Beth preferred to wriggle out of her trousers to show that she was wearing her dance leotard. She slipped on a headband and said she wanted to show off her newly learned aerobics.

"Hi, my name is Benny," said another child, trying out a newly-developed British accent and touching Mary, an elderly woman with a bandage on her nose, the bandage of a skin operation.

"Hello Benny, my name is Mary," she replied.

"Reahlly?" he said—and then giggled. Mary giggled too.

There are four such "inter-generational" care programmes in New York State, and such centres form a rapidly growing trend.'

New York Times.

Handiwork and gardening

Competitions between the aged themselves, between clubs and between towns. Also bazaars and fêtes, shows of handwork, etc.

Clinics for the elderly

These include mobile units.

Paramedical services

Chiropody.
Physiotherapy.
Provision of aids for the infirm such as wheelchairs, walking-sticks, spectacles, dentures, hearing-aids.
Emergency supplies of home nursing requisites, bed-clothes, etc.

Domiciliary services

Home helps.
Meals-on-wheels and lunch clubs.
Visiting Service—including visits to aged in homes and hospitals.
Good Neighbour Scheme (neighbour assists with regular meals, shopping, etc.)
Emergency Call or 'Silver Fish' Schemes (aged person supplied with name of volunteer to 'phone in an emergency'. The volunteer is in turn supplied with telephone number of doctor, details of illnesses, hospital card number, etc. Alternatively a silver fish is displayed in his window by the senior citizen in time of need.)
The Hospice Movement (see p 556) provides long-term home care and emotional support.

Community alarms

This service refers to special telephones which link the client to a control centre which is manned 24 hours a day. In an emergency she can activate the unit either by pressing a button on the unit itself or on a *radio pendant* which she wears. The operator at the control centre will then arrange to have the problem dealt with.

Help the Aged raises £334 for each special telephone. This amount covers the cost of the telephone including VAT and a proportion of the first year's monitoring charges.

Contact:

Community Alarm Dept
Help the Aged
St James's Walk
London
EC1R 0BE
or
The Crime Prevention Officer at your local police station.

Crime Prevention Officers at local police stations give expert advice on making the home safe. They are not usually uniformed. In addition to giving advice on improving home security, Crime Prevention Officers or Permanent Beat Officers will advise on locks and reputable installers of security equipment schemes.

'Simply 'phone or call into your local police station to arrange for an officer to visit you. It is a good idea to join a Neighbourhood Watch Scheme. Your local police will tell you about it.'*

Perhaps the best guard–companion is a loving watch-dog.

Day and night sitters in times of illness.

Transport service—to clubs, hospital, clinic, church, etc.

Help with mending and alteration of clothes.

Provision of radio sets and repairs of same.

Laundry schemes.

It is a good idea to provide duplicate sets of front-door keys for the Community Sister or house doctor.

Entertainments

Christmas and tea parties (for groups or individuals), concerts, film shows, musical evenings, attendance at theatres, dress rehearsals, bus outings, etc.

Youth services

Schoolchildren invite senior citizens to tea at school and provide entertainment. Adopt a 'grandparent'—visit, take posy of flowers, read, help in garden and around home, remember birthday and Xmas, write to them while on holiday, etc.

Assist in clubs and service centres—participate in activities: games, handwork for fêtes, making and setting out of decorations for parties (St Valentine, Hallowe'en, Christmas, Spring, etc) serving of teas, etc.

Groups can undertake repairs to private homes—painting, gardening, etc.

Honour-the-Aged Week

To bring the needs of the aged to the attention of the public and to entertain them as guests of honour during the week-special church services, entertainments, etc.

Holidays

Arranging of group and individual participation in hospitality holidays and exchange holiday schemes.

Preparation for retirement

Lectures and courses, group discussions at clubs and centres, etc.

Pensioners' Link 01 328 2688.

Newsletters and suburban press

Interesting news items concerning the elderly, notices of meetings, news of concessions and old age pensions, etc.

Help the Aged's Advice Line

01 250 3399

* Age Concern, England. November 1986.

An advice line for elderly people, their carers, friends and relatives.

Age Concern is a network of around 1 400 Age Concern groups in the United Kingdom working with volunteers to provide a wide range of community services including day care centres, lunch clubs, visiting for the lonely, as well as transport and many other schemes.

Nationally, Age Concern provides a comprehensive information service, produces an extensive list of publications and runs a wide range of training courses.

Age Concern takes an active part in policy formulation by advising government on legislation affecting elderly people and by campaigning on their behalf.

Further information from Age Concern

Age Concern has a wide range of publications for elderly people and those who work with them. For further information or the address of a local Age Concern group, contact:

> Age Concern England
> Bernard Sunley House
> 60 Pitcairn Road
> Mitcham
> Surrey CR4 3LL
> Telephone 01 640 5431

> Age Concern Northern Ireland
> 6 Lower Crescent
> Belfast BT7 1NR
> Telephone 0232 245729

> Age Concern Scotland
> 33 Castle Street
> Edinburgh EH2 3DN
> Telephone 031 225 5000

> Age Concern Wales
> 1 Park Grove
> Cardiff CF1 3BJ
> Telephone 0222 371821/371566

Psychiatric assessment units catering for elderly discharged patients

Bethlam Hospital, on the outskirts of London (the laudable successor to old Bedlam), which contains several geriatric pavilions for psychiatrically disturbed cases, reports the largest turnover in the hospital—and not to the undertaker either.

Geriatric medication, sometimes complemented by ECT for depression, and intensive vitamin therapy, together with appropriate social and environmental manipulation, result in remarkably successful return to the community. However, prescription of geriatric medicine is a 'tricky business'—patients may over-react or respond in unexpected ways due to reduced metabolism and thus cumulative effect. (p 446)

Dr Len Tibbet in a paper read at a meeting on 'The Role of the Home for the Aged—The Decade Ahead' (1974) stated that the future policy for homes for the aged should provide only for those *in need* of institutional care by virtue of their frailty. With the extension of supportive services to the aged such as meals-on-wheels, laundry schemes, etc. many more old people would be retained in the community. He stressed the need for psycho-geriatric assessment units for those who have been mentally ill and have been retained in the psychiatric hospitals unnecessarily simply because there is nowhere else for them to go.

In his article 'Out from the Geriatric Ghetto', extracted from *Social Work Today* Vol 14 No 20 (25/1/83), Raymond Jack emphasizes the necessity for *avoiding that unskilled and casual assessment of the crises of old age,* which may misplace clients in psychogeriatric wards:

'Because it may be assumed, incorrectly, that there is no treatment for dementia, the elderly person presenting with symptoms of cognitive impairment, lethargy, withdrawal and so on may be regarded as dementing, and little effort made to further investigate the condition or understand the environmental and emotional factors which may be contributing to it. . . . Such a person may be suffering from a reversible physical or emotional disorder—such as a toxic confusional state or depressive pseudo-dementia. . . . Social work with the elderly is not infrequently characterized as "filling in application forms for old people's homes" and is seen as a waste of the qualified caseworker's skills. Untrained part-timers, lacking in assessment skills, may be little better equipped to make appropriate judgements than the relatives and therefore may make the same unfortunate assumptions. . . . [Once in geriatric hospitals] those patients who have recovered from emotional disorders, or who have only mild dementias, are acutely aware of the interpersonal environment. To be intellectually and emotionally sound but confined to the company, 24 hours a day, of the doubly incontinent and the incoherent, the intractably restless and the confused, the socially and sexually disinhibited—is an appalling prospect. The possibilities for these patients of sustaining a recovery from an emotional disorder, in such an environment, are limited, and the consequent relapses ensure their continued confinement. Such patients may rapidly take on the characteristics of their demented fellows—becoming understandably apathetic, withdrawn, neglecting personal hygiene and apparel and even showing temporal and personal disorientation as a result of under-stimulation and poor concentration. . . . Eventually the patient is accepted as "permanent" and the final, possibly fatal, misconception is complete.'

In order to prevent such misplacement and distressing deterioration Raymond Jack presents the following recommendations:

1. *A more flexible approach to the use of residential facilities,* providing for intermittent short stays, often in conjunction with day care and more intensive domiciliary services. (Including Community Nurses—Author.)

2. *Marital counselling* may frequently be required to alleviate the unhappiness of marital disharmony in later life. The disinhibiting effects of strokes or early dementing processes in one partner, can release hostility and aggression in the other. Soon the whole range of emotional sequelae may be exhibited by both partners. The afflicted partner may become uncharacteristically withdrawn, aggressive or violent, sometimes depressed. The spouse will be puzzled,

alarmed and may in her turn, become depressed and resentful at the apparent betrayal of a long relationship previously believed to be mutually satisfying.

The death of a supportive spouse may cause depression or anxiety so great that the client may be unjustifiably institutionalized for the rest of her life.

Once such a dependent person is being cared for in a safe place, he or she loses any claim to priority placement in a home for the elderly, or in a sheltered housing scheme.

Soon negative identification results in deterioration and permanent confinement.

3.   Nurses should be constantly aware of the differing cognitive capabilities of their patients. They should avoid relating to all as though they were demented and lacking in awareness of their physical and relational environments. In the long-term, nursing skills of perception, assessment and relationship involvement provide the most 'dynamic' psychiatric *assessment* and *evaluation* of patients' cognitive status. (The nurses of 'The Crabbit Old Woman' must surely have misjudged her cognitive abilities.)

4.   Area resource panels:

'Multi-disciplinary groups composed of medical, nursing and social service personnel, meeting on a monthly basis, can ensure a unified, consistent approach to the changing needs of the particular client, helping to avoid the destructive last minute scramble for inappropriate institutionalization whenever a life crisis occurs.'

Permanent care

Residential care of the aged is, however, sometimes still unavoidable due to poverty, frailty or rejection by the family.

The essence of such institutional care is the maintenance of *individuality, dignity* and a *sense of usefullness*, which is almost impossible to provide in a large institution. Hence the praiseworthy movements towards smaller residential units. Smaller unit 'homes' allow residents to participate in routine activities such as gardening, cooking, etc.

Occupational therapy, in accordance with goals which the resident *can* fulfil, provides opportunities for satisfying creativity, compensating for prowess now lost. Activities should, however, be based on familiar skills.

The importance of active participation by the elderly (and indeed staff members) in creativity was emphasized in the 'Art in Hospitals' Conference conducted under the auspices of the Edgar Wood Centre, City of Manchester College of Higher Education, 16 and 17 December 1981.

Stimulated by the voluntary participation of artists in a wide spectrum of creativity, this conference exhibition presented evidence that:

Murals bring character and identity to featureless areas of institutions and help patients and staff to recognize their own creativity through involvement and participation.

The 'flying shuttle' brings textiles and crafts to the patients on a colourful trolley relieving stress and boredom as patients learn to master, for example, macramé, patchwork, weaving, spinning and rugmaking, in individual or group activity.

The performing arts are covered by visiting groups, classical ensembles, poetry reading, mime groups, folk and old-time singing.

Puppetry: simple glove puppets, junk puppets, rod and shadow puppets made by the team and residents, are fun to make, therapeutic and informative. Puppets as a medium of communication, catharsis, creativity and satisfaction are certainly not only for children:

'The Hospital Arts Team have brought a number of advantages to the Manchester Area Health Authority. First, and most obvious, the environment has been immensely improved, is less forbidding, more welcoming and interesting, and the staff and patients are interested in the transformation so that the vitality of the whole organization is increased. Secondly, the Arts Team responds to the raison d'être of the organization, eg stimulus given to health education and work concentrating on nostalgia in the Unit for the Elderly.

One volunteer had been concerned that the elderly people, when discussing 'Constable' and his trees, mentioned that they had not been out of the hospital for years, and so it was arranged that a group of them should be taken out to sketch scenes of trees and rivers. This took a great deal of organization with many volunteers. They have also visited Art Galleries using an ambulance with hydraulic lift.'

In attending this conference the author was impressed by the planners' realization that, although now old and frail, *residents differ widely in intelligence, education and cultural background*. To impose simple childlike and unsophisticated tasks and entertainment indiscriminately upon one and all is to risk hurt, diminishment and proud withdrawal.

Occupational therapy, in accordance with goals which the resident *can* fulfil, provides opportunities for satisfying creativity, substituting for prowess now lost. For those who are more cerebrally impaired, however, activities should be based on familiar skills.

Jennifer Moodie, OT at the Highlands Jewish Aged Home, recommends:

'Recreation in the form of simple adapted group games is an important part of an activity programme, being especially advantageous in the stimulation of withdrawn residents. Games use a combination of visual and auditory stimuli with maximum resident participation. Colours, shapes, numbers, words and pictures, dice and ball throwing, and music with hand clapping and singing are all enjoyed, and competitive involvement is encouraged by team games and the use of prizes.'

Reminiscence group psychotherapy with institutionalized cognitively impaired older adults*

On the premise that group psychotherapy has rarely been examined systematically in long-term chronic care settings, Frima Christopher PhD and Herbert H Zaretsky, PhD, Psychology Service, Department of Rehabilitation Medicine, New York University Medical Centre, Goldwater Memorial Hospital, investigated

* Based on a paper presented at the 94th Convention of the American Psychological Association, Washington DC, August 1986.

'sixty-five adults, aged 60 years and older, in a long-term rehabilitation hospital and skilled nursing facility, who had been diagnosed as having organic brain syndrome (OBS). Participants were classified into mild, moderate, and severe levels of OBS via the administration of the Mental Status Questionnaire and were then randomly assigned to one of two group treatment conditions, Reminiscence Psychotherapy Group or a Leisure Group. The groups were otherwise heterogeneous in terms of gender, ethnicity, socio-economic status, and length of hospitalization. Each treatment group consisted of two, one-hour sessions per week for a total of 45 sessions. Measurements of orientation, memory, depression, and functional independence were taken at three points in time (pre-treatment, post-treatment, and three months following treatment).'

Example of awareness procedure

Mrs Jones I have brought you something nice to eat.
Do you know what it is? Yes, it's an apple. You had stewed apple for lunch today.
Did you eat apples when you were a little girl?
Do you remember how they looked?
Let's draw them.
Do you remember how your mother cooked apples—do tell us about it.
Did she cook them any special way at Christmas [or at Passover]?
Do you remember how long she cooked them?
Tell about the times you ate apples at picnics.
Let's make apples from this coloured plasticine.
Did your husband like apples?
How did you cook them?
And your children—how many apples did you cook for them?
Did you cut them in half?
How long did you cook them?
Did they like apples sweet or sour?
Would you like honey with this apple? etc.

Sometimes photos or video tapes were used to stimulate memories and set the client in time and space. By regressing to the more deeply traced, and emotionally provocative, memories of youth the investigators hoped to recall and activate familiar, well-learnt concepts and apply them in the present.

Results

Some clear trends could be identified as worthy of discussion and endorsing the value of group psychotherapy with this population.

1.   Reminiscence was more helpful than psycho-social discussion.
2.   All the patients demonstrated some behavioural improvements. These included reduction in attention deficits, increased alertness, increased ability to interact appropriately within the group, reduced destructive acting out behaviours, and more appropriate mood presentation.
3.   Orientation, memory and functional independence improved and depression decreased in each treatment group.

It is essential that a home provides for *flexibility and personal preferences* in rising, going to bed, outings, etc, as well as, of course, for privacy in rooms, flatlets, etc. More supervised routine care, where unavoidable, should be reserved for the hospital or infirmary unit, and even here with maximum emphasis on independence and dignity rather than safety restrictions and personal diminishment.

Occasionally one comes across a residential facility gone crazy on security . . . or is it the insecurity of the staff? In one home, laudable for its material facilities, on admission of both the able-bodied and the frail, their belongings were inspected and catalogued by the matron or sister. All valuable possessions are receipted and removed to the office for safekeeping. It is difficult to imagine anything more diminishing; or heartbreaking than invasion into one's possessions and removal of status symbols and loved objects of sentimental value. Surely the time comes for a more meaningful 'risk' philosophy! In addition, too much talk of safety precautions may stimulate latent paranoic ideas.

At all costs, *one should avoid the large institution where senior citizens are forced into a routine designed for convenience of administration rather than a dignified personal life*. It is pathetic to see 'tranquillized' residents 'tucked up in bed' as if they were children, in order to facilitate staff routines.

Younger people are often surprised to learn of the sexual needs of the aged. In fact, because old age reduces inhibition and self-control, the *sexual needs* of the aged are often very apparent—especially the more overt sexual needs of the male.

Sexual intercourse may well continue into the eighties. It hardly seems necessary to stress that all residents should be provided with the privacy of their own bedrooms—double-room units being provided for couples. (See Sexual Needs of the Aged, p 459.)

Dearth of *tactile comfort* through the loss of marriage partners, even through the absence of children and grandchildren, constitutes sad deprivation to the geriatric patient. It is for this reason that some progressive residential care centres provide physio-therapeutic programmes for their residents. There is a a laudable move away from 'single' to more flexible 'dual sex' facilities. *Interest in the other sex proves an effective stimulant to the motivation to survive.*

Forced separation due to disproportionate deterioration in one partner is both cruel and detrimental to motivation to survive. Flexibility in care remains fundamental.

Separation from loving pets certainly adds to the burdens and trauma of institutionalization. Avoidance of this sorrow certainly justifies appropriate administrative provision. (See Pets and the Aged, p 460.)

The nurse who is at ease in putting her arm around her patient, holding his hand, or performing procedures with affectionate warmth, is of particular value in the geriatric unit.

'Residential homes often place heavy constraints on the emergence of loving relationships between residents, between staff and residents, and between residents and members of the local community. Indeed, the organizational and physical framework of the home may be designed to prevent them from arising. On the other hand, in the most mature residential centres, a wide variety of relationships may be encouraged.

Unfortunately, not every resident has a family member to whom he or she may relate; not every resident is able to find and sustain a satisfying relationship with someone outside the home. Some residents may be so unattractive, damaged or damaging that, without considerable help, they are unlikely ever to engage in the warm relationships aspired to by most human beings. Yet, life is so arranged that we cannot do without loving and being loved.'

It hardly seems necessary to advise that *family visits and participation in residential life should be encouraged* and facilitated by free, open visiting arrangements.

Very often visitors themselves require guidance and support for

'the role of the visitor is not easy, and we often underestimate the difficulties faced by relatives or friends when visiting in residential establishments. In many instances they are really confronted with the question: "What do you say after you've said hello?" It is unnatural for some people to sit formally for an hour or so, perhaps in a massive lounge with a crowd of other people. It may feel strange to discuss very personal matters in a vacuum and away from the cut and thrust of their day to day shared environment and common experiences.'*

The geriatric ward

The relatively long-term and chronic nature of the diseases here presented renders specially important the *personalized psychological approach in ward administration*.

The infusion of a *sense of being wanted, of relative self-sufficiency, of physical and emotional well-being* are usually of greater import than complicated technical nursing procedures.

There is a special place here for the nurse whose academic potential is limited, but who is content to spend time, effort and personal involvement on routine procedures. The nurse who spends time 'doing' the patient's hair, her face, on bathing and talking to her patient is of special value and should not be harried by the necessity for completing routine semi-domestic chores within the ward. In fact, here, especially, *flexibility in ward routine*, and above all, welcoming and encouraging visitors at any time convenient to themselves, are of primary importance.

A danger in nursing the aged consists in unconsciously encouraging *regression* by doing too much for them: 'Nobody needed me—now I want every one to need me!'' (It is important that the student re-read pages 121-130.)

The nurse who has been unconsciously motivated into her career by a need to have people dependent upon her, perhaps as a compensation adjustment resultant upon feelings of childhood rejection, should be guided into a realization of this motivation. She should realize the necessity for avoiding that regression which may well lead her patient into a permanently dependent state.

There appears to be a retrogressive *tendency to substitute mechanical devices for personalized routine nursing*. Routine catheterization and enemata are frequently utilized rather than bottle and bed pan 'rounds', and astute bedside observation; feeding-tubes are substituted for personalized cup and spoon feeding.

---

* Leonard Davis 'As in Life.' *Senior News* Vol 16 No 1.

Especially in the case of the geriatric patient, this is a policy fraught with long-term and serious psychosomatic complications. The integrity of natural and independent body processes should be safeguarded.

Old people find it very difficult to adjust to change: body processes unused soon become atrophied, and one frequently encounters distressing case histories of patients 'temporarily' catheterized during illness, who are rendered permanently bladder-incontinent due to *loss of tonus* which cannot be regained. Within the context of illness and medication a geriatric patient may well become temporarily partly incontinent, *returning to continence provided natural processes have been preserved.*

It is difficult to believe that, given reasonably efficient, patient and conscientious nursing, a patient will develop bedsores during a relatively short illness. The use of continuous catheterization under these circumstances would appear, very frequently, to constitute a rationalization for easing or speeding nursing duties.

Deprivation of the patient's independent functions soon leads to regression—he becomes more and more infantile in his body patterns, losing the motivation for return to the integrity of independence. As regression spreads, his physical and mental processes atrophy; depression and even death may intervene.

Of special importance is the *emotional distress* suffered by geriatric patients exposed to the *introduction of foreign objects*—metal, plastic, rubber, etc—into their bodies. Their deteriorating cerebral processes, impeded further by medication, delirium, etc, result in *traumatic delusions and hallucinations*, which often constitute a most painful and distressing experience. It is not unusual for geriatric patients to interpret catheters as 'burning, red-hot pokers', enemata as 'menacing guns', etc. In addition, enlarged prostrate glands result in constricted apertures, discomfort and pain. In an attempt to relieve this agony, the geriatric patient may try to remove tubes, etc. To prevent this his hands are tied, he is heavily sedated, and well on the way to a permanently vegetative and confused state.

Careful and intelligent observation of the geriatric patient subjected to mechanical devices frequently reveals psychosomatic complications and physical suffering quite out of proportion to the nursing convenience provided by the devices. He is burdened by loss of independence, humiliation, fear, acute physical discomfort, pain and frequent terrifying delusions and hallucinations.

Realization of the serious implications of inserting mechanical devices should render the decision to institute such treatment a serious one, constituting a 'last resort' rather than a routine treatment, and warranting concerted team discussion. The same would apply to establishing the justification for introducing continuous catheterization as a means of 'intake–output' measurement in preventing pneumonia or restricting patients in cots and under nets.

Food and the geriatric patient

Food is one of the few reliable pleasures which can still be enjoyed by the geriatric patient. In the welter of personal and environmental deprivations to which he is exposed, here is one thing he can still enjoy—provided he has the financial means for so doing, and the food is prepared in an appropriate manner. Individual choice is, of course, of primary importance.

Apart from his need of especially nutrient intake, psychologically food gives him that pleasurable mouth activity which is *associated, from the earliest hours of his mother–child relationship, with mother-love, safety and security*

Here, at least, is a piece of precious, but now departed, mother-love association—proof that he is still loved and wanted; a source of loving comfort.

Frequency of eating, and thus mouth activity, constitutes an important individual need. Many patients are greatly comforted by the opportunity for long-term and frequent eating provided by snacks, sweets, etc.

To quote from Student Nurse Jill Brawley's prizewinning Johnson & Johnson article, 'The Aged Require Attention' (*Curationis* March 1983):

'The most degrading experience is to have everyday natural things done for you. One such example is feeding—the older person can be slow when it comes to eating and often it is assumed that all people of the same age are similar (lack of individuality). Consequently, some nurses go around cutting everyone's food or quickly wiping each bit that misses the mouth. This emphasizes the patient's incapability to everyone else. How degrading to have your neighbour think that you are either a fool or an invalid! People tend to generalize; if the patient is unable to do something physically there must be something wrong psychologically as well.'

Some special problems encountered in geriatric nursing

A basic problem in ward administration consists in the necessity for *distinguishing between patients' delusions and hallucinations and the reality situation.*

Did the nurse fail to give the patient lunch, or is this a time-distinction delusion associated with classic fall-off of recent memory?

Is a nurse inconsiderate and rough in handling procedures, or is this a hallucination resultant upon the patient's tendency towards paranoia?

Clearly *each complaint calls for tactful investigation*—bias towards patient or nurse should be carefully avoided. Especially is this true in the supervision of less intellectually endowed *nurse-aids* who encounter real *difficulty in accepting the involuntary etiology* of patients' failure to co-operate. Such nurses tend towards a simple but dangerous philosophy of punitive patient handling, believing that the patient should be 'taught a lesson'.

In addition, frequently imposed upon by others, they are quick, albeit unconsciously, to *displace* their aggression on weaker patient-figures, thus indirectly achieving status *compensation*.

In fact one of the difficulties encountered in supervising the less intellectually endowed nurse-aid is the correction of her tendency to get involved in personal squabbles with her patient in her efforts to 'establish [her] rights'.

Nevertheless, as stated above, wisely supervised, she finds considerable valuable 'common ground' with her senile patient.

The intelligent *student nurse* also presents with special difficulties in geriatric nursing. Feeling herself far removed from the aged, she encounters real *difficulty in identifying* with them.

Experiencing difficulty in 'putting herself in their shoes', she loses patience with her aged patients, taking their accusations seriously, personally and with annoyance. Finding the work unchallenging and aesthetically displeasing she certainly requires more mature senior staff interpretation, deeper level understanding, emotional-level support and opportunity for catharsis. Her very resentment of her patients, perhaps even her fear of the ageing process, disturb her self-concept and implant *feelings of guilt, anxiety and, perhaps, avoidance.*

Quite often an elderly patient, his appearance, the way he speaks, the sacrifices his condition demands, *link back to long forgotten associations in the nurse's own unconscious mind.* He might remind her of a disliked relation, or an unkind teacher. Involuntarily she finds herself disliking the patient, avoiding him, resenting nursing procedures. Her sense of guilt (illogical as it may be) makes her anxious and unhappy, and she may become quite disturbed should her unconscious wish for his death be fulfilled. The manner in which guilt and anxiety may be *converted* into psychosomatic symptoms is described in the case study reported on page 126. Nurses should be helped to understand, and accept without anxiety, their *ambivalent feelings* towards their patients.

The geriatric team—and this includes social workers, occupational therapists, physiotherapists, nurses, the patient and his family—tries to *motivate towards relative independence and physical integrity,* or at least, towards some form of *happy adaptation.* Each day should provide something special for which it is worth while making the effort to survive.

Much enlightened motivation is undone by nurses who, *in their anxiety to avoid 'blameworthiness' for neglecting safety precautions, and perhaps to offset their own guilt feelings, stifle independence by imposing a network of diminishing restrictions. These can result only in regression to childish helplessness or childish anger.*

'It often appears that life in residential settings is following different rules from those which apply outside. [The stories one hears] suggest that walking into a residential establishment is like passing through a gateway into an alternative universe, operating on different principles. ... One problem for the newly admitted resident must be having to "ask permission" ... permission to do things which only a few weeks or days before, he may have had entirely within his own control; about going out, about coming in, about making a telephone call, about smoking or about his inviting a friend into his bedroom.'*

Rules are usually established to protect the staff. Necessity for rules is proportionate to the stresses imposed upon staff by poor management-communication, inadequate finances, under-staffing and poor training of senior members. Staff interactions based on *power* stimulate within residents the only reciprocal 'fight' responses available to them—*active defiance, or passive regression* to utter helplessness, with the additional staff labour resultant thereupon.

Safety restrictions should take into account that many elderly persons, and indeed their families, would prefer that, at their advanced age, they *take a risk rather than be reduced to the indignity of childish dependence.* There is a strong case for team decisions, including the resident and his family, to *avoid the imposition of safety precautions which stifle, restrict and diminish.*

* Boards and Staff: Sharing the Responsibilities.' *Senior News,* Vol 10 No 1

It is sometimes difficult to impress upon the nursing staff the fact that little pleasures should take precedence over many ward routines.

Familial visits, something especially nice to eat, a film or TV show, the visit of a concert party, outdoor excursions, a beauty treatment, a ward sing-song 'social' or dance, should all be encouraged. *It may well be that her ingenuity, her warmth, her flexibility, her ability to identify with her patients, constitute important ingredients of that general cheerfulness that her work demands of the geriatric nurse.*

Attitudes of the staff, medical, nursing, ancillary, domestic and catering, to elderly residents may leave room for a great deal of improvement. Often decrepit, dejected, disillusioned residents, sitting vacantly staring into space waiting for the inevitable and wishing for the end, are to be seen in homes for the aged. The emotional and psychological needs of residents must be understood and met by not only all staff members working as a team, but by residents, visitors and voluntary organizations all co-operating in providing a stimulating, congenial and happy atmosphere.

In order to achieve a change in attitude it is therefore essential that the staff of homes be encouraged to enrol for a training course . . . especially 'untrained' junior staff.

Summary

The *'senior'* client needs new amended goals which he can fulfil, a feeling of importance and being wanted. Supported and encouraged by the multidisciplinary team, and introduced to community services, he may be *motivated* to a reasonably purposeful and happy life.

Through using nursing procedures in order to talk to her patient, to establish a friendly relationship, the *nurse may show that someone cares, someone wants him to get better, to go on living.* She should try to make her relationship a sample of a better world for which it is worth making the effort to get back into the swing of life. *Identifying* with *her* youth, *her* confidence, *her* hopefulness, he may be motivated to take her hand and cross back over the bridge of life.

Rights of the elderly in nursing homes

The following *Bill of Rights for the Aged* has been endorsed by the Private Hospitals and Nursing Homes Association of Australia, Ltd.*

1. Every resident is an individual to be treated with respect, and should be accepted as he/she is.
2. The resident has the right to quality of excellence in care, environment, furnishings, food and activities, and the home should maintain this standard.
3. The resident's right to privacy must be respected in room, bath, records, personal possessions and relationships. There should be freedom for the residents to choose and pursue companionship with their own or opposite sex, without fear, criticism and censure from staff or other residents.
4. The resident's family should feel welcome at the home and become part of it by visiting and participating in the activities (subject to nursing regulations).

* *Senior News*, March 1980

5. The resident should be encouraged to do as much as possible for him or herself as long as he/she is able.
6. The resident has a right to rehabilitation and resocialization programmes that emphasizes his or her abilities. The resident has the opportunity and responsibility to avail him or herself of these offered programmes.
7. The rationale behind necessary examinations, medical care and in-house changes in both schedule and accommodations should be explained to the resident, consistent with his/her comprehension. The resident also has a right to know medications by name and effect; he or she has a right to refuse treatment and, if desired, should know about his or her condition.
8. The resident has the right to know in advance what appointments have been made or changed, and when and where the physicians are available.
9. The resident has the right to know the home rules and regulations which should include a vehicle for involvement in the decisions that concern his welfare and functioning.
10. The resident should receive all messages or phone calls left for him, and receive and send mail uncensored.
11. The resident has the right to manage his own finances and to examine and receive an explanation of his monthly fee for services.
12. An evaluation of relationship between a resident and a staff member may be made, if there is ongoing friction.
13. The resident is entitled to life, love, moral support and comfort from staff, family and friends.
14. The resident has a right to die with dignity, with strength, with courage and in peace.

Abuse of the elderly

Reporting on 'Granny bashing' at the International Congress on the Elderly (London, 1983) the organisation 'Age Concern' submitted that 500 000 elderly people are at risk in the United Kingdom. Abuse includes physical assault, forced medication, locking away, abandonment in hospital, financial exploitation, sexual abuse, and a wide range of psychological abuse.

Causes

1. Owing to physiological deterioration, confusion, paranoia, etc, some old people involuntarily precipitate frustration and aggression in those who care for them.
2. The lifestyle of the care-giver may render her particularly vulnerable. Precipitating factors include divorce, unemployment, responsibility for additional dependent or handicapped family members. In such circumstances the aged person may become the substitute object of displaced aggression.
3. There is a direct relationship between the extent of dependence and the risk of abuse.
4. Role reversal—There is increased risk where the care-giver has herself previously been abused by the aged person and is now, albeit unconsciously, 'getting her own back'.
5. Cramped housing with little privacy.

Presentation and warning signs

A history of falls, bruises and a care-giver who herself spends a lot of time with her GP, often for psychosomatic symptoms.

Nagging behaviour on the part of either party.

Incontinence.

The aged person is afraid to show anger or to criticize, and is frequently depressed.

Low self-esteem on the part of the care-giver, who reports that whatever she does for the aged person is never good enough.

'Other people's daughters are always better.'

Unemployment and hardship, especially a shortage of food.

Inadequate emotional support for the care-giver herself.

Solution

Involvement of a multi-disciplinary team for support of both key family members.

Specific training for professionals.

Identification of patient and care-giver at risk (nurses should realize that guilt feelings and anxiety may inhibit verbalization of difficulties).

Counselling the family.

Information of available community services.

Support groups.* (See p 613.)

* From a report-back lecture by Pat Meyer, 1983.

CHAPTER 21

EMOTIONAL REACTION TO ILLNESS: PAIN—SLEEP

'Caring is a state of mind, not additional work.'*

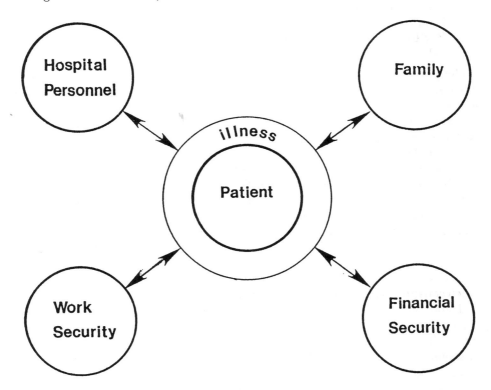

The fragmented world of the Patient

It will help the nurse identify with her patient if she understands the following COMMON REACTIONS TO ILLNESS:

1. *The patient sees his unknown future as endangered*—what suffering, loss of body image and efficiency, financial stress lie ahead?

Frequently for the first time he faces the reality of his own death.

His dreams, ambitions, hopes of fulfilment formerly taken for granted now drift out of reach. Maybe he has no future at all. Only disintegration.

2. *There is a splitting-off or estrangement between the individual and his own body,* the

---

* Wisser, Susan Hiscoe: 'When the Walls listened American.' *Journal of Nursing* **78**(6).

control of which he had always taken for granted. Now this control passes to a disease, an injury. In succumbing to a germ, a spinal injury, a cancer, his body has let him down, abandoned him.

> 'For five bitter years, satirist Adam Leslie ferociously fought illness.
> But he lost the battle.
> He died this week at the age of 62.
> Only a few months before his death he raged against his "traitorous old body" which he felt was letting him down when he needed it most.
> "There is nothing wrong with my mind," he said.
> "I am much wiser now than ever before and full of ideas for the theatre."
> "But I am trapped inside a body I cannot control." '*
> 'What will my body do to me next?'

The patient feels simultaneously angry and guilty as his body is reduced to dependence on others—it is felt, handled, investigated, listened to by those who now govern it.

3. *He is suspended in a timeless limbo* of inactivity, anger, guilt and fear. His very existence becomes simultaneously temporary and endlessly empty. Frightened by his future, he broods about the past and mourns the unknown future.

4. *The barriers are up* between healthy, independent, purposeful and busy family, friends and staff and the patient whose life is limited to the area of his bed. The 'gap' between himself and healthy people increases as he becomes preoccupied with his sickness, his symptoms—his temperature, his blood pressure. Pathology reports, medication, bowel movements which dominate his thinking and control his life are of no consequence to the healthy people who surround him. In isolation, his terror, depression and anger increase. Cut off from normal environmental stimulation, from reciprocal human relationships and confined in the sterile goldfish bowl which constitutes the hospital ward, he becomes obsessed with his body symptoms, food and the deprivation which diet brings; with the unpleasant habits of his ward-mates, the lack of concern and compassion (real or imagined) of the staff. He may well rally his resources to defend his body against what he feels to be the 'onslaught of' surgery and other procedures.

5. In sickness, *frustration of work and study output* constitutes a serious frustration to the ambitious person and the family breadwinner. Frequently justifiably, he fears that competitors will expose his shortcomings, block his promotion, even show him to be redundant. The self-employed professional or company director fears, sometimes justifiably, that his practice or business may suffer irretrievably. A sense of worthlessness or panic spreads into all aspects of his life, financial, social, sexual.

6. *The sick or injured person suffers role reversal.* From being the powerful breadwinner, the controlling family and businessman, he becomes the dependent, tolerated, powerless, even despised receiver. The marital role may be reversed so that his wife, albeit unwillingly, becomes the dominant breadwinner; his children become physically dominant, financially powerful custodians, while he is subjected to the obedient and compliant child role. He may well be subjected to the ultimate humiliation of being fed, washed, and even handled by others in basic bodily

---

* McIntyre, Gordon. *Sunday Times,* 29 April 1979.

functions. *Thus diminished to a piece of suffering flesh, he becomes rebellious, resentful, depressed and, in accordance with his lifelong pattern, resorts to classic defence mechanisms* such as:

> *denial,* rejecting his sickness, refusing diagnostic and therapeutic procedures and demanding discharge (this especially in 'proud' people),
> *introjection* of the expected sick and helpless role
> *regression* to childish dependence, demanding that everything be done for him, to amuse him, to continuously comfort him,

He may resort to childish unreasonableness and fault-finding; *aggression* or *passive resistance* such as refusal to eat, to participate in physiotherapy or occupational therapy, in social intercourse. It is important that his pride in self be built up rather than diminished. *Whatever his reaction, the patient is not a child.*

Post-anaesthetic confusion or 'delirium' is largely resultant upon the temporary toxic effect of anaesthetic agents especially upon a brain rendered vulnerable by old age, alcoholism, drug addiction; underlying predisposition to schizophrenia or depression, and organic pathology such as cardiovascular abnormalities, and infections especially where operations are of longer than four hours' duration.

Women appear to be more vulnerable than men. Because she returns (sometimes precipitously) *to her pre-operative state,* a terrified patient may well return to consciousness in panic, aggravated by her physiological ordeal and possibly mutilated body-image.

This observation, consistent with higher incidence of post-operative 'delirium' in emergency surgery, emphasizes necessity for *effective pre-operative emotional-level reassurance* (unlikely when 'prepping' is allotted to untrained personnel) *and a positive supportive relationship not only as between patient and nurse but very emphatically as between the patient and her surgeon who holds the knife.* Specific agreement on the extent of surgery, and appropriate definition on the 'consent form', are basic to pre-operative confidence.

'What have they done to me?' is the panic query with which, even in the context of a sound surgeon–patient relationship, the frightened patient frequently returns to consciousness.

Many patients would prefer the inconvenience (and slight risk) of a second anaesthetic, to unexpected mutilaton and permanent impairment of quality of life. Some may wish to obtain a second opinion (p 81).

Gillis points out that 'amputations, hysterectomies and mastectomies . . . cause disturbance of the body-image which requires considerable psychological adaptation'. * And that's putting it mildly'!

---

* Gillis, L. *Guidelines in Psychiatry.* David Philip (1978).

A summary of mental mechanisms and other patient reactions to illness appears on page 125.

Pain, being essential in nature's warning system, is intrinsic to man.

It can never be eliminated. In fact were it thus, we could never rejoice with Rupert Brooke at 'body's pain soon turned to peace again'.*

Some pain in illness, injury or childbirth is almost inevitable.

None of us can ever know how pain feels to another: nor can we know exactly how the patient feels about his suffering.

Some mothers are ambivalent about the whole matter of producing a particular baby, and may well express illogical, but none the less potent, feelings of anger and hostility towards the baby, the father and everybody else concerned in the whole matter of delivery. Above all, it is necessary to *avoid the imposition of complicating guilt feelings,* which, by increasing anxiety and tension, will increase pain.

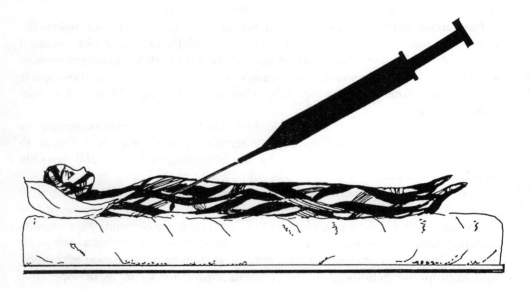

The most frightening aspect of pain being the 'unknown', *explanation and reassurance* can do much to prevent the establishment of the Fear–Pain cycle:†

---

* Brooke, Rupert: The Great Lover.

† Pain — from an illustrated slide presented by Dame Cicely Saunders (see p 556)

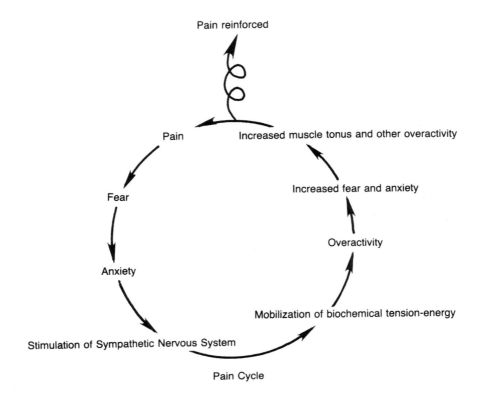

Pain Cycle

Because each individual has his or her *own 'built-in' threshold of pain*, each will vary as to the point at which pain–distress is expressed. In fact, even individual reactions to pain will vary from time to time with competing environmental stressors, conscious or unconscious emotional reactions thereto, general physical condition, etc.

There are certainly physiological bases to varying susceptibility to pain. In his *Textbook of Clinical Neurology* (pp 103-9), David Wechsler points out that the sensory effect of pain is determined by the patient's own individual patterns of sense organs, the number per square centimetre of active sensory nerve fibres, cerebral pain-centre sensitivity, the number and frequency of pain impulses reaching the parietal lobe.

The patient's involuntary reactions to these pain sensations are of course much affected by the intensity or sluggishness of his sympathetic nervous system.

There are various complicated instruments for measuring pain, such as the esthesiometer, algesimeter and algometer.

A person's threshold of, and reaction to, deep-pressure pain can be assessed by compressing (or pinching) a muscle or tendon, or by over-extending the joints of the digits.

An algometer, with a spring which registers deep pressure exerted in terms of pounds, shows a wide variation in the amount of pressure required to elicit a painful reaction in each individual. Similar variations in levels of painful response can be measured by the temperature at which a patient experiences discomfort to a test-tube filled with very cold or very hot water—here degrees Celsius measure the widely varying level at which pain is first perceived in the parietal lobe.

There is thus *nothing praiseworthy nor blameworthy in a patient's capacity to bear pain*—rather is this dependent on his own individual anatomical, neurological and biochemical structure. However much we may want to share it, pain remains the patient's own suffering. It cannot be avoided, sensorily shared, or the fact of its existence denied.

To understand our own primitive reactions to pain, it is helpful to consider pain-expression in a young baby, whose response thereto is *generalized throughout her body*. Her pain-twisted face, thrashing limbs, writhing body suggest that she is trapped in a small world of nothing but pain. Only later, with increased maturity, does pain-reception and recognition specialize out to specific body parts.

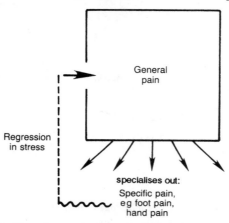

The perceptual disturbances of pain include time perception.

For most people, with individual variations,

the personal past is unchangeable history, tinged perhaps by feelings of remorse and guilt.

The present is limited to present activity.

The future is still to come—its horizons, containing one's expectations, one's hopes.

But where pain predominates, strangling the present, cutting off or blocking the future, then we regress to the guilt, remorse and despair of the past.

In keeping with that search for tension-relief, mother love, safety and security which we know to exist in the mental mechanism of *regression*, the older child, adult, geratric and obstetric patient in pain *unconsciously* regresses to earlier, helpless, all-engulfing generalized pain, and corresponding behaviour. This behaviour pattern did, in the past, bring tension-relief and comfort through direct generalized 'all-over' protest—both physical and verbal.

So in understanding its etiology we should accept without censure, even perhaps welcome, the patient's attempt to find tension outlet and comfort; to *externalize* her pain in the *direct* physical activity of random movements, in crying out, in weeping. Above all we should *not impose feelings of guilt or shame,* thus increasing, via the SNS, biochemical tension, and the intensity and duration of pain; nor force upon the patient that *inhibition which both entraps tension outlet and denies* her that emotional reassurance and supporting comfort which she needs.

We have seen how patients attempt to cope with the tension-fraught pain situation by *introjecting* or unconsciously taking unto themselves those patterns of tension release which, during their formative years, constituted an important part of their individual environment. Thus some patients 'take' pain quietly with a 'stiff upper lip'. Some express their hostility, fear and anger verbally; others physically, in resisting, aggressive, demanding behaviour. No one is a 'good' or a 'bad' patient: all are merely introjecting patients.

Sometimes, to spare her own feelings, the nurse concentrates on *persuading the patient to stop showing pain*—she might even persuade the patient's husband or mother to withdraw from her side 'because she makes more fuss when you are here'. But, in so doing, she:

(a) *denies* the patient the tension outlet, comfort, support and reassurance embodied in someone with whom she has *long, deeply-established associations* of comfort and confidence. To hold the familiar hand of a husband or mother one has long loved and trusted is often more *emotionally comforting* and reassuring than the learned, eloquent, intellectual reassurance of the most eminent surgeon,

(b) *is imperilling all-important human relationships* by allowing the patient to feel, at an emotional level, that her loved ones are abandoning her in her time of need, and so denying their concern and love;

(c) is denying the loving husband or parent the satisfaction which comes with being needed and relied upon, being able to love, comfort and support. For *pain*, like pleasure *shared, can be an enriching human experience.*

(d) fails to realize that a patient who externalizes her pain is more likely to get over it sooner, and will suffer *less long-term psychological trauma*, than one in whom entrapped pain causes festering resentment and anxiety.

We, as adults, often ask children to adopt our pattern of handling pain, e g 'You mustn't cry—big girls don't cry'. In so doing we are burdening them with a code of behaviour for which they are not ready. If they try to act in this developmentally inappropriate way, they will be caught in the additional conflict between fear of pain on the one hand, and the superimposed fear of cowardice and disapproval on the other.

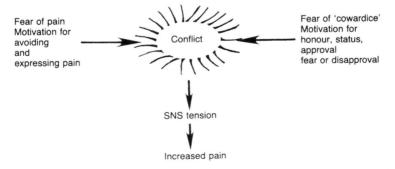

Fear of pain
Motivation for
avoiding
and
expressing pain

Conflict

Fear of 'cowardice'
Motivation for
honour, status,
approval
fear or disapproval

SNS tension

Increased pain

To lie that pain does not hurt, or will not hurt for long, may serve only to deceive the patient, causing confusion, frustration and distrust. The truth may hurt less. <u>The nurse who admits to pain and its distress; who reassures her patient that she is 'standing by her', sharing and identifying herself in her ordeal, endorses and fulfils her professional obligation.</u>

Psychogenic pain, if it exists at all without real organic pathology, is very rare. Psychological factors may lower the pain threshold.

Investigatory procedures, frightening case-conferences, exhaustion, may well cause painful exaggeration of present organic symptoms. Sometimes relief of conscious or unconscious familial, sexual, financial or other anxieties, may reduce aggravated pain. Psychogenic pain overlay within the context of a longstanding pain-reactive pattern may sometimes be distinguished by non-anatomical, flitting distribution—vague 'headaches', 'loss of memory', 'tingling sensations', etc.

All pain symptoms, irrespective of etiology, constitute suffering and warrant careful team investigation.

TELL ME ABOUT YOUR PAIN (*or pruritis or nausea*)

How does the patient perceive his pain?
What does it do to his life? When is it worse?
Does he suffer more in the loneliness of night?

Certainly the patient himself, and his priorities, should be included in his pain control programme.

Psychologial mechanisms for coping with pain

1. Generally, but especially in antenatal preparation, the patient should be 'conditioned' away from the idea of 'coming out', tensed up, to meet her pain, but rather letting it *'flow over her'*.

2. *Impersonal displacement or dissociation:* The necessity to impersonalize the cause of pain is probably related to a need to relieve oneself of the *guilt associations* which are early *attached to physical suffering by punishment* and thoughtless or ignorant adults. Remarks such as 'naughty children who smack their little sisters are punished by cutting their own hands', or 'If you are naughty I will leave you in that hospital'; or, to the adolescent, 'love-making brings pain and suffering' are typical. Where a sexual connotation is present, as in child birth, it is particularly important to try to remove personal guilt from physical pain. The patient's need to 'externalize' her guilt feelings by *displacing* them on objects or other people (including nursing staff) should thus be understood and tolerated.

It is 'the book that fell on my toe' rather than 'I dropped the book on my toe'. Children seem comforted if helped to think: 'Bad table hurt Peter's foot'; 'What a naughty driver ran Mary down!'

Adults like to blame the 'rotten appendix', or, in obstetrics those 'darned' muscle fibres which are interfering with the dilatation of the cervix.

3. *Isolating or 'specializing out' pain reaction:* Even for adults pain regresses to total, all-enveloping, childlike engulfment. In children this reaction is reinforced by their own developmentally appropriate generalized pattern. Both adults and children need help in 'breaking down' pain into specific parts they can handle. Pain can

sometimes be eased if it can be located and identified as 'the burning toe', 'the aching muscle', 'the dilating cervix'.

4. *Tactile comfort:* Physical contact is the medium through which there flows, from one creature to another, warmth and comfort, an emotional level communication, which cannot be conveyed by words. See:

(i) Mother–child relationship.
(ii) Soothing effect of parasympathetic nervous system stimulation: antihistamine secretion resulting in a feeling of physiological well-being (see p 33).
(iii) Levy's puppies (see p 39).
(iv) Harlow's monkeys (see p 43).

5. *Identification* (see p 108): Some are gifted with acute sensitivity, enabling them to creep beneath the skins and into the souls of others. Often this is a matter of intelligence and imagination. Sometimes it can be acquired by devoting five minutes in each day to the exercise of pretending that one *is* a specific patient.

No doubt it is difficult for a young nurse, herself a late adolescent, to overcome her feelings of shyness and embarrassment, to achieve verbal and demonstrative comfort, reassurance and communication with her patient.

As she matures, as she herself establishes relationships outside herself—with friends, spouse, her own children—as she walks with them along the path of life, she will become less inhibited, more spontaneously outgoing, and overtly compassionate.

A youngster who instinctively achieves rapport and meaningful communication with her patient is indeed a 'born nurse'.

Dr Cicely Saunders suggests that a shy, hesitant nurse be assigned to a warm, spontaneous, outgoing patient, who will initiate and respond to tactile communication.

'Pain is only insufferable when nobody cares.'
The role of pain relief requires that the nurse 'stays with' her patient, listening, noting, comforting.

But witness of pain, the feelings of powerlessness and frustration it arouses in attendants, provokes their own frustration, anxiety, even resentment and displaced anger.

'Staying with the patient requires a deep conviction of purpose, of self-giving.'

Dr Cicely Saunders * presents impressive statistics and case histories to support her conviction that when physical and mental pain is relieved, even terminally ill patients who have previously contemplated suicide *want* to continue living fully as long as possible.

Her experience, individual monitoring, and careful scientific research indicate that within the context of

(i) *absolute regularity of medication in anticipation of pain, rather than as a result of 'relief having been earned'* by 'sticking it out', or insistence on an arbitrary degree of pain,
(ii) the application of *individualized, smaller but more frequent dosage to allow for smoother pain-free maintenance,*

---

* 'The Management of Terminal Pain'—a lecture conducted by Dr Cicely Saunder, OBE, SRRI, MRCP of St Christopher's Hospice, March 1979.

DR CICELY SAUNDERS, OBE, SRN, MB, BS, FRCP, MA(OXON), ON MANAGEMENT OF TERMINAL PAIN AND THE PROVISION OF CARING SUCCOUR FOR THE DYING AS PRACTISED BY THE HOSPICE SYSTEM, WITH PARTICULAR REFERENCE TO ST CHRISTOPHER'S*

The suffering of the dying is total—physical, emotional, social.

Hospices operate on the principle that when orthodox and active medical and surgical treatment show diminishing return for the pain and discomfort involved, they should be withdrawn, and replaced with a caring system of pain relief and emotional support.

Factors lowering the pain threshold, and thus detracting from effectiveness of analgesics, together with corresponding Hospice policy designed to counteract negative emotional experiences:

Problem	Hospice Policy
Anger	Removal of unproductive and uncomfortable apparatus, painful treatment and procedures.
	Control of pain.
	Preservation of dignity, self-decision and freedom of the individual.
	Verbalization, catharsis—acceptance of anger by the team; insight preventing attempts to 'reform' the patient or ganging up against him.
Social pain—unfulfilled responsibilities, eg young children, loneliness, loss of dignity, feeling of worthlessness	Catharsis, reassurance.
	Support and environmental manipulation by social worker and team as a whole, to assure the provision of family and community facilities.
	Communication and reassurance by loving, supportive relationships—all wards are 'open' to family and friends, who continually surround the patient, especially as his needs mount.
	Visits by loved ones are not confined to a 'frantic half-hour visiting time'; rather are they encouraged to participate in constant interaction and comfort.
Guilt feelings	Positive steps are taken to bring teenagers into loving and supportive relationships, even when their inclination is to take 'flight' and stay away. Group and team interpretation, catharsis and support.
	Religious support and comfort.
Pain of parting	Sharing identification; religious support and hope; constant presence of loved ones with the aim of making the most of living moments, rather than centring thoughts and attention on future parting. Celebration of birthdays, anniversaries, Christmas, etc, entertainments, poetry and art workshops, etc.
	The family are *not* kept at arm's length by intervening apparatus—rather are they encouraged to participate in loving, supportive tactile experiences—indeed some establishments provide privacy for marital intimacy during terminal *illness*.
	'There is no panacea to the dreadful pain of parting, but you can change its nature—we encourage our patients to *live* until they die peacefully.'
Isolation and loneliness	The hospice is a 'community'.
	When a patient arrives he is met in the ambulance by the matron 'Welcome Mr ———. I am sure you will be happy with us.'
	The patient, his family and staff share 'around the clock' in wards, lounges, garden, chapel, etc. The 'community' eats together in an informal dining-room.
	Tactile comfort bearing proof of emotional involvement is encouraged.
	50% of hospice patients are cared for in their own homes.
	'District' hospice facilities extend into the home, supporting, guiding and sharing, to death if possible; otherwise until pain and crisis in the home indicate admission, virtually of the whole family unit, into the hospice situation.
	Rooms have large windows looking out on people, changing, living views and nature.
	'The deepest sharing of all is with God.'
Provision of privacy	is respected and individual personality needs catered for.
	Zigzag window-facing cubicles are designed to provide privacy.
	Private rooms are available, usually with a blind on the passage, permitting choice of privacy or participation in 'passing life'.

(iii) 'the utilization of *flexible liquid* di-morphine as opposed to wider-spaced more traumatic injections,

all terminal pain can be controlled.

Of 3 362 patients monitored from 1972 to 1976, only 1% presented with 'Pain difficult to control'.

Slides screened by Dr Saunders illustrate the *manner in which terminal patients experience their pain*, viz a ball of red fire piercing into the blue peaks of body tissue; a mass of interwoven scarlet and black, tied to a mattress, upon which picture is superimposed a black syringe; red-beaked rodents drilling into a tree trunk, symbolic of the patient's body.

Spiritual pain, especially anger; social pain due to feelings of unfilfilled responsibility; pain of parting, isolation and loneliness; lack of privacy, and failure to find sharing support were largely responsible for this 1% of suffering patients, and do indeed constitute important factors in lowering the threshold for pain.

A community study conducted in London of 270 bereaved relatives, as reported a year later, showed gross *persistence of guilt feelings and stress* as a result of having witnessed terminal pain in their loved ones.

Pruritis, nausea and other characteristics of terminal suffering also require individualized monitoring and control.

In their study 'Mediators of Pain and Depression in Rheumatoid Arthritis' Gregory K Brown,* Perry M Nicassio, Deborah A Abraham, Barbara Strudler Wallston and Kenneth A Wallston of Vanderbilt University investigate

(1) The causal relationship between pain activity and depression in patients with a chronic history of rheumatoid arthritis
(2) possible mediators such as cognitive helplessness, social support, and behavioural pain-coping style

Sample

Their sample comprised 322 patients (75% females and 25% males) who were diagnosed with definite or classic rheumatoid arthritis by rheumatologists practising in the middle-Tennessee area. The mean duration of illness was 3½ years (range: one month to 7½ years) with 7% of the sample reporting a diagnosis of less than one year.

Measurement

Their measures were a visual analogue scale of pain intensity over the past month, the Pain subscale of the Arthritis Impact Measurement Scales, and the number and intensity of arthritis flare-ups. Depression was measured with the CES-D.

Method

Subjects completed and returned by mail three questionnaires every 6 months.

---

* This study was presented at the 94th Convention of the American Psychological Association, Washington DC, August 1986. All correspondence should be sent to the Health Care Research Project, School of Nursing, Vanderbilt U., Nashville, TN, 37240.

Pain and depression were assessed at all three time intervals and the mediators were assessed at the second six-month period.

Results suggest that

(1) patients with RA are more likely to become depressed if they have experienced a high level of pain intensity and flare-ups at an earlier point in time. This emphasizes the effect of pain anticipation.

(2) in order to alter the pain–depression cycle, it may be important to improve the quality of social support, reduce thoughts of helplessness and decrease the frequency with which RA patients use passive pain coping strategies i e do nothing actively to relieve their situation. (See also Psychosocial Aspects of Arthritis p 455.)

Structuring a 'pain clinic'

In her paper 'Coping in Context: Adaptation Group for Chronic Pain Patients' presented at the 94th Convention of the American Psychological Association, Washington DC, August 1986, Ann Marie McLaughlin, PhD Bryn Mawr Rehabilitation Hospital, Malvern, Pennsylvania describes the structure and content of their *Adapt Group's Didactic (teaching): Discussion Format.*

Sample Themes slected for groups (handouts)

• Purpose of the program and group—

> emphasis on *coping*, not cure; discuss impact of pain behaviour on self, activities, relationships; teach stress management, offer support, confront mind- sets which interfere with improvement; rehearse functional activities in supportive context.

• Goal Attainment Scale—Participants identify target problem behaviours in several areas: individual (personal, interpersonal, vocational, family, functional activity) and specify goals. This is a very difficult task for most patients.

• Chronic Pain Information—Videotapes are used as basis for discussion. Patients open up more readily, initiated by the anonymous video participants.

> 'Managing Chronic Pain' (Encyclopeadia Britannica Education Corp); includes chronic pain patients discussing steps they had to take to successfully manage pain.
> 'Nature of Pain' (Harmarville Rehabilitation Hospital) educational information about the physiological basis of pain, placebo effect, endorphins, role of positive attitide.

• Parable of Two Pain Patients—2 sample cases, one successfully managing pain, one not managing pain. Discussion of 'ingredients' in the successful case. Discussion of the importance of identity and attitude change.

• Family relationships—impact of pain behaviour. Stress caused by *both* sick and recovering role changes.

• Stress Management—4–5 sessions

1. Overview of stress: Sources of stress, physiological responses, cognitive, behavioural, emotional indicators, stress related diseases.
2. Identifying sources of stress in your life: 'The Social Readjustment Rating Scale' (Holmes & Rahe, 1967).
3. Type A behaviour: Behaviour Rating Scale (Journal of Chronic Disease, 22).
4. Pain and stress—setting limits in relationships. Avoiding the secondary pain pitfalls of anxiety and depression reactive to pain.

- Assertiveness—2–3 sessions

Because chronic pain patients need to learn to manage stress better, learning to comfortably express their needs is important.
Exercises, vignettes from the *Relaxation and Stress Reduction Workbook* (new Harbinger Publications) are used.
Differences between passive, assertive, aggressive behaviour highlighted.

- Coping Techniques—3 sessions

1. Various relaxation techniques are practised including proper breathing, progressive muscle relaxation, coping imagery, glove anaesthesia (tape) across 3 sessions.
2. Cognitive-behavioural approaches are discussed including self-talk, irrational beliefs.
3. Importance of exercise (OT-led) as stress reducer.

- Defence Mechanisms—A handout describing and giving examples of defence mechanisms is used as a discussion stimulant. Participants identify their styles; ways in which defences can provide a healthy way of coping are reviewed.
- What the Experts Say—3 sessions
  These sessions prompt active, sometimes heated discussion and stimulate peer confrontation both of each other and of the health care system.

  'Madison Scale' (Hackett)—characteristics correlating with the psychogenicity of pain.
  N Hendler's categories: 'Coper, Moper, Malingerer, Exaggerator'.
  Participants complete 'How much pain do you fel? A test for Pain Victims' which identifies their 'label'.
  'The need-to-suffer patient', 'The overwhelmed patient',
  'The psychogenic patient', 'The assigned patient'.
  From (Gildenberg and DeVaul, 1985).
  'Ailment Aegis: A no-fault response to psychosocial stress' by D J Herbert. Pain patient describes pain as 'holding him together' . . . helping him 'take time out'. Discussion of pay-offs from the role of being a pain patient.

- Lifestyle—Discussions about diet, nutrition and their role in pain and stress reduction.

Research findings

Identity Resolution among Chronic Pain Patients in Group Therapy

ie the relationships between individual long-standing personality coping patterns (chapter 4) and specific pain response.

Identity Status ie personality pattern	Pain Perspective	Primary Affective Response	Nature of Group Participation
Rigidly maintains former self-image but without goal pursuit	Denies/avoids chronic nature of pain	Anger at others, self-blame Pre-occupied about legal, medical, employment systems	Peripheral or self-focused inter-actions Dismisses psychological strategies 'Yes but' response to peer suggestions May withdraw from group
Sick role, views self as dysfunctional	Pain incorporated as significant focus of identity	Depressed and helpless May deny psychological distress	Passive stance Compliant but with minimal insight May be avoided by peers who feel helpless toward patient
Unable to describe goals Stripped of former roles Unable to define identity	Uncertain, confused about chronicity of pain In transition	Depression with anxiety May express hopelessness Grieving lost 'self'	Expresses anxiety, confusion Seeks peer support Responds well to confrontation Relatively open to suggestions
Adopts new lifestyle Redirects goals	Accepts pain as a reality around which to plan Takes exacerbations in stride	Moderate reactive depression Positive adjustment	Endorses attitude change as key to pain management Offers peer support Acknowledges role of personality change Goal-oriented

Author—Caution. The professional should beware of counter-transference, projecting upon her patient her own normal feelings of inadequacy, depression and anxiety. A blaming or judgmental attitude should be avoided.

Anxiety—see chapter 1, pp 32-36 including Panic Attacks

Anxiety, Depression and Obsessional Compulsions occur especially frequently and painfully in serious and/or progressive illness

Any situation that threatens the well-being of the organism is assumed to produce a state of anxiety. *Anxiety* consists in diffuse apprehension which is vague in nature and is associated with feelings of uncertainty and helplessness. It is an emotion without a specific object, subjectively experienced by the individual and communicated interpersonally. It occurs as a result of a threat to the subject's being, self-esteem or identity.

Most people feel anxious from time to time in response to appropriate stimuli. Psychoanalysts maintain that unconscious conflict and guilt feelings increase underlying anxiety and, hence, psychosomatic stress. Certainly, predisposed by hereditary(-anatomical and physiological factors), reinforced by an unfortunate fear-provoking life-story, one may develop a *generalized anxiety stress underlay, providing fertile soil for free-floating anxiety of all sorts*. The subject is easily frightened and tries to cope with his generalized fear by attaching it to, and eliminating it from, one stress situation after the other.

The mother is afraid her child will run in front of a bus on the way to school; fall and break his leg in the playground. She may check to see whether any of these catastrophes has happened, and then fear her husband has lost his job; that she has a heart murmur; that robbers have raided her home. She is involuntarily hounded by free-floating, diffuse fears amongst which fear of injury, of dying, of rejection, frequently predominate. Technically she is said to be suffering from 'anxiety neurosis'; we know her as a 'nervous, highly strung' person. In times of real anxiety-provocation, her customary debilitating and distressing fear may mount to a crescendo of terror. Sometimes real dangers are easier to handle.

Anxiety disorders may be:

(a) episodal, as in panic
(b) chronic or persistent, as in generalized anxiety

Managing anxiety (see also Stress Management chap. 2, p. 32)

1. Ask the patient about the reasons for his anxiety (ventilation catharsis—the relief that comes with 'talking out', p 65).
2. Restate known information and reassurances applicable to the patient's fears or illness. Show faith in his treatment programme.
3. Explain, in simple terms, how anxiety is aroused and its psychosomatic sequelae.
4. Communicate with other staff or departments the nature of the patient's worries, e g delays in pathology reports, fears of X-rays or cross-infection.
5. Provide relaxation training to counteract ANS arousal and help the patient break into his tension cycle (Chap. 2 p 32-36).
6. Encourage and plan distracting and enjoyable thoughts and activities; stimulate positive thoughts towards the patient's circumstances.

7.   Remind him that his anxiety will pass—rational discussion (even at an intellectual level) can help counteract negative anxiety stimuli. It is of course important to try and understand unconscious fear association.

8.   Encourage him (health permitting) to find a congenial direct outlet for biochemical tension energy in sport, walking, aerobics, etc.

Depression (see also p 591)

Depression which occurs in response to a life blow, crisis, loss or illness is called *reactive* depression (as opposed to unprecipitated and probably constitutional *endogenous* depression).

Reactive depression presents with *marked and persistent change* from the individual's norm. Clinical symptoms are divided into:

Somatic symptoms

sleep disturbances, especially 'early morning waking'
some patients sleep more than usual
vivid, disturbing dreams
anorexia—loss of appetite
changes in gastro–intestinal functioning—constipation or when depression is mixed with anxiety, diarrhoea
 loss of sexual desire.

Cognitive signs

the patient describes himself as 'depressed', 'sad', 'hopeless', 'without a future'
obsessional thoughts—repetitive thoughts or actions (p 119); in illness these thoughts perseverate on death, pain, symptoms real and imagined, infections
guilt feelings, especially about illness as punishment
loss of self-esteem—feelings of being 'unclean', 'contaminated', "unwanted"
lack of concentration, slowness of thought
inability to cope with the smallest tasks or decisions
irritability and pessimism
crying spells
talk of suicide—to be taken seriously (chapter 25).

Behavioural signs

passivity, inactivity, procrastination
slowness of speech and movement.

Treatment

(i) Psychological—for milder depression: investigation, catharsis, support, reassurance ('Depression always passes'); alleviation of environmental precipitants, such as isolation or, alternatively, lack of privacy.

(ii) Medication—for more serious cases: the patient should be assured that

(a) medication is not tranquilization, neither is it detrimentally habit forming. It will not reduce his control, his self-determination. It provides the body with something it needs, comparable to insulin for the diabetic.

(b) medication takes from 14–21 days to work.

Warning to staff

Nothing is as contagious to fellow patients, family and staff as depression—so recognize your symptoms and seek immediate catharsis or distraction.

Countering Anxiety and Depression in Serious and Terminal Illness p 508

Obsessions (p 119)

Obsessional thoughts may be so vivid as to border on hallucinations. Anxiety is a cornerstone of depression.

In illness, especially life-threatening and progressive conditions such as AIDS and cancer, obsessional thoughts are turned inwards towards painful, persistent, ever-widening mental checking or a physical ritual in which patients anxiously feel for lumps from head to foot and then back again.

The AIDS patient's rituals are emphasized by his guilt or guilt and anxiety concerning 'forbidden' homosexuality with which he may still be struggling to come to terms whether he has done anything, even inadvertently, to expose his loved ones to infection. This may become a painful ritual of reliving actions from the first sexual partner through to the last, over and over again. Often obsession and anxiety are inerwoven with depression.

Treatment of obsessional thoughts where actual compulsive behaviour is absent may include the following:

1. *Reassurance by a trusted professional* that specific symptoms are not indicative of progressive deterioration. Indeed, some symtomatology, such as faint rashes, vague pains, visual disturbances and lethargy described by PGL patients, may actually be psychosomatic stress symptoms. Explanation and recognition of anxiety symptoms may forestall the compulsive cycle. 'Tumors' and 'lumps' may be normal tissue undulations caused by fat deposits or tendons. Patients may require *repetitive reassurances* which, being at the intellectual level, give only temporary relief. Often that is the best the patient, compassionate professional can do.

2. *'Thought stopping'*, in which the patient is taught to recognize and interrupt the obsessional thought as it begins. The patient is helped to *select a thought blocker* which is potent, harmless, pleasant and strongly distracting, such as a happy memory, a scene from a film, preparation for an anticipated journey. As the compulsive thought enters consciousness the *predetermined, harmless thought is pulled out, grabbed at, 'held on to' for a few minutes until the dreaded compulsive thought recedes.* Substitute *'intrusive thinking'* may both counteract obsessions and lower precipitatory anxiety.

3. *Avoidance of exposure to other patients' negative experiences or to media coverage of AIDS, cancer,* or other progressive diseases: Patients who, through professional help and

'worry work' or intellectualization, are in a stage of reasonable calm, often find their confidence shattered and their terror reinstated by bad news, true or false. In some overpowering situations 'flight' is a better mental mechanism than confrontation.

4. In chronic cases, where relief provided by other methods is sadly short-lived, intervention may be complemented by *medication* with antidepressants such as clomipramine hydrochloride or tranquillizers such as Ativan.

In cases where <u>obsessional thoughts are accompanied by compulsive behaviours</u>, interventions described above may be complemented by techniques of *response prevention*.

Typical symptomatology in cases of dreaded progressive illness is *compulsive, apprehensive searching and self-examination* for bodily evidence of, for example, AIDS infection or recurring cancer. The deeper and wider one is compelled to feel, the greater the possibility of misinterpreting normal tissue—and the greater one's terror.

The core of this method is *limitation of the amount of time given over to bodily checking*, thus minimizing disruptive behaviour and, hopefully negative, intrusive thoughts. Professional and patient may together agree on:

> checking for only three minutes (later two and one minute) and in one specific location, such as the bath followed by the new goal of no checking at all.*

Sometimes, however, nothing relieves one's fear but *presentation of the terror area to one's trusted professional,* and his forceful reassurance that the offending tissue is normal.

Guilt concerning demands on one's professional may lead to the 'wounded healer' anxiety syndrome (p 200).

Post traumatic stress disorder

This disorder occurs in response to overwhelming

(a) events outside the range of normal human experiences, e g disaster, crisis, army battle trauma,
(b) psychologically traumatic experiences, e g divorce.

Characteristic symptoms: Re-experiencing the traumatic event through nightmares, daydreams and dissociative states, withdrawal and depression, depersonalization and anxiety.
(See Crisis and Disaster chapter 24 p 563)

Obsessive compulsive neurosis (see p. 119)

Munchausen's syndrome

This is an obsessive neurotic condition in which the patient craves operations and anaesthetics.

---

* Miller D, Weber J and Green J: The Management of AIDS patients. MacMillan Press, London, 1986.

Miss S H, aged 24, appeared in the Shrewsbury Magistrate's Court where she was charged with reacting violently when a hospital orderly informed her she was about to be discharged. While in court custody she had mutilated herself, apparently hoping for readmission to hospital.

During the previous five years she had undergone forty unnecessary operations.

Apparently the accused's *need for involved attention,* or a *self-imposed need to suffer in order to assauge guilt or remorse,* was so strong that, after a genuine operation to remove an ovarian cyst, she attacked orderlies, threw a fire extinguisher down the corridor and hurled a chair through a window.

Rather than sentence Miss S H to a prison term, attempts were made to admit her to an institution willing to undertake treatment for a condition that may not be as rare as one would think.

Phobias

Phobias are *persistent and excessive fears attached to objects or situations which are not, in reality, a signifiant source of danger,* e g

Paralipophobia—fear of precipitating disaster by having omitted or forgotten.

Mysophobia—fear of contamination by soiling with dirt or contagious material.

Pyrophobia—fear of causing a fire through negligence.

Aichmophobia—fear of pointed objects.

Agoraphobia—fear of open spaces.

Claustrophobia—fear of closed spaces.

Erythrophobia—fear of blushing.

Necrophobia—fear of death.

Pantophobia—multiple obsessive fears, e g drowning, being run over, infection.

Zenophobia—fear of fear itself.

Taphephobia—fear of being buried alive.

Intrusive Thoughts—fear of life disruption by involuntary personally and socially destructive thoughts.

At an intellectual level the sufferer knows his fear to be unwarranted. Yet he experiences overpowering anxiety which he tries to diminish by *'flight' or persistent mechanism of avoidance,* i e he tries to keep way from the object or situation which frightens him, and in so doing his relationships, work comfort and pleasure are interfered with. The specific fear may have been conditioned by unfortunate experience for example, claustrophobia—initiated by having been locked in a cupboard. At a deeper level phobias represent repressed anxiety which is displaced, transferred or attached to another object or situation.

They may be so vivid that the patient may confuse his fears with actual hallucinations.

Treatment usually involves (i) insight (ii) interpretation (iii) catharsis (iv) gradual reintroduction to phobic area in presence of supportive professional. (p 162-164)

Sleep

The neonate alternates frequently between sleeping and waking. Gradually sleep periods consolidate and become less frequent, until at about 10 years, day and night rhythm is established.

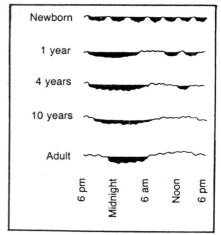

Development of the sleep pattern

The shaded areas represent periods of sleep. Note that the newborn's frequent short periods of sleep gradually coalesce and eventually become the single night–day cycle of the adult. (After Kleitman, 1963.)

Data abridged and adapted from *The First Five Years of Life* by Arnold Gesell *et al.* Copyright 1940 by Arnold Gesell. Reprinted by permission of Harper & Row, Publishers, Inc.

At the same time, allowing for fairly <u>wide individual differences</u> in sleep needs, there is a drop in total number of hours required.

Sleep patterns become set with the years. Experiments conducted on young adults whose sleep was shifted from night to day (sleep period 11 pm–7 am shifted to 8 am–4 pm) showed that *quality of sleep did not change, but there was a deterioration in skilled performance tests* (Webb, Agnew & Williams 1971). This investigation is of interest to nurses in night duty switch. Initial fall-off in speed and quality of skilled visual-motor tasks should be expected, but counteracted by increased voluntary concentration and the allocation of more time per task.

Stages of sleep—as gauged by the EEG (Electroencephalograph)— show 5 stages of sleep pattern, namely:

Stage 1 and 2 as waking passes into sleep marked by a fairly flat, regularly undulating graph pattern.

Stages 3 and 4 presenting with regular, slow, Delta wavelength, during which sleep is deepest and awakening hardest. During these stages the sleeper does not awaken easily to general external stimuli, but does respond to personalized stimuli such as his name, own alarm clock, individual household noises, etc. Thus if it is necessary to awaken the patient or while he is coming round from an anaesthetic, it is wise to use his name as a personalized waking stimulus. Stages 1 to 4 are classified Non–REM ie NREM.

Stage 5 features Rapid Eye Movements, together with a flat, regularly and gently undulating electroencephalograph (similar to that at Stage 1 when the patient begins to fall asleep). REM were thought to indicate a similar period of lighter sleep and easy wakefulness. However, Stage 5 REM differs from Stage 1 in that the patient does not awaken easily. As this is the period of dreams, some researchers believe that dreams actually safeguard sleep, rendering REM 5 a period of restfulness.

Sleep distribution is cyclic, usually at 60–80 minute intervals (Dement 1972) and apparently regulated by an internal 'pacemaker' rather than random external environmental stimuli. Hence for the first 50–60 minutes of a sleep cycle the subject falls deeper and deeper into sleep. The period 50–80 minutes—usually of approximately 20 minutes' duration—consists of REM waves marking a period of lighter, but still effective, sleep in which dreams abound.

SLEEP DISTURBANCES

Somnambulism

Sleepwalking occurs in approximately one to six per cent of the population and there is evidence that sufferers tend to 'grow out of' the condition. There is usually complete amnesia for the incident, consistent with the belief that it occurs during deep Non-REM (NREM) sleep. Remember to use the sleeper's name if you want to awaken him.

Handling: Attempts should be made to ensure that the child does not injure himself by sleepwalking. Dangerous objects should remain out of reach, and stairways and open windows guarded. Persisting into adulthood, sleepwalking may reflect psychological problems warranting professional attention.

Insomnia

Difficulty in falling asleep, and intermittent, wakeful periods during the night constitute a lonely and sometimes stressful condition.

The very fear of sleeplessness may initiate a vicious tension cycle. It is important to reassure the sufferer that individual sleep requirements are very flexible, and loss of sleep does not usually impair daytime functioning. In fact, many people put wakeful hours to good use by creativity and pleasant memories. Sometimes sleeping pills themselves may set up a vicious circle of increasing dosage and should be utilized only in times of pain and overwhelming stress or grief. Sleeping pills tend to repress REM sleep and thus dreams. When the pills are removed the patient is exposed to 'REM rebound' sometimes resulting in disturbing nightmares.

Persistent, disturbing insomnia may be associated with psychiatric illness, especially depression (pp 590-2). *Behavioural treatment involving specific and voluntary relaxation* and auto-suggestive techniques is often helpful, e g

switch on gentle music or think of one specific soothing note;
lie comfortably on your back or in the S shaped 'fetal' position. Tell yourself your shoulders, arms, thighs, knees, feet feel heavy . . . your back feels heavy, sinking through the mattress;
tense all your muscles and let them flop one by one;
focus your eyes strongly on a slit of light;
your eyelids are heavy . . . heavy . . . you cannot keep them open . . . your eyes are closing;
you are breathing heavily, slowly . . . heavily . . . slowly;
you are on a rubber mattress floating gently out to sea towards the setting sun. You are floating, floating, heavily floating into sleep . . .

A cycle of persistent wakefulness may be interrupted by walking round the room, attempting to complete some task, only returning to bed with a feeling of sleepiness.

In contrast *Narcolepsy* and *Apnea* constitute an uncontrollable tendency to fall asleep even while dancing or lecturing. In *Cataplexy* gross relaxation and loss of postural control result in physical collapse dirctly into REM sleep.

Nightmares	*Night-terrors*
Occur at any age.	Usually occur in children, who tend to outgrow these distressing experiences.
Normal phenomena, consisting of a frightening dream, usually *remembered in some detail* on awakening.	Content of the dream or other experience is *seldom remembered* on waking.
Manifestation: There is usually little overt evidence that the person is experiencing a distressing dream.	*Manifestation:* Typically, there is gross and often distressing, overt evidence of the child's fear and suffering.
Content: If a particular dream persists, it may constitute a reliving of a frightening, feared or disturbing experience which emerges when the inhibitory power of the Conscience is reduced in sleep.	He usually emits a piercing shriek before sitting up in bed, his eyes wide open, his expression terror-stricken. His heart beat increases. He perspires freely, and often holds out his hands as if seeking to protect himself from a dangerous onslaught. Although his eyes are open, it might prove difficult to awaken him properly. His terror state is usually of one or two minutes' duration, after which he falls asleep again. When he awakens he is probably unable to recall his experience.

Handling

1.   It is advisable *to awaken* the child from his distressing experience, being sure to talk to him *reassuringly* while holding him close in a warm embrace.
2.   If he is able to do so, he should be encouraged to *verbalise* his experience in the immediate 'hot' situation where he can deal most effectively, at an *emotional level,* with his still available traumatic experience.
3.   If night-terrors occur frequently, or if a particular nightmare *persists,* these sleep-disturbing phenomena may constitute reliving of a frightening, feared or disturbing experience such as surgery, the traumatic death of a close relative. Psychotherapeutic intervention, aimed at defining, analysing and reliving the dream, or suspected terror-association, at a conscious level, in order to counteract its frightening power, may be indicated.

   As in all psychotherapy, one seeks to reconcile the 'conscious' with the 'unconscious'.

CHAPTER 22

REHABILITATION

AFTER MAJOR BODY LOSS, CANCER, MYOCARDIAL INFARCTION, CEREBRAL INSULTS ALSO SUNDRY REHABILITATION PROGRAMMES

'The disabled are not a race apart, they are not a group of people made totally abnormal by a single diagnosis of "disability". The disabled are ourselves as we could have been if catastrophe had fallen on us yesterday, ourselves as we may be if catastrophe befalls us tomorrow.'*

A *disability*, in terms of the World Health Organization definition, is an impairment, loss or abnormality of physical structure, or physical or psychological function, *with which an individual cannot cope.*
Rehabilitation consists in helping the individual to cope by providing relevant personal support and skills, or by intervening in the environment on which his disability rests.

Rehabilitation has been defined by the World Health Organization 1969:
'The combined and co-ordinated use of medical, social, educational and vocational measures for training and retraining the individual to the highest possible level of functional ability.'

MUTILATION OF THE BODILY EGO OR SELF-IMAGE DUE TO SURGERY OR TRAUMA (see also pp 78-85)

The lifelong image which the individual has of himself is seated deep in the intimate self-conscious. By losing part of his body, especially when it is externally visible, the individual will consider himself incomplete and mutilated—this is a traumatic experience which requires a period of adjustment, identification, comfort and support.

Deep in 'group consciousness' (Jung, p 80) the deformed and ugly symbolize evil and untouchability. It is easy for the mutilated patient to see himself as the rejected outcast: the evil hunchback; the beautiful good fairy.

Phantom limb

'Phantom' limbs are not only due to persistent CNS-parietal afferent images but also to the unconscious *need of the patient to cling to his own original body image.* This is especially true following amputation and similar traumatic loss after the age of 5 years.

The amputee will often feel the entire amputated extremity (or breast) with various unpleasant and painful sensations. She experiences unpleasant images of flesh cramped in odd positions.

---

* Hamilton, A. 'The Sexual Problems of the Disabled.' *Br J Fam Plan* **4**: 12–13. 1978.

Although vestigial afferent cerebral receptors and destroyed body image are contributory, etiology of phantom pain is largely unknown (Loon & Inman) and no treatment methods—including nerve blocks, reamputation or hypnosis—have been found successful. The most promising method so far has been immediate post-operative fitting of a plaster socket and pylon while the patient is still in theatre. Phantom limb pain usually subsides to some degree with the wearing of a prosthesis, but may never completely disappear.

Phantom limb sensation is not a psychotic hallucination, but a fact of amputation surgery about which the patient should not be frightened and which should gradually diminish.

The author has been impressed by the number of amputees and paraplegics who report repetitive dreams of running and dancing, swimming and normal sexual participation.

An American survey (1978) referring to psychological problems in women who underwent mastectomy for cancer found that one in four had suicidal ideas after the operation, and more than half 'phantom breast' symptoms.

A similar survey in Britain found that one woman in three who underwent mastectomy had either ceased sexual activity or did not enjoy it. (An analysis of husbands' true feelings in sexual activity was not reported, but would probably have swelled the incidence of maladjustment (p 82).) One in four of the group surveyed required specialized psychiatric treatment for anxiety and depression.

The authors conclude: 'Many women who undergo mastectomy seem to be paying a high price emotionally for the possibility of survival.'

(See page 81ff for recent work on alternatives to mastectomy.)

Strong in intention to emphasize respect for the human body by the soul that inhabits it, as well as by those who tend it, the sayings of the Prophet Mohammed require that any limb parted from the body should be cleansed and buried with the love and ceremony which will one day attend the body that is for ever diminished by its loss.

The patient mourns a lost limb as if it had been a beloved relation. Some, indeed, are comforted by the knowledge that it was given a decent and loving burial.

So deeply engrained and intrinsic to oneself is one's body image that *even* a desired change, such as removal by *plastic surgery* of a cosmetic *deformity*, may result in acute and classic mental shock and post-operative depression.

This 'shock' reaction may to some extent be offset by pre-operative preparation. It certainly requires the support of the professional team, family and friends in order that positive aspects of the operation may be absorbed and accepted at deeper emotional levels.

Many patients exhibit a sort of *hypomania* (excitability and deceptive optimism) as a *defence mechanism* against severe depression and loss. It is in the patient whose defence mechanisms are inadequate to hide his deep sense of deprivation, loss and anger that we glimpse the real emotional anguish which is almost certain to be experienced by patients undergoing amputation surgery.

> 'Pre-operative and post-operative interviews with amputees show that despite the existence of an irreversible and incurable pathological condition in an extremity, one inevitably requiring amputation either as a lifesaving measure or to promote better function, the prospective amputee has a strong

emotional attachment to all the parts of his body. He is *unable*, without sympathetic preparation, *to see the pathological portion of his limb through the eyes of the surgeon* in order to realize that the prosthetic device to be furnished him following surgery will actually, despite all the problems of an artificial device, be better than the diseased or deformed extremity from which he is being surgically parted.'*

The most helpful approach in easing the impact of amputation of limb or breast lies in helping the patient to adjust to his loss as if it were a beloved relative or friend.

Reaction to amputation and thus destruction of body image

Mutilation of one's body image is impossible to imagine.

Disbelief that the patient will actually have to lose a part of his/her body often continues after surgery despite surface level acceptance ... hence great grief, anger, denial and depression occur even after 'preparation'. Some believe they will awaken from a terrible dream.

Those who actually allow the full loss-impact to come into consciousness may become agitated and self-destructive: spend phantom insurance compensation or become abusive to hospital team and family.

Generalized anger in response to the cruel blow fate has dealt may crystallize out in personal anger against the hospital team, and the surgeon in particular. It is thus very important that the patient be convinced that every effort was made to save the body part.

Guilt

In a society featuring body or mutilation as punishment for 'evil in thought, word or deed', there is a tendency for the patient to torture himself with guilt feelings lest he himself has contributed to his loss.

Self-reproach will increase the distress of the smoker with a circulatory disease, or the driver whose reckless speed has brought him into the casualty department.

Throughout, care should be taken to *avoid blaming* the patient for his terrible predicament.

Depression: 'After the mastectomy she sat for days under her bed, weeping'†

As the impact of loss and disablement is realized, the patient may become hyperactive and aggressive in his desperate misery, or silent, withdrawn, anorexic, immobile. He may wish to weep but pride prevents this tension release. Anti-depressant medication may be indicated, but the most meaningful comfort, support and source of motivation lies in human relationships—amongst which the intense *nurse–patient relationship* is certainly very important.

To 'shrug off' the emotional shock of mutilation as 'expected' will not help the sorrowing patient. He needs opportunity to ventilate his deep and personalized fears, anger and depression.

---

* Mital & Pierce. *Amputees and their Prosthesis*. Little, Brown and Co.

† Student nurse in class discussion.

The role of the nurse

Pre-operatively the nurse should be emotionally supportive helping her patient believe that although an artificial limb cannot completely replace his own, it will be better than the pathological limb which is to be amputated.

The nurse should try to encourage her patient to verbalize fears about amputation. She should also help him realistically anticipate his future abilities and limitations, increasing her knowledge of these factors by conferring with other members of the team.

Post-operatively she should work to help the patient attain the *goal of feeling the prosthetic limb to be psychologically a part of himself*, and not simply a device such as a crutch, or a spoon to be used and set aside.

Having forgotten that he no longer has two legs on which to stand, two hands with which to grab and hold on, especially when he is experiencing phantom limb sensation, the patient may fall.

In the case of female amputees, a female nurse who is able to identify may be particularly supportive in allaying or coping with the patient's fears concerning cosmetic results of amputation. Unlike the male amputee she cannot cover an arm with a shirt sleeve or a leg with a pair of trousers. In addition, the female sex partner is expected to be more beautiful and complete than the male.

Patients will need much help to counteract the ugliness of artificial hands; in fact, from almost all points of view, amputation of upper limbs constitutes a more emotionally traumatic situation than lower limbs.

The nurse should encourage (but not force) socialization with other patients, and should avoid regression by promoting independence in mobility and self-care.

Aiding acceptance

In some cases the patient may be helped to understand that the prosthesis will actually be superior functionally to the deformed or diseased member of which amputation will deprive him. (This consolation does not apply in breast amputation where there has been no pain, function is satisfactory and amputation will deprive the woman of her sexual self-concept, and erogenous organ, and impose stresses and doubts in the marriage union—inhibited or overt.) Prostheses are usually such ugly and cumbersome objects that it is no wonder many *patients consider them a mockery of their own bodies*. (See The Nursing Process—illustrative case, p 228ff.)

It is only when the client is able to accept his prosthesis as part of his own body—to absorb it into his self-concept—that it fulfils a worthwhile purpose.

In dealing with *the parents of an amputee*, the nurse should try to identify with their grief in witnessing the permanent disfigurement, and suffering of one whose body they love more than their own. Parents need sympathy, catharsis and hope. Of special importance is emphasis on compensation status activities, and ability to see their child as a whole functional human being, and not just an empty sleeve or trouser leg. (See The Physically Handicapped Child p 286.)

Cerebro-spinal injury

The disabled speak:

In response to my invitation to write a few comments on his hospital experience a paraplegic man aged 27 years, injured two years previously (October 1979), wrote thus:

Three weeks after I had an accident, the P.T. told me that I was never going to be able to walk again and the more I realized it the better. I felt so bad I couldn't even cry. I began to think about my future. I had been a sportsman and was still young. My life had really only just begun. Now what was I going to do without the use of my legs? In this strange place, I was faraway from my parents and friends. Nobody was there to just talk to me. Nobody knew how I felt and they probably weren't even interested. After many weeks on my own, I thought the best thing to do was to get a hold on my life.

Now that I am a paraplegic, noone has come to ask me how I feel about being one. I was shown how to handle and look after my body. Once a patient had a disagreement with a male nurse. The male nurse said, "You must keep your mouth shut and take what you get because you are just a patient." My reply to this would have been that everyone is treated like a patient and not a person. A grown-up man is treated like a child. If the nurse were talking to me I would have been treated the same.

Although the sister asks for any complaints, she doesn't expect them. If anyone does complain they are regarded as a weakling and treated as one. A good patient never complains and always takes what comes his way. It seems that a patient has no choice because there is always someone else who knows what is best for him.

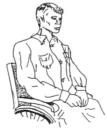

Obviously experiences differ, and one would hope that this man's ordeal is an exception.

At the 'Independent Living Seminar' convened by the National Council for Cripple Care, Year of the Disabled (1981), a survey of client opinion required participants to list their worst fears. In the result, their fears were ranked in the following order:

1. Fear of dependence, physical, personal and financial.
2. Fear of falling.
3. Fear of not being accepted as an equal by hospital staff, family and society.
4. Fear of being stared at.
5. Fear of employer prejudice.

The consensus was that at least *two to three years are required* before a paraplegic can be expected to achieve significant emotional-level acceptance of his drastically changed body image.

There was conviction that *more frank and imaginative attention should be given to sexual compensation* satisfactions and alternative techniques.

Frank discussion with the patient's family is helpful in providing moral support, and increasing the number of persons around him who, understanding his problems, will be able to help him to accept his loss. A particular source of diminishment, *anger and dissatisfaction emanated from clients' exclusion from case conferences* at which they were discussed and decisions affecting them taken:

'Secondhand reports are just not good enough—we are as sensible and as "grown up" as they are. This should not be a "we–they" situation.'

On the subject of family and chronic illness and disability, Professor Duane Bishop, Brown Hospital, Rhode Island, USA opines that the *'uncooperative' patient and his family sometimes benefit* from the ego defence mechanism of *denial*.

By refusing to accept and deal with 'realities' they were more open to challenge, applying attack, ingenuity, and defiant determination, often with surprisingly fruitful results.

> 'Professionals and the public tend to expect the handicapped to assume a "disabled role", in which they are seen as permanently dependent, accepting an almost childlike role in their physical, emotional and sexual needs. This role implies the stigma of deviance and inferiority. At best they are encouraged to form their own groups or clubs in order to achieve understanding, acceptance, catharsis and motivation from "their own kind".'

In fact avoidance of regression to the introjected Learned Helpless Role is a major function of the rehabilitation team. It should be stressed from admission that the client is a whole, adult, self-determining person with rights and abilities. Rehabilitation commences on admission.

There is strong suspicion that society's motivation to segregate and stereotype the disabled stems from a *primitive, fear-induced taboo*, setting apart the handicapped as contagious, displeasing, evil and dangerous; or at least so discomforting and guilt-provoking that they should be in some way 'ghettoed'.

The disabled on the other hand, especially the young disabled, *see themselves as self-determining adults*, determined to resume normal or compensatory personal and work roles, at maximum capacity, as soon as possible.

Within the context of intact motivation, they are determined to remove the stigma of dependence and diminishment from themselves and their disability.

Determined to vindicate their claim that the disabled, as a minority consumer group, are diminished, segregated and discriminated against, the angry, young and articulate have formed their own self-help group:

British Council of Disabled People
Telephone: 01 854 7289

'Our Bodies Disable Us But Society Handicaps Us'

In the quest for equal opportunity and full participation the organization challenges the traditional approach which results in isolation from the mainstream of society.

It calls upon professionals and volunteers in the field to recognize the full human status of people with all disabilities and to work WITH them towards the achievement of equal rights.

The Disabled Peoples 'Bill of Rights' is based upon that of the American Coalition of Citizens with Disabilities.

DISABLED PEOPLES' BILL OF RIGHTS

All people should be able to enjoy these rights, regardless of race, creed, colour, sex, religion or disability.

1. The right to live independent, active and full lives.
2. The right to the equipment, assistance and support services necessary for full productivity, provided in a way that promotes dignity and independence.
3. The right to an adequate income or wage, substantial enough to provide food, clothing, shelter and other necessities of life.
4. The right to accessible, integrated, convenient, and affordable housing.
5. The right to quality physical and mental health care.
6. The right to training and employment without prejudice or stereotype.
7. The right to accessible transportation and freedom of movement.
8. The right to bear or adopt and raise children and have a family.
9. The right to a free and appropriate education.
10. The right to participate in and benefit from entertainment and recreation.
11. The right of equal access to and use of all business, facilities and activities in the community.
12. The right to communicate freely with all fellow citizens and those who provide services.
13. The right to a barrier free environment.
14. The right to legal representation and to full protection of all legal rights.
15. The right to determine one's own future and make one's own life choices.
16. The right of full access to all voting processes.

Professionals accustomed to or, for personal reasons, *needing an authoritarian Adult–Child relationship* (p 179) with their clients, tend to feel threatened by, and thus on the defensive, in their relationships with *financially independent, more sophisticated clients*. Tense, and thus lacking empathy, they fail to identify with clients' real needs of advice and emotional support, albeit within an Adult–Adult consumer type partnership. Unfettered, personally secure professionals are able to tolerate, and even enjoy, more 'demanding' clients within a relationship sometimes facilitated by an invitation to use first-name communication.

Communicating with wheelchair users*

1. Do not automatically hold on to a person's wheelchair. He is *not* a baby in a pram.
2. When talking sit so that you have eye contact.
3. Be alert to architectural barriers when selecting a place to visit.
4. Push a wheelchair down a kerb by placing your foot on the tipping level at the rear of the chair and take firm hold of the handgrips. Tip the chair backwards and lower gently down the kerb, lower the wheels and proceed.
5. Push a wheelchair up the kerb by putting your foot on the tipping lever, lift the chair off its front wheels and on to the kerb.

Communication and co-operation between members of the multi-disciplinary rehabilitation team vis-à-vis community resources is a long-term necessity. Experience with the physically handicapped emphasizes the waste of time and effort spent on physical rehabilitation at the expense of, or without reference to, educational needs.

Co-ordinating physical treatment with education

How often one hears words to the effect 'Just as I was ready to write my end-of-year examination I had to go to hospital for another operation'! In consequence of *failure to dovetail physical treatment with education*, frequently aggravated by *long terms in hospital* or other institutions with their deadening effect on emotional development and independence, we find many people of normal intelligence entering adult life with middle rather than senior school education which would have equipped them for a truly independent and fulfilling life career. There is a need for educational authorities to realize their indispensability in rehabilitation. Liaison with social workers should reassure teachers that arrangements *can* be made to prepare the handicapped child, the physical environment (toilet facilities, rails and ramps, etc) and the other children, for the fruitful integration of the physically handicapped youngster into the normal classroom situation. Commenting on enrolment of an 'open heart' sixteen-year-old, just over a metre tall and weighing 19 kg, Jack's headmaster reported:

> 'We were a little worried about him coming to a large school filled with boisterous schoolboys.
> But we have found in the past that the boys tend to protect rather than tease someone they can see is in need.
> We had a boy here last year who had no kidneys and it was remarkable how the boys looked after him.'

Sexual rehabilitation after spinal-cord injury

> 'Relatively few disabilities totally preclude intercourse or fertility, very few destroy libidinous drive, and none destroy sexual identity. No disability precludes closeness or intimacy.'†

Causing permanent sexual impairment, and occurring frequently among the young at the peak of their sexual performance, *spiral-cord injury* may have a devastating effect on those individuals who have always been reasonably interested in sexual fulfilment.

---

* From *Communicating with Disabled People* compiled by Co-ordinating Committee for the International Year of the Disabled.

† Sapire, K E. 'Disease, Disability and Sexuality.' *Continuing Medical Education* vol 1, May 1983.

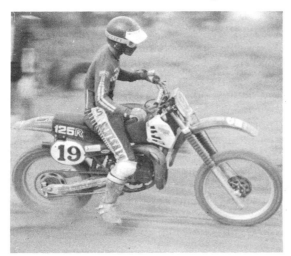

HANS

'The worst was the hell of the day they lifted me into a wheelchair for the first time. In the hospital bed I had the feeling it was all temporary, that I'd get well and be able to go surfing again.

'But when they lifted me into the wheelchair I looked the world square in the face again. That day I realised for the first time I could move only my head, that I couldn't move my upper body at all. I would never be able to walk again.'

The depression that followed was indescribable. 'People often say they know how we feel. But no one knows.'

SHARON

'I went through the same trauma as Hans because I was as sports-mad as he was. I lived for my gymnastics and it was also in my wheelchair that I realised for the first time I'd never be able to jump on a trampoline again.

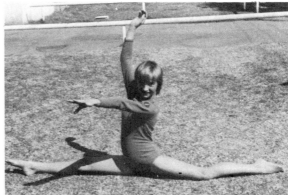

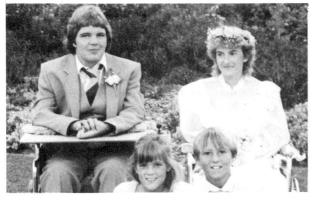

'Don't pity us and treat us like children. Although we can't walk around like you and play rugby, we think and feel just like you. There's nothing wrong with our minds. We can also work, cook, go to church . . . and be loved. That's why we married.

'Does one ever "accept"?' 'Should one ever "accept"?'

The author extends her special thanks to Hans and Sharon Heuschneider who let her into their private world 'in the hope that it will assist nurses to understand others'.

Thanks are also due to Edward Parker author of the article 'Then we'll Dance Until Dawn—You and I'.

'YOU' Magazine August 25, 1988.

Opportunities should exist to express concern over sexual function and to receive an explanation of the effects of the disability.

Above all, the effect of an altered body-concept associated with disfigurement—the image of being half a person—may certainly be one of general loss of self-esteem and depression. Moreover, the anxiety of being rejected by an established or new partner may result in withdrawal and depression. (For self-help support groups, see p 613.)

Fortunately, human bonding is not as fickle as some may assume and sex partners, especially women, are often motivated to a high degree of sensitivity, tolerance and ingenuity.

As with all forms of sexual enlightenment, it is important to realize that *no sexual practice is 'wrong' between partners as long as it is enjoyed by both*. In fact there is nothing intrinsically 'wrong' with ego-directed sexual practices such as sexual self-arousal and satisfaction through 'masturbation'.

What specific substitute techniques can one offer to those suffering from spinal-cord injury?

Alternative sexual activity

Residual function should be carefully assessed and interpreted.

'Caresses with lips and tongue can be very effective and oral-genital stimulation (and orgasm) may be one of the most important options for a paralysed or impotent person . . . the couple are encouraged to seek out and nurture new erogenous zones. *When sensitivity is reduced in one part of the body it may become greater in others.'**

Moonay *et al* write*
'Sensations can be transposed from an intact part to another part of the body that has less sensation by using imagination or magnifying sensations. Phantasy and recreation of intense feelings may possibly result in mental orgasm.'
If both are stimulated simultaneously, feelings from, for instance, the hand, may, with purposeful concentration be transferred to the penis.

Preparation for coitus

This may involve emptying the bladder and bowel, making a towel available in case of accident and catheters taped out of the way, while for personal preference drapes or cloths may be applied over an emotionally sensitive area such as an ostomy bag.

Some feel freer making love under the shower.

Artificial aids

Just as spectacles improve vision, so artificial aids may improve sexual function in both the whole and the handicapped.

Such aids may include the use of lubricating jelly, support from pillows, a vibrator, a splint-like implant prosthesis or a water bed.

* Mooney, T O, Cole, T & Chileren, R A. *Sexual Options for Paraplegics and Quadraplegics*. Boston: Little Brown, 1975.

When all else fails, one wonders about re-experience of previous sexual (and other) satisfactions under hypnotism. Reproduction may require artificial insemination or local rectal stimulation.

Coital positions

The four basic positions (sitting, lying, kneeling or standing) have many variations, depending upon personal preference and the physical difficulties involved.

Intensive sex therapy may be necessary to help couples overcome their inhibitions and enhance their self-esteem.

As the rehabilitation of the client is not likely to be complete or successful unless sexual rehabilitation is catered for, this is an area which should not be avoided or played down.

Sapire*, in her sensitive article quoted above, speaks thus of the general aura of support, insight and initiative which the professional should extend towards both partners:

> 'Successful treatment and rehabilitation involves consideration of the effects on *a partner's support* for the latter [i e the spinal-cord injured] in their loneliness and anxiety and in their new roles at work and at home, and an understanding of their fears about their own sexual needs. The partner becomes a nurse and lover and may fear causing pain, or feel revulsion towards the spouse's altered body. Therapists must be aware of the mourning and distress that the partner undergoes, and it is important to recognize the need for both parties to explore and come to terms with the "new" body in privacy.'

Griffith & Trieschmann† recommended the availability of a private room in hospitals where couples can be encouraged to spend time together as soon as the partner is well enough to establish closeness and intimacy. Before being exposed to the home situation, difficulties can be more comfortably handled in the hospital environment with supportive counselling.

Support group

Association to Aid Sexual and Personal Relationships of Disabled People (SPOD)
286 Camden Road
London N7 0BJ
Telephone: 01 607 8851.

The Community Nurse should be able to recapitulate reassurance and systematically check on understanding and emotional acceptance. She should also be available for support and advice in the physical set-up of the environment to which the patient will return.

The patient's regression, feelings of insecurity and dependence may result in 'role reversal'.

---

* Saphire, E: Further information available from author.

† Griffith, E R & Trieschmann, R R. 'Sexual Training of the Spinal-Cord Injured Male and his Partner.' *In: Human Sexuality and Rehabilitation Medicine.* Baltimore: Williams & Williams. 1983. 119–133.

The dominant father becomes the clinging child; the passive, dependent mother is forced into the role of decision-maker and breadwinner. 'Now I'm the only adult in the family'. 'I didn't bargain on having *two* children'. Clearly such a 'role reversal' causes humiliation, anger and distress in the diminished; insecurity and resentment in the formerly protected. It is important that the temporary dominant role be not exploited nor the client's personality diminished. His every responsibility and adult decision should be preserved and nurtured; his opinions asked and respected.

Interpretation of the etiology and (within the context of successful rebuilding of ego-strengths) temporary nature of role reversal constitutes an important aspect of rehabilitative family therapy.

Mechanical and electronic equipment play a major role in the achievement of independent living. In order to disseminate information about the ever-growing range of equipment on the market an international movement towards Independent Living Centres has recently emerged.

In Britain the Disabled Living Foundation (01 289 6111) provides an accessible display of equipment and appliances for people with varying disabilities, as well as a wide range of other information pamphlets. The centres are under the supervision of a qualified occupational therapist whose role is to discuss the extent to which specific equipment may reduce or eliminate an individual handicap, to demonstrate it and to supply information as to its availability and cost. The Psychology Department at Keele University has invented a remarkable, computerized bionic arm capable of feeding, and perhaps related tasks. Literature and videos are available. Enquiries to: Mike J Topping, Department of Psychology, University of Keele.

Adaptable model for introductory communication with the physically handicapped

The following Parkinson's Questionnaire (patient) was designed by Carter R E and Carter C A and presented at the 94th Convention of the American Psychological Association, Washington DC, August 1986: Symposium on Marital Therapy with Chronically Ill Patients—A Bio-psycho-social Approach.

1. Since I found out that I have Parkinson's Disease my marriage has ....
   ....
2. With regard to my illness, the things I worry about the most are ....
   ....
   ....
3. Adapting to my disease has meant that we have had to change ....
4. I would advise a person who has just found out that he/she has Parkinson's to ....
5. Since my illness my doctor has ....
   ....
6. The biggest help to me with my illness is ....
   ....
7. Since I found out that I have Parkinson's my children have been ....
8. Since my illness our marriage has improved/deteriorated/remained unchanged.

9. Since my illness our friends have ....

10. To a person who has Parkinson's a good marriage is ....

....

11. In a marriage Parkinson's ....

....

12. Since my illness, my spouse and I have talked a lot about ....

....

On a scale of from 1–10 please tell us how you liked filling out this questionnaire by circling the number that best fits your feelings, where 1 means LITTLE LIKING and 10 means LIKED A GREAT DEAL.

1 2 3 4 5 6 7 8 9 10

little   great deal

An amended form is provided for the unmarried.

Such questionnaires often provide a useful 'springboard' to significant areas of emotional and social function. In this case so great was the need for catharsis, that 7 in 10 clients used the opportunity to express themselves on the back of the page.

The role of the physiotherapist:

Clients are touchy about 'being assessed'. One should emphasize that body function and not personal qualities are 'under the microscope'

The physiotherapist is responsible for assessment of the patient's general overall muscle strength and the strengthening of all musculature used in stressful and tiring specific movement of the artificial limb or other prosthesis. It should be remembered that unlike pre-operative automatic afferent-efferent responses, each individual movement must be thought out, planned and purposefully achieved.

Every intact physical movement protects the integrity of the body concept. Research involving amputation of useless or deformed limbs in order to improve mobility has proved ill-conceived: loss of body image was more emotionally destructive than immobility! While the body is overtly intact there is a fantasy of hope. And how motivating is acceptance *without* hope?

The role of the social worker/community nurse

Social casework features in catharsis, emotional support, interpretation and acceptance.

The intake interview, preferably prior to amputation, assesses the patient within his family, social and work situations—his developmental history, his family background, financial status, cultural milieu, educational level and goals.

His established patterns of dealing with stress and sorrow; his vulnerable areas are important in assessing his predicament, resources and needs.

It is not uncommon for patients from middle and upper socio-economic strata in spite of their emotional needs, to reject what they misinterpret as 'interference' by welfare workers. In such a case the social worker should merely show her interest and state that she is available if needed.

The social worker should try to identify with her client, sharing his impaired body image and self-concept. She should be careful not to make her client's decisions nor to take over this life to the extent that he regresses to childhood behaviour patterns, or alternatively becomes hostile and rebellious at being deprived of his adult status. A *particular source of resentment among patients is their exclusion from case conferences at which they are discussed and decisions are taken about their lives.* (See also resentment of the disabled role p 506 and role reversal p 512.)

The role of the occupational therapist in avoiding regression and depression and its interpretation to the nurse (This model of early activity participation and programming is also applicable to other conditions and team members)

Is there a need for occupational therapy in the acute phase of illness or injury, particularly if the patient is not short term (ie will require ten days or longer in hospital)?

In her presentation, 'Audio-visual Equipment and Tasks for Patients in Difficult Functional Positions' Ilse Eggers (September 1980) presented a strong affirmative answer.

Inactivity to such a person means arrested or suspended physical activity in the context of acute and distressing mental awareness—left unassisted he will *regress*. This regression may seek an outlet in various ways, for example:

(1) Search for help from the patient's 'support system', eg his visitors, whose help may be limited by lack of professional knowledge.
(2) He may become frustrated, agitated, aggressive; filled with feelings of helplessness, soon sinking into unmotivated depression.

In contrast, if we are able to reach him and motivate communication through the utilization of his intact auditory and audio-visual intake; review and discussion output we may be able to help him retain his personal integrity.

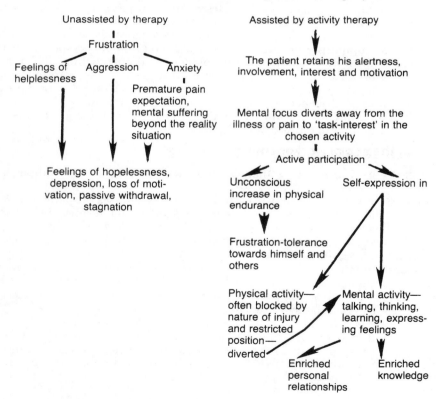

It is highly desirable that the patient be *immediately* introduced to auditory-oriented activities *before* the 'rot' of physical inactivity sets in, and eliminates former participation-satisfaction behaviour patterns.

Using psychodrama as a 'patient–student' learning experience, Mrs Eggers extracted from it:

(i) the need for identification with the discomfort and irritation of restricted uncomfortable positions. Role-players emphasized the frustration and diminishment flowing from the inability to see speakers, to control annoying noises, to gesture away unwanted stimuli, etc:

'I wish you would all experience my difficulties, then you would understand why patients in difficult positions are agitated and unco-operative';

(ii) Difficulty in eliciting from the patient his interests and tastes. 'Patients' were resistant to expression of their feelings to strangers, finding their persistence an encroachment on their privacy.

(iii) That, in their anxiety to help, personnel attempt to *impose* tasks upon patients. While they paid lip service to natural resistance and inevitable depression, 'staff' became frustrated, aggressive, or withdrew their involvement.

(iv) 'Staff' failed to realize that what a 'patient' had found interesting and stimulating in his state of healthy independence, he often failed to tolerate in his state of physical and mental shock. It was necessary to suggest simpler, tuneful and repetitive musical themes, undemanding poetry, familiar religious music and reading, etc.

When themes were appropriate, 'patients' did tend to focus away from their discomfort, becoming more relaxed and involved.

As therapy progresses, the patient will gradually move into a more active phase of involvement, based on 'feedback'. He may be invited to record his opinions and reactions to taped material, thus stimulating self-expression.

It is important that, *even in the acute post-operative or port-trauma stage*, the occupational therapist *conveys to her patient that his rehabilitative programme is commencing.*

Within the team situation, of which, provided he is not grossly brain-injured, the client–patient himself should be an active participant, she would be well-recommended to adapt the **nursing process** to her own science, based on

1. Data collection

This includes affected and intact physical and mental powers, and potential for bodily care; dressing, household tasks, recreation, gainful employment, social independence, etc; family support, social and peer group; work supports; pre-trauma personality assets and difficulties, education, etc.

2. Diagnosis (Assessment)

The client's health status is compared with the norm in order to determine whether any deviation from it may be termed:

normal or abnormal;
temporary or permanent;
the extent, impact and permanence of his capabilities, limitations, etc.

The OT diagnosis is related to, and judged within, the context of diagnoses made by other caring professions.

The diagnosis concerns

(a) aspects in which the client's health may need to be promoted,

(b) areas in which he requires help in adapting to, and overcoming, his physiological-psycho-social handicaps.

Most such diagnoses are based on the deviation between the client's resources and his goal-attainment possibilities in terms of Maslow's Hierarchy of Human Needs (see p 100).

3. Planning

Consists in

(a) following up the goals mutually identified and accepted by professional and client;

4. Implementation

(a) compiling the time-programme in which goals may be expected to come to fruition within the patient's own limitations and resources;

(b) activities, social experiences, use of prostheses, etc are matched to mutually agreed goals, and the specific therapeutic experiences by which these goals may be implemented are specified by the client and his team. Patient involvement is essential.

5. Evaluation

This is the 'feedback' phase. Together the OT and patient assess progress, or lack thereof, as measured by his current goal attainment.

In the client's opinion, are OT actions improving the long- and short-term quality of his life?

Are timing expectations reasonable?

Have the client's goals changed etc? (See Chapter 9: The Nursing Process.)

Orthopaedic technician

The *orthopaedic technician* should familiarize herself with psychological implications of limb loss, including the patient's emotional rejection of the appliance constructed so painstakingly in the workshop. *He may see it as a hideous mockery of the beloved body part he has lost.* His impatience at fittings may reflect his resentment of body contact with his prosthesis, and he may displace his anger on the technician.

Complaints about discomfort may mask total prosthesis rejection. In fact, observation shows the extent of effort and ingenuity amputees are prepared to apply in order to avoid use of their prostheses, which frequently hang uselessly on their attachments. The orthopaedic technician who has considerable contact with his patients requires a level of insight, tolerance, compassion and patience seldom associated with work-bench vocations.

Facial and skin disfigurement

Because the skin is the envelope of the body, its disfigurement carries the extra burden of constant exposure to the public—there is 'no place to hide'. Sometimes, as in the case of psoriasis, unsightly stigmata provoke fear of contagion, soon communicated to the sufferer who feels himself to be unclean and untouchable. These special problems have given rise to the psoriasis support group movement.

Special medically prescribed cosmetics may help avoid feelings of inferiority, revulsion and avoidance. But the most meaningful therapy is the conditioning of inner ego strengths.

Communicating with the blind

1. Always identify yourself; don't assume they will recognize your voice.
2. When being introduced, take their hand to shake . . . they can't see yours.
3. Don't shout. They are blind, but they can hear!
4. Guide them verbally offering your arm; don't grab theirs.
5. Give directions clearly and specifically. Don't use use hand signals.
6. Show them to a chair by placing their hand on the chair back.
7. Don't distract their guide-dog.
8. When you leave their company let them know you are doing so—don't leave them talking to themselves.

Communicating with the deaf

1. Have their attention when you are speaking.
2. Look directly at them. Make sure your face is in the light so that they may lip-read.
3. Don't speak with your back to them.
4. Speak slowly and clearly.
5. Don't speak with anything near your face or in your mouth: this distorts sound and makes it impossible to lip-read.
6. Don't shout. If they are totally deaf, this won't help; if they are wearing a hearing aid, shouting will distort the sound.
7. Use hands or gestures if necessary.
8. Use pencil and paper if all else fails.

Communicating with those suffering from speech impediments

1. If you create a relaxed atmosphere they will be able to speak better.
2. Keep out extraneous noise by shutting doors and windows.
3. Allow the person to finish sentences himself, unless he is totally stuck.
4. Don't pretend you have understood when you have not—it only increases frustration.
5. Avoid the impression of hurry.

Stuttering

Etiology

In spite of a mountain of data, etiology remains a mystery.

Risk factors appear to be determined by

(i)   genetic elements interacting with environmental stress triggers;
(ii) an underlying psychoneurological basis similar to minimal brain dysfunction
      and associated with late speech: 'dyslexia' featuring
         right–left confusion and 'mixed dominance'
         hyperactivity
         abnormal EEG especially in the left temporal area.

Aggravating factors lie in

(i)   parental over-reaction to non-fluency
(ii) social pressure leading to frantic attempts not to stutter and thus establish-
      ment of a self-reinforcing stress cycle.

Stressful precipitating situations include:

   meeting strange people
   talking about stuttering
   an anxious expression on the listener's face
   speaking to a stranger on the telephone
   job interviews
   remarks such as 'You're not speaking properly', 'Stop and repeat',

'Take a deep breath'—which action eventually becomes part of the stutter. 'At
school it was at its worst. Teachers and other children lacked compassion and
spotlighted my embarrassment. I escaped from school as soon as possible.'

Treatment depends upon age of presentation:

Infantile non-fluency involves work with the family. With the child, therapy in
a play setting is designed to reduce communication stress, and teach that speaking
is fun.
   Speech hints include:
      'Talk a little slower—stretch our your long words, eg "Give back *Jennifer's*
      doll." '
With the older child treatment provides situations where the stutterer
experiences reasuring fluency and positive learning experiences. Helpful techniques include:

   singing
   whispering
   prolonging difficult words in a sing-song lilt
   control at a slow rate—breathing *out* half-way
   reading a passage, with appropriate eye contact, and in time to a metronome
   the 'Edinburgh master' which makes a noise at special times may break into
   the stutter build-up
   use of a tape recorder, the earpiece being placed in left ear leading into the
   more active temporal lobe.
   a mirror for self-monitoring smooth mouth movements.

In difficult cases the most realistic relief comes from *learning to stutter more fluently*—the subject learns to 'desensitize' his speech—to analyze his problem and work out a modification plan for an easier way of stuttering.

It is important to carry out *procedures designed to reduce apprehension*. When the stutterer feels he is going to stutter he should let himself *stutter slowly* by delaying his auditory feedback, eg 'I am *going* to town.' Hearing his own voice in delayed time, he learns to monitor his speech.

The stutterers speak:
>   'Some people try to help but they say the wrong things. Nevertheless I want people to help. Some stutterers don't want help—it's an individual thing.'

How does it feel to be a stutterer?
>   'Awful—strained—helpless.'

What the listener can do when the stutterer gets into a 'word block':
>   Reassuring remarks such as 'That happens to all of us' help break the stress cycle.
>
>   Especially with children, substitute physical activity. Don't hush up the rest of the family or hurry the stutterer—insist everyone gets his proper turn to speak.
>
>   Positive identification helps. Famous and achieving stutterers include Moses

and King George VI, who won his way to his people's hearts as he battled through his broadcast speeches.
>   'Remember that tolerance is the most important encouragement for fluency in those who speak with words whose wings are broken.*

The left-eyed child in Western culture

Constructive steps to reading skills

Improving right lead eye-movements impaired by minimal cortical injury or 'mixed dominance' and counteracting the 'reversal' tendency

(1) Red markers (i) about 2,5 cm wide and 20 cm long (the marker slides from left → right under the line just ahead of the pupil's reading focus); and (ii) in perpendicular position on right margin. A torch-bulb attached to writing utensil, so providing useful right-directional target, is also helpful.

(2) Single lines of very large writing may be isolated on charts or the blackboard so the pupil can practise left to right eye movements on isolated focal lines. *Isolation facilitates concentration on the material in hand*.

(3) A card with a horizontal slot is covered by a movable cover-piece which can be slipped off so that only a few words are revealed at a time and the eyes are directed to each part of the line in a left → right direction.

(4) The Metronoscope is a useful triple shutter short-exposure tachistoscope.

(5) The Controlled Reader: a moving ribbon film, exposes words and sentences, with increasing speed, in a left → right direction.

Authorities agree that a child should not be asked to read individually in the class until he can do so with reasonable efficiency and confidence. Exposure of poor skills predisposes him to feelings of inferiority, anxiety, disorganization and depression.

---

* Charlewood, Carol. 1986.

Constructive steps to writing skills

(1) Encourage paper cutting, holding the scissors stationary in the dominant hand and moving the paper with the secondary hand only. Colour in and cut out fruit, houses, people, etc.

(2) Drawing and writing with large coloured chalks on a blackboard or large piece of paper.

(3) Crayon work on paper.

(4) Pencil work on paper, using a thick pencil of about one-half the usual length.

Again word tracing is of importance, as is the use of a free-flowing ball-point pen.

Where visual motor skills are grossly impaired, but intellect reasonably intact, it is often advisable to teach *typing from an early age*. This is certainly preferable to continuous, frustrating inhibition of mental output by the complicated neurological processes involved in writing.

Rehabilitation and the cancer patient

The Damocles Syndrome

Because the cancer patient lives his whole life under real threat of reoccurrence, cancer is a *physiologically, psychologically, socially and vocationally chronic illness*. The paraplegic patient, struck down by traumatic assault, at least knows his injury will go no further. The cancer patient at a conscious or unconscious level, and in keeping with his basic personality structure, *does not know where within his being the dreaded disease is spreading its tentacles, nor where, and with what agonizing death* it will emerge. If his cancer is deep within his body he is constantly frightened by real or imagined physiological sensations.

The woman with breast cancer fears to touch her body, lest normal undulations and connecting tissue feel hard and rigid. The further and deeper her fingers wander, the more she fears the tissue is abnormal. If she has suffered a mastectomy, the mutilation of her body bears constant testimony of its vulnerability.

Fears may escalate within the context of other stresses such as migration, bereavement. Even happy events may stimulate fear that anxiety may invade and spoil long anticipated joy.

We live in *a cancer-terrified society*.

In 1981 the American Cancer Association conducted a survey which revealed that:

> 1 in 2 Americans agree 'the very word cancer scares me',
>
> 1 in 3 consider the disease to be 'the worst thing that can happen to a person'.

Especially if he has undergone hospital treatment, and watched other patients shrivel and die, it is no wonder the apparently successfully treated patient undergoes the 'Damocles Syndrome'*

He is afraid to hope or plan for the future.

'How do I know I will be alive to see my grandchild?'

As every 'check-up' approaches, protective 'denial' defences disintegrate and the patient's terror of recurrence escalates.

---

* In Greek mythology, Dionysus, to show how precarious is a ruler's happiness, seated the tyrant Syracuse at a banquet, suspending over his head a sword held by a hair.

For most, intervening periods are marked by mounting *episodes of symptom fear*. Every time he learns of the suffering or death of a cancer victim, he identifies negatively. Non-pathological and aggravated psychosomatic symptoms escalate, and, unless he has a *strong, confident relationship with a doctor or nurse he has learnt to trust, and who can tolerate his necessity for frequent and repetitive reassurance,* he is doomed to a life of high- or low-level terror.

The patient frequently requires reassurance to counteract his deeper-level, conscious or unconscious, apparently irrational fears lest, in being close to those he loves, he is actually infecting them with what is, in many ways, still a mysterious and terifying disease, or he fears infection by others.

Current theories that stress undermines immunity may cause another spiralling fear.

Therapeutic rehabilitation

Of primary importance are *long-term relationships with professionals* who combine real medical skill with that long-term empathic identification which is able to:

> invite admission of fears;
> provide strong, authoritative and repetitive reassurance;
> bear the strain involved in the patient's repetitive demands for reassurance of both understandable and tangible, and emotionally slanted and intangible fears;
> cope with the patient's own shame and guilt at having to lean so heavily upon her support system—she even fears lest, in burdening him too far, she may offend or wound her healer (see The Wounded Healer p 200).

Because they constantly demand reassurance, patients fear rejection by their all-important support system. They may adopt subtle, indirect and sometimes irritating bids for reassurance. They may bring unwanted gifts.

They may put on a show of bravado or irrelevant chatter before being able to express their fears.

Sometimes it is difficult for professionals to tolerate *the duration of a patient's need for frequent examination and reassurance*. Indeed the more intelligent the patient, the more interest he takes in his disease, the more acutely is he aware that he is a long-term 'bad statistic'.

> 'I know I am doing well to have been free of symptoms for ten years, but a little voice inside me keeps saying "Ten years! How much longer can you expect?" '

It is sometimes possible to help the patient become more emotionally independent by supporting her while her stress waves recede, thus spreading her reassurance sessions gradually further apart, eg intercession telephone calls: 'There's nothing to worry about . . . this fear, too, will recede.' While one may reward such increasing independence by praise of her coping mechanisms, it is nevertheless important to avoid guilt should the stress wave become too burdensome and emotionally destructive.

> Some patients experience frightening spirals of imagined misunderstanding even as they leave the consulting room. Some are reassured by *written notes* to the effect that all is well and contradicting specific fears. Some prefer to bring *a relative to reinforce reassuring witness.*

Some may be comforted and strengthened by taking away with them a short *tape recording* of the professional's reassurance.

It is important that the professional understand, and not take offence at the patient's efforts to cope with a disease so fraught with justifiable terror.

In certain personalities *Compulsive Thoughts* of new symptoms with repetitive body searching are a painful complication.

In her paper 'Sexuality and the Cancer Patient', presented at the 4th International Conference on Cancer Nursing, organized by the American Society of Nurses in Cancer Care and delivered at the Hilton Hotel, New York City, September 1986, Margaret Lamb, School of Nursing, University of New Hampshire, described the use of *creative interpretation and prognostic information* when working with children, the educationally underprivileged and the anxious:

> 'Drawings, clay models and slides are all utilized. The nurse uses stuffed toys or plasticine to show the haemophiliac patient "good" blood cells are returning.
>
> The patient's emotional needs are deep, and individual understanding and information, together with freedom for catharsis of even the most apparently ridiculous "fears" are encouraged.
>
> An interim *telephonic support service* is also of value in bearing the stressful times "between". Certainly isolation increases the terror of anxiety.'

For some, according to their long-term personality structure, identification and catharsis within *self-help support-groups* help ease burdens of long-term mutilation and fear. Others resent group participation or find it imposes negative identification with advanced or relapsed members.

Sexual rehabilitation is also dealt with on p 508 and in the section Stomotherapy and Rehabilition p 524.

Extracting from Margaret Lamb's address quoted above:

Sometimes for fear of offending her patient, the nurse fails to reach real areas of misconception, discomfort, isolation, rejection fear and diminishment.

In *taking a sexual history* the nurse should try to understand her patient's long-term and newly traumatized personal experiences, circumstances and values.

Partners may also wish for information about the patient's disease, treatment, temporary and permanent sexual handicaps (see also p 82). Some cannot help fearing that cancer is an infection. '*The nurse should not allow her personal discomfort to prevent focus, and verbalization of feared or real alterations to sexual fulfilment.*'

Beginning with less threatening aspects, by bringing up delicate subjects the nurse shows she is interested in her patient's sexual satisfactions. 'Try unloading the question *by taking sexual activity for granted.* "It is important to avoid fatigue when first returning to sexual fulfilment." ' Hence it may be possible to broach the subject of new positions, warm baths, massages or analgesic poultices to avoid pain.

It is important to stress to *all* patients including adolescents, 'singles', married, divorced, widowed, the aged, homosexuals that they are entitled to the physical and psychological satisfactions of sexual fulfilment, even though this may require amendment of technique (pp 508-11, 526ff). The nurse should, of course, keep up to date in areas of reconstructive surgery.

Especially where there has been mutilation of a specifically sexual nature, as would apply in mastectomy and penectomy, the nurse's ability to accept anger and rejection, misery and despair—together with her ingenuity, patience, optimism and deep affection are needed to restore the patient's body image, self-esteem and confidence in his sexual role and desirability.

Reintegration into society

Cancer patients returning to society are often confronted by unexpected traumatic events such as termination of personal, accident and medical aid insurance.

Socially, they may be avoided by those who fear lest association with this dreaded disease prove either frightening or even physically, contagious.

Their presence at social gatherings may cause involuntary embarrassment, fear and avoidance, all of which are 'introjected' by patients, compounding their feelings of personal, social and physical rejection.

Vocational rehabilitation

Perhaps the most disconcerting obstacle to social rehabilitation is impaired employability.

Impaired employability

In studying 17 350 post-cancer patients, Bell found that although recovered patients often had better work records than their colleagues, only 55% were still working after five years. Employers' reasons for reduced employability included:

> fear of contagion;
> physical and cosmetic disfigurement.

A Californian study reported by Patricia E Greene, Assistant Vice-President for Cancer Nursing, American Cancer Society, at the 4th International Conference on Cancer Nursing, New York, 9 September 1986 *(Reintegration into Society)*, found that of recovered *'white-collar' workers reintegrated into society* reasons for non-employability were as follows:

> 54% identified problems due to:
>> hostility;
>> exclusion from promotion—employers lacked confidence that training and increased responsibility were justified due to the possibility of recurrence.
> 22% had experienced job application rejection due to:
>> ineligibility for insurance;
>> anticipated absenteeism;
>> applications screened away because employment of former cancer sufferers 'is not company policy'.

'Blue-collar' workers:

> although 45% could show an average absence from work for treatment not exceeding nine weeks, and

45% show no absence from work thereafter,
35% felt discriminated against;
23% were rejected from previous employment;
13% were denied new jobs.

'Very clearly the extent of social and business prejudice against the successfully treated cancer sufferer is deep, real and widespread. It involves emotional reactions on the part of employers and colleagues requiring educational and propaganda campaigns, directed towards both tangible and intangible fears.'

STOMATHERAPY AND REHABILITATION

In a society so obsessively cleanliness-oriented as ours, in which the all-important mother-figure, from the earliest days, attaches feelings of disgust and rejection to the processes, products, sounds and odours of elimination, the trauma of finding oneself reduced to an externally-sited mobile lavatory is a devastating one. Irrespective of *intellectual* insight into the need for a stoma, the patient is swamped by *feelings* of self-disgust, which he *projects* on to others, convinced they also conceive of him as a 'dirty' and maldorous 'bag' . . . as indeed, some involuntarily do!

Katherine Jetter, Rehabilitation Counsellor, Arlington, Virginia, USA, (1980) summed up the predicament of the stoma patient thus: 'It is beyond description what incontinence does to a man's ego and dignity.'

'In childhood', Sister Mara Ferreira of the Red Cross War Memorial Children's Hospital, submits 'it is essential that we understand the developmental stages of the child. We must help him adjust, stage by stage, from babyhood, through his schooling and into the teenage years.'

In the context of appropriate maternal education, a child may be discharged within 14 days post-operatively, thus avoiding the mal-effects of maternal deprivation.

The continuity of *out-patient and home visiting care* should provide an opportunity for increasing rapport, support and self-confidence, through the realization that someone will always be available to help.

The hospital serves child ostomates over a wide area. Mothers and children from far-flung places are brought into town, where they are taught, advised and supported in coping with their problems.

Most children requiring stomatherapy are born with anorectal abnormality or with Hirsch Sprung's disease.

Although ectopiabescia occurs only approximately once in 40 000 births, this does not reduce the plight of children suffering from this condition.

Sister Ferreira conducts a very individualized and long-term programme to help these children. She realizes the necessity for encouraging free discussion of cosmetic and psycho-social aspects.

Comforted by identification, and his inhibitions relaxed, the child is able to communicate his problems, obtain catharsis, insight and information; to become aware of his developing sexuality, and throughout his life to seek help in plastic surgery, psychotherapy, establishment of heterosexual relations, etc. A commonly verbalized anxiety-area in parents pertains to their child's capacity for normal sexual development, participation, reproduction. Sister Ferreira finds that fathers are most concerned with their child's ability to reproduce, and mothers with participation in the sex act. She records their relief when girls begin to menstruate.

The ostomate child needs to be helped in many social areas. Spending a night with a friend becomes a major problem. Although one does one's best, the child still misses out in many aspects of his social development.

(See also The Physically Handicapped Child, p 286.)

Sister Prilli Stevens, Principal Stomatherapist, emphasizes the difficulties encountered by schoolchildren in disposing of stoma bags:

> 'They are obliged to make themselves conspicuous by obtaining special permission to leave the room. They must stand in queues to use public toilets, many of which flush insufficiently. These matters should be discussed with the child and his teachers, the latter being asked to allow adequate time and opportunity to change bags and to keep spare ones available.'

The effects of ostomy on intimate relationships

Katherine Jetter emphasizes the necessity for ongoing sex and marriage counselling. She points out that

> 'having an ostomy may cause severe strain in marriage. Even if we are not qualified for marriage counselling, we should still listen and have empathy, since this is the beginning of counselling. Marriage problems are rampant in cases where a baby requires an ostomy, since the mother usually gives most of her attention to the child and the husband is neglected. The rest of the family are also affected by a lack of attention.'

Owing to specific feelings of uncleanliness and humiliation, the rehabilitation of the sexual self-image of the ostomate is a particularly sensitive area, but is not to be avoided. Patients worry about the sight, smell and sound of the stoma during intercourse. What is the risk of dislodgment and soiling?

The risk of dislodgment

> 'In a survey of 20 male ileostomates after panproctocolectomy for ulcerative colitis, interviews were conducted 1 month and 3 months after operation. This study indicated a significant improvement in the rate of partial impotence between these two periods. All patients were being seen regularly by a stomatherapist and had received pre-operative counselling.'[*]

For a more detailed discussion of sexual rehabilitation after an ostomy, refer to Rehabilitation after spinal-cord injury (p 508).

Penectomy certainly requires sensitive reassurance of a man's capability to satisfy his partner to orgasm through manual and oral-genital stimulation (which clitoral stimulation, according to Masters & Johnson, in any case produces a more intense response than that produced through intercourse).

---

[*] Immelman, E J (professor of surgery). 'Surgery and sexual dysfunction.' *Continuing Medical Education* Vol 1, May 1983.

It is important, for this reason, that the partner be aware of alternative erogenous zones, such as the mouth, the nipple and inner thighs.

Stomatherapy and the cancer patient

Bridget Breckman, clinical specialist in stoma care at the Royal Marsden Hospital, maintains that a warm and caring environment, where patients feel safe to expose strong fears and emotions, is essential to individualized care of the ostomy patient.

One mourns the loss of an important body-part as one would a loved relation. 'It is not sufficient for the care-givers to know about surgical and chemotherapeutic techniqes. Explanations should be tailored to meet the individual's needs, in reducing fear and promoting trust between the patient and the care-giver.'

Discussing problems with nurses who can listen and advise helps to minimize the depression that many patients feel at some stage during treatment:

> 'The greatest compliment a patient can pay his care-giver is the *trust that she would not abuse his vulnerability* when he shares his fear and feelings with her.'

The Royal Marsden Hospital carries over its ostomate care to district or *community nurses*, who go out to visit patients, assess their needs and then report back to the hospital clinic.

Amid the pain, terror, life-threatening illness, and general aura surrounding cancer diagnosis, the patient may consider it inappropriate to enquire about sexual function. Yet despite their fatal illness, people do continue to be interested in sex, and should be encouraged to enjoy the bonding, the comfort and the closeness of sexual intimacy, even, if possible, in hospital.

Vocational rehabilitation

Norma Gill, Director of Enterostomal Therapy, Cleveland Clinic (USA) and President of the World Council of Enterostomal Therapists, herself an ostomate, is cautiously optimistic about public opinion in the United States:

> 'Even 10 years ago, employment for an ostomate was a disaster.
>
> Today the USA has a vocational rehabilitation service, partly state-funded, which reviews, and where necessary, re-educates the ostomate for an alternative job at his present place of employment, or with another organization.'

Stomatherapy and the Muslim community

Special difficulties are encountered by Muslims in a community which has strict and *specific taboos pertaining to hygiene*. These involve the ritual purification of one's body, garments, and place of prayer five times daily prior to performing religious duties.

> 'Before each of these prayer-times ablutions have to be performed. The discharge of any substance—even gas—from the anus, urethra or genitalia, makes ablutions compulsory. To the ostomate this means removing the bag if

soiled, cleaning the stoma and re-applying a new device 5 times a day, since he may not go from one prayer-time to another without undertaking ablutions.'

Besides the inconvenience, this is very expensive unless covered by National Health.

If one or both natural openings are closed, a substitute *made below the umbilicus* is treated as a natural opening, and any substance passing out nullifies ablution. This prevents a person from performing salaah and, especially to the orthodox Muslim, is a major problem interfering with the core of his life. If the opening were made above the umbilicus, this would not nullify ablution, even where the natural openings are blocked.

The advent of stomatherapy is to be welcomed because it helps counter the belief that the ostomate is an 'unclean' person who should be disqualified from performing salaahs. Despite the problems, there has been much progress in the Muslim community, where there is growing acceptance that an ostomate, being a person with an illness which may befall anyone, should be accepted in the performance of salaahs.

There is in Enterostomal Therapy emphasis on the deep-lying, and persistent, emotionally crippling effects of mutilating surgery—mal-effects which may fester at conscious or unconscious levels long after the patient presents with overt 'brave' and 'conforming' behaviour.

Myocardial rehabilitation

In their paper 'Multidisciplinary VA Cardiac Rehabilitation: Preliminary Results and Treatment Efficacy'* Edward J Hickling PsyD, Susan S Daly PhD, Maria-Paz Alfonso MD and Kurt Euller PhD report on the physical and psychological effects of a programme directed towards an older, generally retired Veterans Administration group of 44 males aged 48 to 79 years, over the period May 1981–85. Twenty-one subjects had undergone bypass graft surgery.

The programme consisted of 14 sessions comprising:

1. *A physical exercise programme:* individualized exercise programmes were followed by comprehensive evaluation.
2. *Lifestyle modification sessions* of one hour's duration.

These emphasized lifestyle changes and risk factor modification, education about heart disease, and supportive counselling.

'Emphasis is placed on dealing with the loss of personal roles, adjustment to lifestyle changes and developing a supportive group atmosphere which fosters individual growth and positive change. These sessions also offer an opportunity to reinforce positive health behaviours and identify participants who may need individual psychotherapy.

Spouses and family members are encouraged to attend the group sessions and are specifically invited to attend sessions dealing with diet, the effect of

* Presented at the 94th Convention of the American Psychological Association, Washington DC, August 1986.

heart disease on the family, and problem behaviours such as overeating or smoking. All groups are led or facilitated by a team of psychologists.

A multidisciplinary team approach is used, and invited speakers include a psychologist, social worker, dietician, recreation therapist, nurse, physician and corrective therapist. Teaching methods include lectures, audio-visual materials and group discussions.'

The pre- and post-treatment measurement instrument was the New York State Heart Assocation functional Classification Ratings.

Results

1. 'Significant improvements were found on all treatment measures. Of the 44 patients studied, 35 (77%) demonstrated improvements in NYSHAFC functional classification, 9 remained at the same level (23%) and none (0%) worsened. These changes across treatment were statistically significant, $t(43) = 8,45$ p $< 0,001$.'
2. It appears that this treatment programme is effective despite variations in initial cardiac status.
3. This improvement extends to a number of important physical, educational and emotional factors.

The latter were as follows:

Hopkins Symptom Checklist
Mean Raw Scores Across Treatment

Subscale	Pre	Post	t	Alpha
Interpersonal sensitivity	10,94	9,56	2,667	p<0,05
Phobic anxiety	14,62	13,31	1,167	n.s.
Retarded depression	24,25	23,00	1,091	n.s.
Anger-hostility	20,25	19,00	1,212	n.s.
Somatization	33,62	29,75	2,175	p<0,05
Obsessive compulsive	10,94	10,25	1,090	n.s.
Agitated depression	19,31	16,81	2,236	p<0,05
Psychoticism	10,94	10,50	0,499	n.s.
Total score	144,88	132,19	2,568	p<0,05

N = 16, df = 15

4. Some risk factors appear to take longer to change than others. Smoking is one such example. Of the five patients who smoked in this study, two stopped after the ten-week programme supported by continued intervention from the psychology staff. 'It seems reasonable in our older, more resistant population, not to expect them to be able to change everything at once.'
5. Lack of change in the weight of patients has resulted in a more concerted team approach to weight loss and greater behavioural intervention by the psychology staff.

Sexual rehabilitation

Myocardial infarction may affect sexual function largely through fear of recurrence, pain or death, or as a result of side-effects such as depression and anxiety.

Although intercourse is considered ill-advised for the first six to eight weeks after the attack, and until the patient can comfortably climb two flights of stairs, intimacy through touch, caressing and other loving gestures should be encouraged, even in the hospital. Therein lies comfort, emotional growth and hope for the future.

Reference: Nursing Times, June 1980, and *Congress Report.*

REHABILITATION IN HANDICAPS RESULTANT UPON CEREBRAL IN-SULTS—congenital, obstetric, CNS infections, cerebral haemorrhages, cerebral tumours and haemorrhages, motor and industrial accidents, etc.

Many significantly disabled people never seek welfare service assistance. Physical disability *alone*, especially where it occurs in people under approximately 30 years of age, is seldom comprehensively devastating. Throughout school-going years there is increasing emphasis on integrating the limb-deficient and CNS impaired pupil of normal intelligence into ordinary school facilities. But where *cerebral injury has occurred, the client frequently presents with multple impaired areas,* e g

frontal lobe organic brain damage featuring fall off in speed, recent memory, new learning, and mental flexibility with resultant rigidity and 'flatness' of thought processes leads to

→ reduced intellectual output calculated by *Net Deterioration Index.* N.D.I. is obtained by statistical comparison of

'*Hold*' abilities: comprehension, vocabulary, social insight

with

'*Don't Hold*' abilities—recent memory, speed of new learning; occipital-spatial discrimination, visual-motor organization

→ fall-off in specific areas of intellectual functioning, preserveration,

→ the larger *the N.D.I. the greater the probability of significant organic cerebral loss*

→ anxiety

→ feelings of inferiority + reduction of inhibitory power, seated in frontal lobe

→ aggression, anger, sometimes paranoia-like symptoms, reduction in self-control, over-reaction

→ personality deviation.

It is these changes in intellectual processes (net DI) and personality rather than physical symptoms which hamper rehabilitation.

Client characteristics

Where the person of *reasonable intellectual potential and emotional adjustment*, ie IQs 90 upwards, Mental Age approximately 16 years (consistent with normal expectancy), lower fourth form and above attainment, does seek special training, rehabilitation services should be designed to provide:

Specific assessment techniques

Aptitudes	Interests	Personality
General learning ability	Outdoor	Preference for
Verbal–Language	Computational	Group participation
Numercial	Mechanical	Stable routine
Spatial creative	Scientific	Ideas
Form perception	Persuasive	Concrete things
Clerical	Literary	Avoiding conflict
Motor speed	Musical	Controlling others
Fine finger dexterity	Social service	
	Clerical	
Manual dexterity		

Projective Techniques involving storytelling, drawing, etc reveal deeper level emotional functioning.

Programming

Specific Job Training
1. Skilled craftmanship.
2. Amended job training, eg qualified mechanic with head (motor neurone) injury leading to right-hand paralysis. Use of alternative processes and equipment, and supervision of an unqualified assistant.
3. Development of Predominant verbal-numerical-clerical skills (some left-hemisphere injuries impair speech).

The implementation of this programme requires

(a) specialized 'shortcut' specific *educational procedures*. The long parth of orthodox educational requirements is time-consuming and discouraging. One hopes for development of audio-visual *crash courses* in office calculating machines and typewriters—business administration, accountancy, business communication, etc within restructured work situations.

(b) Public speaking—telephones and switchboard—shorthand and dictaphone typing. Office grooming and manners, filing, duplicating.
Office relationships—how to manage without boring or burdening other staff members with the specific problems of the handicapped.
Training requires audio-visual equipment—films, slides, dramatization, comic representation . . . all within a reproduced clerical-administrative-retail setting parallel to workshop working model.

Where cerebral involvement has reduced intellectual potential or the *client has only rudimentary education and below average intelligence*—of whom a high proportion present at rehabilitation centres—an especially difficult rehabilitative problem results.

Assessment: Borderline or Mild Mental Handicap (or Learning Difficulty/ Dysfunction)

IQ 50–80 ultimate Mental Age 8 to 12 years relative to normal cerebral maturity at Chronological Age 16:

The client's Aptitude Pattern is assessed relative to standardized job requirement patterns.

In spite of a long history of academic failure, clients IQ 60–80 (and their parents), expect to 'learn clerical work because I am crippled'.

The unrealistic ideas of the client and his family (frequently uncorrected by welfare agencies) result in heavy reliance on rationalization (excuse making).

Long periods of hospitalization, or other institutionalization, have (a) impeded formal education, and environmental learning, (b) resulted in blunting of the personality and dependence expectation. These clients require specific audio-visual and reality model training in the existent environmental orientation—outlay of the city, location and utilization of public transport, places of entertainment and cultural development; how to find one's way around and utilize supermarkets. Clearly this programme should be extended to evening and other after-hour activities.

Limitations

Owing to their intellectual limitations such clients will always

(a) lack social judgement;
(b) lack sufficient discretion for economic independence, or for more than marginal social success. Their naïve judgement may produce unfavourable conduct;
(c) require some form of protective environment, preferably within the community.

It is thus apparent that they will rarely be able to compete on the open labour market and require permanent sheltered employment facilities.

Usually such persons can be divided into two areas of vocational training in accordance with areas of relative cerebral integrity:

(a) reasonably intact upper motor neurone and occipital-visual integrity: metal and wood preparation—sorting, assembling
stitching; soft goods assembly; assistant role in cooking, baking, confectionery, domestic and janitor services, eg cloakroom attendant;
(b) some integrity of frontal lobe intellectual function and Clerical Perception IQ 75 upwards: very simple routine checking, packing, sorting, stencil labelling.

This group also requires modified environmental orientation programmes detailed above.

Post cerebral haemorrhage, tumour and other brain-injured clients present with multifaceted handicaps of which, in general, physical crippling presents less long-term impediment to rehabilitation than do personality and intelligence defects. Typically personality changes include mood swings, agitation, reduced self-control and concentration, or, in contrast, loss of mental shift, *persecutory ideas. Sometimes emotions are flat and motivation blunted.*

In June 1983 Judge Deborah Rowland granted a divorce to Oscar winning actress Patricia Neal because of her husband's alleged 'unreasonable behaviour':

> 'The couple, who have four children, married in July 1953. The marriage has been described as one of the greatest love stories of the present day.
>
> The way he fought to bring her back to normal living, after she was left a near-vegetable by the strokes, has been immortalized in a film starring Glenda Jackson and Dirk Bogarde.
>
> But the woman who "came back" was said to have a different personality to the one he had known and the couple parted. He returned to his Buckinghamshire home and she to her home in the United States.'

Certain cerebral functions are complex and interwoven. Among others, Syren Johnstone of the Department of Experimental Psychology at the University of Oxford (1988), reports research indicating that:

1. Functions of the temporal lobe extend beyond auditory discrimination and balance.

2. Although the occipital lobe is concerned with basic aspects of vision, it is primarily a relayer (rather than a processor) of visual images to the *inferior temporal cortex*.

    "Indeed, this latter site represents the highest level of visual processing, its neurons dealing most effectively with information about the *synthesized* shape and colour of objects, words, etc."

    In association with projections to the limbic structures, the temporal lobe subserves processes related to *visual attention, recognition and memory*. Thus, damage to, or dysfunction of the *inferior temporal lobe cortex* may result in failure both to *synthesize and recognize objects*, although their parts may be identifiable, eg the patient may recognize individual letters but not word shapes. (*Remediation* may harness intact substitution processes such as parietal kinaesthesis and motor movements—tracing, clay modelling, etc—in order to bridge and rebuild word recognition.)

3. *Parietal cortical processes* extend from touch, pain, body temperature, etc, to information concerning the *location and motion of objects in space*. Thus lesions or dysfunctions of the parietal lobe may lead to defects in locating and following objects in the visio-spatial spectrum, such as a football or flowing traffic. Such loss may also result in *sensory loss including the reception and processing of warning pain*.

A complementary and multifaceted, interwoven team approach is thus fundamental. In fact, the more deeply one probes beneath a veneer of adjustment, the more one realizes the extent of underlying flat wasteland or emotional complications and suffering. At best, the client is learning; at worst, there is churning within him anger, confusion at impaired memory and personal orientation, distressing job and personal unproductivity, the threat of poverty for himself and his family, and a feeling of having been diminished. One answer appears to lie in acknowledging, and catering for, many-faceted handicaps, widely diverse ability and personality patterns, and socio-economic environments.

The policy keynote is to restore a reasonably *healthy self-concept* by providing tasks within the client's ability in which he is likely to succeed, thus accumulating success experiences and, hopefully, restoring self-confidence.

In their paper 'The Value of Group Psychotherapy in a Young Adult Head Injured Population;, Carper and Rosenthal (Tufts University School of Medicine, Boston, Massachusetss) describe the use of group psychotherapy and its potential value in the overall psychosocial rehabilitation of the severely head-injured. Six head-injured young adults participated in a once-weekly, one-hour psychotherapy group for a period of five months. Each patient rank-ordered 60 statements from Yalom's list of curative or therapeutic factors in group psychotherapy. Analysis of patient rankings reveals that their primary concerns were for each other's progress and adjustment to their disabilities and, more broadly, for developing social skills. The results suggest that head-injured patients *can* participate in traditional group psychotherapy, and identify factors which they feel are important in accepting and coping with the consequences of their injuries. Implications for further research are discussed.*

---

* This paper was presented at the American Psychological Association Convention, Washington DC, August 1986.

CHAPTER 23

CARE OF THE DYING
AND THE BEREAVED

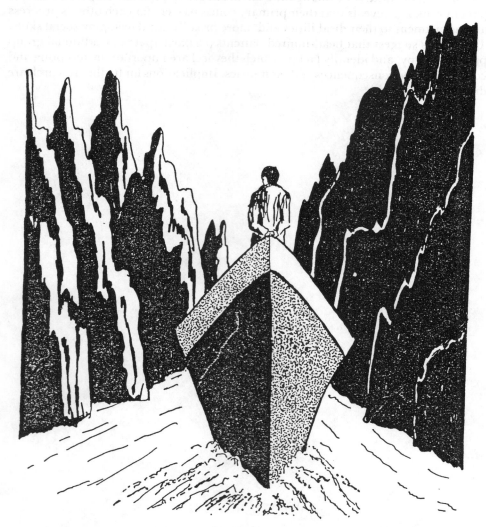

The Lonely Voyage into the Perilous Unknown* — from St. Christopher's Art Room.

'The aim is to make dying a little easier,
not to apply a dogma of always divulging
the truth.'—John Hinton *Dying*.

* Inspired by a lecture-demonstration delivered by Dame Cicely Saunders, March 1979 (see p 545).

The science which covers the problems, for patients, relatives and hospital staff, surrounding death is termed thanatology.

In dealing with the Motivation to Survive (see p 97) we have considered how the hospital team may strengthen this motivation in its conflict against motivations to escape from pain, emotional stress, etc, in death.

But what happens when death seems inevitable?

To tell or not to tell

'I would like to think that should I ever be suffering from a mortal illness, I will be told and would want to be told. It would be nice to think that one can say one's goodbyes. But at the same time do any of us know how we would react if in fact it was happening to us? Would you really want to know?'*

The team is familiar with the apparently mature, sensible and philosophical patient who claims to be capable of ' "taking" the truth'. Many doctors succumb to this type of persuasion—after all, the truth appears less trouble than does a sustained subterfuge. It may well also appear more principled to tell the truth.

The weakness of this argument lies in the *impossibility of foreseeing how he will manage to bridge that gap between intellectual understanding and emotional acceptance or feeling reaction to which we have already referred* (see p 66).

Granted intellectual-level philosophy, how can we, or he foretell how he will really react, at an emotional level, in his new, untried situation? How can we foretell the unconscious terror associations and depression his new situation will elicit?

I remember a priest, a man of deep religious faith and devotion, to whom his vocation had been a source of great joy. How many had he helped across the river of no return! I met him after his second coronary—and never have I seen anyone so frightened to die. He told me how, since his illness, he had been unable to 'shake off' a memory-picture of the expression of terror and agony on the face of his grandfather as he died—of the terror he had experienced at being obliged to see his grandfather's body as it lay in the coffin—memories long submerged, and now recalled to consciousness by his constant thoughts of death.

It is well known that patients want to gain the approval of medical staff. At an unconscious level, they may even feel that this approval will obtain for them the best of medical attention. They put on a brave front to others; but what of their hours alone, of their thoughts at leaving their loved ones? What of the family trying to comfort, and take leave of, their loved ones—all of them without hope under the sentence of death?

Some members of the hospital team maintain that a patient's constant doubts are more painful to bear than knowledge of forthcoming death.

However, it may well be argued that the patient's constant questioning is really a *bid for reassurance that he is not going to die.*

Proponents of the 'tell all' school claim that radiotherapy, chemotherapy and mutilating surgery are in themselves evidence of fatal illness. 'Patients are not fools—they know.' Yet even those told the cold-blooded truth retreat to denial and rationalization when the reality is too terrible to bear.

---

* Taken from David Alexander 'Last Word'. *Social Work Today* Vol 14 No. 7. Quoted in *Senior News* Vol 10 No 1.

Perhaps we should consider the matter from another angle. In view of the terrible suffering imposed by current cancer treatments, is the medical profession not beholden to show more sensitivity in selecting only those patients who really do have a reasonable chance, leaving others to deny where possible, or to 'go out' floating on a sea of comforting drugs as the end of the journey approaches?

Above all, can there be justification for telling patients their treatment has failed, the manner in which the disease is spreading, and the hopeless suffering that lies ahead? What benefit lies in anticipation of hopeless suffering, personal disintegration and heart-rending partings?

The case against the death sentence is well put by David Miller, Clinical Psychologist at St Mary's Hospital, London:

> 'Much discussion inevitably centres on the prognosis. Where possible, the staff should avoid attempting to give a prognosis, particularly estimates of time left to live. Such estimates could well be quite wrong, and they tend to take hope away. Patients who have been told they will be dead in so many months or years will usually 'accept' this information, and the incentive to fight for life, or even a better quality of life remaining, can be destroyed by the apparent certainty of the medical authority. Dwelling on the statistics of mortality is similarly unhelpful, and can lead to helplessness and pessimism. General statistics are not relevant to individual cases, and although many patients will be aware of the bleak prognosis associated with particular illnesses, the emphasis should be more on prospects for maintenance and recovery. Replies should be honest and constructive, not destructive. In these circumstances no one can honestly say when a patient will die, and the job of the staff is to promote health—not to pass death sentences!'*

The facility with which even intelligent patients 'grab at the straw' of hope embodied in a reassuring rationalization illustrates the manner in which 'hope springs eternal in the human breast'. *Are we justified in killing hope?*

The relief on the face of a patient when he is reassured that radiotherapy is for arthritis rather than for cancer evidences the strength of the motivation for personal survival.

How can the nurse handle constructively the patient's frequent questions which reflect his anxiety concerning death? To advise the patient to hold back his anxiety until the doctor's ward round is often impracticable—he needs long-term reassurance by the whole team.

The following handling of such a situation may well constitute a useful pattern:

Patient: Nurse, am I going to die?

Nurse: We are all going to die—no one knows when. I, or your doctor, may be killed in a motor-car accident tomorrow. I suppose in a way we begin to die when we are born. It's part of nature's plan; but no prophesy *when* an individual is going to die is silly and pointless.

Patient: But what of my illness—I don't feel as if I'm getting better.

Nurse: What makes you think you are going to die?

Patient: Every day I feel a little worse. And all these treatments. . . .

---

* Miller D, Weber J and Green J. *The Management of AIDS Patients* (MacMillan Press, London 1986).

Nurse: You are sick—there is no doubt about that. But you are in the capable hands of a very experienced hospital team. Everyone is doing his best. The way medical science progresses nowadays it is impossible to make rash calculations about anybody's life-span. But would you like to talk about death—the way you feel about it . . . about your experiences with dying people?

In her article 'Communication with the dying—a Christian perspective' Frederika de Villiers (1986) advises thus on answering the questions of the terminally ill:

'First find out why he asks the question, perhaps by asking him a question, such as "What do you think you have?" or, "What have you been told?" After that, find out what he knows, what he has been told and by whom.

It is not safe to assume you know what the person wants before you have made the effort to find out from him in detail. If the person asks whether he is dying, even more care should be taken to find out just why the question is asked. Again the best reply might be another question: "Do you think you're dying?" If he says "Yes" then find out who told him, how he knows and what exactly was said (Birrer, 1979:5)'

Many people experienced in the handling of serious illness have found *the general truth more comforting than the specific death sentence.*

The patient may *want to talk about death.* If we prevent him from so doing we are emphasizing our own fear in this area, and denying him the opportunity for catharsis.

In inviting the patient to talk about his ideas of illness and death, we are *afforded the opportunity of gaining insight* into his anxieties, sadnesses and phantasies. Such conversation is of great import, affording an opportunity to help the patient in those areas which are so important to him.

Realizing the *emotional isolation and personal distress,* albeit hidden, in which the dying patient may, all too often, find himself, there has, in recent years, developed a movement which claims *to help achieve acceptance* and thus relative peace of mind. Among the writings upon which this school is based are *Dying* by John Hinton (Penguin Books, 1967) and *On Death and Dying* by Elizabeth Kübler Ross, (London Tavistock Publications, 1970). They describe the following anticipated stages of patient reaction in response to confirmation of expected death:

1. *Awareness*

The first stage of awareness includes feelings of shock, unreality, emotional numbness, anxiety, panic, and sometimes uncontrolled weeping.

To the nurse trying to help her patient in this terrible predicament Federika de Villiers recommends:

'The personal relationship between us and the dying person functions very strongly. By our loving attitude and compassion we must make him feel that he is accepted and free to express all his feelings of distress. (De Klerk, 1971; Venter 1972; De Villiers 1976.)

When he begins weeping, we must maintain an attitude of warm acceptance and stay quietly by him. Some people want absolute privacy, even from their own family. In this case we should leave him alone for a while and then return.

When he stops crying, we must be available to listen to him if he wants to talk. A leading question can initiate or encourage a conversation, such as "Is there anything I can do to help?" or "Would you like to talk about it?" But be careful not to force an explanation (McGreevy, Van Heukelem, 1976:21)'*

2. Denial

Freud says 'no one believes in his own death', and that 'in the unconscious everyone of us is convinced of his own immortality'.

This may well be Nature's defence in the face of the unacceptability of total personal decay and extinction.

As a defence mechanism denial carries the disadvantage of alternating with anxiety. However, even Dr Judith Landau, a convinced exponent of this school of thought, concedes 'denial may occur at any point, and people often need to retreat to a state of denial and hope, even after reaching acceptance. One must be sensitive to this need and allow it to happen, provided it does not become overwhelming. Despite the knowledge that it is a façade, the world of daydreaming may, at times, be an essential consolation.'†

3. Anger

'He experiences an intense and increasing fury, which is all the worse for not having any logical object. He may blame the treatment staff, his friends and even his God and dearest relatives. This is the time to be gentle and understanding, when one is least capable—for anger hurts all the more when one feels helpless. It often takes great effort to allow the patient to express his anger while remaining relatively unscathed oneself.'

Handling of this reaction to serious illness requires real intelligence and compassion. Where the hospital staff retreats into cold aloofness or into retaliatory aggression the patient's anger twists into self-agonizing fury against anyone who is whole, healthy and with a prospect of a good life to come.

4. Bargaining

In the book of Job it is written 'All that a man hath would he give for his life'.

But deep in his heart 'each man knows that, in reality, life and death are not for trading'.‡ The patient who is exposed to these stages towards death is especially prone, at this stage, to search his heart for causes why *he* should be singled out for such a fate and in this search he will inevitably encounter 'reasons' for mounting guilt and anxiety.

* De Villiers, Frederika. Communicating with the dying—a Christian perspective. September 1986.

† 'Truth or Lie to the Terminal Patient', a paper delivered by Dr Judith Landau at a conference on death, June 1976. (Details available from author.)

‡ Ibid.

'Free expression of feelings by the patient must be encouraged by empathetic listening, so that feelings of rebellion, guilt and despair can be expressed. We must be patient with the patient and realize that he is miserable and that aggression is not meant personally.'*

5. *Anxiety and fear sometimes mounting to terror*

There are few predicaments more terrifying than the knowledge that no one—neither one's most beloved nor those one respect most—can help one.

Anxiety and fear of death are not the patient's alone, but are shared by his family, friends, doctors and nurses. In 'abandoning' their patient to death, the doctor and nurse encounter their own fears of failure, their own guilt feelings.

The patient's anxiety is not always overt. The classic picture of panic, tremor, palpitations and other manifestations is not always present. The patient may even project his anxiety on others: 'Are you sure my child's all right?'

Sometimes his fears may recede, to re-engulf him later.

It is in exposing their patients to death's terror association and depressions that the exponents of this school encounter conflict with those who have long struggled, often in vain, to *bridge the gap between intellectual understanding and emotional acceptance.*

The world's greatest psychotherapists, in spite of long, intense and highly skilled psychotherapy, sometimes fail to achieve changes in *feeling* as opposed to intellect. *Even were such facilities available to every dying patient, there would remain the great danger of 'fixation' on distressing terror, anger and depression, rather than hoped-for arrival on the serene shore of 'acceptance'.* To expose the patient to the terrors and depression of death and then rely on psychiatrists and psychologists to 'put him back together again' is indeed dangerous. Specialists in human emotions and behaviour are not magicians!

There is something very ironic in the healthy telling the ill how to die!

6. *Depression and grieving*

'At this time the person enters a period similar to that of the people who are losing someone they love. In fact, it has often been suggested that the stages of dying are very similar to the stages of grieving.

We always think of those who grieve as the family of the dying person. We ignore the fact that the dying person has the same, if not more, cause for grief.

He faces the loss of not one, but all his loved ones. And he faces also the loss of himself and all the things that are important to him.

If we don't see evidence of grief in a dying person he may be managing to keep it hidden from us and probably others.'†

There is realism in the attitude of Islam:

'The terminally ill patient may often be in a state of anxiety and even depression, but there is nothing that relieves the anxiety and depression. The

* De Villiers, Frederika. Communicating with the dying—a Christian perspective. September 1986.

† De Villiers, Frederika. Communicating with the dying—a Christian perspective. September 1986.

recitation of the Holy Qur'an, in the sweetest manner in this most solemn way, will help him sooth the pangs of dying.'*

Depression incorporates the loss of all hope. It follows poignant realization that the patient's life holds no future. He will not see his children grow up; he will never again walk in the sunshine. Even while he decays in the dust, the world will go on living, loving as if he had never been. After the respite of sleep he faces anew the spectre of his doom and the agony of leaving loved ones.

> 'Depression is a very lonely place and while one dwells in it there appears to be no door. There is no loneliness greater than that of the dying person if he is allowed to isolate himself, or, as still sadly happens, is isolated by those around him, who cannot handle his dying within themselves, or who have already started to mourn, thereby commencing the process of separation. Unless an enormous effort is made, isolation is inevitable. This is therefore one of our most important roles . . . be available, not only caring, but sharing, person to person.'†

The personality of the patient may appear to disintegrate . . . one part battles to live, the other seeks to die. This latter death-seeking avoidance mechanism may present in various ways, such as varying degrees of mental withdrawal, attempting to starve oneself to death, or actual infliction of self-violence.

7. 'Acceptance'

Although life is always sweeter than the unknown disintegration of death, acceptance *may* sometimes be easier for *the elderly* who have moved into the final stage of their lives prior to the onset of terminal illness. *Children*, still near the intermingling of earthly reality and imaginative heavenly concepts, may appear to have some acceptance of death. They are still in that stage of life which believes death to be a reversible process followed by a return to life, mother and home. For the *young and middle adult* acceptance is very difficult.

Sometimes a patient's behaviour is very deceiving. Overtly, he may discuss his terminal illness with orderliness and courage.

Then he will suddenly stop in his tracks, only sometimes verbalizing his disbelief and horror:

> 'What am I talking about! Who has cancer! I haven't got cancer! *I'm* not going to die.'

The idea is quite unacceptable in its horror. Throughout this book the difference between *intellectual understanding* and *emotional acceptance* (feeling) has been emphasized. Informing the sick of the inevitability of their approaching death may indeed prove a hazardous process.

PATIENTS ARE SO APT TO FIXATE ON THE PRECEDING DISTRESS-ING STAGES OF DEATH ANTICIPATION, THAT ONE MUST HAVE

---

* Ismail Jubeda. The care of the dying patient in Islam. (Article available via the author.)

† 'Truth or Life to the Terminal Patient', a paper delivered by Dr Judith Landau at a conference on Death June 1976.

GRAVE DOUBTS OF THE WISDOM OF SETTING THEM DIRECTLY ON THIS PAINFUL PATH.

From a nurse's point of view, of course, a depressed patient is often easier to 'handle' than an anxious one.

General practitioners whose lot it is to assume long-term care of the terminally ill ask 'For how long do we place the patient in the shadow of his death sentence?'

Surely in the beginning he is entitled to some hope! At the end he is in any event, so medicated that he is little aware of his predicament. Probably nearer the patient's real need is the observation of John Hinton:

> 'The aim is to make dying a little easier, not to apply a dogma of always divulging the truth.'*

While quoting, with respect, from Dr Landau's presentation, I do differ with her on the supposition that most patients can be led to a comforting acceptance of death.

There can, however, be no argument with her submission that

> 'It is also of great importance to prevent the wrong person talking to the patient about his own death. Clumsy honesty can cause catastrophic distress. Only people with experience, trained in the field, and who really care, would be able to assess the patient's personality, strength and weaknesses, and be able to listen and to talk appropriately at the right time. The general findings are that, if possible, the person who becomes involved in these discussions should remain available to the patient and should never hand over to anybody else equally skilled. . . . The minister of religion plays a traditional and very important role in preparing both the patient and his family for death—giving of himself as both man and minister. The members of the team looking after the patient should be trained in the care of the dying and taught to send for the minister sufficiently early for him to give continuous help to the patient and his family throughout.'†

There are of course, many patients and families, of deep religious faith, who are thus comforted—but even here there is frequently a *'splitting off' between religious belief and the personal fears of the dying*. It is my conviction that religious advisers of the dying tend to *project their own religious faith upon patients*, assuming this to be much deeper than is, in reality, the case.

If the patient does come to accept his death, he may well *abandon the motivation to live*. Goals and their achievement carry no challenge or satisfaction. Without motivation he lacks even that elemental SNS tension-energy—stimulants and blood sugar—which is essential for the maintenance of body processes. Lacking motivation he atrophies physically and mentally, 'turns his face to the wall' and dies earlier than anticipated, usually in a state of sad, withdrawn depression. Or, when all hope is gone, he may choose The *Hemlock Solution* borrowing a quote from Shakespeare: 'Is it a sin to rush into the secret house of death 'ere death dare come upon us?'

---

* John Hinton. *Dying* (Penguin Books, 1967).

† Op cit. See the note on p 537.

The Hemlock Society, contends there are at least two forms of suicide—emotion, or 'irrational' suicide, and justifiable, or 'rational' suicide.

Members endorse 'rational' suicide for people who have carefully thought through their options. 'For many people in unbearable pain, or grave, intolerable physical handicap, just *knowing* suicide is possible may be a great comfort, even extending life.'*

The stages of denial, anger, terror and depression are intrinsically so painful that one wonders why the patient should be subjected to such emotional trauma. In the last stages of most terminal illnesses he is, in any case, so weak or heavily medicated that he is *unaware of or detached from the imminence of death.* Why, then, should he, and his relatives be subjected to exposure to the death sentence? Rather than spend time thinking of ways to accept death, which will probably come in a state of extreme physical weakness, heavy medication and reduced consciousness, it would appear *wiser to concentrate on making as happy as possible the patient's conscious moments* . . . encouraging both patient and family to live for the day, the hour, the moment, attempting to fill each with some little pleasure—a creative activity, a visit; favourite food, participation in friendship; a film; music. Always something to look forward to—always the conviction that 'tomorrow is another day'.

An eminent, much respected surgeon believes in gradually revealing to his adult patients the fact that they are going to die, and supporting them through their trauma.

Yet, in the very distressing situation of a child with a cerebral tumour, he allows the parents to enjoy the benefits of a 'shunting op', without warning them of a reassertion, within a varying period of time, of the symptoms.

He maintains that to do so would 'spoil' the last period with their child. It would appear to me that the validity of his argument extends to the adult patient and his family, who in the context of the distressing, frightening loneliness of the death threat, regress to the immature and frightened responses of children.

Medical staff are often cross-questioned by clients who apparently seek truthful answers, only to be accused later of destroying any hope that they may have enjoyed and plunging their last months into depression. In an effort to handle pressure and guide personnel Dr Spencer Jones, a chest physician in Folkestone, England, selected 183 patients suffering from terminal lung cancer.

All were told that, after investigation to exclude various diseases including cancer, they could, if they so wished, receive truthful answers concerning diagnosis, prognosis, etc.

If they did not wish to know their diagnosis, all they needed to do was not ask: <u>Ninety patients asked for their diagnosis and 93 deliberately did not ask</u>.

Of those 90 who did ask:

Ten 'denied' their diagnosis and talked as if their life expectation was good. They used vague diagnostic terms such as 'lung congestion'.

---

* 'To be or not to be' An ethical discussion. *Cope Magazine for cancer patients, their families and physicians.* September 1986. 12600 W. Colfax, Suite B–400, Denver, CO 80215 1–800–343–COPE.

It was surmised that these, and perhaps other patients, in asking, were confident they would receive good news. When diagnosis were bad, they resorted to the mental mechanism of 'denial'.

Of the 93 patients who did not ask.

> some explained that they simply did not want to know, while 43 later gave signs that they were aware of the nature of their illness—possibly because of the treatments prescribed—but apparently preferred uncertainty to the 'sentence of death'.

The investigators concluded that absolute policies of telling all patients, or telling none, could never suit more than half.

It is Dr Spencer Jones' conviction that terminal patients should *not be encouraged to ask for their diagnosis*, though most of them can be given an opportunity with a simple question such as:

> 'Is there anything more you would like to know?'
> 'By avoiding the conviction that everyone (or no one) should be told, or that anyone has the power to perceive who to tell, it should be possible to approach the theoretical ideal where patients accept, or even approve, of what is said, and where only the fewest possible need the safety net of "denial" because the truth is too much to bear.'
> 'Some patients really do prefer uncertainty and no-one would care to be guilty of aggravating their suffering.'*

A BBC panel under the chairmanship of Professor Hugh Dudley, consultant surgeon at St Mary's Hospital, Paddington, discussed the topic 'Should doctors tell the whole truth?' (April 1983). Younger members of the panel disapproved of the professor's non-committal approach to the terminally ill. In contrast they advocated an honest prognosis.

Striking a more cautious note, Dr Frank Tovey, a consultant general surgeon, cautioned: 'Those of us who would wish to be told the bad news of our illness exactly equal those who wouldn't.'

But the last word in the debate went to listeners who wrote in their opinions to the BBC. Ninety-five per cent preferred professor Dudley's more old-fashioned euphemisms to the more honest approach of his young and healthy colleagues. When one considers that, in spite of careful, tactful and reassuring responses to death fears on the part of the hospital team, many patients actually read their death sentences in their folders, the gap between conscientious professional behaviour and the expediency of administration becomes glaringly and destructively apparent.

> 'It's not for everyone.† *Some patients signal they don't want to know.*
> Some verbalize "I want to know", but what they are really saying is "I don't want to know".
> The professional working with the terminally ill needs to become *sensitized to the individual personality* of the patient with whom he is dealing ... her

* *British Medical Journal,* August 1981.
† Prof. Lyn Gillis.

long-standing needs and reaction patterns. This type of "metacommunica-
tion" may give clues to the patient's real needs, and if appropriate, most
suitable method of communication."*

Because of the complex nature of individual reactions to fear or knowledge of
death, <u>nurses should not feel guilty nor disappointed at their inability to carry their
patients through the death stages</u> and to reach the alleged goal of 'acceptance'.
Sometimes the path is inappropriate and the goal unattainable.

Counteracting depression resultant upon realization of serious, chronic terminal illness (see The chronically ill or disabled child p 286; Bodily loss p 503; AIDS p 347)

Typically, anxiety and depression overlap. Where early morning awakening
with heavy sadness, loss of interest in previous pleasures and marked inactivity
predominate, depression is probably a major problem.

Counteracting moves may include:

1. <u>Increase in the patient's physical activity</u>. This promotes metabolism and
   releases fight-flight survival-motivated tension energy. Understanding of
   biochemical energy output usually promotes co-operation:
   'The more active you are, the better you'll feel.'
   A programme of increasing exercise stimulates most people and helps them
   feel more in control of their situation. Moreover, participation helps prevent
   withdrawal into snowballing depression.

2. <u>Counteracting the gloom</u>. 'What's the use? I'll soon be dead anyway.' patients
   may be asked to *list despondent thoughts*. Together with the counsellor/nurse they
   are helped to consider and challenge the basis of their defeatist thinking—
   'Why cancel the vacation just because you may have to come home a bit
   earlier?' *It is important to remind all depressed patients that the present depression, like all
   other episodes, must pass.*

3. <u>Helping the patient feel that she, and not her emotional burden nor physical
   illness, is in control of her life</u>. She is a person, not a statistic, to turn off her
   motivation for survival, and thus her tension energy, just because the
   computer tells her her time is up.

Imagery technique: the 'Simonton' method (1978)

'Imagery techniques, such as the "Simonton method" (1978), <u>imagine</u> the
[<u>cancer or AIDS</u>] <u>virus being crushed</u> and dissolved by the "life force"
within your body. Similarly, in the treatment of <u>anxiety</u> accompanying
depression, patients are trained to imagine their anxiety or despair is a black
cloud enshrouding the future. They then visualize blowing the cloud into a
small, manageable box set to one side of their imagined landscape of the
future. Here the cloud rests in a concrete but not so pervasively destructive
form. In short, the extent of the anxiety and despair is limited significantly

* Dr David Rabinowitz, Senior Psychiatrist, Groote Schuur and Valkenberg Hospitals.

and the patient is allowed to do other things without these suffocating black clouds hanging over him all the time.'*

4.   Introducing an activity programme to counteract passive withdrawal and to promote increased involvement in routine and pleasure. Encourage the patient to
     (i)   list his pre-illness activities;
     (ii) devise a programme for return to realistic, albeit amended, activities, both routine (to encourage perseverance) and pleasurable (for modified goal-setting and realistic reward):
           I will get dressed.
           Then I'll make myself a cup of tea, eat my favourite biscuit and read my newspaper.
           I'll visit old Mrs Smith next door, then I'll have a whisky and watch telly. (Self-talk: 'You've done well! You're beating it!')
           Tomorrow I'll feel strong enough to go shopping.

     The role of the counsellor/nurse: The patient may try to displace the activity on the professional. By doing too much for him one may encourage regression. It is important to encourage, reward by praise and recognition, and thus reinforce activity achievement.

5.   Encouraging socialization by involving 'significant' people; asking his help in community projects such as the Easter church service; introducing to a self-help support group (taking care to avoid negative identification with more 'advanced' or anxious patients).

6.   If possible, encouraging the patient to resume work. Occupational regime involvement, and achievement as well as social contact, help break into distressing preoccupation with negative thoughts and fears for the future.

7.   Complementing the treatment programme by anti-depressant medication (probably tricyclics). This may be necessary where the patient is unable to emerge from his overpowering depression and especially where his misery is increased by obsessions and perseveration on suicide. More intense psychiatric observation and treatment may be required in the 14–21 days before medication takes effect. Programmes will require amendment in accordance with individual differences in physical condition, education, social background and personality.

Terminal agitation

Among the worst fears of the dying are isolation, pain and suffocation.

Patients eager to please kind staff may well present with a false front. Tranquillity cannot always be assumed from direct observation. For this reason Dr Cicely Saunders† trains her staff to glance back as they depart—in that instant the

---

* Simonton O C, Mathews-Simonton S and Creighton J C. *Getting Well Again*. Bantam Books, Toronto 1978. Quoted in Miller D, Weber J and Green J. *The Management of AIDS patients* (MacMillan Press, London 1986).

† Dr Cicely Saunders, OBE, SRRI, MRCP, from her lecture on St Christopher's and the Hospice Movement. March 1979.
Reference: *Care of the Dying*. Macmillan.

mask falls and they may observe depression, terror, agitation.

(*Author's note:* In addition to involved identification, comfort and distraction, terminal agitation must surely involve sedation.)

Verbally, and in their paintings, *patients 'see death as a lonely, sad and dangerous journey into the unknown'.*

A common theme in painting death associations shows a little ship sailing towards a precipice, into unknown, black, jagged mountains.

Dying is acknowledged to be very hard, but patients are encouraged to *live* until they die peacefully. To keep them in touch with the comforting reality of their 'assumptive world' patients are encouraged to bring with them books, handwork, photographs, cushions, rugs, etc which usually abound in easy disarray.

Flexibility, programming of pleasures and fulfilment so that every day contains something to which the patient can look forward, motivate him to enjoy living rather than to dwell on sorrows and fears of dying.

It is a policy at St Christopher's that each patient's file contains *a weekly observation sheet* in which everyone surrounding him—the hospital team, family, even ward maids, are invited to record their feelings about the patient's total reactions—his verbalizations, actions, joys, griefs, fears. This unstructured record-sheet is basic to weekly case conferences and team participation.

Communicating with the terminally ill

Commenting on the work of Elizabeth Kübler Ross, Dr Cicely Saunders emphasizes the former's great conribution in the care of the terminally ill. As pertaining to the six 'stages' of dying (denial, bargaining, anxiety, depression and, hopefully, acceptance), described in her book 'On Death and Dying'. Dr Saunders maintains that *Kübler Ross never intended the impression that the dying, and their loved ones all do, or should, go through these stages.* Rather does she intend to convey to her readers the kind of experiences suffered in these circumstances.

How much does one tell a terminally ill patient?—Saunders

Dr Saunders believes in allowing the patient 'to mark the way he wishes to make his lonely and frightening journey'.

Considerable *intuition, and certainly sensitivity to the needs of the individual, rather than any dogmatic formula are indicated.*

(It should be remembered that Dr Saunders works with a Christian religious milieu.)

Remarks such as 'I'm not going to die and that's that', or 'I don't want to know—I'm letting everything take its course', indicate that the patient 'wishes to close the door that leads to this dead-end corridor, or the lonely journey which lies ahead. *Closed doors should be respected.'* Patients should not be deprived of their defensive denials or phantasies.

Queries and statements such as 'We are not incurables are we?', 'Do they know what is wrong with me?', 'They told me this is a convalescent home', do not indicate readiness for learning of approaching death. Rather do they suggest a *combination of reassurance, and introduction to the possibility that the patient's illness is serious, but that everything possible is being done to ease his burden.*

'If only I could see my daughter again.' 'I'm afraid I won't see another Christmas.'

The cancer patient who says, 'I have fought so hard, and lost every battle on the way—I just can't go on fighting like this'.

Such verbalization *may herald the onset of some level of acceptance, but may also indicate deep-seated depression.*

'The person in deep communication with the dying should be sensitive to the way he talks about his illness, rather than to any thought of a death timetable.'

Dr Saunders reports the case of a young married couple, increasingly estranged as the husband's terminal stage approached. He felt his wife's failure to communicate verbally or affectionately with him to be symptomatic of love withdrawal. His fears, conveyed to the social worker, led to a confrontation, in which the wife (to whom a hopeless prognosis had been revealed early in the illness), admitted to great stress, depression and fearful isolation. *Fearful to communicate meaningfully, she had withdrawn from her husband.* When her predicament was interpreted to him, he summed up his complaint: 'Not that I should have been told more, but that she should have been told less.'

Does one leave a patient with hope, even though one knows this hope to be false?

In respone to this query Dr Saunders quoted the case of a terminally ill young woman warned of serious illness, who was determined to 'fight back' and live on, even to the extent of insisting on embarking on a pregnancy. The staff did not presume to remove her motivation to live, and were currently supporting her through the pregnancy.

> 'In dealing with those facing the mystery of death, we are with people facing the loneliest of experiences. For each individual it is the end of the road he can see. We must walk with him, supporting and sharing with him where he leads.'

Dr Saunders believes that many patients are strengthened and reassured by witnessing the peaceful death of their fellows. So dying patients are not, by routine, screened. (One wonders about the real danger of negative identification with the dying.)

Constant tactile comfort, an embrace, a loving hand to hold, constitute emotion-level comfort and support.

In order to permit close support, the nurses at St Christopher's are permitted to sit on the patient's bed.

> 'What does one talk about with a person who is dying? Too often we forget that the dying person is a living person. He has both a past and present history, his own talents, his unique interests and viewpoints. Dealing with him should be viewed as getting to know him and appreciating him as a person.'*

Specific communication difficulties in terminal paralysis

The long-standing inability of the patient to express his fears, his needs; to communicate both verbally and physically his loving feelings towards those important to him, constitutes an added barrier requiring astuteness and ingenuity, as well as patience, on the part of those surrounding him.

* De Villiers, Frederika. Communication with the dying—a Christian perspective. September 1986.

Trans-cultural communication

> 'Islam lays down principles for the care of the dying person; the caring of
> the terminally ill by the family with kindness, respect and dignity; the
> recitation of the Holy Qur'an, prayers, invocations and the attributes of
> God; keeping the patient in a state of purification, including the private
> parts; keeping the patient physically comfortable; the encouragement of
> medical therapeutic means that brings relief to the patient; allowing the
> patient to die naturally if there is no cure.'*

Interpreters are, of course, important, but more direct contact and support are
required. Saunders says:

> 'Remember that everything you do with your face and body means
> something to somebody else. A smile, touch—loving, reassuring, supportive,
> soothing—constitute international communication.'

Some nurses encounter considerable difficulty in *achieving ease of tactile communication*. Dr Saunders suggests that the shy or somewhat inhibited nurse be helped
towards ease of tactile communication by assigning her to patients who will
respond to her touch:

> 'Success and gratification in tactile communication will encourage and
> reinforce, until spontaneity is achieved. One never stops learning from
> patients.'

Although some stay much longer, even returning several times, the average stay
at St Christopher's is fifteen days. *Does segregation in an establishment for the dying lead
to panic and depression?* This is a distinct possibility which St Christopher's attempts
to counteract by:

(i) stressing that 'not everybody is dying'. There is purposeful inclusion of the
 geriatric frail accommodated, sometimes in couples, in bedsitting rooms;
(ii) extending its services into community home-care and neighbouring general
 hospitals.

> 'Although we try to alleviate suffering, and to fill life with every possible
> pleasure, parting is still very sad. By providing pain relief, efficiency in
> comforting, individual dignity, and assurance that we will stand by lovingly,
> we do believe we are able to assuage grief and ease the lonely journey of the
> dying.'

The dying child

In the tragic situation of a *dying child, infliction* of the truth upon the mother may
well constitute an emotionally unbearable situation.

'The child usually senses something is wrong as soon as the parent is told of the
diagnosis.' In order to preserve the integrity of her personality in the face of her
child's needs, and to render as happy as possible the closing period of his life, it is
probably best to warn the mother that her child is very ill, but to reassure her that

---

* Ismail Jubeda. The care of the dying patient in Islam. September 1986.

everything is being done, and that no one can be sure of the outcome of the illness. *Naturally she should be allowed to spend every possible moment with her child, both for his sake and for hers.* This is an exhausting experience, but she would be even more devastated were she deprived of the closing stages of this precious relationship.

'Terminally ill children suffer most from separation. After that comes distress caused by medical procedures and then hospital events such as the death of another child in the ward. . . . The child's understanding of death varies with the age group. Before the age of 5 most distress is caused by separation from the mother. Between 5 and 10 death is seen as a person in the form of a vague, ghost-like figure, and fear is largely physical.'*

It follows that the child should always feel safely protected by God, religious symbols, his parents and other surrounding adults. Sedation is also indicated. After 10 years children's attitudes to death approach emotions introjected from the adult environment.

Claire Irwin summarizes the child's developmental concept of death thus:

3–5 years

Research indicates that children first become aware of death around three years where it is viewed as reversible sleep.

'You are dead, then you are alive again, you are awake; or like going away, you are gone and then you come back.'

5–9 years

'The second phase in the understanding of death is between 5 and 9 years old. Children are able to accept that someone they love has gone away and will not come back for a long time. They accept this view of death but *in terms of other people*, it is something that happens to someone else but not to them. Mary, 7 years old, worried who would look after her mum when she got sick in Heaven. At this stage, death is personified, *becoming a person*, e g God, bogeyman, the Devil.'

From the age of 10 children are beginning to form abstract conceptions, and gradually begin to perceive death as nothingness, as eternity, as a permanent separation.

'Over 9 years, we find both *mutilation and death anxiety*. Death anxiety is defined as the apprehension the child feels in relation to his existence, his identity, his future.'

This anxiety may be expressed in several ways:

- 'physiologically: symptoms such as nausea, anorexia, vague pain unrelated to the reality of procedures, the illness itself, medication;
- behaviourally: the child becomes hyperactive or withdraws from activities and people, regressing to inappropriate age behaviours;

* Dr J Anderson, Senior Psychiatrist, Red Cross Children's Memorial Hospital on 'The Care of the Dying'. 1979.

- symbolically: in drawing or in play, e g the persistent use of dark colours, the playing out of his phantasies in play concerning his illness, e g a 9-year-old dying of leukaemia drew his fear of being eaten up by sharks;
- verbally: stating. "I am worried", "I feel frightened", "I feel sad", "It's sore".'

If the adults really listened:

'they would learn that children who lie in a hospital ward for any length of time can tell you the diagnosis, the symptoms, the procedures carried out, the medication, and life expectancy of other children in the ward. The children listen to the groups of doctors standing around their beds or whispering at the bottom of their beds. They talk to each other and pass on the information they have seen and heard. Each morning they check to see who's still alive, who went out into the night. They don't ask, they just listen and observe, picking up minimal cues. They become very aware of the significance of a particular side ward or a special kind of machine or procedure. Each child identifies with the very ill, the dying child. When a child dies, the one that still lives is relieved it is not he who died, but also feels guilty at feeling such relief.

The life experience of the child also influences his concept of death. Anthropologists have shown how cultural and religious beliefs and tradition influence attitudes towards death. It is important to be aware of all these factors if we are to understand the child's reactions to his own dying, and to be able to answer the three main questions children want to know about death:

- What is death?
- What makes people die?
- What happens to people when they die?'*

'We members of the multi-disciplinary team caring for the dying child must be astute to cues reflecting anxiety and provide opportunities for discussion of feelings.'

Sally aged 11:

'I'm so frightened—and my mummy must also be frightened because she doesn't want to talk about my illness and my pain—sometimes I think she doesn't love me when I'm sick and just wants to run away home to the well children.'

Sally's mother to the social worker:

'I have an awful feeling the more I love her the quicker God will take her from me—and I can't bear to see her suffer so I talk about something else or run away.'
    The role of the professional includes that of mediator

 (i) to help both parties uncover their feelings, show each other their needs;
(ii) suggest ways of reaching, comforting and reassuring each other.

Dr Cicely Saunders, pioneer of that movement, feels the hospice does not contitute a suitable environment for the dying child. Growing opinion supports children dying at home in their natural environment, 'on the sofa in mother's arms'.

---

* Irwin, Claire. The dying child. September 1986.

The efforts of Ida Martinson, a senior nurse in Minnesota, supervising an area of 400 square miles, follow a policy of identifying a good district nurse and providing her with guidance and support. In these circumstances '70% of children die comfortably in their own homes'.*

The dying adolescent

'Faced with the dying adolescent most adults are unable to gain a concept of the anger, frustration, depression, the feeling of having been cheated of fulfilment of life; the fears aroused by "What happens when I die?" At a time when the problems of dying and eternity would normally evoke anxiety, the adolescent must come to some solution for himself. Dying deprives the adolescent of the time to find out who he is, where he is going, and why he is here at all.'

A dying child or adolescent presents the whole family with a crisis situation. Clearly avenues of *communication* and *support* in following through the *classic stages of crisis* (chapter 26) are imperative if the suffering of the youngster and his parents is to be assuaged.

Siblings of the dying

If there are *siblings*, it is important that they be frequently reassured by their parents to the effect that *they are in no way responsible* for the illness of their sister or brother.

Sibling relationships are almost always complicated by rivalry, hate-swings of ambivalence, aggressive death wishes and alternating love-swings.

Where a sibling is threatened by death, brothers and sisters, caught up in the 'love-swing' of ambivalence, may well be convinced that *the death threat is a fulfilment of their previous death wish*. They suffer consequent serious feelings of guilt and anxiety, and may establish a guilt pattern constituting a life-long burden. Siblings should thus be encouraged to talk about their relationship with the patient and the casues of death, achieving that clarification and catharsis which come with verbalization. *Emphasis is thus on support of the whole family.*

When death is imminent, who copes and how?

Some hospital personnel wish their patients a dignified, quiet death free of tubes, wires, artificial resuscitators, etc. Others prefer to continue treatment, even past the moment of death . . . a course of action which may counter despair in the patient and guilt in his family.

A patient with any appreciable level of consciousness is aware when his treatment stops, the curtains around his bed are drawn, and 'important' medical personnel are no longer 'interested' in him. He may well panic when he realizes they are no longer trying to save him. He feels himself alone, a pariah cut off from the rest of humanity.

If treatment is stopped before death, the family may, at an emotional level, be

* Dr Cicely Saunders 'Death and the Family'. March 1979.

permanently haunted by the fear that more could have been done, that his life may, in fact, have been saved . . . an omission for which they may, within the context of those guilt feelings which classically accompany death, mercilessly blame themselves for the rest of their lives.

This observation is of import in handling relatives from whom consent is requested for switching off a 'life-giving machine' or for taking donor parts.

Although they may, at the time, be convinced, at an intellectual level, of the inevitability of death, they may afterwards develop very persistent and distressing feelings of guilt and anxiety. *Feeling* that death *may* have been avoided without such consent, they may well be subjected to most distressing guilt, anxiety and self remorse. This applies most strongly in post-traumatic death. *In general the most comforting compromise probably consists in the maintenance of that treatment which does not cause disproportionate pain and discomfort.*

The love-hate swings of ambivalence stalk every close relationship.

Guilt feelings stalk death. Doctors, no matter how irrationally, feel guilty at their failures, often taking to 'Flight'. These feelings are *introjected* by nursing staff. The ward sister may *rationalize* that her time is wasted in caring for the dying. So she too takes flight to the care of the living. If the senior nurse is able to do so, she may well *identify* with the sister, leaving the dying patient and his distraught relatives in the inexperienced hands of the frightened junior nurse, or to the usually somewhat limited intellectual resources of the assistant nurse. The latter is usually horrified, frightened, embarrassed or quite at a loss as to how to handle the situation.

In response to a desperate query 'Is my husband dying?' she may blurt out: 'It looks like it, doesn't it?'

David Miller, Clinical Psychologist at St Mary's Hospital, presents a moving picture of the nurse's role in the imminence of death:

> 'When death is imminent, the nurse needs to provide comfort and distraction. Favourite music and videos may be used at the patient's discretion. He needs to be given only simple choices and decisions, and not many of them. It is often more acceptable for the nurse to hold the patient's hand, stroke his hair or offer him a well-chosen prayer than expect him to converse with her. . . . The patient is often silent and socially unresponsive. Care must continue to be given unconditionally. The patient is usually more dependent on the nurses for activities of daily living, so the total nursing requirement is increased.'*

At the deathbed the nurse becomes part of the family. They desperately need her *identification*, her participation, her emotional-level support.

When the waiting press confronted Mrs Washkansky, widow of the first heart transplant recipient, she told them tearfully, but gratefully: 'Even the sisters were crying.' Very clearly their emotional-level identification meant much to her.

Without causing confusion or panic, or losing their dignity, the nursing staff may well share in the caring grief of the family, for, as we have learnt, in identification comes emotional-level support.

---

* Miller D, Weber J and Green J. *The Management of the AIDS Patient*. MacMillan Press, London 1986.

As pertaining first to the patient, and then to the family, *tactile comfort* (the emotional-level communication that comes through holding a hand, or placing an arm round a shoulder) may be more meaningful than the spoken word.

Cerebral areas die at a varying pace. The *temporal lobe,* responsible for auditory interpretation, usually last longer than does the *occipital lobe.* Thus the patient *may hear destructive or supportive remarks after he has ceased to 'see'. The parietal lobe,* usually the toughest, will probably endure the longest, so that he will *feel tactile support*—his hand held, an arm around his shoulder—long after he has ceased to understand, to see or to hear.

The patient should not lie in a darkened room, on the flat of his back ,staring aimlessly at a blank ceiling. If possible his head should be raised to a pleasant view, and to ease his human communication.

That he should *not* be left alone as death approaches is surely obvious. There can be nothing as lonely as the isolation imposed by approaching death.

Until about 50 years ago, death was a common event in the home. Today it is virtually banished to institutions, having become the responsibility of a small group of professionals.

It is important not to isolate the dying from the living, and to give as much physical and spiritual support as possible. If he is not deeply unconscious, the patient will probably wish to have his dearest ones beside him.

The author remembers being deeply impressed by the sight, in a faraway mission hospital, of an old gentleman dying peacefully, surrounded by a loving family group. The hospital had fed and housed the family (who came from a barren mountainous region), for the past five days.

It is tactful to ask a patient if he would like to see a certain visitor—some, no doubt, are unwelcome.

Should a confused patient call in vain for a special loved one, the compassionate nurse may well pretend to be her.

I was very touched by a student nurse's story of the manner in which the ward staff helped to support a 19-year-old boy dying of leukaemia.

That he was terrified of death was obvious. He lay for long hours clutching his mother's hand. So distraught was he when circumstances forced her from his bedside that, during these short but important periods, the nurses took turns to dress themselves in his mother's clothes. Thus disguised, they sat beside him, holding his hand, sharing with her the sad but comforting ritual.

HELPING THE BEREAVED FAMILY

Nurses are frequently nonplussed by the overt, even fierce, mourning reaction of a relative who, during the patient's illness, was clearly negligent in her duties. She, who seldom visited, 'throws an hysterial mourning tantrum' on learning of the death of her mother.

In fact, she is now caught, by the 'love swing' of ambivalence, in violent feelings of guilt and anxiety, in which distress she requires comfort rather than reproach. People need to mourn overtly. Lacking this outlet, their grief, guilt, anxiety and distress are often channelled 'underground', resulting in psychosomatic illness or long-term neurosis.

'Grief discussion groups' may well assist the bereaved to achieve rehabilitation. Having learnt through the ages of the healing processes inherent in group identification, support and catharsis, several religions have extended their rituals thereunto—as is witnessed by the Irish Catholic wake, the Jewish Shivah week and African group mourning.

Helping the bereaved parent—death of a child is the ultimate loss

It is helpful to speak naturally about the child.

Friends should make themselves available to listen, run errands, help with other children, etc.

Tell the bereaved how sorry you feel and encourage them to speak of their pain.

Do not suggest to parents that they should be grateful for their living children or that they can always have another child: They cannot replace the child they have lost.

Reassure the parents that they and the medical personnel did everything possible to relieve his pain and save his life.

It is not disloyal to a child to let other children share clothes, toys and personal possessions. Parents are beginning to make progress when they are able to do this. Neither is it culpable to resent other children for being alive when one's own beloved child is dead . . . one is only human!

Grief adjustment, like other growth, does not proceed in a straight line, but is vulnerable to pain-precipitated regressions. School holidays, birthdays and other anniversaries are times when parents and siblings, through past associations and engulfing longing, are especially overwhelmed with grief. Remembrance of happy times may help.

In fact one never really 'gets over' the death of a child, and although, in time (a *very* long time), the rawness may recede, the agony will always be there. Parents should not feel guilty about their persistent grief—nor about those times when they will again experience happiness.

There is a current tendency to believe that *preparation* for death can help assuage grief. But the reality is *so terrible that it is unthinkable*—and, at an emotional level, the truth must, for survival, be 'denied'. So when tragedy strikes, the grief of loss is terrible and overwhelming. *Little wonder that many parents react with desperate denial, fury and wild grief.* It is important not to add to parents' burden the imposition of feelings of guilt and shame at the externalization of distraught grief—perhaps their catharsis is, in the long run, healthier for them.

Attempting to cope with the core problems of devastating loss of a child, and the many escalating personal and family disruptions flowing therefrom, parents in the United States have formed themselves into *self-help groups.*

'The main formal organization for bereaved families is "Compassionate Friends", a British initiated group that now has 22 chapters in the States, and expects soon to double its American membership.

In Babylon, a district in New York, 150 families belong to the Friends. Once a month they gather in a room donated by a local bank. Each meeting opens with an affirmation of personal tragedy in the style of Alcoholics Anonymous:

"My name is Ernie Freireich, and I am a bereaved parent.

I lost my son Mark in an automobile accident."

Such families are in desperate need of help. By one estimate, 90% of their marriages run into serious trouble, and many end in divorce.

Alcoholism and sexual dysfunction abound among adults; the husband may think his wife has allowed herself to drown in her grief; she may think him unfeeling and uncaring. Surviving siblings frequently take their parents' anguish as a sign that the dead brother or sister had been by far the best beloved.'

Some phone calls will get Sarah Berman, wife of comedian Shelley, out of bed late at night, and send her driving to a hospital in Beverley Hills in answer to a cry for help or comfort from a parent whose child is terminally ill.

Sarah and Shelley know the agony and grief of losing a child. Two years ago their 13-year-old son Joshua died from a brain tumour.

'To lose a contemporary—a brother, sister, or long-term friend— is to lose a part of your past. But to lose a child is to lose a part of your future. . . . It's the things you know you will never see or experience with your child, which makes the loss so hard to bear. The knowledge that you will never share the excitement of him learning to drive a car, bringing home a girlfriend, growing up and making a happy marriage. I try to help people who are suffering in the best way I can simply by being around.'

Support groups

MacMillan Nurses 01 402 8125

Cancer Link 01 833 2451

St Christopher's Hospice 01 778 9252.

If a mother becomes pregnant soon after the death of her child, it is important to remember that the new baby can never 'replace' the lost child. To expect in him some mystical reincarnation of his dead brother or sister is to impose upon him the impossible task of becoming a compensatory 'carbon copy'. Both parents and child would then grapple with an over-idealized ghost of the past, failing to see, enjoy and love the new child for what he himself is.

'The bereaved have to do ("grief work") which may run through various phases of *anger* against God, the hospital, medical and nursing staff and even relatives and friends, *deep depression* and often feelings of loss of meaning in life. The objective is to *help adjust to the loss*. . . .

In a family it is not only the spouse who has to do "grief work"; the children also have to work through their feelings. If this is not done the family may become paralysed in a situation frozen around the loss of a loved one. . . . Survivors of disasters often share common features. These include the death imprint—the wreckage of the life pattern caused by the event, a sense of guilt at surviving when others died, psychic numbing—being unable to feel anything—and resentment towards rescuers.'*

GRIEF WORK encourages catharsis through

---

* Nash, Eleanore. From a lecture on care of the dying. March 1979.

1.   expression of strong emotions—crying, cursing, threatening, verbalizing anguish and guilt feelings.
2.   comfort and release experienced in reliving memories, recent and long buried.

'Linking objects', such as photographs, letters, clothes, may provoke memories, anecdotes and even significant areas of conflict, anxiety and agonizing remorse, eased by ventilation, sharing and reassurance.

Persistent avoidance and pain may call for formal psycho- or behaviourist therapy.

A useful technique confronts the client with those reminders which she finds especially painful and stressful.

The _aim_ is to exhaust the emotions, just as one would confront a phobic with his feared situation. Painful and traumatic areas include

(i)   real or imagined guilt for things done, or not done, to and for the deceased; real or imagined neglect or anger felt towards the deceased
(ii) conflict arrears or 'unfinished business' . . . last communications which remain unmade.

These can be confronted and ventilated in the 'third-chair' technique in which the bereaved establishes 'a dialogue' with the deceased who is 'called back', explained to, questioned, asked forgiveness of, or whatever needs to be said.

Finally, some sort of symbolic leave-taking may be necessary, to cement the acceptance of the death.*

As painful feelings intensify before the recede, a supportive environment of relatives and friends is essential.

Therapy generally does not last more than two months, but the patient is seen intensively two or three times a week. Such therapy does not resolve the grief completely; it pushes the bereaved through the phase in which he or she is stuck.

   'To improve does not mean to forget—as the shock of raw grief recedes, the memories of people we love get stronger.'†

Dr Cicely Saunders, founder of the Hospice Movement (01 778 9252):

   'When anyone dies, all around him die and lose something of themselves— something of the 'assumptive world'' they have for so long taken for granted.' Some families draw together.

Sometimes death releases antagonism and anger long smouldering, such as sibling rivalry, or hostilities between a child and a step-parent.

Long silences are broken. Even these feelings may be utilized for good, providing greater reality of interaction, catharsis, the growth of deeper mutual supportive feelings and other growth experiences. The role of the care-giver includes:

(i)   deep involvement;
(ii)   'cushioning' intense family hostility and recriminations;
(iii) catharsis;
(iv)   support.

---

* Hodgkinson, Peter E. Senior Clinical Psychologist, Bexley Hospital, Kent. Abnormal Grief and its Therapy. _Psychotherapeia and Psychiatry in Practice._ August 1984.
  † Dr Murray Parkes, _Herald of Free Enterprise_ 1st Anniversary programme. BBC 4 March 1988.

Sometimes there is no reconciliation within the family, and we see persistent anger and hurt in arguing over wills, blaming each other for neglect, and often irrational displacement of guilt feelings on other family members.

Bereavement in old age

Death in old age may find the survivor too old and too lost to start life again. 'When two old sticks lean against each other, and one falls, it is frequently not long before the other too falls to the ground and passes on.'

Parkes *et al* (1969), observing some 4 500 British widowers for a period of six months after the death of their wives observed

high rates of illness and depression
a mortality rate 40% higher than expected for their age.

How may we comfort a bereft old person? We may suggest it would have been worse 'had it been the other way around, and he had been left unable to cope for himself'.

'The measure of your loss is the measure of your love.'*

However, even in old age one sometimes sees remarkable endurance, a tenacity for some sort of new life. Group identification with the bereaved person's own generation sometimes 'sees him through' to some form of new life.

Bereavement in middle age

Death in middle age when one would have expected so much to look forward to, makes the wrench for both the dying and the surviving almost unbearable.

Financial problems; children to raise; the menopause in women, cosntitute very real grounds for social work and community support.

Yet, those who have lost have much to give the world in comfort, in the strength that comes with identification, and in service sublimation.

Comfort lies in the reminder that divorce or desertion, burdened by guilt, failure, remorse, feelings of rejection, loss of self-concept and dignity, are much harder to bear than unavoidable separation in death. For women, there are added burdens of financial insecurity and loss of status, together with the painful knowledge that another enjoys a loved one.

Sometimes the grief, resentment and guilt feelings of young adults are aggravated by new responsibilities in caring for the bereaved spouse.

Social work involvement of community services, and introduction to similarly placed young people's groups, may do much to alleviate emotional and physical burdens.

Twenty years of grief-work have convinced Dr Colin Murray Parkes that grief by loss is the greatest single cause of non-psychotic psychiatric illness.

'Harvard Project', surveying a group of widows younger than 65 years, showed the *two most significant sorrow-alleviating procesures* to consist in:

(i) memory of a loving farewell;
(ii) observing participation to the end.

* Dr Cicely Saunders, March 1979.

It is the conviction of hospice staff that *the pain of bereavement is increased by deprivation of sharing support and mutual expressions of love*. The bereaved are comforted by memories of shared, 'last' loving words and caresses. The intimacy of this experience is a precious one, not to be frustrated by impeding apparatus and arbitrary time restrictions.

Sipping soothing cool water in the arms of a loved one is more mutually comforting than an impersonal mechanical drip.

Teenagers in bereavement

Against the background of conflicting emotions and the insecurity characterizing physical, emotional and social transitions of adolescence, loss of comforting and supporting parental figures is felt very keenly. The girl loses the model with which she identifies, and is frequently called upon to prematurely assume maternal responsibilities whilst herself needing protection; the boy loses his father model and, in the midst of his own adolescent anxiety, is expected to assume the protective role of 'paterfamilias'.

In the throes of 'Oedipus revisited' (p 316), in which opposite-sex parents have become transitionary role models for developing heterosexual phantasies, parental death can cast the adolescent into terrible guilt and anxiety. Is his father's death his punishment for his 'incestuous phantasies' of his mother?

Caught in the typical conflict of adolescence, these young people mourn their parents, but, at an emotional level, experience anger and suppressed aggression at having been 'deserted', albeit in death.

'Why did she go and die and leave us?'

Classic guilt feelings and distressing anxiety accompanying death are intensified. As a result of adolescent difficulty in coping with, and expressing acute, conflicting emotions, these are internalized, impeding concentration on mounting demands in education and examinations. As oprhans, they feel 'different', conspicuous and deprived among their peers, at just that time when the need to identify with 'the gang'.

Comfort in gang-identification may well be channelized into productive group therapy.

Children in bereavement

Kaffman & Ellzur (1979) and others have shown that approximately 50% of children under 17 are significantly impeded in everyday functioning, even beyond three years of paternal death, by anxiety, depression, behavioural problems and learning difficulties.*

The younger child, lacking time concepts is terrified lest mommy die and leave him as granny did; or lest he die like mommy. He may even fear mommy died because he was a 'naughty boy'. Bereft by surrow, fearful and guilt-laden he suffers

---

* M Kaffman & E Ellzur. 'Children's Bereavement Reactions following Death of the Father.' *Int J Fam Ther* **1**: 3, 203–29.

intense maternal deprivation. He is cross with mommy for having left him. If *she* abandoned him thus, who can he trust! He longs for her physically and emotionally, and is angry with other women for not being his real mommy—for continuing to live while she is dead. (Just as parents experience aggression towards other children when they have lost their own beloved child.)

The child's egocentric view of his world is developmentally appropriate. Thus he feels himself to blame for every bad thing that happens to his family.

The bereaved child wants to express his guilt feelings, anxiety and grief but because he lacks appropriate vocabulary, his distress festers within him.

In order to study the effects of opening up communication about the dead parent and thus to facilitate cathartic mourning, Dr Dora Black (1983) devised a controlled study in which therapists used techniques (toys, drawings, etc) to enhance emotional confrontation and abreaction, thus promoting weeping.

Among her conclusions were the following:

1.   In both treated and control groups a favourable outcome was associated with 'the child crying about and talking about the dead parent, particularly amongst the older children'. Over fives who cried more had fewer and less serious behaviour and emotional problems.
2.   Parents in the treated group, although exposed to only six therapeutic interviews, showed fewer health problems and mood swings than the controls.
3.   While within the first year after bereavement 25% of the control group sought professional psychological help, none of the treated group 'felt the need for anything other than our intervention. . . . I think we now have modest evidence that an intervention designed to promote expression of grief in children and enhance communication in families can help prevent short term distress following bereavement and appears to be free from harmful effects.'*

The child should have free access to dying adults, who will almost certainly find his presence pleasantly distracting and comforting.

It is better for him to see his parents ill, than taken away to hospital, never to return. In the latter predicament he is liable to feel deserted, which is even more painful than unavoidable loss.

A child may well be frightened at his ambivalence on the death of a sibling. Almost inevitably he will feel a certain pleasure and relief at the removal of his 'rival'—emotions soon swinging into guilt and anxiety. He may even feel that his sibling's death is a result of his own 'death wish'—the 'crime' punishable by his own death. (See p 64.)

It is important that, even if he does not verbalize his guilt and anxiety, he be reassured that love and hate are both acceptable emotions—that the death was nobody's fault and that nobody will be punished.

We have seen elsewhere that it is kinder for the child that he dies in his mother's arms in his own home. This may also be more natural for siblings. If the child does die in hospital Joan Goodall recommends that the staff take a photograph of the dead child, that his siblings may one day be comforted by his peaceful and normal demeanour.

---

* D Black. 'Bereaved Children—Family Intervention.' *Bereavement Care* **2**(2). Summer 1983. Cruse House, 126 Sheen Road, Richmond. Surrey. TW.

Death is a frightening intrusion.

Fearing that they themselves or their parents may die, children often cling and refuse to separate even for short periods. In that it is usually comforting—and in the long term even constructive—that the whole family go through mourning together, separation is probably unwise.

Forced separation will only aggravate anxiety and the conviction that the surviving children are not loved as much as their dead sibling.*

Should children attend funerals?

On this controversial point, even Dr Saunders, in spite of much experience, is unable to offer firm advice. She feels a harrowing funeral with open coffin is best avoided—a religious memorial service stressing love, peace and resurrection may, in certain situations, be acceptable. Certainly no child or adolescent (or adult for that matter) should feel forced or obliged to attend a funeral. Loving involvement in life is certainly more important than dutiful presence after death.

No matter how cushioned, death of a loved one is characterized by:

emotional numbness—inner sorrow and longing result in refusal to accept heartrending change, and a search for the dead in his possessions and environment; through religious and other spiritual contact;

feelings of rejection—giving way, when all searching roads lead to dead ends, to realization that the loved one is never coming back, and hence feelings of *hopelessness*.

Within the context of sharing support and loving memories, knowledge of love returned and fulfilled, the bereaved may eventually come to terms, and 'in spite of permanent chinks in the armour against grief, participate in new activities and relationships'. (For self-help support groups, see 613ff.)

How can the staff themselves be helped and strengthened in this most distressing task?

Discussion and mutual sympathetic 'group support', catharsis and guidance may provide a source of reassurance and supportive identification to counteract guilt feelings, distress and isolation.

Group therapy is important for staff, both with the whole team and within their own 'peer group' in which they are able to 'let off steam' about senior members.

St Christopher's seldom advertises for staff. When it does, an average of two in three applications are turned down after hour-long interviews with the matron and social worker.

Many, through that intensive sharing identification and deep caring which are the keynote of hospice care, do need 'a moment of desperate crying'. Little can be gained by waiting for the group therapy situation.

'*It is essential to see who is in trouble, and help them there and then.* . . . When they witness pain turned to peace, comfort of patient and family, conversion of

* Dr Joan Goodall, in a lecture sponsored by the Hospice Movement, 1983.

terror of dying to satisfaction in daily living, and a more peaceful attitude about death itself, the staff are rewarded and motivated to go on. . . .

The hospice movement has shown that ordinary people, as well as highly qualified medical scientists and people of religious vocation, can help ease terminal illness.'*

Ward discussions (including doctors) may well *cover the possibility of a particular patient's death*, the role of individual staff members in handling the situation, the patient's expected level of consciousness, the role of medication, the expected family reaction, and how these may be most profitably handled.

Much has been said in this book about the nurse's own *ambivalence* towards her patient. This is a natural phenomenon, frequently increased by the involuntary associations set up by the patient. He may remind her of a kind grandfather whom she loved, thus setting in motion a pleasant association chain-reaction to deeper level feelings; conversely he may remind her of a schoolteacher whom she hated, setting up a negative association link to submerged feelings of hate, hostility, anger—and, at his death relief, guilt and anxiety. In reliving personal trauma she may develop illogical, but powerful feelings of anxiety, lest she herself be in some way responsible for his death—as in the case of the young nurse who developed anorexia nervosa on finding herself in this position (see p 126). Some develop illogical, but distressing, anxiety lest they administered an erroneous injection or medicine. *Most conscientious members of the hospital team suffer guilt feelings when a patient dies.* In many cases, especially when death comes to the young, the nurse may become deeply distressed. At such times it is essential that there be available to her that *intersecting staff-identification* described on page 110ff.

The nurse who, in vain, has shared with the mother of a dying child many nights of sad debilitating vigil, and ultimate failure and grief, should feel free to approach the ward sister, to verbalize her feelings of guilt, grief, aggression, despair—her motivation to take to physical flight. The sister should be able to provide catharsis, to identify with her, to reassure and comfort.

'I know it is terrible to lose a patient. I know how hard you tried and how much this child meant to you. I know how sad, hopeless, angry and defeated you feel—I know you want to run away—I feel the same. But we shall go through this thing together. Tomorrow, perhaps, we shall be able to save a patient, and things will be more hopeful, and the sun will shine again.'

Only in meaningful identification, irrespective of 'rank', can the nursing staff give each other that deep emotional-level support without which it is impossible to fulfil their role in the care of the dying.

The young nurse is of course very distressed at having to LAY OUT THE DEAD—especially where she has had a close relationship with her patient. One wonders how many sensitive, intelligent and compassionate girls have been lost to the profession due to lack of support, imagination, tact on the part of other staff members, especially senior staff members, in this matter of laying out the dead.

The newcomer may well be protected from this ordeal, then introduced gradually, in an assistant role, in performing the last offices for a patient she does not know very well. She should certainly never be asked to do so alone. Many

* Dr Cecily Saunders, St Christopher's Hospice, March 1979.

remember with gratitude, for their whole nursing careers, those senior nurses who brought to their introduction to these sad offices their own comforting philosophy.

Others remember with horror, or sadness, the silly, giggling or coarse behaviour which was only later realized to constitute an immature 'defence mechanism' and outlet for tension and anxiety. Many are distressed by rough and callous handling of bodies committed to their care by porters and mortuary attendants.

The young nurse is often helped by reassurance, by discussion, and by verbalization that this is no longer the patient she cared for efficiently and tenderly, but the cast off, pain-ridden and useless remnant of an earthly existence now happily terminated. The nurse's need for catharsis after her vigil by the bedside of the dying, her ordeal in laying out the body, is frequently intense. She needs support, interpretation, reassurance, encouragement and finally distraction by a happier task.

> 'Give sorrow words; the grief that does not speak
> Whispers the o'er fraught heart and bids it break.'
>
> *Macbeth*, Act IV

CHAPTER 24

DEALING WITH CRISIS
AND DISASTER

Freud has described the naked distress of the Ego, foresaken by the protective powers of the Super Ego.

The integrity and *independence of physiological, ethical, psychological and growth mastering self* have given way to the disintegration of the self-concept. One is a fragmented pawn of death!*

Definition

When the strength of environmental blocks causes frustration so great that no established adjustment mechanism can contain nor channel off biochemical tension-energy, and the fulfilment of Maslow's needs are so hopelessly thwarted that homeostasis is impossible, the individual is said to be in a state of crisis.

A crisis is thus an internal disturbance or loss of equilibrium resulting from an actual overwhelmingly stressful event, or a stressful set of circumstances, seen as a threat.

Crises may be divided into the following three classifications:

1. *Maturational crises* in which the individual is caught in the conflict between a stultifying but safe, familiar developmental stage and the unknown but challenging threats of a subsequent developmental stage (see Erikson, p 245). Maturational crises therefore result from internal homeostatic disturbances, intended to lead to growth.
2. *Adventitious crises* result from gross environmental changes affecting Maslow's *fundamental physical safety and security needs* (tiers 1 and 2 of the Hierarchy), such as the disasters of war, fire, earthquake, severe drought, flood, plague, etc, and are thus resultant upon external factors. Examples are the Great Fire of London, the Blitz, the sinking of the Titanic, the more long term nazi holocaust.
3. *Situational crises* are more personal, occurring when *a specific external event throws out the psychological equilibrium of an individual, or small group.* Typical precipitating situations threaten Maslow's personal security, love, belonging and esteem needs (see p 100—tiers 3 and 4). They include the loss of a loved one, physical mutilation, divorce, school failure, job loss, psychiatric illness, etc.

Reaction to crisis—Hirschowitz's model

Typical of an *adventitious crisis* is:

A disaster causing the overwhelming fragmentation of an individual's physical, emotional and social personality. Even his most elemental human needs are beyond his reach and he is reduced to the fulfilment of his most basic physiological/safety needs—cf Maslow's Hierarchy (see p 100).

---

* Ventress, K.D. Further information from author.

His physical needs are imperilled—Deprived of physical need-fulfilment: food, sleep, air, water, and normal physical activity—all of his higher needs recede. Unlike the newborn child, he *knows* he has lost the fulfilment of his safety and security needs, his love and belonging needs. He is bereft of *primaeval* safety and security. He is unloved, rejected, friendless, abandoned.

He is in crisis. Thus the underlying philosophy of disaster medicine lies in insight into, and successful handling of his immediate needs *in the here and now*.

RECOMMENDATIONS IN CRISIS INTERVENTION

'If I learnt one thing from the Herald of Free Enterprise ferry disaster it was the importance of intervention—as soon as possible—by one strong disaster leader who knows what he's doing.'*

'Although 193 people died, the rescue of another 367 passengers and crew was achieved largely because of excellent planning by the Belgians . . .

Mr Vanneste, the Belgian provincial governor . . . had a plan for a catastrophe, had the power and the authority and organized the ferry rescue. . . .

When the Herald turned turtle, Zeebrugge was waiting with plan, Catastrophe OH. At his home a dozen miles away, Mr Vanneste was watching television. It was 7.45 pm. . . .

A voice said simply: "Catastrophe Plan—Zeebrugge Harbour." The governor asked no questions because the plan forbids them. "Asking what or why wastes time. I knew I just had to go," he said.

When he reached the crisis centre in the port office, pre-ordained by the plan, fire and police chiefs were already present. It was 8.02 pm. By 8.10 pm, the governor had set his operation in motion. In the next 20 minutes he was able to accomplish much. . . . He scrambled a police helicopter in Brussels to head for Antwerp to collect army divers stationed there and fly them direct to the Herald.

He was able to commandeer 500 blankets from the military base and send out a call for lights, ropes and ladders.

He set up reception centres for survivors in a local naval base and in a community hostel and accepted a hotel's offer to become a third.

"Doctors advised us that wet people, in shock, must not be kept on the quay. It was two degrees, very cold. . . . The Zeebrugge experience is that what was most needed for people in shock was beds . . . (for nursing procedures and for 'regression' to the comforting warm womb"—author)'.†

GILLIS presents the following facilitator for successful crisis intervention:
    'As easy as PIE:
Proximity—be close to the person involved, and stick with him.
Immediacy—intervene in the heat of the situation, even if it is only by being there or listening.
Expectancy—provide hope and maintain confidence.
    The enemy to beat is psychological denial.
    To deny is to avoid reality or acknowledgement that we need help.'‡

---

* BBC 1st Anniversary programme, 4 March 1988.

† Tom Dawe and Brian James 'One-man show was key to tackling ferry capsize'. *The Times*, London 4 March 1988.

‡ Gillis, L S. *Guidelines in Psychiatry*, p 208.

Specific handling of the three phases:

Phase 1: Impact Phase

Usually the majority of survivors are temporarily *cushioned by Nature's stunned behaviour.* They may well take second place to those presenting with *disturbed emotional behaviour,* especially those who *panic.*

Panic presents in loss of self-control, blind and irrational flight, fear of being trapped and feelings of powerlessness. 'Contrary to general opinion, panic reactions are relatively uncommon, but they are contagious so it is necessary to act quickly.' Panic reactions may be controlled by separation, physical restraint, calm firmness and clear directions. 'Your own controlled and purposive behaviour is the best corrective.'

Other acute emotional reactions consist in over-activity, interfering, anger, argumentativeness, distractibility and wild, random hyperkinetic behaviour.

Dealing with acute emotional reactions:

Calm, firm, control; avoidance of arguments; allot a specific task such as fetching water, cleaning rubble, issuing food, rescuing others, etc.

Returning to the stunned 'emotionally anaesthetized' group:

Having lost the framework of their lives, these victims regress from denial to childhood feelings of confusion, isolation and babyish helplessness. Their need is for personal contact (empathy), reassurance, tactile comfort and provision of basic life essentials. Most should, within a relatively short time, return to some form of functional self-sufficiency.

'*In summary,* the principles of psychological First Aid at the time of the impact phase are:

(1) Adopt a leadership role because people are without a rudder; establish priorities for action.
(2) Gather the survivors together; identify those who need special attention and concentrate on them; issue clear and easy-to-follow directions and stifle rumours.
(3) Give them something material—food, clothes, blankets, etc; the act of giving helps to personalize people.
(4) Look to your own defences. Are you also emotionally wounded? Do not try to be all things to all survivors or waste time blaming or emoting. Rescue workers clearing the crash of the Boeing disaster near Paris developed depression and other psychological reactions after their work was done.'

The role of the professional

Addressing the Fifth National Congress of the Association of Child Psychology, Psychiatry and Allied Disciplines, April 1985 Dr Vera Bührmann quoted research ranking *the most important features of effective 'hot', on-the-spot, impact phase intervention* to be as follows:

   (i) The quality of the initial 'here and now' assessment. (The full psycho-dynamic assessment comes later.)

  (ii) Promptness: 'because entrenched ego defence mechanisms are disturbed, the psyche is more available'.

 (iii) The awareness and sensitivity of the facilitator: her ability to identify with, and share, suffering; to enter into the sufferer's life-situation, his social and cultural processes.

 (iv) to listen effectively.

  (v) to encourage ventilation.

Tasks of intervention facilitators include:

(a) involved comfort;

(b) reduction of overwhelming fears into manageable portions;

(c) assistance of the damaged and vulnerable ego towards reality orientation: prevention and counteraction of spiralling phantasy; encouragement of reality-orientated verbalization: What can be done to relieve the sorrows and stresses of the 'here and now'?

Warning

Because disorientation, confusion, amnesia, etc may be due to actual cerebral trauma, exposure, blood loss, sleep deprivation, etc, these elements should not be ignored.

Phase 2: Turmoil—Recoil Phase

This phase is characterized by relatively long-term (at least some weeks) emotional disturbance.

Etiology

    'Oh God—look what's happened!'

Realization of the destruction of life's framework and the loss of loved ones who formerly gave purpose (motivation) to living; disappearance of security and identity symbols; all these leave victims heartbroken, disoriented and vulnerable.

Presentation

Powerful primitive emotions are laid bare; fear, anger, guilt, loss of confidence, avoidance–withdrawal, dependency and apathy, all these distress and debilitate.

Stephen Wrottesley, reporting on a town washed away by sudden flood observed: '. . . Some people are still trying to recover what they can from the remains of their homes. But a form of apathy has struck others. Some of them sit around in the tent city, the emergency area for many of the homeless, and do nothing. It is this apathy that worries people who wish to reconstruct the town. They fear it may turn to despondency and that eventually the people will leave. Coupled with this is the fact that the emotional crutch of the townsfolk—"imported" welfare agencies—will not stay here for ever.'

Psychosomatic ailments frequently constitute a plea for provision of caring comfort.

Programming for effective help

The 'emotionally lost' should not be left unsupported. In order to 'work through' grief and emotional disturbances victims require catharsis—to show their feelings rather than to suppress them—and to re-experience (in the context of loving, caring support) the horror and terror of the event.

Impact Phase

> 'When (we) first arrived in the flooded town people were wandering around the streets in a daze or wild distress. We were giving them tranquillizers to calm them and help them through their traumatized state.'

Turmoil and Recoil Phase

> 'But now they have to talk things through with us. It was necessary that the victims pass from denial to recognition of the negative elements, mourn their loss, recognize the necessity to reconstruct their town and their lives.'

Phase 3: Emotionally Wounded Phase: The Survivor Syndrome

When acute reactions have subsided (allowing for some overlapping) the victim enters the *survivor syndrome*.

Concentration camp survivors remain haunted by death, damage and dismemberment. Loss of loved ones, loved places, loved objects; destruction of one's life pattern—all these lead to realization of universal vulnerability to tragedy—and terror that it can happen again. 'I wouldn't have believed it could happen to me—what next!' Unrelated events precipate terror anticipation.

The victim has undergone a massive psychological trauma which has damaged his sense of self and which may burden him with lifelong neuroses, psychosomatic disorders and permanent personality change.

To a lesser but still painful and potentially destructive degree the immigrant undergoes crisis trauma.

To a lesser, but still painful and potentially destructive degree, the older, uprooted immigrant undergoes crisis loss and terror anticipation.

Characteristics of the survivor syndrome are:

> *Death anxiety*—as a result of the Death Encounter in many unrelated circumstances death threatens him and his loved ones.
> The mental pictures conjured up by the <u>disaster imprint</u> are so frightening that the victim
> (i) relives his original ordeal
> (ii) escapes by 'flight'.

Of the approximately 40 crew who survived the capsizing of the Herald of Free Enterprise, few returned to the sea. Those who did found seagoing associations terrifying:

> 'Every time the ship rolled to one side I clung to the rails in terror, seeing again the huge sheets of water, hearing the horrible cries of the drowning.'

By the first anniversary (4 March 1988) only two crew survivors were still at sea.*

Psychic numbing—in order to prevent pain and risk of loss, the victim avoids new experiences and new relationships. Dull survival leads to a half-life devoid of enthusiasm, spontaneity and pleasure.

Survivor guilt—unable to forgive himself for having survived while his loved ones perished, the victim is tied for ever to the dead. His guilt feelings, his pre-occupation with the dead; his fearful reliving of the death imprint, haunt him and prevent him from moving on to new relationships and experiences.

Impaired human relations—excessive, in fact unbearable, psychological dependence, moodiness, over-reaction and unco-operativeness impair personal, loving and vocational relationships. Victims demand support, and when this is forthcoming reject and destroy it.

'When is my real husband coming home? This is a different person.'†
Much forebearance is required in order to weather the victim's need for solace and support.

Hopelessness and despair—to be a victim of circumstances is dehumanizing. Because nothing can be trusted or meaningful, life is barren of support and motivation. *Feelings of stigma, uncleanliness and untouchability* classically result from tragedies such as disease epidemics and nuclear explosions.

The survivor syndrome is a deeply ingrained and persistent emotional disturbance requiring more intensive, skilled and long-term therapy than that provided by 'psychological first aid'.

Alleviation is the task not only of the multi-disciplinary psychiatric team but extends to community organizations.

It should be noted that rescue and support workers, as well as victims, characteristically suffer from the survivor syndrome. They also have to work through their survivor guilt: *'Why them and not me?'* It will be hard; there will be many scars and it will probably take years to get over what has happened.

'I live it over and over again. I cannot help it. And I keep thinking what I omitted to do—what I could have done better.'‡

'There are not only a hundred corpses, but a hundred families to think about, and even people who were not there at the time but are related or connected will show effects.'§

For this reason social workers attempted to trace every survivor and every victim—and every family affected by the Herald of Free Enterprise ferry disaster.

Commenting on the Boeing explosion disaster at Lockerbie (December 1988) and basing his projection on his study into the long-term effects of the King's Cross tube station fire (November 1987) Dr James Thompson, senior lecturer in psychology at the University of London predicts that *when the immediate impact of the disaster wears off many of those who lost loved ones, relatives or friends or who were involved in the gruesomeness of the accident will suffer symptoms of stress and need help.* 'They will

---

* BBC TV anniversary programme, 4 March 1988.

† Wife of a Herald of Free Enterprise disaster survivor. Group therapy. BBC TV.

‡ Salvation Army officer praised for his rescuer role in the Herald of Free Enterprise disaster.

§ Gillis.

experience a lot of *anxiety* and many will be *unable to sleep*. They will find *difficulty in concentrating* and will be socially *disorganized*.'

'People's immediate reaction after the horror of what they have experienced at Lockerbie will be to say "I am fine", but within a few days the symptoms of the stress they have experienced will start to emerge.'

The essential need was to <u>link social services and health services closely together</u> and to draw up a <u>register of those at risk of post-traumatic shock</u>. A disaster which affects a whole community has the advantage that everyone understood their neighbour's problem, but the disadvantage that because everyone is involved each had less energy to help.

Anniversaries may be mini-crises. The victim's disaster imprint mounts. He *relives with special intensity his terror, grief, loss, guilt and despair.* Yet in confrontation, catharsis and supportive identification there may be healing.

Reporting on the first anniversary of the Zeebrugge disaster (6 March 1988) The Evening Standard wrote:

. . . 'There were many . . . reunions in the makeshift chapel set up on board the Baltic Ferry. . . . A new flame of friendship burned brightly at Zeebrugge yesterday as survivors of the disaster were reunited with Belgian heroes.

For 15-year-old Nicola Simpson [whose mother drowned in the Herald of Free Enterprise] the emotional first meeting with the nurses "who brought her back from the dead" was overwhelming:

She collapsed crying tears of happiness and gratitude into the arms of Sister Cecile Aerds, head of the intensive care unit at Brugges' St Jan Hospital.'

Some people, however, due to immaturity, festering anger, oversensitivity or simply an unbearably long sequence of debilitating misfortunes, may attempt to seek refuge and relief in *long-term withdrawal or avoidance*. Albert died of typhoid fever in 1861 . . . for the next 40 years Victoria, Widow of Windsor, was rarely seen in public. The ultimate avoidance is, of course, suicide.

Grief work, pp 555–7

Caution:

The 'tightrope' between *identifying involvement* and *objectivity* is threatened by arousal of the facilitator's personal psychic trauma and the vulnerability of her own ego defences. Hence the need for team support.

It is important that the team *avoid judgement or condemnation* of an individual's reaction to crisis. It is easy but insensitive, even destructive, to measure one person's reaction against another's. Each must cope within the framework of his own individual personality—his physiology, his heredity, his life story. One is no more 'worthy' than the other. For one paraplegic a way of life within the protection of his own home is as great an achievement as Olympic basketball participation for another.

Some *withdraw* into silent isolation; others unconsciously *'displace'* or 'take out' their anger on family or hospital team.

This is no time for nurses to react with disapproval, to retreat into their own status isolation, or to 'team up', against a 'difficult' patient.

Even if he appears to reject human approaches of warmth and support, he needs them desperately, and every means of communication—verbal, tactile, facial— through food, warmth, spirituality, should be grasped and utilized.

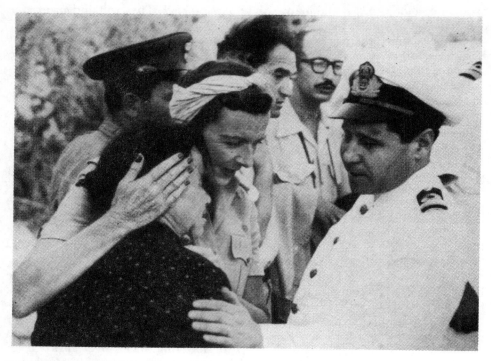

Lady Mountbatten in Greece
—After an earthquake she brings material relief and human sympathy.

Courtesy of Museum and Library, The Order of St John, London and The Lady Edwina Mountbatten Trust.

In the context of constitutional predisposition, shock may even trigger off manic-depression or schizophrenia.

To quote Frederika de Villiers (1979):

> '*The family* is a basic rescue group. During a disaster one first looks for one's dear ones. They shelter together and try to encourage and protect one another. If the members are separated the social disruption is much worse (Strümpher 1975: 55–57). A child's reaction is largely determined by the supporting and comforting presence or absence of the parent. The principle in coping with disaster must therefore always be directed to allowing the parent to accompany the child. The child must, like the adult, assimilate the experience; one must allow the child to ask questions, to talk about the events, including those he is afraid of and allow the child to mourn out such events. He may also be allowed to visit the debris and play his disaster games. (Strümpher, 1975: 48, 52–9; Fritz, 1961: 683–4; Wolfenstein, 1957: 59.)'

Helping the person to face his crisis

'Now that such-and-such has happened. . . .'

He should be helped to think about his predicament, his sorrows and dangers. The expression releases his pain, his fears, his angers. He should understand that catharsis heals rather than breaks. The necessity for 'putting on a brave face' or adopting a 'stiff upper lip' often serves only to increase tension, grief and isolation. Sometimes grief comes in waves each time the sufferer faces his tragedy anew.

'The truth shall make you free'—the ability to face facts often reduces them to a perspective at which one is able to handle them more successfully. It is better to learn that one has lost one eye than to imagine oneself blind.

Support of a terminal patient, for whom there is no hope, is a unique situation. Individual circumstances differ and the truth does not always serve as a positive growth experience. The student is referred to chapter 23 'Care of the Dying'.

The important sense of involvement and physical comfort emanating from *tactile communication* should not be forgotten—a hand held, an arm round a shoulder, impart a *feeling of love and security* deeply rooted since the supportive mother–child relationship.

It's nobody's fault

In avoiding the truth one *projects* one's feelings of anger, guilt, stress and despair on to others—and more distressingly on to one's self. This would occur for instance when one parent blames the other for a child's motor-car accident or worse, torments herself with self-reproach.

Easy does it—One cannot 'take' too much at once

Postponing for too long coming to grips with loss or other distress may serve to magnify crisis and reduce the patient's confidence in coping. Yet it should be remembered that some sorrows and losses do seem almost too much for flesh and blood to bear.

Mobilizing Resources, Personal and Communal (see also p 565)

Crisis limits resources for indispensable daily tasks such as shopping, paying the rent, cooking meals, etc.

This is especially true in large, somewhat impersonal urban situations where there is little meaningful long-term personal and group support.

The value of material help is enhanced by assuming a token of affection, involvement, caring and sharing.

However, one should be careful not to 'take over' the person's freedom of decision, authority and adult self-image.

Dr D Dickman, associate professor, Department of Psychiatry, Universityof Toronto, stresses the importance of *timing*. The first priority is to 'mobilize as much support as you can—don't try to be an omnipotent god'.

Especially in this type of work, *speed comes before detailed quality performance*.

There is no time for obsessive perfection in method or achievement.

The nurse cannot expect too much of herself, her co-workers or her patient. She should reassure the sufferer that this is a time when all efforts will be concentrated on him, his problems and means of alleviating them.

In order to concentrate all efforts on relieving suffering, nurses are well advised to work in a team of two—one working with the family, the other supporting by taking records, telephone calls, mobilizing the team and in general 'backing up' her colleague whose attention is focused on the person in crisis.

Dr Dickman reminded his listeners that clients are coming into the unknown—the hospital should provide a pleasant place, privacy, coffee and sandwiches (mouth comfort).

Crisis intervention should not take place in 'public reception'—a whole string of people may increase crisis by introducing elements of unsympathetic curiosity, confusion and darting distractibility of staff members.

It is important that family members be seen in their own natural environment. A home visit is very important in assessing vulnerable and strong areas.

Clearly, effective crisis intervention requires a multi-disciplinary approach, providing inter-personal support of those affected and the team members themselves.

The Jewish Shivah week, in which family and friends fill the house constantly, coming together to talk of the dead, to mourn, to weep, illustrate, throughout the generations, the healing power of supportive identification. It is customary to bring to the house of mourning sweet foods to succour and to provide mouth comfort—symbol of mother, love, safety and security. Jewish funerals accept, even ceremoniously include, the rending of garments and the swaying of bodies. But when one leaves the cemetery it is customary to wash one's hands as a symbol of washing away grief and returning to life. On returning from the funeral one eats eggs in salt water, a symbol of rebirth through tears.

There is frequently also indication for environmental therapy.

Crisis intervention as a nursing process

Crisis intervention aims at offering the *immediate help* that a person in crisis needs in order *to re-establish his equilibrium*. It is an inexpensive, short-term therapy which focuses on solving the immediate problem *'in the here and now'* and is relatively independent of past development problems.

The goal of crisis intervention, which usually lasts about six weeks, is to help the client return to his pre-crisis level of functioning or as near to it as possible.

1. *Data collection—Death of husband—a "situational" or more personal crisis*

One encourages expression of strong feelings (abreaction or 'affect') by *asking the client how she feels* about the situation, recent events and significant people within the crisis situation. Open-ended questions provide opportunity for reflecting back the client's feelings.

Weeping and angry outbursts reflect valuable catharsis.

Caution:

> When feelings threaten to burst beyond control and into extreme rage or despondency it may be wise to discourage abreaction and switch to thinking processes, returning later to the emotional approach.

For example, if the client threatens suicide it may be better to switch from encouraging free expression of self-destructive feelings to a more intellectualized consideration of the consequences of self-destruction.

2. Nursing Diagnosis (Assessment)

Identifying precipitating events:

An accident→guilt and shock.
A long-term disease→long-term stress, psychosomatic involvements, survivor guilt, exhaustion, neglected relationships, etc.

Assessment of deviation from the norm of the client's most immediate physical and interpersonal needs; is life insurance or workman's compensation money available? Is there money for rent, fuel, food, etc? Is there someone to perform these survival-business tasks?

How can the client's support system, including family, neighbours, communal services, community sister, religious minister and home-help, be mobilized so as to defuse gross deviation from the norm?

Community Nurse: are there medicines to be fetched from the out-patient clinic? Is a general practitioner to be informed? Is liaison with schools to be arranged?

Identification of the client's previous strengths and coping mechanisms, tendencies towards depression; anger; withdrawal and relief in active participation.

Assessment of the nature and strength of the client's support systems—familial, vocational, communal, religious, etc.

What would one expect to constitute:

the most serious impediments to rehabilitation?
the most promising, ie constructive factors?

Sometimes even at the early stage of assessment, reflection of the client's emotions, needs, goals and values may enable the nurse to motivate rehabilitative goals.

In fact, as in most applications of the nursing process, there is considerable overlapping of therapeutic stages.

3. Planning

Because crisis intervention is geared towards solving immediate crises, the professional worker and the client should *together explore and evaluate alternative solutions*, eg administration of the husband's estate; increase of family income by utilization of the client's professional or other qualifications; arranging daytime care of children; moving from a house to a flat; taking in a boarder to ease financial stress; involvement of the extended family; establishment and extension of social contact through 'singles clubs', extra-mural (ie Summer School) courses, etc; planning a holiday, treats for the children, etc.

It is important to remember that the crisis situation is *neither* the place nor the time for *self-analysis or modification of the client's long-term pattern* of adjustive mechanisms. One should rather seek to work within her existent personal and social norm. It is important that the worker communicates with confidence that her client is able to overcome the otherwise crushing misfortune which has beset her.

The planning stage is designed to help the client towards a better understanding of the development and precipitation of her present feelings and how these may be alleviated. Even though understanding is an intellectualized rather than emotionally meaningful process, *insight may help* the client to accept her anger, sense of loss, fears, etc. One should, however, remember that within the personal fragmentation and overwhelming distress of crisis it is seldom possible to reach and handle long-standing unconscious mental processes.

4. *Implementation*

This consists in the specific structure of a mutually agreed *programme in which the client's resource-support system may be mobilized*, e g

> Within a week the client's mother will be able to spend afternoons with the children.
> The possibility of a professional refresher course will be investigated.
> Within a month the client will
>
>> apply for a part-time job;
>> investigate advisability of moving from the house to a flat;
>> begin to visit friends on Sunday afternoons.

Significant planning occurs when adaptive behaviour patterns are discussed and reinforced by agreement, praise and the reward of feelings of increased self-sufficiency.

Realistic acceptance of the permanent loss of marital companionship may well lead to plans for sublimation in other relationships.

At this stage the professional worker may utilize mechanisms such as

> *suggestion* in influencing the client to strengthen her feelings of self-esteem through achievements of increasing significance such as the opening of her own bank account, self-decision of children's education, etc;
> *identifying* with others who are learning to weather loss in singles groups, summer-school courses, etc.

(The value, and also the danger, of identification with self-help groups are discussed within the context of specific stress, sorrow and body-loss situations, Chapter 26, p 613 et seq.)

The professional worker should remember that reinforcement of positive behaviour occurs most successfully *within the context of warm, meaningful relationships*, not least of which should exist between client and professional worker.

5. *Evaluation*

The client should be helped to evaluate her return to pre-crisis effectiveness within the context of a realistic upward *cyclical* rather than continually upward *'recovery'* gradient.

During this phase, the professional worker and her client together evaluate the effectiveness of intervention:

> To what extent has the client returned to her pre-crisis level of functioning?
> Which of her imperilled needs can now be met?

To the loss of which must she adjust permanently?
Has her usual pattern of coping mechanisms begun to function again?
How reliable is her personal support system?

It is important that the client feels that ultimately she herself will manage to overcome her crisis and rebuild or amend her resources and goals.

Post-Traumatic Stress Syndrome occurs in the aftermath of both cataclyisms, and more elongated disasters, such as the sustained horrors of war, or watching a loved one in terminal illness. Untreated, it can last for years. It consists of the psychological injuries the victim carries with him through the motions of living.

Symptoms may recur after many years, precipitated by personal crises such as bereavement; psychoneurological changes of the climacteric and ageing; anniversaries. Many researchers have reported delayed post-traumatic stress disorder in long-term studies of concentration camp victims and prisoners of war.

Typical symptoms are:

Death imprint and anxiety.

Feelings of *pervasive helplessness* . . . the victim can do nothing about his suffering or his quality of life.

Psychic Numbing—glib, lack of emotion until catharsis relieves stress.

Anger at his helplessness, people, and life in general.

Grief and mourning for the dead,
                    for the familiar, protective world . . .
                    one's home, community, loved pets and objects.

Feelings of loneliness and frightening isolation. . . . lack of comforting identification even with fellow victims. These feelings are even worse in more personal 'situational' disasters.

Survivor Guilt . . . loved ones have perished.
What could I have done to save them?
Did they die because of me?

Depression

Psychosomatic stress symptoms: sleeplessness, loss of appetite and concentration, or other overt symptomatology are indices of internal suffering.

Special additional features of post-traumatic stress in relief workers are:

(i) *compulsive reliving of guilt feelings* . . .
    'What more could I have done to help?'
(ii) *'Did I train and prepare my team well enough?'*
(iii) Introjection from victims of feelings of contamination and uncleanliness.

A corner-stone of therapy is opportunity for catharsis as soon after the ordeal as possible (see below).

The flood disaster referred to above emphasized *the helpers' need for help.* Rescuers were daily exposed to searching for 'swollen, decaying, stinking bodies and pushing them into plastic bags'. Despite the fact that these men had been toughened by sixteen training courses they none the less sought tension-relief in bawdy jokes, in constant repetition of their traumatic experiences, and ultimately became physically ill.

All helpers experienced survivor guilt, and felt contaminated by tragedy, death and decay. They phantasized purification rituals, such as diving into the pure waves of the sea.

'We were the rescue group that worked in the mortuary at Zeebrugge. Nothing—not all the training videos we had experienced—could have prepared us for the sight of all those rows of battered and drowned corpses. We had to look after each other.

Each evening before we turned in, our group leader got us together. Without blaming anyone, he wanted to know who wasn't coping. It was a litany of grief.

But we didn't go to bed until we'd talked it through. You belong to an exclusive group—we did it together!'*

Long-term after-effects

'Among other disasters, the nazi holocaust has shown that the repercussions of disaster-experience can reverberate for several generations.' Dr Nash presents the following *factors rendering an individual vulnerable* to long-term post-disaster psychiatric disorders:

  (i) Loss or *separation from loved person.* By association, the loss of prized possessions is also deeply mourned (see Bowlby *Attachment and Loss*).
 (ii) *Physical mutilation and infection, and feelings of stigma and untouchability* are factors emphasized in interviews with survivors of the Hiroshima atomic bomb explosion.
(iii) Factors precipitating psychiatric breakdown among victims include *anniversaries*, and *repetition of the same or similar experiences*, which resurrect old memories and reactions; personal crises such as retirement, loss of spouse or children leaving home, emigration.

Therapeutic handling should emphasize prevention on three levels, namely:

 (1) *Primary prevention*—prompt on-site 'hot' crisis intervention—sharing supportive relationships should seek to prevent the establishment of denial and other maladaptive response-patterns. It is necessary to face and work through the pain of loss from the beginning when defences are shaken and the ego exposed to therapeutic intervention. This may help keep the frightening painful imprint within real and manageable proportion. Professionals seeking to help concentration camp survivors note exclusion by this exclusive group who resent outsiders unable to identify with their horrifying experiences.
 (2) *Secondary prevention* should seek to face, and avoid secondary maladaptive mechanisms such as escape through alcohol; the search for 'safety' in obsessive neurosis, aggressive displacement in parent–child relationships, etc, by the *availability of appropriate psychiatric resources*.

Interviews with members of CRUISE, The Herald of Free Enterprise disaster support group, in the BBC TV first anniversary programme broadcast on 4 March 1988, recounted that throughout the year, their emotional pain—their 'loneliness', 'emptiness' and 'longing'—had escalated.

---

* BBC TV anniversary programme, 4 March 1988.

'At first I was shocked and numb—then the suffering set in—and got worse as the year progressed.'

Therapists believed that mourning would culminate on this first anniversary and then begin to heal.

(3) *Tertiary prevention*—through the provision of psychiatric and community preventive and therapeutic facilities.

Pastoral (religious) care in disaster situations

John Vaughan, Hospital Chaplain:

The apparent absence of God in the midst of disaster and cruelty evokes a cry of despair. The religious point of view is that God does not desire or cause suffering; that He is not a callous spectator but experiences history with us. *The biblical God combats, with man, the negative powers of suffering and death.*

The pastor should be empathetically *attuned to the needs* of those in distress and have *sufficient knowledge of psychology* to judge when those who are suffering are in a defeatist stage or on the way to recovery. The pastor should also be able to judge the degree of the receptivity of the person. Pastoral care is not only the application of psychological methods. It also includes 'acknowledgement of a Presence and an awareness of the fact that this *Presence can be personally experienced*'.

Disaster causes people in distress to grapple with the problem of *guilt*. 'Their problems should be handled in a sensitive manner and should not be negatively exploited.'

Actual *physical distress* should not be ignored. It is not enough to evoke gratitude for being alive in spite of everything. Physical care should include an awareness of God and his desire to alleviate suffering. *Superficial attempts to find a reason for suffering should be avoided.* That God's plans are good should be a personal discovery, and not given as a palliative: Dull acceptance is not in accordance with the Scriptures.

The Church should give serious consideration to the *actual suffering of mankind*. The distressed should be given the opportunity to express their suffering and the Church should, unlike Job's friends, lend an ear without trying to justify suffering or to defend God in this world of suffering and injustice.

Help should be given in time of need. The Bible tells us that food and clothing are often of more value to the needy than sermons and admonitions. *Aid should not be limited to people of the same denomination.* It is essential that ministers be trained in handling crisis situations.

They should also be sensitive to the needs of the rescue team where they are under stress. They should have a knowledge of *group dynamics*, as people often have to be treated in groups. Trained, clearly identifiable and dedicated ministers should form an integral part of the whole concept of disaster medicine.

Frederika de Villiers stresses the importance of sensitivity towards the emotional and spiritual needs of the victim:

'It is important that the rescue worker should allow the love of God (1 Corinthians 13) to take gestalt in his life; this is embodied in:

(a) the disposition of warmth, tenderness, empathy, genuineness, respect radiating from us, serving as if it were a transfusion of courage, power and strength to the victim;

(*b*) the ability to listen creatively to what he says, but also to that which he does not say, eg by his attitude and behaviour;

(*c*) the discussion in which sincerity is the central moment; lack of sincerity is the unnatural way of trying to reassure him. Sincerity exists in our helping him in assimilating his anxiety and distress by verbalizing this; it is concrete sentiment which releases him from his isolation; accept that everyone has a right to express his feelings in his own manner; and

(*d*) a loving look and therapeutic transfer, to touch or take his hand or stroke his hair.'

To Rabbi Harold Kushner fell the tragic ordeal of watching his son die of 'premature ageing'.

What could be worse for a parent than to see his beloved child grow old, waste and die before his eyes . . . As Rabbi Kushner watched his son become cut off from his generation, grow bald, wrinkled and arthritic, he wrestled with the Bible and with his own soul:

'I could not respect a God who made an innocent child suffer. (I'm too compassionate to do that to somebody's child. And I don't think I'm more compassionate than God.)'

More than a year after Aaron's death, when Rabbi Kushner was 'beyond the point of self-pity', he began to write his book, '*When bad things happen to good people*'.

'Aaron's death was a tragedy that had no purpose or meaning. It was a freak of genetics. The painful things that happen to us are *not* punishments for our misbehaviour, nor are they in any way part of some grand design on God's part.

Bad things happen to good people because *God does not control free will: because natural laws—like accidents and illness—treat everyone alike* . . . .

Because the tragedy is not God's will, we need not feel betrayed by God when tragedy strikes. We can turn to Him for help in overcoming tragedy precisely because we can tell ourselves that God is as outraged by it as we are. . . .'

For Rabbi Kushner the power of God comes through when He summons

'friends and neighbours to ease the burden and fill the emptiness. We were sustained in Aaron's illness by people who made a point of showing that they cared . . . people like that were God's language. If I could choose, I would forego all the spiritual growth and depth which have come my way because of our experiences and be what I was 15 years ago, an average rabbi, an indifferent counsellor, helping some people and unable to help others, and the father of a bright, happy boy . . . but I cannot choose.'

A mine explosion

Four young miners who were still capable of communicating sat in a corner, their eyes staring ahead, their expressions blank. Holding their heads in their hands, they appeared *unable to comprehend the details of their situation.*

The explosion being less than an hour past, they were clearly in the *impact phase*, still stunned by the terror of their death encounter.

How does the therapist enter and reach out into their situation?

This is a place with no rôles. All you can do is to throw everything you've ever learnt out of the window, and *meet with a human being completely stripped of his defences.*

You must enter with him into his psychic numbness—and that is frightening.

Identifying with them, I felt their *defencelessness* in their terror of death.

You can't just say, 'Let's chat about it'.

I sat quietly, *feeling* with them their helplessness and their despair. Even comfort seemed irrelevant. A knife-edge from death, or undersized egos faded into irrelevance.

Only by demonstrating my feeling-with (empathy) could I enter into their situation, to achieve a measure of intervention.

Intervention

Support in performing a mundane, familiar and comforting action may intervene into psychic numbing—a shared cigarette, a cup of tea.

Eye contact reveals relief and amazement that such anchors to familiar security actually exist!

Within the context of a supportive, caring relationship there is encouragement to experience catharsis. The *emotional storm* acquires treacherous and *gigantic proportions*, and one feels one's relationship to be a dimunitive canoe over a tidal wave without direction—all one can hope for is to keep the canoe afloat, the trapdoor open.

Many try to close the trapdoor—the dead, numb state is preferable to terrible reality. *Freud has described the naked distress of the Ego, foresaken by the protective powers of the Super Ego*—its monitoring of the traumatic, its values and its self-concept.

The victim's illusion of his own immortality has been shattered. The life-sustaining images which, since his earliest years, have protected his personality from the threat of total destruction, are torn from him. He knows that the strong, loved people, and the supports in which he has always trusted, are as powerless as himself in the face of death's onslaught. Comforting bonds with his nurturing religion, mother, peer groups, ideals and historical forces have been replaced by separation and isolation.

The integrity and *independence of his physiological, ethical, psychological and growth-mastering self* have given way to the disintegration of his self-concept. He is a fragmented pawn of death!*

Re-orientation 'First Aid'

1. *Personal re-integration of the fragmented self* becomes the therapist's primary goal.

    It is necessary to mobilize untapped 'Ego' resources such as courage, insight and curiosity, that he may re-integrate, and move forward from maladaptive to adjustment processes.

    At a conscious level one *mobilizes* correct and appropriate *cognitive perceptions (dynamic reasoning, 'insight')* in order to help fill in gaps between pre-trauma

---

* Ventress, K D. National Psychology Congress 1981.

security and post-trauma disorientation. One attempts to *tell him what has happened, objectively, to his body* and *subjectively, to his mind.*

In order to *decrease his unstructured confusion and boundless panic*, one tells him who he is, where he is, what has happened; what one's relationship to him is, thus redefining where he belongs in the shattered jigsaw puzzle of his traumatic experience.

2.   *One tries to help him define and express his feelings*—the catharsis of talking and of crying, within a supporting, caring relationship relieves distressing and disorganizing tension, terror, guilt and anger.

3.   There is an urgent need to *replace symbols* of love, support, ideals and religious faith damaged by the intrusion of death. One tries to send for his next-of-kin, his doctor, his religious minister.

4.   One attempts to *initiate new feelings and coping patterns* appropriate to new losses, and at the same time find new caring supports, strength, etc.

Pertaining to the supportive role of *long-term introjection of religious belief*, Ventress has found a somewhat surprising negative correlation:

The 'non-prayer' tends to be more fatalistic about personal disaster than the 'prayer' who finds himself in conflict with his religious faith in individual protection. He feels guilty and anxious as to the reason for desertion by his religious supports: 'What have I done wrong to be thus afflicted?'

Immediate, 'hot' and effective crisis intervention offering skilled help within six to twenty-four hours after exposure to disaster, ie before personality disintegration sets in. At this stage the behaviour pattern is still sufficiently flexible for movement from

Impact Phase 1 through to
Recoil and Turmoil Phase 2 to
Emotionally Wounded Phase 3 and
Adjustment and Reconstitution Phase 4.

In hospital

When admitted to hospital the victim is often in a state of severe shock, in much pain and possibly faces an operation. Many confusing and distressing things have happened between the time of his injury and his being settled in a hospital bed.

Emergency medical procedures, makeshift transport, many strange faces in foreign environments, together with his pain cause him not only to feel *anxious*, but *emotionally isolated*. His *future is uncertain* and he is *incapable of doing anything* about the situation. This helplessness further increases his anxiety.

From this anxiety there emerge *attempts at adjustments, defence, mechanisms*, prominent among which is *denial*. The victim denies that it is tragic to have lost his leg, or that his friends have died. On the surface he appears nonchalant and unconcerned, even jocular. While he is sorry for his next-of-kin he claims that he has 'accepted the situation'. Avoiding the issue, he fails to come to grips with it.

Regression—there is constant need for the physical presence and reassurance of another person, and he is frequently dependent on tactile comfort.

Aggression—the maimed patient has pent-up feelings of aggression against invisible forces responsible for his injury. Finding himself constantly surrounded by the kindness of those upon whom he is dependent, there is no-one on whom he can *displace* his aggression. Often next-of-kin constitute his displacement objects, requiring insight into etiology. The most unhappy of aggression displacements is in-turned upon the victim himself, causing guilt feelings, anxiety, self-diminishment, and disintegration of confidence and motivation. 'How could I have been such a damned fool! Look what I've done to myself!' Illogical self-blame for deaths of friends increases his burden.

Depression—just as one mourns the death of a loved one (survival guilt feelings p 576), one mourns the mutilation of one's own body image (see pp 81, 501). Distress is of course compounded by pain.

Negativism is characterized by non-co-operation, self-isolation, refusal to carry out medical prescriptions, criticism of all and sundry—all these constitute the victim's endeavour to fight for his self-preservation, his identity, his personal dignity.

Efforts should be made to meet his need for privacy.

Other reactions consist in *phantasy escape mechanism, fear of pain, anaesthetic anxiety, disturbed sleep and nightmares, hypersensitivity to sudden loud noises and the reactions of others to his injury.* These and many other factors aggravate the victim's *despondency, depression and anxiety.*

Next-of-kin suffer shock, hysteria, grief, anxiety, anger, remorse, denial, confusion. Natural ambivalence, aggravated by emotional trauma and displaced aggression by the patient, may well lead on the relatives' part to unconscious feelings of rejection, conflict and hence a vicious circle of guilt and anxiety. 'I'm here to see him every day and I try to be cheerful and loving, but he gets so cross with me. What on earth am I doing wrong?'

Therapeutic handling

Stage I: Provision of

(a) *Catharsis*—suppression increases the potency of tension symptoms. The patient and his next-of-kin require opportunity to 'unload' their feelings. The provision of two 'therapists' allows repetition of the victim's story without fear of imposition on the listener.

(b) *Crisis intervention* (see p 572): During the first few hours following upon hospitalization, the patient and his next-of-kin usually hear the worst news, e g that a foot must be amputated or that he has lost an eye. The emotional impact of this period should never be underestimated, the whole psychiatric team being intensely involved.

Stage II: During the following weeks or months, feelings, perceptions, emotions, experiences of the patient and his next-of-kin 'must be worked through'. Attempts should be made to gain insight, interpret feelings, achieve acceptance and new reaction patterns, as well as to prevent self-diminishment by role reversal (see p 512).

Preparation for discharge

Intense individual and corporate interviews are needed in order to prepare the victim and his family for the effects on familial social and vocational life resultant upon maiming.

The varied reactions of people to his injury, and the effects thereof upon his own adjustment, are discussed with the victim and his family.

Because one cannot gather the whole community together to educate them, the client should be equipped to handle, with understanding and *increasing immunity* possible social reactions. Role play (p 626 et seq) is often helpful.

In cases of permanent disfigurement, a social worker may endeavour to accompany and support the client beyond the protective hospital environment. It may be necessary to extend the rehabilitation programme into community services such as those provided by vocational counsellors, community sisters, occupational nurses, etc.

Victim support schemes

The National Association of Victim Support Schemes
17A Electric Lane
Brixton
London
SW9 8LA
Telephone: 01 737 2010'

Local schemes offer support and advice to the victims of crime. Also support groups detailed in Chapter 22.

CHAPTER 25

SUICIDE

When an individual can find no adjustive mechanism to cut through the stressors constituting his crisis, he may resort to the ultimate Flight-escape of suicide.

According to the World Health Organization (WHO) there are 3 million unsuccessful suicide attempts in the world every day, and each day 25 million people in all corners of the world find themselves in a suicide crisis.

Those closely involved with the problem can predict the pattern of suicides. There is a steady number up to Christmas and New Year. Then the rate peaks sharply when the bleak reality sets in after the holiday season. These predictions are based on international observations made through the years. Almost every nation seems to have its own brand of seasonal blues. In Israel the suicide season comes after Rosh Hashana and Passover, and in Japan there is a marked increase in the spring.

Men usually commit suicide on a Monday. They use more violent methods than women and two men commit suicide for every one woman. Very often their work situation plays a major role in the crisis.

Women, on the other hand, usually take their lives at weekends, when they seem to have an increased awareness of their emotional insecurity, and they begin to question their worth as women. For single, unattached women it is a time of intense aloneness.

In both sexes the suicide peak age range is 40–59 years—the years when one encounters 'the moment of truth'—the turning-point in life's hopes and dreams. These are the years when many people must face family break-up. However, lately there has been a very marked increase in suicides among *teenagers*, often as young as 12 and 14.

A study of 24 countries by WHO has reported suicides among children under 10 years of age, and it blamed adults for giving youngsters the wrong impression of death.

> 'Children may not regard death as permanent because they see actors die in films or on television, and later appear again. . . .
>
> Adults add to this confusion by referring to death as "going to sleep" or "passing on". The idea of death as a state which is not permanent is strengthened.
>
> Suicide already ranked second or third in several European countries as the cause of death among people aged between 15 and 24.'

The study shows that of the 24 countries surveyed, Hungary had the highest suicide rate for all ages in 1969. The rate there was 25 times higher than the lowest national level, that of Malta.

Many successful and attempted suicides occurred among people under the influence of alcohol or drugs.

But the study added that more important factors in self-destructive behaviour among young people were <u>mental illness</u>, *social change* and the *<u>breakdown of the family</u>*. Then there is the <u>excessive pressure to 'achieve'</u>.

In many homes children are under **enormous pressure** from their parents **to come out on top of the class or do well in sport**. They are forced into competitive situations, and if they can't make it they would rather destroy themselves than face their parents.

In a survey conducted at Edinburgh University, Dr James Hemming found that the suicide rate among girls had doubled since 1968. The worst affected age group is between 15 and 19.

Dr Hemming believes that girls get upset when their lack of knowledge about sex leads to breakup with their boyfriends. He said that boys relieve their sexual aggression in crime, violence and vandalism.

These alternatives are not open to girls, who turn aggression inwards upon themselves. That is why the number of suicide attempts among them has soared.

Experts agree that <u>loneliness</u> can be one of the strongest immediate motives for suicide, especially among elderly people who often live alone in flats and houses, with neighbours whose names they don't even know. Loneliness also threatends young people, divorcees and others who live all by themselves. A profile of the typical victim reveals that he or she:

> is unlikely to be very religious. Protestants have the highest suicide rate of all religious groups; Catholics are second and Jews are third;
> is likely to be either in one of the professions (burn-out) or in a totally dead-end job;
> is probably not married;
> has attempted suicide before or spoken of so doing.

The nurse should *not* be misled by the old adage that he who threatens suicide seldom executes the deed.

Etiology

A desperate need to escape physical pain

Painful physical illness, especially involving frightening treatment and a poor prognosis, is a significant cause of suicide, especially when it occurs outside the context of loving familial support. The patient, perhaps quite logically, doubts the value of strugling on, and the motivation to survive gives way to the motivation to escape.

Psychological etiology

(a) The manifestation of extreme *hostility inwards towards the patient himself*—often due to guilt feelings; self-remorse; the pain and desperation engendered by the *failure of obsessive attempts to relieve tension*; guilt, stress and depression. Some ambivalence does however usually persist, affording opportunity for positive motivation of the will to live.

(b) A desperate cry for help in the face of acute and long-term feelings of failure, *loss of love and above all rejection*, especially within Erikson's maturational crises of

adolescence and the mid life crisis (see pp 249–53). *In old age*, often faced with increasing physical weakness, financial burdens and familial and social rejection, suicide may present as the only solution. The AIDS sufferer who attempts suicide seeks to escape from rejection, isolation, terror and, later, pain (see chapter 16, p 347).

3. Psychoses

(A) Schizophrenia—a psychotic mental condition marked by:

(i) Disturbances of thought processes or reasoning are fundamental to the diagnosis of szhizophrenia, giving rise to other symptomatology, such as isolation, delusions, hallucinations; inappropriate emotional reaction, bizarre behaviour, etc.

In fact, on this hinges a fundamental distinction between

Manic depressive psychosis characterized by gross *disturbances of mood and feeling.*	*Schizophrenia* characterized by *thought disorders in which logic is distorted, thoughts fractured.*

Thought intrusion: It would appear that the schizophrenic is *overpowered by an influx of thought processes which he is unable to filter out, classify or control.* To free himself from 'messages over the ether waves/ he may try to drown himself.

(ii) The patient's emotional reactions are not appropriate. He may weep when 'Santa Claus' brings him a present and laugh at a death in the family. Sometimes he overreacts with disproportionate elation or irritability. Frequently he presents as dull and apathetic irrespective of the reality of the environment.

(iii) Involuntary withdrawal from his real social and material environments. Enclosed in his cubicle of unreality, *preoccupied with his delusions and hallucinations,* he loses interest in and contact with people and events.

So complete may his withdrawal become that he remains silent and immobile for hours, even days, responding to nothing.

(iv) Sometimes highly suggestible, usually *completely unmotivated* by his surroundings, his stance becomes statute-like, sometimes robot-like. His movements become awkward and stiff, his mannerisms stereotyped.

(v) Frequently he curls up in bed, unaware even of his bodily functions. Where this presentation predominates the patient is said to be suffering from catatonic schizophrenia.

(vi) A consequence of his withdrawal is the patient's classic autism. Absorbed by his inner phantasy life, his reactions become self-orientated, the term 'autism' deriving from the Greek *autos* meaning 'self'.

(vii) So complete is his break from reality that he is lost to the natural limitations imposed by time, space and other reality dimensions. His hand can be burnt by the surface of the sun. He can fly through time—or through a window! In this phase of his illness he is clearly a suicide risk.

(viii) Delusions and hallucinations usually emanate from the schizophrenic's conviction that *external forces* are attempting to govern his thoughts. These delusions of *influence* persecute, harm, plot against him. Delusions of *persecution* predominate in *paranoiac* schizophrenia. *Believing his 'enemy' plots to kill him, he gets in first and kills the enemy. Or he may poison the demon within his own body.*

Delusions are false, impossible beliefs. It is common for delusions and hallucinations to centre on distortions of body function and body image. The patient may have a fearful delusion to the effect that, should he defecate, he will pass all his internal organs. So he may attempt to cut them out. Or seek to escape by death from his terrifying delusions.

Hallucinations involve unreal sensory perceptions. They occur when the patient actually 'sees', 'hears', 'feels' and 'smells' the figments of his imagination. In hallucination, this same patient may actually see in the lavatory pan his heart, liver, stomach and lungs. *He may obey messages heard from the archangel Gabriel by killing himself.*

(ix) <u>Bizarre behaviour</u>—probably emanating from his overpowering phantasy world; the patient presents with *grossly inappropriate or peculiar behaviour* including gestures, words, movements, all of which make no sense to the onlooker. (While neurotic phobias may be very vivid, they are distinguished by the patient's 'gut feeling' that they are not real.)

Etiology

The etiology of schizophrenia is indeed complex and remains the subject of much research. Researchers are agreed on the existence of a *basic vulnerability to schizophrenia,* built on varying combinations of the following predisposing and precipitating factors:

(i) hereditary predisposition
(ii) biochemical—it would appear that the patient inherits a susceptibility, under certain circumstances, to metabolic deficiencies. Incomplete metabolism causes the formation of *toxoids* which, *affecting cerebral function,* results in cortical perceptual misinterpretations and clouding of frontal lobe functioning, much in the same way as fever or post-anaesthetic confusion
(iii) hormonal disbalance
(iv) neurological factors
(v) psychological factors.

Treatment of schizophrenia

Punitive handling, rewards, appeals to reason, even psychotherapy fail to penetrate the incarcerated mind of the psychotic in the acute phase of his illness.

Electro-convulsive therapy (ECT) may be helpful during the more acute stages of the illness, when given in association with drug therapy.

It is, however, *drug therapy* which has revolutionized treatment of the psychotic.

Psychotropic drugs

Phenothiazines are most frequently prescribed in controlling the symptoms and behaviour of schizophrenia. Within the context of

(i) regular compliance in medication—promoted by the patient's realization that conformity is not addiction, but rather supplementation of the body's natural requirements;

(ii) treatment within the therapeutic environment followed by;

(iii) community support.

most patients can return to some form of satisfying and productive life. He will, however, probably always suffer from persistent vulnerability in more subtle areas of pervasive functional performance, eg decision making and maintaining relationships.)

(B) Manic-Depression and Endogenous Depression

The affective (manic-depressive) disorders present as *extremes of mood or feeling*, and develop from the concept of *manic-depressive psychosis*. The patient presents with wild elation and overactivity (hypomania or mania depending on the degree of activity) or, at the other end of the bipolar 'see-saw', with unwarranted deep depression. It would, in fact, appear that both extremes are interrelated manifestations of the *same illness, featuring lability, or mood swings beyond the range of normalcy*. Some distinguish between *'bipolar' affective* illness manifesting both extremes, and *'unipolar'* illness when symptoms settle at one end of this psychotic 'see-saw'.

The 'Manic' Swing

HYPOMANIA—In this milder form the patient is over-talkative and presents with quick, jerky movements. He is enthusiastic to the extent of over-excitability and unrealistic in his self-appraisal. He formulates grandiose schemes, frequently to the detriment of his studies, business or personal relationships.

HYPERMANIA is characterized by wild ravings, continuous undirected moving around, singing and shouting, often obscene in content. The patient's *hallucinations may drive him to prove that he possesses special powers of flight—which he may dangerously attempt to demonstrate.* His special 'healing powers' or religious 'relations' force him to harangue all and sundry with his political or religious messages, sometimes even frightening and threatening his audience. While most manic phases give way to depression, a normal period or another outbreak of mania, untreated or chronic cases may continue thus for years.

Etiology

'Scratch a manic and you'll find a depressive' is an adage emphasizing the 'other side of the penny' that is part of the manic-depressive syndrome.

Independence of precipitating factors, and the almost *inevitable cyclic nature* of presentation, *emphasize organic, probably hormonal etiology.*

Psycho-analysts on the other hand consider mania to constitute a psychological defence against the agony of depression.

They believe mania to result from an unconscious motivation to cover up an inner void.

The patient appears to seek feverishly for distraction in new objects and experiences, none of which succeed in achieving inner peace.

Treatment

Currently the most useful medication consists in lithium carbonate. Phonothiazines are also profitably utilized. Psychotherapy may constitute complementary treatment.

Depression—The 'depressed swing'

A. DEPRESSION AS A PSYCHOSIS (ENDOGENOUS DEPRESSION) is characterized by

(a) absence of significant external precipitation,
(b) eventual spontaneous lifting of symptoms,
(c) almost invariable recurrence in a cyclic pattern.

SYMPTOMATOLOGY falls into two types:

(1) *Depression as mania*—Feelings of hopelessness, unworthiness and misery, panic, guilt and self-reproach are *expressed in the hyperactivity of desperate agitation.* The patient wrings his hands, cries out loud, tears at his clothes, bangs his agony out on objects. Sometimes his activity of desperate misery is turned inwards upon himself, the patient smiting his breast, banging his head and attempting to 'punish' or destroy himself by self-mutilation such as self-flagellation, slashing of wrists, burning, and even amputation of extremities. At the time of self-onslaught the patient appears to suffer little physically, but experiences great pain thereafter. THE ULTIMATE DEPRESSIVE SELF-ONSLAUGHT IS SUICIDE.

The painful anger of depression may also be *projected outwards on others*, aggression increasing isolation when the patient most needs supportive relationships. IN DESPERATE, FRUSTRATED OVER-ACTIVITY HE MAY KILL THOSE HE LOVES MOST.

(2) *Depression as the antithesis of mania*—the patient's loss of self-esteem, his *feelings of rejection, isolation, defeat and hopelessness*, illogical though these may be, *result in loss of motivation.* He lacks Autonomic Nervous System stimulation, with resultant diminished supply of stimulants (adrenalin, histamine) and energizing chemicals (blood sugar). There is a *slowing down* of voluntary and involuntary physiological processes. Pulse rate and blood pressure drop, digestive processes diminish. In his *indifference to his present and future* he ceases to eat, to speak, sometimes even to move. Anorexia, constipation and loss of weight are evident.

Alternatively, in a desperate bid for mouth comfort, he may eat compulsively and indiscriminately.

Endocrinological sluggishness leads to loss of sex desire and impotence. The patient is heavy with misery and despair.

The patient exists in an aura of facial and overall stolidity, sadness and 'oldness' beyond his years.

Early morning awakening (diurnal fluctuation) is typical.

Sometimes there are psychotic symptoms such as loss of contact with reality and delusions. His conversation, if there is any, dwells on his misery, his wickedness and unworthiness. Delusions are more frequent than hallucinations, but he may actually *see* germs and rottenness exuding from his body. Fearing this evil product of his body may contaminate the world, he may be driven to attempt suicide.

Death seems preferable to, and the only escape from, his utterly miserable and burdensome life. In fact suicide presents a real danger.

Melancholia: lack of pleasure in all activities
                  lack of reactivity to pleasure, pain
                  3 of the following:
                      depressed mood
                      worse on awakening
                      early awakening
                      no interest in eating—weight loss
                      guilt: excessive and disproportionate
                      psycho-motor flatness or agitation

Etiology

Reinforcing the *neuro-hormonal etiology* of endogenous depression are its *irrelevant* presentation, *cyclic* recurrence and special *vulnerability at periods of endocrinological imbalance* such as adolescence, premenstrually, after child-birth, at menopause (involutional melancholia) and in senility.

Metabolic etiology

The biochemical changes characteristic of endogenous depression are more clearly definable than those associated with most psychiatric conditions.

There appears to be some disturbance in osmosis, water content of the body shifting from extra to intracellular compartments. Resultant electrolyte redistribution effects a change in cellular activity, and appears to stimulate adrenocortical activities.

Intracellular bone sodium is increased by as much as 50% in depression and 200% in mania.

On recovery normal body chemistry is restored.

Genetic etiology

Research suggests endogenous depression, together with its 'see-saw' complement mania, or hypomania, to be traceable to an autosomal dominant gene.

Variations of the condition are more common in relatives than in the general population. An especially potent genetic link is said to exist through the maternal line, probability of inheritance from mother to daughter being ± 24% as against ± 12% for other relationships.*

Psychological precipitation

Although endogenous depression appears without apparent psychological deprivation, there are those who believe it may be precipitated by psychological trauma such as bereavement or surgical mutilation. Psychoanalysts believe ambivalence, conflict, guilt, remorse (especially involving inturned aggression and

* Prof. J Angst, University of Zurich. 1979.

self-punishment) fruitless efforts to recover a lost person or body image; anger and a protective withdrawal are important ingredients of all types of depression.

Therapy

The greatest impediment to successful therapy—and even to suicide prevention—is *denial* by the patient, family, the community and sometimes even by the medical team, *of the physio-psychotic nature of the illness.*

Tied to prejudices of the past they are unwilling to admit to psychosis, attempting to rationalize environmental pressures, 'nervous breakdowns', lack of co-operation by the patient, etc, as predominant percipitating factors. Time and effort are wasted on palliative treatment such as tranquillizers and psychotherapy, exposing the patient to the agony of his depressive illness and the danger of suicide.

In the case of endogenous depression where there are *no specific environmental pressures to be relieved,* predominating treatment is by anti-depressant medication such as tricyclic compounds of the imipramine group, Tophranil and Motivan, sometimes complemented by ECT. The latter may also be helpful in freeing the patient of painful recurrent thoughts.

Alternative anti-depressant medication consists in mono-amine oxidase inhibitors such as phenelzine (Nardill)—this latter medication requiring careful monitoring of blood pressure.

DURING THE ACUTE STAGE OF HIS ILLNESS, AND ESPECIALLY AS THE EMERGING PATIENT GATHERS THE ENERGY TO COMMIT SUICIDE, HE REQUIRES VERY CAREFUL OBSERVATION; there are no grounds for believing that he who threatens suicide does not fulfil his intention. In fact, very often he does just that.

It is important that the nurse use her relationship in order to stimulate *motivation to live* by gestures of involvement, friendship and affection; by placing individual preferences and pleasures before ward routine; by welcoming familial and other relationships which the patient holds precious. It is important that his Sympathetic Nervous System be motivated to produce histamine, adrenalin and blood sugar of which *some* quota is necessary. Without them he becomes emotionally dead, motionless, almost paralytic. Communication establishes individual needs and goals. The possibility of goal-fulfilment within the hospital situation reinforces motivation.

Famous comedian Spike Milligan (70) of Goon Show fame, wants to tell fellow victims that 'being a manic depressive need not be all darkness', so he has just agreed to become patron of the Manic Depression Fellowship.

While praising new medication he pleads with psychiatrists 'before you administer medicine, manic depressives must be surrounded by three things: love, understanding and sympathy.'

B. DEPRESSIVE NEUROSIS

This occurs as part of a more general neurotic syndrome associated with ambivalence, *unconscious conflict, guilt feelings and anxiety. Painful obsessive rituals and other fruitless neurotic attempts at achieving homeostasis fail to give relief, and the hopelessness of the patient's suffering leads to depression, even unto terminating his misery in suicide.*

Presentation is similar to reactive depression and *treatment* consists in psychotherapy, mild sedation, environmental manipulation and, in more severe cases, anti-depressant drugs. In order to gauge its effects, drug therapy should be continued for a minimum of 10 days to 3 weeks.

The patient requires companionship, support, social involvement and distraction. His *condition is involuntary* and he would give much to be relieved of his unhappiness. Thus to chide and rebuke with exhortations to 'snap out of it' or 'think of others for a change' is both fruitless and destructive.

Swamped by his utter misery, the patient needs to be reminded that his acute depression, no matter how painful, *does always pass*.

'This bout, like others, will recede.'

Depression is an 'infectious' condition easily spreading to the hospital team themselves.

The nurse herself should seek hope in her own future. The bleakest times, like the best, do pass.

C. REACTIVE DEPRESSION

This occures in response to a grievously disturbing outside influence, resulting in *personal loss or other stressful change in the individual's life*.

Infection and other physical illness reduce resistance to the emotional upheavals of life.

Mutilating surgery such as mastectomy or limb amputation; psychological trauma such as death of a loved one, a broken love affair; failure in an examination, battle trauma, financial loss are all classic precipitants of reactive depression. (See Post-operative depression, pp 78–84.) Uprooting in emigration involves terrible loss of support systems and personal identity.

Reactive depression following real trauma such as the death of a loved one, cancer realization, mutilating surgery, etc *can* be acute, distressing, long-term. It may lead to neurotic depression, even THREATENING THE MOTIVATION TO SURVIVE. The nurse should have available a working knowledge of what has come to be termed 'CRISIS INTERVENTION'. Indeed nurses are often in the 'front line' of crisis. (See Crisis intervention, pp 563–82).

Depression in the elderly—see chapter 20.

Methods of suicide

Suicide results from many and ingenious methods, including gas poisoning and drug overdose (particularly barbiturates); less frequent methods are jumping off bridges and under trains, hanging, drowning, shooting, self-electrocution, jumping off high buildings—a favourite method in the hospital situation—and cutting of wrists or throat. This latter method appears to be associated particularly with obsessions of guilt and self-destruction. It is a method often used by adolescents, clearly in a desperate effort for reassurance, acceptance and love.

Warning signs

(*a*) History of a recent attempt. Most suicides contact a doctor within a week before they take their lives and most have been known to suffer from depression for approximately six months—these disconcerting facts result from research in the UK and are reported by Potocnik (p 450).

(*b*) There are strong features of *general depression*. When warning occurs it often consists primarily in the patient's extremely *miserable expression of despair and despondency*. In *contrast* the face may assume an air of *'smiling'*, *'accepting'* depression. The patient's appearance is usually unkempt and untidy.

(*c*) *Conversation*—usually conversation is *extremely stilted*, almost monosyllabic. The content of such minimal conversation may include delusions or hallucinations of unworthiness, guilt, desperation and rejection. CURRENT TALK OF SUICIDE INDICATES RISK 'TEN TIMES AND POSSIBLY A HUNDRED TIMES AS GREAT AS IN ITS ABSENCE'. Questions such as 'How do you feel about the future?' may lead to significant verbalization (Priest, R G. Recognizing suicidal patients. *Psychotherapeia*. November 1984).

(*d*) *Mood*—is one of utter and *complete sadness*. Sometimes there are moods of *desperation*, melancholia being complemented by verbalization of suspicion.

The patient is sometimes withdrawn and apologetic, verbalizing his belief that he is a 'nuisance', 'unwanted', a 'burden', 'too much trouble'—this especially in cases of menopausal and geriatric depression.

However, the nurse should be warned that a difficulty in preventing suicide may flow from its presentation within *quick mood changes*—success of suicide often results from its suddenness.

It should be noted that during the depths of depression the patient is frequently too lethargic to exert the physical effort required. *Suicide is more often attempted during the period leading up to depression or during the convalescent period.*

(*e*) *Intellectual functioning* is slowed down. Attention span and concentration are impaired—the patient's miseries are certainly too great to allow concentration on other matters, and he presents with much poverty of thought.

(*f*) Life habits. Eating: the appetite is classically very poor or non-existent. Sleep: the lowest point, or nadir, of mental operation usually occurs on waking, usually in the early hours. On emerging from the temporary relief of sleep, he is confronted by his problems, sadnesses and burdens, and may soliloquize: 'Oh God, another day to live through! How am I going to face its sadnesses, its emptiness, its horrors?'

(*g*) *General health*—all physical functions are conspicuously slowed down. There may be conspicuous loss of weight, eyes may lose their sparkle and the skin becomes coarse and dull.

Conversely, there may be marked compulsive eating in an effort to overcome anxiety and depression by mouth satisfaction. A general slowing-down of body processes may be reflected in sluggishness of bowel movement, and thus in constipation.

Prevention of suicide

1. Care should be taken to prevent exposure to electrical appliances and sharp instruments.
2. For a patient in a suicidal mood, even a plate, by breaking it, becomes a potential weapon.

3. In hospitals, drugs, chemicals and disinfectants should be carefully controlled.
4. The nurse should take precautions against her patient's storing his medication—a wise precaution being to crush tablets, before giving them.
5. *However, the most important preventive of suicide remains human contact.*

On the professional side there is virtually always a remnant of ambivalence—a swing of *wanting to live*. The client really wants to put an end to his suffering—not his life. This is the professional's lever back to life.

Although, during his most depressed stage the patient may appear to reject overtures of friendship, staff should persevere. Although the patient may not possess the motivation or energy to respond with words, it is very likely that our approach to him, our verbalization, our tactile communication, are not wasted.

When an actual *suicide attempt appears imminent* it is essential that the patient be *not left alone* but remain supported by the physical presence of the nurse, whose verbalized approach should be strongly reinforced by tactile reassurances. An arm around his shoulders, a hand held, will do much to convey *feelings of identification* caring and emotional-level support.

If the patient asks to see any special person it should be realized that the latter occupies a major place in his emotional constellation and may well provide something of that caring, reassuring support he craves. He may even have the power to provide the stimulus of life-saving motivation to survive.

Frequently suicide attempts arouse *hostility* and *frustration* in family and medical personnel, especially where the patient has failed to respond to their attempts to assist and guide. To protect themselves from guilt feelings and social censure they *deny* that the patient is seriously mentally ill usually in a state of serious endogenous or reactive depression, and thus requires intensive psychiatric treatment, including anti-depressant drug therapy, possibly ECT and psychotherapy, certainly intensive supportive care and team rehabilitation.

It is most important, in dealing with all types of depression, that *the staff avoid being 'infected' thereby*—in fact, because it finds a fertile corner in every personality, depression may spread quickly through the ward.

IT IS ALSO IMPORTANT TO REMIND THE PATIENT CONSTANTLY THAT THE DEPRESSION *MUST PASS*. ALSO THAT SUICIDE IS NOT THE ONLY WAY OUT—HE HAS *OTHER OPTIONS*.

It is gratifying to observe how impressively the crisis *is* often passed. The nurse who has established a warm, close and supportive relationship as a motivating path back to life is indeed herself rewarded.

Attention is drawn to the organization 'Lifeline' which, in larger centres, provides 24-hour emergency 'First-Aid' support to the potential suicide. It is a 'last ditch' service via which he may appeal for *help, reassurance, acceptance and an alternative 'way out'* without finally resorting to the suicide deed, about which the *psychogenic patient is to some extent ambivalent.*

Because a suicide threat does constitute A LAST DESPERATE PLEA FOR SOLACE AND LOVE, this very poignant need warrants our urgent attention.

For effective suicide prevention:

1. hospitals should have trained anti-suicide teams of medical and paramedical personnel operating on a 24-hour roster;
2. hospital treatment should be followed by home visits.

A potential suicide should know there are people who genuinely care and who are willing to help him solve his problems. A handful of tranquillizers is simply not enough.

Patients and teams should be aware that the urge to kill oneself does not last very long. If someone can intercede between the person and his lethal pills, jump or gun, there is a fair chance of averting the lonely tragedy.

Experience in Vienna shows that suicide is most frequent in the few months after an unsuccessful attempt. Follow-up treatment of would-be suicides should continue for one year after any failed bid. Indeed the person in deep depression is usually too motivated to attempt suicide which usually occurs as he emerges into convalescence.

It is essential to treat any underlying mental illness.

Thus medication, possibly ECT, psychotherapy, the therapeutic community (in either in- or out-patient facilities) and other therapeutic techniques (chapter 26) should precede or dovetail with anti-suicide counselling.

Self-Help Group: The Samaritans   01-4392224.

SUICIDE IN CHILDREN AND ADOLESCENTS

'Sorry to do this to you and Mum', wrote a 14-year-old Manchester boy to his father, 'but you did not believe me about my pain, and I can't stand it, so I am going to shoot myself.' Then he bequeathed his few possessions to friends, and took his life. . . . For every child's suicide, experts say there are about 100 attempts, and these are often unreported because of social taboos. Many parents cannot face the reality of suicidal behaviour.

Etiology

Most suicides among youngsters are the end result of an accumulation of worries too heavy to bear, perhaps culminating in failed exams, parental reaction and reaction by peers.

The *multifactorial etiology* of suicide is illustrated by the case of a 15-year-old Leeds boy with a long history of difficulty in making and maintaining social relationships.

He stole £2 000 from his father's safe and bought a motor car. Attempting to gain social recognition, he took his classmates for a spin and smashed up the car. He sought help from his father but was turned away. The terrified, lonely boy hanged himself.

Precipitating factors

Youth's most stressful problem appears to lie in *loneliness*.

1.   *Parental divorce frequently robs the child of companionship* by the departure of father and the fact that mother is forced to work outside the home. Often there is a move away from familiar school, neighbourhood and peer-group support, with the aggravating necessity of making new friends while self-esteem and financial resources are still in crisis.

     Many children feel superfluous—both parents may seem too busy for the child, even taking out their own anger and frustration on him, diminishing his self-value.

2. It is easy for physically or emotionally isolated children to *identify negatively* with morbid pop-songs such as 'Rock and Roll Suicide' or 'I think I'm Gonna Kill Myself'.
3. *Conflict with parents or step-parents,* is often related to constitutional inability to meet parents' academic demands and justify their financial sacrifices.

    Punishment thought to be too severe, both at home and at school, is certainly a precipitant of gross child-adult conflict.
4. *Harping criticism,* leading to a feeling that 'nobody understands me', and *repetitive failure* in a society in which children are expected to be 'status achievers', escalate until the child feels himself to be an incurable, hopeless 'loser'. In a desperate attempt to restore his feelings of self-worth, to ease his loneliness, he may *seek* and *cling to 'love'.* Disillusioned, he may feel his last bulwark and purpose in living are gone, and so he attempts or commits suicide.

Warning signs

Deep down, there is ambivalence in suicide. He really wants to put an end to his suffering, not his life.

So, consciously or unconsciously, he puts out certain warning signs in a last-ditch plea for help.

Some young people *hide their desparate depression* in 'bad' behaviour such as stealing, running away, truancy, bullying and accident-prone 'near misses'.

Boredom, restlessness, fatigue, loss of concentration, inexplicable behaviour changes, poor appetite, withdrawal, insomnia, aggression; general sadness and indifference to things which usually please; obvious anxiety, attempts to escape into alcohol and drug abuse; disposal of valued possessions, last wills and testaments, all constitute *help-pleas which should be taken seriously.*

So should remarks such as 'Who'll miss me when I'm gone?' or 'What's the good of living anyway?'

Prevention

1. In the long-term prevention lies in the *establishment of strong, supportive relationships based on reality of the child's potentials,* both *academic* and *vocational,* and on *acceptance of him as he is,* as a person to be loved and repected.

    Most important is the ability to *'show him'* that *he is loved and accepted for himself* as a person worthy of love and belonging. This is his right as a human being.
2. One should *utilize public and private crises* facilities such as hospital psychiatric casualty services, Suicides Anonymous, church ministers, and registered clinical psychologists.

    Almost anybody who *cares* can help avoid the tragedy of suicide. A cornerstone of prevention techniques is to persuade *the youngster that his problems can be solved and that suicide is neither the only nor the best way out.* He has options.

    To get an adolescent *to explain why he wants to commit suicide* is in itself therapeutic; and from there it's only a short step to *convince him* that his parents *love him*—that God loves him. But we must show him that we care.

    'I've been noticing you becoming so much quieter lately. I'm concerned for you—would you like to tell me about it?'

At the Symposium 'Youth Suicide: Prevention, Intervention and Postvention', 94th Convention of the American Psychological Association, Washington DC, August 1986, Lisa B Mayer, High Point Hospital, Port Chester, New York, presented the following suicide *high risk factors* which may be overt or covert; masked by apathy, boredom or psychosomatic involvement:

Losses in life—parent, boyfriend, even pet
School Failure, especially during the first 24 hours thereafter
Child Abuse
'Base to base' Removals: family transfers, sent away to boarding school, camp, etc.
Closed Family System—rigid and inflexible, in which members are not allowed to manifest anxiety or depression—'where the message is to maintain or restore homeostasis (p 103) of the family at all costs.'
Substance Abuse
Truancy
Physical injuries
Environmental stresses: marital discord, academic pressures, etc
Morbid preoccupation with death
Changed behaviour: Isolation from friends, refusal of social activity, etc

'Suicide is an effective cry for help—it is better than drugs; it doesn't need long explanations or expose the youngster to nagging. Nothing works like suicide!'

Treatment

Hospitalization

(i)   keeps the youngster safe;
(ii) structures his environment;
(iii) holds him for evaluation, interdisciplinary team investigation and feedback.

The evaluation period at Dr Mayer's hospital consists of at least one week in a locked unit.
Nursing checks on each individual are made throughout the day.
The therapeutic programme includes psychological testing, family interviews, assessment of medication needs, etc.

Psychotherapy, group and individual—

(i)   establishes strong bonds;
(ii) improves frustration tolerance;
(iii) teaches coping mechanisms and realistic goals.

It is *important that the youngster admits* to his suicide ideas, which <u>therapeutic step</u> is reinforced by praise and approval.
Planning for discharge includes a detailed support system and continued treatment plans.
William Reulbach, Pelham Family Services, New York, addressed his presentation to the necessity for *preventing* 'linked suicides and the "<u>Romeo and Juliet syndrome</u>' " within school and community services situations.

He recommended:

1.   Recognition of 'the need to face it yourself—denial and guilt will bury and prolong the danger period'.

     This recognition should be at four levels namely:

     administration;
     support services: guidance-teachers, psychologists, school nurses, etc;
     teaching faculty;
     para professionals.

2.   Staff should be notified immediately, and told what has happened, and what led up to it.

3.   Don't use the public address system. Rather assign stable teachers to tell children in small groups in 'crisis rooms' for at least one hour per session. This provides opportunity for the expression of grief, invites cathartic conversation, squashes rumours and enables opportunity for staff feedback.

4.   *Don't romanticize death or the deceased. It is important not to create a role-identification figure.* Avoid impressions such as: 'I went to Emily's funeral and they said marvellous things about her—I'll make them do the same for me.'

5.   Network with Mental Health agencies in the community. Encourage formation of an 'Adolescent Suicide Task Force'.

6.   'Bury hatchets' and avoid displacing guilt on others.

7.   Identify 'high-risk' students for special catharsis, guilt reduction and counteraction of the 'living will' syndrome.

     Counteract (a) guilt association situations such as: 'Tommy can have my football—I won't be needing it anymore.'

     (b) Morbid identification stimuli such as: 'Peter left me his love—and a message always to cherish it.'

     It is important that 'Romeos', 'Juliets' and 'rejectees' learn that *life satisfaction is not dependent on one relationship;* there is no guilt nor disloyalty in 'moving on'.

8.   Call an evening meeting for all parents, to inform, provide opportunity for catharsis, and discuss the general response to suicide and how to handle grief.

9.   Do not hold a memorial service. Rather allow small-group 'psychological autopsy' sessions with friends, relations, teachers. These should aim at healthy identification figures, guilt reduction and comfort.

10. Identify causative factors such as drug abuse.

CHAPTER 26

THE PSYCHIATRIC NURSE

The therapeutic community

Because sharing the poignant experiences of illness is an important therapeutic factor, every aspect of the hospital—its structure, its function, the behaviour and attitude of its staff and fellow patients—all have a potentially therapeutic or destructive effect.

Evolution of the 'democratic' hospital structure

An important first step in the construction of a therapeutic community was the *amendment of the formerly authoritarian attitude* of the governing body and its superintendent, followed by the formulation of a new administrative policy to include all members of the community, staff and patients. Relaxation of authoritarian administration may vary from equal voting rights of all members to a policy where patient-decision may, in fact, be relatively limited, but the atmosphere of *administration by participation* is accepted as the keynote. It has, in fact, been found that overall participation usually results in overall increased standards of personal and social behaviour, and responsibility. The 'they' attitude, formerly the butt of aggression and destruction by the patient, now gives way to the 'we' attitude, where there is motivation to direct energy in a constructive manner for the benefit of the whole community.

The nurse–patient relationship

'Humanized' care—care enhanced by the dignity and autonomy of the patient. Specific components of humanized care are:

(1) Perception of the patient as a whole being, unique, and worthy of the carer's concern.
(2) Empathetic handling by the staff, every member of which is accountable for the welfare.

Traditionally the nurse is seen as the protector of the patient against himself, other patients, the community, the family, etc.

> 'Within the treatment model the nurse, because she spends most time with the patient and is thus especially available to him, is in many ways the main determinant of the quality of service the community health service is able to offer.'*

Confused, frightened and diminished by the torments of mental illness, the patient is dependent upon the sense of safety and personal dignity conveyed by the nurse.

A community depends largely on the availability of *free channels of communication*

---

* Bruwer, Ms A M, The Role of the Psychiatric Nurse — further inquiries to author.

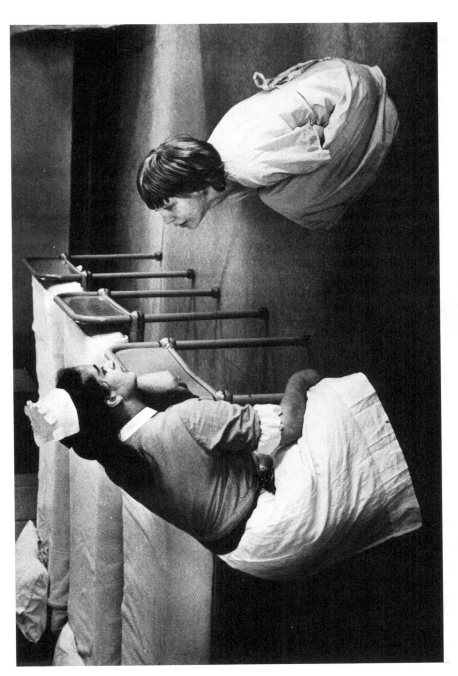

NURSING THE MENTALLY ILL

Reproduced by kind permission Camera Press, Ltd, London.

Photograph by Lord Snowdon

upwards, as well as downwards. A keynote of this communication is the establishment of a *vehicle for group dynamics* through the conduct of *group sessions or meetings.* Such meetings may vary between sessions discussing the business of running the institution, or more correctly the community, and those providing a vehicle for the observation and therapeutic interpretation of human behaviour. Problems are discussed, grievances aired and sometimes decisions reached. Responsibilities of participants in routine activities are discussed and patients assisted in the difficult task of reaching decisions. Nurses, accustomed to the more authoritarian attitude which still prevails in some general hospitals, may encounter difficulty in establishing with patients, individually and in groups, an attitude of friendly concern, support and guidance rather than instruction.

Within the more long-term and intimate situation prevailing in the psychiatric unit, a nurse must give much of herself; in fact the *relationship* between patient and nurse is at least as *important as the administration of technical skills.*

In the psychiatric ward, as in geriatric nursing, it is the relationship between the patient and his nurse which may well *motivate* him to embark on the difficult course back to normal familial and community life. If she cannot *show* her caring, her support, her identification, she is unable to assume the subtle role of a Psychiatric Nurse.

A Psychiatric Nurse is expected to <u>spend much more time in building her relationships</u> with her patients, whether this be through individual comfort, group discussions, debates, dancing, general 'over tea' chats, walks in the garden, outings into the community—in fact in a wide range of situations in which ingenuity, flexibility and freedom from her own obsessions with routine, are all of primary importance.

So intimate is the relationship between the psychiatric nurse and her patient that she herself may require *special group sessions* in order to balance her personal integrity with the demands of her patients, while at the same time maintaining effective identification, compassion and support.* The nurse may, for instance, need advice, guidance and support, in judging whether, and to what extent, a post-hospital relation with a patient should be encouraged and conducted, and how, constructively, to wean the patient—and sometimes herself—from such a relationship. (Colleague case 'supervision' and review, p 232.)

Professional 'burn out'

Psychiatric nurses are especially 'at risk' for professional impairment or 'burn out' (pp 200–204). Special stresses to which they are exposed include:

(i) the subjective, often intangible illnesses of their patients;

(ii) the frequent necessity, in diagnostic and therapeutic relationships, to enter the distorted, terrifying world of their patients, balancing on the knife-edge between healthy reality and sick phantasy;

(iii) the necessity to forego the satisfaction of cure for the more modest achievement of alleviation, and to accept the disappointment of frequent relapse; to tolerate the 'revolving door' patient without recrimination or self-blame;

* Diagram overleaf p. 601.

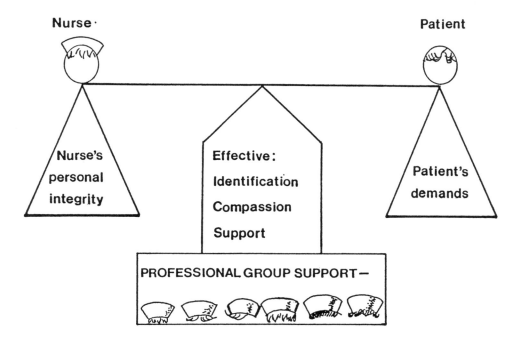

(iv) the necessity to tolerate without personalization psychiatric symptomatology such as the unjust accusation of paranoia; the aggression and manipulation of psychopathology; the hopeless dependence of catatonia and asthenia; the displaced aggression of frustrated and guilt-laden families;

(v) possible residential requirements with their inherently stressful inescapability, intimacy and isolation;

(vi) the constant high confidentiality of patients' illness, symptomatology, cathartic content and prognosis which creates a barrier with all but, and sometimes including, colleagues.

This strict ethical secrecy isolates the nurse emotionally from meaningful communication, cathartic release and the support of friends and family.

Statistics for psychiatric nurses are not to hand, but it is not surprising that while the suicide rate for unmarried female physicians over 25 years of age is 4 times that for the general age-group population, that for similarly placed psychiatrists is 6 times the general rate.

Dealing with complaints

Because the psychotic patient is known to suffer from delusions and hallucinations, it is easy to misinterpret a legitimate complaint as a misjudgement.

A classic case is that of a patient suffering from paranoic schizophrenia who frequently complained to the ward sister that a junior nurse was 'digging lighted cigarette butts into my back'.

In the knowledge that he suffered from persecutory delusions and hallucinations, the sister sympathized with the patient but did not accept the reality of his complaints—until, temporarily admitted to a general ward, his back was found to be pitted with cigarette burns!

Another area of complaint encountered in the psychiatric ward is that pertaining to homosexual approaches by other patients or by the staff, some in phantasy, some in reality.

Maintaining balance between reality and phantasy in the psychiatric ward (as in the geriatric ward) is difficult, but the ward sister should be very aware of both aspects, superfluous investigation being preferable to casual dismissal of complaints.

One cannot overstress the importance of establishing free channels of communication between all members of the hospital community, with the assurance that such communication will not, under any circumstances, lead to punitive discriminatory retaliation on the part of the staff.

Ward reports

Because the nurse enjoys long-term and intimate contact with the psychiatric patient, her keen and intelligent observation of his mental processes, as reflected by his long-term behaviour, is of primary importance. Both oral and written reports should be full, highlighting those areas important to the individual case. Observations may be classified into:

A. *Positive observations*

1. Unusual or emphasized *facial expressions:* fear, confusion, blankness, suspicion, furtiveness, sadness, depression and preoccupation.
2. *Body movements*—were they slow and depressed? Were his reactions quick, disconnected, hyperactive, aggressive, timid, stilted, defensive?
3. His *social relationships*—was he aggressive, self-ingratiating, lethargic, suspicious or very excited?
4. His *conversation content*—did he discuss suicide, his hallucinations, complaints about other patients; anxieties about his home, his family, his job? Did he seem interested or disinterested in his present condition or his future life?
5. *Personal functions*—Was he content? Did he eat? Did he sleep? Was he reasonably tidy or obsessively compulsive?
6. *Care of and interest in his appearance* constitute a valuable index of progress.
7. *His reactions with his family during visiting hours*—without prying and depriving his patient of privacy, it is important that the nurse make some observations as to this important index of family adjustment.

B. *Negative observations*

Negative reporting highlights something which might have happened but did not, eg a decrease in epileptic seizures, in compulsive neuroses, in aggression or depression, or absence of usual participation in social or sporting activities.

Structuring the therapeutic situation

Admission

An extremely important aspect of the psychiatric situation emphasizes the fact that treatment is transitory, the hospital stay only a means to the end of personal readjustment, and a full, responsible life within family and community.

Most patients and their families have been exposed to lifelong association of a psychiatric hospital with long-term, prison-like doom—a rotting away, an end to purposeful life.

In order to counteract this conviction, it is important that, from the time of admission, the therapeutic programme emphasizes preparation for discharge.

Even though, on admission, the patient may be oblivious thereof, mention of plans—social, financial and vocational—on discharge, will constitute an important reassurance to his family, and hence to himself. In any case, usually some feature of the conversation does penetrate and this attitude is a most constructive one. Clearly, the nurse, the social worker, the occupational therapist, in fact, the whole psychiatric team, should find ways of communicating to the patient and his family that every step in treatment is an optimistic stride towards a normal future. The patient's worst, and most destructive, blow consists in loss of status and self-determination.

The following is a valuable and sensitive dramatized learning experience aimed at achieving audience involvement in the predicament of a psychiatric patient subjected to standard admission procedures:

Audience participants were invited to the stage, blindfolded and taken through procedures prevailing at a psychiatric hospital—admission, physical and mental assessment (eg 'Tell us about your sex life'), medication, etc.

Staff members demanded, exhorted and pleaded: Trust me! Responses in these normal people, who were aware of the transitory nature of their predicament, varied from terror to physical aggression. This 'brought home' the devastating ordeal of *unfamiliarity, helplessness, status loss* and *personal diminishment* experienced by those for whom the situation is 'for real', ie real-life patients.

The Nursing Process

1. *Data collection*

Most historical data, expertly collected, and collated by other health professionals will be available in the file. For her particular insight into the patient's problem in the 'here and now' Stuart & Sundeen* recommended that the nurse equip herself with the following problem-oriented information:

'How is the problem perceived by the patient? Is it interpersonal, somatic, or sociological? When was the problem first noticed (onset)? How long has it lasted (duration)? Does the patient have any ideas as to the possible causes of the problem? Has it become worse (progressed) or changed in degree? If so, when did the change occur? Has the patient found any solution or obtained any type of relief?

---

* Stuart, G W & Sundeen, S J. *Principles of Psychiatric Nursing.* St Louis: Mosby. 1979.

In eliciting this information from the patient, the nurse would look for other factors related to the current problem of which the patient may not be consciously aware, such as a change in personal relationships, job, financial condition, and other circumstances surrounding the initial occurrence.'

Should she be a primary history taker, the nurse should try to cover:

Related family data;
Relations who have suffered from the same or similar illness.

Patient history

Duration of presentation.
Previous presentation:
    frequency, intensity, treatments, outcome.
His usual capacity to form and maintain relationships.

Childhood memories

—first or second hand
—right back to obstetrical details
—family visitors
—family relationships
—school successes and failures
—relationships with teachers and fellow pupils
—conflicts: nail-biting, enuresis, nightmares, etc?
—adolescence: 'facts of life'—his source of information
—attitudes of parents, teachers, friends
—extended family
—own feelings
—sexual feelings and conflict
—social successes and failures
—religious feelings
—hobbies
—escape mechanisms: drugs, alcohol, etc (avoid judgemental attitude)
—goals: success, failures, re-education
—sex and marriage history
    fulfilment and loss areas
—what are his main life-goals?
    does he think he will achieve them?

Very clearly such an exhaustive and intimate history can reach fruition only within the context of a respectful, warm and non-judgemental relationship. The patient's withholding of information should be respected, perhaps to be re-approached as the nurse's relationship with him develops.

2. *The nursing diagnosis (assessment)*

The nursing diagnosis is based on
    (a) The extent of deviation between
        (i) client health status relative to the norm,
        (ii) goals set and obtained,

      (iii) client goals and norm goals;

(b) The nursing diagnosis relative to that of the team;

(c) Aspects of mental health to be promoted: aspects of environmental stress to be modified.

However, standardized, accurate laboratory procedures are not always applicable. Thus diagnostic procedures, dependent on client revelation, often merge with therapeutic procedures as inner dynamics become more readily available through catharsis projective and other techniques, etc.

3 & 4. *Planning and Implementation*

The physical environmental of the hospital is, of course, important. Many consider it unwise to isolate patients in large psychiatric hospitals, physically separated from the community into which they are to be rehabilitated. An easier flow of communication and acceptability between the patient, his family, his work and his community may result from integration of the psychiatric unit within the local general hospital than if he is 'sent away'.

Carrying this concept of freedom of movement and communication with family and community to its ultimate, modern psychiatric administration places great emphasis on avoiding, as far as possible, that 'hospitalism' which is associated with institutional isolation (p 46). The patient's 'in-patient' stay is curtailed as much as possible. 'Graduation' to 'night hospital', 'day hospital', 'half-way house' hostel, 'out-patient' and group therapeutic situations constitutes an important aspect of the psychiatric treatment plant.

A bar-windowed ward, containing a long row of dismal iron bedsteads, bereft of privacy and aesthetic appeal, a cross between prison and a benevolent concentration camp, is unlikely to impart to the patient feelings of self-respect, happiness and optimism.

Most modern psychiatric hospitals consist of ward or pavilion units, individual cubicles or rooms—permitting of vision from without—day rooms, occupational therapy rooms, family visiting rooms and feature taped music, brightly coloured furnishings, etc. Tact in the administration of any environmental restrictions such as locked doors is of primary importance. So is the provision of as much variation and stimulation in daily routine as possible.

During hospitalization every effort should be made to *motivate the patient back to reality*—a reality for which it is worth making the effort to get better. Long stay patients are now being placed in the community within small-group, supportive facilities. It may fall to the community nurse to prepare the community to receive the mentally ill and mentally handicapped into their daily living.

The Psychiatric Nurse should be a participating colleague in the multidisciplinary team.

The psychiatric team

The *Psychiatrist* is a medical specialist who conducts individual or group therapy. Because he studies organic components of psychogenic processes, he is able to prescribe medication or conduct other physical treatments. The psychiatrist is usually the team leader and unit administrator. He is also frequently a community educator.

The *Clinical Psychologist* defined as a 'specialist in human behaviour and mental processes' measures the patient's intelligence and ability patterns. He calculates deterioration of intellectual processes due to ageing, physical trauma, etc. He conducts tests of personality structure, emotional functioning and interpersonal relationships. The clinical psychologist may also conduct psychotherapy.

A specialised Diploma in Clinical Psychology (or its equivalent) and registration with the British Psychological Society is required for participation in the National Health Service.

The *Occupational Therapist* provides therapeutic occupation. The tangible, concrete nature of these activities helps bring the patient back to reality from his mental withdrawal and abstract fears and conflicts. A wide range of activities to meet individual personalities, interests and educational levels motivates satisfaction in creativity and provides group support.

Creative and social tasks are also designed to provide specific healing. A withdrawn patient, frightened to emerge from his shadowy, muted isolation, may well be given opportunity to contact, and work with artistic materials of increasingly bold colour, providing opportunity for both tangible and symbolic contact with more outgoing media. Hence he may be encouraged to participate in group artistic or drama projects.

A patient obsessed by the necessity to perform cleanliness compulsion rituals which shield him from contact with 'forbidden' 'gooey' sensuous material may be encouraged to participate in gently graded, supported therapy consisting of contact first with the pastel-coloured crayons, through freer, less-structured and larger movements with finger paints, to black and brown starch-reinforced paint resembling 'forbidden' childhood media such as excreta, to strong tactile contact with mud, clay, etc. Contact with these media reduces the stress they provoke.

Some patients are able to participate more fully in sound media, progressing from quiet bell-like background instruments through release in aggressive drums, to more balanced musical participation.

The patient's creations, in painting or sculpture; in movement; in music or 'psychodrama', may well serve as revealing *diagnostic projective techniques*, and *records of progress*, as well as a means of *catharsis and reintegration*.

In cases of amputation, neurological trauma or illness (such as cerebral palsy or cerebral haemorrhage) the choice and administration of appropriate therapeutic neuromuscular activity frequently falls to the occupational therapist. Her responsibility extends to the supervision of appropriate equipment and its use in the home situation.

The *Social Worker* conducts case-work designed to:

(a)   investigate the case history and operant environmental pressures;
(b)   provide a therapeutic-supportive relationship with the patient and his family and carry out family therapy;
(c)   reduce stresses intensified by maladjusted family relationships, financial and job pressures, overcrowded housing, etc;
(d)   mobilize community resources such as youth hostels, geriatic clubs, group therapy, etc, for her patient's long-term welfare.

Functions *(c)* and *(d)* are termed 'environmental manupilation' and constitute an important aspect of sound social work.

Post-graduate qualifications in medical and psychiatric social work are available to her. The latter qualification extends to conduct of individual and group psychotherapy. It is important that nurses refer appropriate patients, and extend to social workers the fruits of their personalized contact in nursing procedures. Not only the poor require the help of social workers.

The *nurse's* cheerful respect, support and identification (her willingness to give relief by caring and sharing) create a *relationship* which eventually imparts to the patient the belief that perhaps his problems are not so insoluble, nor life so miserable after all. The nurse, by virtue of the *long-term and intimate contact* occasioned by nursing procedures and ward routine, is in an especially favourable position to create a supportive relationship, to provide catharsis and, very important, to *observe and record accurately* the patient's reactions and progress. Whether he seems remotely withdrawn, excitable, depressed, aggressive, resentful, frightened, obsessed by ritual; whether his expression is blank, suspicious, tight-lipped, vague, friendly; his appetite; all these constitute information of the greatest value to the psychiatric team.

The nurse is traditionally associated with relief of suffering. The fact that she is able to provide *comforting physical care* gives her a *special vehicle* for establishing active communication or rapport with her patient.

The Psychiatric Nurse

The psychiatric nurse's specialized patient-care and therapeutic skills will enhance his status and active participation in the psychiatric team. His longitudinal and intimate patient contact renders him a very special team-member. He participates in both psycho-dynamic and behaviour modification therapy.

The *Community Sister* provides community psychiatric *observation* and *support* in a medical orientation. She is able to administer (under medical supervision) *therapeutic drugs*, and to assess the *patient's response* to them. She is the *communicating link* between psychiatric ward, out-patient unit and community services which extend into the patient's own home and work situations.

In these days of curtailed hospitalization she plays an important role in keeping the patient in the community, returning him thereunto as soon as possible. Moreover, she is in a favourable position to prepare his family and community to receive him back with insight and sympathy.

A merely supervisory role is oppressive for the patient and boring for the nurse. With increasing specialization in psychiatric training the nurse is assuming a more independent and specific therapeutic role. (Those conducting behavioural psychotherapy are advized to complement their reading of relevant sections of this book by giving attention to Techniques facilitating Communication, pp 188–9.)

DIAGNOSTIC-THERAPEUTIC TECHNIQUES

Behaviour modification therapy (for theoretical background to Conditioning see chapter 6, p 152).

Token Economy Systems are positive reinforcement programmes utilize to reward, and thus reinforce, socially acceptable behaviour patterns in chronically hospitalized (frequently psychopathic) patients:

Desirable behaviour   → is rewarded by → a desired token reward constituting pleasurable
experiences → reinforcement

Undesirable behaviour → is punished by → removal of desired token, reward or privilege →
elimination

Accumulated tokens may be spent on sweets, outings or whatever is highly desirable to the patient.

SPECIFIC ROLE OF THE NURSING PROCESS IN BEHAVIOUR THERAPY

(1) *Data collection*

   (a) observe patient
   (b) help him develop his hierarchy of fears, painful and unacceptable behaviour

(2) *Diagnosis (Assessment)*
   compare his behaviour deviation from the norm, and having established the extent thereof, define new behaviour goals, preferably with the patient's active participation

(3) *Implementation*

   (a) teach the patient the nature of behaviour therapy and establish mutual goals.
   (b) help him practise reinforcement exercises in the form of therapy and in 'homework'—eg Today, if I can cut down handwashing to five times, I'll give myself a sundowner whisky. If I can't, it will be a soda only.
   (c) reinforce desired behaviour in daily living situations.

(4) *Evaluate* with the patient and psychiatric team any decrease of painful behaviour responses, and the extent of reinforcement of new positive behaviour responses.

Evaluation of behaviour modification therapy

The most important *contribution* of behaviour therapy appears to lie in elimination of specific fearful, painful, obsessive, ritualistic behaviour and psychopathic behaviour. Because it does not require much insight this technique is used widely in rehabilitation of the mentally handicapped.

An important *criticism* of this method lies in the fact that one works *with the environment rather than the patient* who, if he changes, may do so without his direct co-operation and knowledge. And there are ethical questions: Who assesses the therapeutic value to the patient himself? Does one human being possess the right to control another by either individual conditioning or by mass media conditioning? The nazi regime emphasized the horrible possibilities of mass conditioning. The answer appears to lie in the free dissemination of information pertaining to the methods, use and possible abuse of behaviour modification techniques. For, as in biblical times, 'the truth shall make you free'.

Specifically there should be *conviction that the therapist's goals are the same as those of her client.* (See also Desensitization by relaxation or hypnosis (p 164), Assertiveness Training (p 165), Aversion Therapy (p 165).)

Stuart & Sundeen* prescribe the following criteria in assessing ethical justification for behaviour modification therapy:

(1) Treatment should be preceded by informed consent and mutual agreement as to procedures, goals, etc.
(2) Treatment should include ongoing client self-assessment.
(3) Treatment should be relevant to the client's adjustment to his natural environment.

Of importance to the psychiatric nurse is the article 'The Psychiatric Nurse as a Behavioural Engineer', presented in 1959 by Ayllon & Michael.[†] In her article 'An Adjunct to Training Psychiatric Aides in Behavioural Modification Techniques'[‡] Lee discusses effective teaching techniques at a state hospital.

Psychotherapy

Psychotherapy and psychoneurosis

Psychotherapy is useful but unlikely to achieve a complete 'cure'. In fact, due to the complexity and interweaving of environmental and personality factors, psychotherapy, and psychiatry in general, seldom speak of 'cure', rather being thankful for symptom relief in the case of psychoneurosis, and establishment and maintenance of a reasonable way of life in psychosis.

As pertaining to psychoneurosis, the usual treatment of choice is psychotherapy based on the definition of suffering therapeutic thought association, catharsis, interpretation, re-experiencing, transference 'symbolic undoing', emotional-level reorientation, etc (see pp 64–67).

It is essential that the neurotic patient understands that his psychiatric team will *never be critical nor moralistic, even if he confesses to his most intimate, 'shameful' feelings*. It is very important that in his everyday life, his illogical but powerful fears and guilt feelings about sex, infection, aggression, etc, be accepted, and his personal dignity, integrity and self-concept be assured.

An important contribution to the patient's peace of mind lies in *reinforcing his capacity to 'live with' his symptoms*. Reassurance to the effect that everybody suffers thus in varying degrees provides comforting, positive identification and some feeling of hopefulness.

Faced with inability to overcome or live with mounting, painful ritual, psychoneurotic patients may become *depressed at their inability to relieve their suffering*. Psychotropic drugs and other anti-depressants may well be indicated. Electro-Convulsive Therapy may also be helpful, although ECT may, to an extent, defeat its own purpose in imperilling the subject's all-important self-concept.

Care should be taken lest the patient, finding no relief, seeks to end his suffering by suicide.

* Stuart, G W & Sundeen S J. *Principles and Practice of Psychiatric Nursing.* St Louis: Mosby. 1979.

† *Journal of Experimental Anal Behaviour* **2**: 323. 1959.

‡ *Journal of Psychiatric Nursing* 169. July–August 1969.

Reference: Cantela, J. 'Behaviour Therapy.' *In:* L Herschel (ed) *Your Psychotherapist.* New York: Appleton-Century-Crofts. 1970.

The nurse should realize that *overpowering neurotic disturbances* and distintegration of normal mental functioning are *involuntary*, and that the patient is *suffering intensely*. The neurotic patient is *acutely aware* of the uselessness of his symptoms, and of his deteriorating personal, social and job status. He may well possess intellectual-level insight into the cause and implications of his illness, and is deeply frightened and depressed thereby; but he is powerless to control his fruitless, recurring intrusive thoughts, painful fears, guilt feelings, obsessions. His suffering is intense and prolonged. Much research is still required into the etiology and treatment of this so common and yet so painful condition. Moralistic appeals such as 'pull yourself together', 'think of others for a change', and punitive threats such as 'you'll really drive yourself mad if you go on like this' will only increase his guilt and his terrifying anxiety.

On the contrary, the patient should be comforted by the reassuring information that *the etiology of his primarily psychogenic neurosis is quite different from that of organically orientated psychosis*. One does not deteriorate from one condition to the other.

Owing to the complex interplay of personality and environment, the neurotically ill patient may need the concerted, long-term help and support of the multidisciplinary psychiatric team.

(See pp 605ff.)

Even the long-term, energetic, non-stop and intensive psychotherapeutic communication attempted by Rosanoff failed to penetrate his psychotic patients' cubicle of unreality. A simplification of the essential processes involved in psychotherapy appears at pages 64–67 above. *Psychotherapeutic procedures are certainly basic to the treatment of neuroses* (those mental disturbances in which the etiology of the patient's anxieties, crippling feelings of inferiority and rejection, obsessions and other distressing symptomatology are fundamentally psychogenic, linked to his past experiences, and within the realm of his intellectual reasoning) as opposed to those organically orientated *psychotic conditions* in which the patient's hallucinations and delusions are frequently without connection with his own life story. Rather are psychoses associated with cerebral infection, trauma, hereditary factors, metabolism, etc.

However, psychotherapy may well constitute a *rehabilitative process* by which the psychotic patient, after he has been helped by drugs and other methods to emerge from his isolated cubicle, may be relieved of psychogenic contributors.

	Neuroses	Psychoses
Etiology	psychogenic: linked to past experiences within the realm of intellectual reasoning, although emotional reactions elude change	predominantly organically orientated: heredity, cerebral trauma and infection, metabolic faults, etc; hallucinations may be independent of life experience
Treatment	psychotherapy environmental manipulation	by medication—probably to restore metabolic cycle; perhaps ECT may be complemented by psychotherapy

Rufus Peebles, a Cambridge psychotherapist, refers to '*body-orientated psychotherapy*'.

Touching puts people on the same 'wavelength'. Peebles feels that working with touch adds empathy, clarity and direction to a process which can be very evasive when words are the only communication medium.

'The body doesn't always speak the truth, but it speaks the truth more often than the rest of us.

A deadening loss of contact with our physical selves certainly increases feelings of emotional isolation.'

Body and other techniques may help to bridge that gap between insight and feeling which hinders psychotherapeutic processes.

Ericksonian psychotherapy*

Unlike Freud, **Milton Erickson** (1901–80) *considered 'the unconscious' not as a cesspool of forbidden thoughts and feelings, but rather a storehouse of learning*—a knowledge resource upon which man can draw for the solution of problems in the 'here and now' . . . a powerhouse of healing strengths.

'When you were a little child of six or seven, you were able to learn fifty-two complicated letter and number shapes—just think how knowledgeable and powerful are your unconscious resources now.'

For Erickson the task of the therapist is not so much exploration and interpretation of psychopathology, as the *search for resources and an innovative programme* for overcoming problems in the 'here and now'.

Emphasis on past experiences often causes inhibitory uneasiness in the client. In order to compile the individual's 'programme for change' he adopts an *eclectic approach*, utilizing, with resourcefulness, the contributions of all schools, and that communication with the deeper self offered by *hypnosis*.

The cornerstone of Ericksonian psychotherapy is the establishment of *strong, intimate and deeply involved rapport* with the client.

Briefly Ericksonian psychotherapy is structured around the following stages:

1. *The establishment and prescription of clear therapeutic goals.*
   'What do you want to change in your life?'
   'What do you want to be?'
   'What has stopped you changing on your own?'
   Even the definition of the patient's problems and goals fulfils a therapeutic function.
   It is the therapist's role to meet the client 'where he is at' and define ways of reaching his goals.
2. *Formulation of a solution to the impasse in which the client finds himself.*
   It is necessary to take cognizance of the client's 'embedded' messages, and through a 'deep feeling relationship', work out a programme providing 'additional choices out of the emotional trap in which he is stuck'.
3. *Erickson believes in action—it is important to get the client to **do** something different* rather than insisting on insight.

---

* Barker, Professor Phillip. 'Milton Erickson's Contribution to Psychiatry.' A lecture delivered to the Groote Schuur Hospital Psychiatry Discussion Group, 1 November 1986.

'The therapist, not the client, needs insight—if the client does not learn to *do* something different with his life, he is imply a neurotic who has insight into how he got that way. For example, Mr and Mrs Brown's marriage was imperilled by their conflict as to who should make the business decisions. Erickson insisted that Mrs Brown allow her husband to reach work every morning before she did. Soon Mrs Brown found herself getting to work later and later, her husband making the decisions and the business profiting thereby. . . .'

(*Uncommon Therapy* edited by J Haley, 1973). By 'creative' and often small interventions this therapeutic method claims dramatic changes.

It is important to meet clients 'where they are at', . . . not to confront them initially with a mountain (or cesspool) of past trauma, mistakes and impending tasks.

4. *Presentation of additional choices out of the habitually dysfunctioning behaviour pattern in which the client is stuck.*
Past problem-solving techniques no longer being applicable, therapy should offer other more profitable ways to behave.

5. *Therapy should be broken into stages*—becuase even tiny steps forward can start a new path to adjustment, each should be recognized, praised and shown to relieve tension.

6. *It is necessary to use indirect methods of communication when direct methods fail.*

   (a) *Body language* from therapist to patient is as important as the converse.
   (b) It may be necessary to *communicate in the strange media offered by clients*. Haley quotes how Erickson learned a patient's 'word salad' communication code in order to reach him 'where he was at'.
   (c) *Hypnosis* offering a direct pathway into the client's deeper self may be helpful with any patient who accepts this medium.
   (d) Communication often involves *indirect therapeutic methods* such as:

      (i) Insight into the client's *embedded statements*.
      (ii) The use of *paradoxical injunctions*: 'Tell me the opposite of what you want
         —what you hate, how you don't want to be.'
      (iii) *Metaphorical stories and anecdotes*: objects, tasks and rituals important in your life.
      (iv) *Parables*: a relatively safe and impersonal method of teaching new ways to overcome personal problems. Jesus taught by parables.
      (v) *The Greek chorus*: A therapeutic team on the other side of a one-way vision screen watches and intervenes when the therapeutic process is stuck. The 'chorus' offers messages of congratulations when a hurdle is overcome.
      (vi) *Content rephrasing*: involves altering the meaning of troublesome behaviour or emotions.
         'You say your child has troublesome temper tantrums. Could we say, instead, that you are having difficulty in gaining control of his behaviour? Could we say that this sense of powerlessness is your problem rather than his?'
         'All behaviour can be useful in a certain context. Lying can be a

good thing—novelists lie for a living. Let us move from this point, to rechannel this talent into more valuable creativity, such as the phantasizing of desired goals and acceptable methods of achieving them.'

'It is frequently profitable to rephrase problems as challenges. Every life has calm and happy moments—let us find tools and gadgets to reach such moments again.'

(vii) *The tag:* the 'sting in the tail' which reveals the absurdity, the unproductivity, the alternatives in the client's dysfunctional tangle. 'I accept you're feeling very depressed—that things look so bad you're considering killing yourself . . . and that you don't know how long you are going to feel this way.'

The therapist's embedded message conveys that this burdensome mood will not last forever. . . .

(viii) Humour is a valuable and universal communication path, and a great leveller between therapist and client.

Group therapy and self-help groups (see also p 64)

Yalom has discussed eleven factors which he termed 'curative' (1975)* or 'therapeutic' (1983)† His view is that therapeutic change is a complex process which occurs through an interplay of various guided human experiences. These factors constitute the core of therapy even though group therapies may differ in their structure. Different groups may accentuate different clusters of these therapeutic factors, and different patients in the same group may make use of different facts. According to Yalom, all groups share these basic mechanisms of change:

1. *Instillation of hope.* Therapy groups instil hope in patients who are not optimistic about therapy; this factor's premise is that these patients become more optimistic by watching others improve.
2. *Universality.* This factor's premise is that patients come to feel less isolated in their distress; they learn that they are not the only one with a certain problem.
3. *Guidance.* Groups may provide specific information or guidance explicitly, as in Alcoholics Anonymous via didactic training, or implicitly in less structured groups via clarification of the meaning of symptoms, interpersonal and group dynamics, and the basic process of psychotherapy.
4. *Altruism.* Helping others is an important part of strengthening one's own self-esteem.
5. *Corrective recapitulation of the primary family group.* By reliving family issues in the group therapy situation, patients can learn to recognize and change maladaptive behaviour patterns developed in early family-life experience.

* Yalom I. *The theory and practice of group psychotherapy.* 2 ed. New York: Basic Books.
† Yalom I. *Inpatient group psychotherapy.* New York: Basic Books.

6. *Self-understanding.* Encouraging individuals to recognize, integrate and express previously 'dissociated' parts of themselves is important in psychosocial rehabilitation.
7. *Catharsis.* Patients learn to express held-in feelings appropriately, and find that the expression of feeling does not necessarily lead to social isolation.
8. *Identification.* Patients learn positive behaviour from other group members.
9. *Existential factors.* Patients learn to face the meaninglessness of life. Anxiety, in the existential point of view, stems from the individual's confrontation with existential concerns, ie death, freedom, isolation and meaninglessness. Individuals learn that they alone can come to terms with these dimensions of life.
10. *Cohesiveness.* Feeling accepted by a group and sharing may be very therapeutic and may be the single most necessary precondition for therapy (Brown and Yalom, 1977). Interpersonal and intrapersonal changes can be facilitated after supportive and caring atmosphere has been established.
11. *Interpersonal learning.* Patients may learn to modify their interpersonal relationships by receiving feedback from others. Yalom further divided this category into two parts: 'input' (feedback gained from others regarding the impact that one's behaviour has upon them) and 'output' (learning to relate to other group members).*

There are, however, 'introverted', 'private' people, often highly educated and from upper socio-economic groups, who cannot tolerate public emotional denudement, profiting only from individual therapy.

Katz and Bender (1976, p 9) present the following *definition*:

'SELF-HELP GROUPS are voluntary, small group structures for mutual aid and the accomplishment of special purpose. They are usually formed by peers who have come together for mutual assistance in satisfying a common need, overcoming a common handicap or life-disrupting problem, and bringing about desired social and/or personal change. The initiators and members of such groups perceive that their needs are not, or cannot be, met by or through existing social institutions. Self-help groups emphasize face-to-face social interactions and the assumption of personal responsibility by members. They often provide material assistance, as well as emotional support; they are frequently "cause" orientated, and promulgate an ideology or values through which members may attain an enhanced sense of personal identity.'

Key elements of this definition are
    face-to-face interactions
    personal participation
    relating to each other sympathetically and empathically

---

* Carper, Mark (Greenery Rehabilitation and Skilled Nursing Center and Tufts University School of Medicine), Rosenthal, Mitchell (New England Medical Center Hospitals and Tufts University School of Medicine, Boston, Mass). The Value of Group Psychotherapy in a Young Adult Head-Injured Population. Presented at the American Psychological Association Convention, Washington DC, August 1986.

extension beyond socialization to overcome a life-disturbing problem
provision of a source of reference
the group arises spontaneously from a position of powerlessness.

Types of self-help groups

Katz and Bender (1976) suggest five categories based on group focus or purpose:

1. Personal growth.
2. Social advocacy.
3. Creation of alternative patterns of living.
4. Outcast havens.
5. Other or mixed groups.

Levy (1979) distinguished four types based on composition and purpose:

1. Behavioural control.
2. Stress coping.
3. Survival orientation.
4. Personal growth.

The self-help group process

Katz and Bender (1976) suggest seven processes at work in self-help groups:

1. developing and sustaining a coherent view of the world;
2. learning new and more gratifying behaviour;
3. tapping unconscious feelings;
4. fortifying self-image and pride;
5. achieving more environmental mastery by discovering and using competencies;
6. increasing coping abilities by graduated steps;
7. advance members to new levelsof self-perception and status.

Gartner and Riessmann (1977) emphasize *the helper process* occurring in the self-help group. The person with a problem finds himself helping others who have similar problems. In becoming the teacher the helper convinces himself of the usefulness of programmes. He is less dependent than a patient. He can view his own problem at a distance, and he gains self-esteem by being socially useful. The helper in contrast with a professional relates on a *feeling* basis with others, identifies, and becomes personally involved. His knowledge comes from experience rather than a researched body of information.

Antz (1979) places a significant emphasis on ideology. In his view the success of the self-help group lies in its developing *an ideology* which effectively combats the chief elements that lead people to fall into certain problems. The ideology breaks the destructive pattern and allows the person to deal effectively with life again.

Gartner and Riessmann (1977) present—

A comparison of professional and self-help groups

Professional Groups   Self-help Groups
are at opposite
ends of a continuum

Stress: *objectivity* with the professional in a superior role.

Stress: the equal relationship between the 'helper' and the 'helpee'.

The helper is personally involved and relates to the helpee at an *emotional* level.

The professional relies on a body of special procedures and *technical knowledge.*

The knowledge of the helper comes through the *personal experience* of having faced the same problem as the helpee.

Numerous self-help groups have been started by professionals.

Some self-help groups have arisen because professional services:
(i) ignored their critical problem;
(ii) were beyond the means of those who needed them.

In some cases self-help groups are an integrated part of a total care plan developed by professional services.

The professional role in self-help groups

Gartner et al recommend that the professional should relate to the group by:

1. encouraging its formation;
2. providing skill-training for leaders who will in turn train members;
3. providing backup consultative services for self-help leaders;
4. giving technical information to groups so they can understand the latest developments in treatment or diagnosis;
5. making referrals to the group to establish its legitimacy;
6. offering evaluative advice which would enable the self-help group better to reach those in need, and to improve methods of assistance.
   The professional needs to develop methods of *assessing the critical needs of newcomers* who seek a self-help group. Out of this analysis the nature of the self-help process can be created, or altered, to meet the needs, beliefs and activities appropriate to each referral;
7. preparing literature which will assist self-help efforts.

At the same time they warn of the following pitfalls in professional-group interaction:

1. The professional should not seek to avoid professional responsibility by displacing upon the group inappropriate tasks.
2. The professional should not try to make his services resemble or usurp the seslf-help model.

3. The professional should not seek to dominate the self-help group so that it loses its own vitality or innovativeness.

In his paper 'Models of Self-help Groups for Family Caregivers of the Aged', presented at the 94th Annual Convention of the American Psychological Association in Washington DC, 25 August 1986, Robert I Cassady Jnr, Inmate Management Administration, Arizona State Prison Complex, Florence, Arizona 85232, tells how, for private reasons, he was drawn into the formation and conduct of the 'Generations Group'.

His valuable model, detailing role participation, may well serve as a guide for other caregiver groups facing the long-term problems of physical or mental handicap, or more transitional life-disruptions through death or disaster.

'*Phase I: The Newcomer*

The caregiver who seeks a support group is having problems with his responsibilities. This problem is not going to be solved quickly unless the situation is temporary. The caregiver is focused on the situation, and how he must manipulate it. He has *accepted the responsibility* role and wants to carry out the tasks that need to be done. The underlying cause of the *problem is the manner in which the caregiver approaches the situation, and how he exercises responsibility*. To help the caregiver move to self-assessment the support group must provide several things. (1) The group must listen to the newcomer's tale with empathy for the feelings expressed. Newcomers will vary on how fast they find acceptance and begin to conform to group norms. (2) The group will provide advice to help the newcomer over some immediate crises. However, (3) the group must carefully reiterate the belief that the problem does not reside in the situational factors but *in one's habitual approach* to the situation which cannot be changed quickly. This belief prepares the newcomer for Phase II.

Phase II: The New Member

The newcomer becomes a group member as he is motivated to follow the group norms that encourage him to explore *the four processes which lead to his bad feelings*. He comes to see that *much of his responsibility activity is an attempt to avoid having bad feelings*. Now the group emphasizes the belief that the member will continue to experience bad feelings *until a new behaviour pattern becomes comfortable*. This belief enables the member to bear the pain of the feelings as they experiment with new patterns in the next phase. Otherwise the need to avoid the bad feelings will defeat any attempt to do things differently. The member becomes able to use the knowledge gained from others to help remedy some of the elements of his own situation.

Phase III: The Helper

To solidify gains made in the previous stage the member should take an active role in *helping others*. He can ask *questions which will facilitate self-exploration and share with the group the insights from his own self-assessment*. To further his own growth he can *plan group programmes* which bring in expert knowledge or skill building in areas where he feels ready to try new behaviour patterns. The helper may volunteer for special projects such as developing group advertising literature, or working on an information referral publication on help for the elderly, or speaking to political bodies in support of legislation assisting the elderly or their caregivers. *The proclamation of the group norms and beliefs now falls on the helper.* Through these activities the helper strengthens his commitment to attempt to deal with responsibilities in a manner which is compatible with his strengths and limitations. *He learns to find new satisfactions in carrying out his responsibilities and no longer does it to avoid bad feelings.* During this phase emphasis is placed on the belief that assuming responsibility will continue to be a problem area, and that one must use self-assessment and others to keep control.

Phase IV: The Adventurer

The situation that brought the caregiver to the support group may or may not be continuing. Certainly at this point *the member has begun to learn to handle the responsibility in a more reasonable fashion.* If the elderly person requires more care than the caregiver can provide, then alternative management has been explored and employed. The person is balancing the number of responsibility commitments more sensibly. Group activities are less important. *The person may attend less frequently, but will be able to share more permanent behavioural changes that have been accomplished.* The belief learned in the third phase warns the member transitioning away from the group that *he may have this problem again in another situation.* The skills learned in this situation may help avoid it, but he is prepared to join new self-help groups or to ask the others' assistance when a new crisis appears. This phase encourages the person to move away from dependency, but not to avoid it in the future where it would be appropriate.'

Self-help Groups—their purpose, motivation and organization

Loneliness and isolation are two important reasons people become mentally ill. Human beings need the company of others to thrive, to feel good about themselves and to feel happy. 'For years I thought I was the only person to feel like this—to know that someone else feels the same as me gives me amazing sense of belief.' Self-help groups are usually set up by people sharing a common experience, need or problem.

They provide:

a chance to share experiences of grief, depression, compulsive thoughts or behaviour; addiction to drugs or alcohol, and many other forms of stress and suffering;

mutual emotional support, showing the important part members can play in helping each other through whatever difficulties they are experiencing.

'Talking about our problems and sharing our feelings in an atmosphere where we feel cared for and supported, helps to break down feelings of confusion, shame, self-blame, guilt, loneliness, mistrust, fear, loss, which in turn allows us to feel closer to each other and a valid member of the group.

It sometimes looks like swings and roundabouts—one day you help someone, another day you receive help. Helping each other in whatever way we can is a very good reminder that no matter how low we feel, we don't deserve to be written off as useless.'

Tips for running the group

It is important that the *'facilitator' or group leader* stress that

1. Everything said within the group *is strictly confidential* and cannot be repeated to anyone outside the group setting.
2. *Every member should be afforded an opportunity and encouragement to speak*—to 'find her voice', explaining the situation in her own words.
    Time should thus be shared approximately equally among participants.
    If anyone appears in crisis, or too inhibited, distressed or uneasy to participate, some individual help is clearly indicated.
3. 'Openers'—
    'How have you felt this week?'
    'What have you enjoyed about the week?'
    Particular issues such as insomnia, panic attacks, marital conflict may emerge as key issues.
    It is important that the facilitator air the relevant topic but avoid imposing judgement or solutions, which should emanate from the group itself.

Ending the group session:

Stick to the agreed time, avoiding stress emanating from other responsbilities.
Close on a positive note.

It may help to ask each member what they found helpful about the session—what they've learned about themselves, or other options for coping with life's stresses.

Facing and revealing deep emotional problems *may constitute a painful and frightening experience.* Yet catharsis usually provides a sense of relief.

'It really helped to get it all off my chest and have a good cry.' Others will soon learn that *expressing and sharing emotions in this way brings the group closer together.*

It is of course important to reassure individuals, and the group, that *we all have areas of poignant stress, sadness, loss and hopeful mechanisms* for rebuilding our lives.

Some material requirements for a successful group experience:

1. The motivator or professional group 'facilitator,' once aware of an important issue or problem, may advertise for participants at the local newsagents, shops, laundrette, school library or anywhere where people gather.
2. The meeting place: each other's houses, a community centre, a health centre providing a bright, airy and cheerful room on a good bus route, protected from interruptions, such as telephone calls, people passing through, etc.
3. A crèche or child-care centre is helpful.
4. Tea, coffee, biscuits provide mouth comfort and reduce stress.
5. A small 'kitty' to pay for tea, coffee, postage, etc.
6. Shared responsibility help bind the group.
    Functions, including refreshments, opening the room, arranging chairs in a circle, selecting the topic for the week, may well be rotated.

Advice for setting up a self-help group is obtainable from 'A Woman and Mental Health Self-Help Project', Bristol Settlement, 43 Ducie Road, Barton Hill, Bristol BS50AX. Tel: 0272 556164. This section is based on the projects pamphlet.
'Setting up a Self-Help Group'

Perception

Efficiency of senses and accuracy of neurological input and interpretation are not, of course, always the whole story. Interpretation of information is often subjectively coloured by our emotional experiences.

In chapter 5 we learnt that *attitudes* and *prejudices* are *introjected* from one's environment, predisposing an individual to react in a characteristic way to any object or situation.

Encounter groups (T groups or sensitivity groups)

The therapeutic community

Every aspect of the therapeutic community should be part of a dynamic healing process. There is nothing so wasteful and stultifying as a group of people amongst whom nothing is happening.

Although amendments and adaptations are no doubt indicated, many aspects of Encounter Therapy—personal responsibility, responsible concern, honesty, reality confrontation, catharsis and support—may, especially in rehabilitation, bring deeper-level significance and structure to group interaction.

An important keynote, however, is the assertion of protective and balanced supervision of the Encounter programme.

This consists in an expansion of group expression and support in the revelation, and resolution of those powerful, deeper-level attitudes and feelings usually inhibited by the necessity for personal and public conformity. Sometimes the individual, abandoning hope of conformity and success splits off from these demands and seeks fulfilment in short-term, self-satisfying behaviour destructive of personal relationships.

In the isolation, alienation and inhibition characteristic of our society, there is an increasing need to find ways of relating openly and honestly with each other.

These groups usually consist of 12 to 20 individuals. The frequency and intensity of their involvement varies from weekly sessions, intensive weekend sessions to the type of maximum enclosed residential group involvement conducted until recently at 'Centrum' for persons with *personality disturbances and drug dependency*, where the average stay was nine months. This facility was discontinued because administrators considered it so harsh and confronting as to risk unjustifiable 'ego' destruction. The model may, however, suggest modified alternatives.

The objectives of a well-conducted Encounter Group are not as sweeping as those claimed by less responsible and less self-critical exponents.

They should aim to 'stimulate an exchange that is not inhibited by defensiveness, and that achieves a maximum of openness and honesty'.*

Encounter Groups emanate from the work of psychotherapist Carl Rogers, who in 1970 described the typical pattern of change inherent in Encounter and T therapy:

---

* Hilgard, Ernest R, Atkinson, Richard C & Atkinson, Rita L. *Introduction to Psychology*. Harcourt Brace Jovanovich Inc. 6th Int Ed.

(1) *Confusion and frustration* when the 'facilitator', 'expeditor' or group leader clarifies that he will not assume responsibility for directing the group. Rather is his role of that catalyst, guide and support.

There is also *resistance to exposing intimate feelings* to the group who may criticize or 'attack' the member for their content.

(2) *Gradual exposure and expression* of feelings and problems encountered outside the group.

(3) *Strong discussion of inter-group relationships:* Frequently the first feelings expressed are *self-critical* or *hostile to the group* or its members.

There is interplay of emotions in response to such criticism. If a member finds the emotions he has expressed to be acceptable, an atmosphere of trust and support may develop.

(4) As the group progresses 'members become impatient with defensiveness, insisting that the individual be himself. The tact and polite cover up that are acceptable outside the group are not tolerated within it.'*

'Centrum' Therapeutic Community presented its basic concepts as:

(a) *Personal responsibility*—'We believe that every person, except if he is psychotic, is responsible for himself. A person lands himself in problems, whatever the causes and background may be, and only he can get himself out of it.'

(b) *Responsible concern*—'Because we are concerned about our fellows and friends, we take the responsibility of pointing out to them when they are going wrong, or being destructive to themselves.

In this way we can see ourselves for what we really are, and put pressure on each other to change. We do not believe in being sorry for each other.'

(c) *Honesty*—'If we want to change our life, we need to make a clean break. We cannot make a clean break if we have anything to hide.'

(d) *The community*—'We do not have the situation of conventional clinics or institutions with doctors giving treatment, and patients receiving treatment. We all take responsibility: we all give and receive and no one is called a patient. We are residents in a small community of people living and working together, helping each other to make a better life.'

(e) 'There are only two actual rules of programme which form the sole bases for expulsion. They are:

  (i) no drugs including alcohol
  (ii) no physical violence directed at self or others.'

Queries to the Senior Expeditor (senior staff member) revealed other forbidden indulgences to be sex relations and withdrawal from the group—no member is ever allowed to be on his own. All the girls sleep in one communal dormitory, all the boys in the other.

THE PROGRAMME

This was of at least one month's duration, varying with the requirements and response of the individual. The average stay was nine months.

* Ibid.

The following activity descriptions result from a generous invitation to visit Centrum:

(a) *Introduction*—anybody wishing to join Centrum undergoes the introduction programme consisting of a number of interviews spread over a few days. This will reveal the real motive of the candidate. ('We will not be used as another escape, or some boarding house.')

Members introduce themselves; demand to know salient points of the applicant's background; face him with the reality of his own responsibility in his inability to adjust to life. They demand that he plead—to the point of crying—for admission.

(b) *Therapeutic community* consists of the following aspects:

(i) 'Work programme—most of the time in Centrum is spent working, doing various jobs . . . with the idea of learning about ourselves and others in all possible situations.'

Work conditions are structured to demand *absolute obedience*, even in the face of apparently pointless or exhausting tasks imposed by demanding fellow members. This aspect of the programme is *designed to exert frustrating pressure* . . . with the purpose of forcing reactions—regression, aggression, compliance, co-operation. Carelessness, inefficiency, irresponsibility, lack of motivation, defiance or assertion of personal judgement are severely reprimanded in *Group Meetings*.

Indeed these meetings serve to confront members with their overt and deeper emotional reactions—their anxieties, obsessions, irresponsibilities, aggressiveness, etc.

Tommy was asked to stand on a small dais while members hurled at him reproaches for his slovenly appearance and untidy clothes.

'You don't care—'You just think of yourself'—'You have no self-respect'—'Untidiness is offensive to us'—'You're disgusting'.

Voices were raised; the clothes were hurled at him.

Finally he was praised for having completed some other task, and the group enclosed him in comforting, loving and reassuring arms.

One girl put her arms around him, holding him tightly to her body, providing tactile comfort to reassure him of fundamental loving acceptance. In fact, members appeared to spend almost as much time in conveying warm physical gestures of loving reassurance by tactile closeness in each other's arms, as they did in recrimination.

'The strict discipline and control is backed by real concern and caring for each other.'

(ii) *Encounter groups*—'provide opportunity to explore and express our emotions and relationships with other people . . . we can say whatever we want, to whomever we want.'

Members are required to achieve catharsis by total emotional and physical participation in their reactions, protests, sorrows and aggressive feelings.

'The encounter' takes place on foam rubber mattresses placed on the floor and interspersed with cushions.

John asked the group to help him express his anger towards his parents and brother which was festering within him.

'Go on—shout at him—show him—hit him—hurt him—here you can *do* whatever you feel—he teased you—he got all the privileges at university—he got the degree—your parents gave him all their attention—he got all the presents—he got everything—you don't have to feel bad—you're OK man!'

Provoked, John banged his fists, and then his whole body against the cushions. His legs and arms flailed in the air as he hit out. One member gave him a large stick to hit the cushions which clearly represented his brother.

When the cathartic outburst was expended they took him into their arms, hugged him close and reassured him by their emotional and physical presence.

To reinforce insight into their behavioural shortcomings and goals, some members were obliged to walk around with sandwich boards announcing their change-need. An obsessive neurotic youngster carried a placard declaring 'Efficiency is good—perfection is sick'.

The Centrum programme was complemented by:

— Creative programmes: expression through any form of creativity was stimulated.
— Dramatized social skills programme: 'preparing ourselves for difficult social situations later on—like saying "no" to our old friends, handling problems in the family, job interviews, etc.'
— Family work: 'parents are invited to a special meeting every fortnight, when they can discuss their side of the problem, and also look at their own responsibility.'
— Speaking programmes: 'many people find it very difficult to express themselves verbally, especially in front of an audience. For this reason we have special evenings to practice talking to people.'
— Physical training programmes and physical contact encounters such as blindfolded tactile mutually supportive experiences.

Centrum's overall programme certainly aroused emotional reactions within the context of close group direction, identification and reassurance. One was, however, struck by the *possibility of sado-masochistic activity* at the hands of less able and well-adjusted 'expeditors' than those currently employed.

The dedicated innovator and administrator of Centrum, revealed that 60%–75% of members left before he considered them ready to do so. Yet, he maintains that independent assessment studies show the majority, even of this group, to have profited from Centrum's encounter programme.

How impressive are more widespread evaluations of Encounter Groups? Many raise doubts about the extent and durability of behaviour changes.

Libermann, Yalom & Miles (1973)[*] followed up 200 college students who participated in encounter groups conducted by well-qualified leaders.

Basing their findings on self-reports and ratings by close friends, they concluded:

$\frac{1}{3}$ showed positive changes

$\frac{1}{3}$ showed no change

---

[*] Libermann, Yalom & Miles. *Encounter Group—First Facts*. New York: Basic Books. 1973.

$\frac{1}{3}$ displayed negative changes—they either dropped out because they found the encounters too disturbing or later found this group experience aggravated rather than resolved personal problems.

Widespread opinion sees a *danger in 'damaging those whose self-esteem is too tenuous to withstand group criticism and pressure'*.* Hilgard, Atkinson & Atkinson mention suicide and the development of undiagnosed psychoses as important dangers.

General conclusions indicate that encounter therapy does offer opportunity for identification, disinhibition, catharsis and group support. It is not, however, as effective as individual therapy in achieving emotional and thus behavioural change.

Family therapy

Involving the whole family, this therapy is designed to help members to

(1) clarify and express their feelings in emotional interplay;
(2) develop greater mutual understanding;
(3) work out more effective ways of relating to one another;
(4) solve mutual problems.

Family members are seen separately and together, therapists being chosen for individual group members, usually according to their identification and transference needs.

There are usually two therapists—one of each sex.

Therapy proceeds on the assumption that the index patient's problems are symptomatic of, and reflect, a more general family maladjustment.

Family members should be seated in a circle and at least an hour set aside for each session. The therapist should make contact with each family member, verbalizing his or her intention to avoid taking sides with any one member.

It is important that each, even the youngest child—who may thereafter be diverted by toys, painting, etc—speaking for himself, sharing his ideas, opinions, complaints and feelings with other family members and with the therapist. Both verbal and non-verbal communication should be noted. As part of the therapeutic process the therapist should:

(i) single out significant statements
(ii) identify—

    (a) the role filled by each member in family interactions and dynamics;
    (b) the strength and nature of emotional attachments;
    (c) repetitive mental or coping mechanisms.

In order to illustrate and work on destructive reaction patterns it may be useful to draw a geneogram (p 419) on a blackboard.

Therapeutic skill lies in the creation of a climate of mutual problem-solving and motivation of a programme of 'homework' or between-session tasks.

---

* Hilgard, Ernest R, Atkinson, Richard C & Atkinson Rita L. *Introduction to Psychology*. Harcourt Brace Jovanovich Inc. 6th Int Ed.

Tact and sensitivity are required to avoid permanent hurtful damage resultant upon premature and excessive exposures. Slowly does it! Praise is also helpful.

Special techniques include:

videotape recordings to confront family members with their interactions, home visits,

the 'empty chair technique', where individuals are invited to address, and behave towards the chair as if it were occupied by another family member in a controversial or emotion-laden confrontation,

'role reversal' acting out—members confront each other with their projected feelings about family reactions, acting out the role in which they see each other, e g the oppressively disciplined child projects or acts out how he sees his disciplinary parents.

'Brief Focal Family Therapy'*

In London, the Tavistock Clinic, under the direction of Dr A Bentovim is developing an abbreviated family therapy programme in response to diagnosis by a professional panel. The family's 'maladjustment focus'—or *the basic core of dissension*—is identified, and therapy limited to 20–25 one-hour sessions, usually at two-weekly intervals, is designed and conducted.

Families are given inter-session therapeutic 'tasks' such as allowing all members to speak uninterruptedly, democratically organizing household chores, withholding from physical violence, etc.

In a study of 22 families, 19 showed 'some' or 'much improvement'. Other studies show therapy to be more successful for the index referred patient, while family units improved in approximately half the families referred.*

A grown woman, plagued by persistent cleanliness compulsions was invited to 'act out' a childhood boarding-school incident when a nun had allegedly shamed her publicly for enuresis. The patient assaulted the therapist (acting her former teacher) with considerable venom.

Psychodrama

Developed and described by Merino, a social psychologist, psychodrama is an effective diagnostic and therapeutic individual and group technique. Patients are invited to 'act out' important episodes in their lives, and in so doing *reveal* for therapists, and themselves, traumatic experiences, emotional conflicts, unresolved aggression, hallucinations and delusions, as well as their growing reorientation and readjustment.

Psychodrama is especially useful in achieving *catharsis learning new methods* of establishing and maintaining social relationships. However, in inviting the expression of strong, emotionally-fraught interactions, therapists may arouse considerable 'transference' aggression, requiring skilled handling.

---

* Bentovim, A & Kinston, W. 'Brief Focal Family Therapy when the Child is the Referred Patient.' I, II, *Journal of Child Psychology and Psychiatry*, vol 19. April 1978.

Role play therapy (and self-assertion therapy)

Both psychodrama and role play are *action enactment* orientated therapies. The methods may, however, be distinguished thus:

Role play	*Psychodrama*

involves:
    self-observation,
    social insight skills,
    desensitization.
	is a *psychoanalytically* orientated process aiming to lead subjects into deeper layers of developmental, unconscious trauma and conflicts.

Within a repetitive, *behaviourist-orientated learning process* in the *here* and *now*. This method does *not* delve into the past to find developmental reasons for emotional disturbances, but rather tries to teach *practical* techniques for dealing with specific situations in the present and in the future. It does not aim at exposing unconscious conflict and trauma, but tries to deal with burdensome material *'on the spot'* by providing *insight* and *solutions*. Should disturbing material come into consciousness, it attempts to provide *supportive catharsis*.	By revealing, exposing and interpreting *subjective* material, it provides opportunity for therapeutic catharsis.
Insists on *directive structuring of objective* practical, programmed situations on the basis of their specific purposefulness. 'The therapist should always assess: "by confronting the subject with *this* situation am I making him feel emotionally better, and helping him cope with his immediate problem". '*	It is a more 'in depth', individualized, and *non-directive* method of freeing the subject from his painful past and disturbed present. To do so it encourages random, unstructured association.

In role play, therefore, the approach is
    concrete,
    practical,
    structured,
and in terms of its behaviourist learning basis, repetitive. Re-inforcement is by rewards of praise and personal satisfaction.

Example

In preparing psychiatric patients for discharge:
Confrontation with the objective problem of accounting to friends for absence in hospital—

---

* Nicholls, Lindsey & Psychiatric Occupational Therapists, Using Role Play in Psychiatric Treatment—A Lecture Demonstration with Video, 27 October 1986. For further details refer to author.

Pre-session preparation involves:

> identification of specific patient needs,
> drama structure,
> role allotment,
> relevant props consisting of everyday furniture and equipment.

In order to limit stress:

> theme and role choice are limited,
> it is wise to introduce a humorous, fun element,
> provide 'warming up' verbal, acting and social games such as charades, word finding, etc.

Therapist:	Joan, in the supermarket you meet a friend, Sally, who asks you where you've been the past two months.
Joan:	I've been on holiday.
Sally:	That must have been fun, where did you go?
Joan:	Brighton.
Therapist:	How do you feel in this situation?
Joan:	I feel awfully uncomfortable.
Therapist:	Try it again with a different approach.
Joan (with	considerable hesitation and stress-revealing body language): after Peter left me I couldn't cope—in fact I got so bad I had a breakdown, and had to spend some time in a psychiatric hospital.
Sally:	I'm so sorry to hear that. Please do let me know if I can do anything to help. Why don't you come to the book-club meeting Wednesday morning. We'd love to see you again.

The drama session is discussed and repeated until increased learning, and consequent confidence, reduce stress and increase fluency.

Complementary techniques include:

Doubling

Peter (ex-husband) visits Joan who is centrifugal to this emotionally charged situation. She is 'doubled' by, and, when appropriate, speaks through less-involved Betty.

Peter:	Hullo—I hope you don't mind my visiting.
Joan:	What do *you* care what *I* mind!
Peter:	I wanted to show I'm concerned for your welfare.
Joan:	Isn't that nice—all of a sudden you care! Well don't bother.

Enter Double Betty who now assumes Sally's role.

Peter:	Hullo—I hope you don't mind my visiting.
Betty:	No of course not, I'm pleased you came.
Peter:	I wanted to show I'm concerned for your welfare.
Betty:	It really does give me support and encouragement to know we can still be friends.

Joan repeats Betty's role until she feels more comfortable therein. Having been shown an alternative reaction pattern, and words to express her conflicting feelings, Joan 'introjects' (p 107ff) Betty's responses.

Feeling more comfortable, the new reactions and behaviour pattern are repeated and reinforced, teaching better adjusted and more profitable social interaction.

Mirroring

Joan applies for a job. She hesitates, fidgets and stammers. Betty, her 'mirror', copies Joan's behaviour as closely as possible.
Therapist to Joan: How does she come across?

Joan   (who has been watching in a relatively detached role): I don't look confident, and I didn't tell him anything that would make him want to employ me.

Therapist: If you fight harder you will overcome your communication obstacle. Let's do it again until you feel and act more positively.

In discussion Joan admitted to other osbstacles. She sees herself as shy and unattractive: But people have always said I'm a good listener.

Therapist: The shyness has to do with the damaged way you see yourself. You are learning better self-esteem. But you really can't feel good in that same old jersey.

Joan: Yes, I must get the courage to go out to the shops and choose something else.

Therapist: We'll act that out too until you feel more comfortable in *asserting yourself*, so that you purchase what *you* really want.

Role reversal

Graham: Mother, this is Steven—we're going on the adventure trail tomorrow.

His over-protective mother: But it's such a stiff climb—and the weather is so uncertain—and you've not got over your cold yet . . .

Graham: But it's a safe Grade A track!

Mother: I'll worry myself sick.

Roles are reversed:

Therapist: Now you're Graham. How do you feel about your mother?

Graham: Embarrassed and irritated—she's treating me like a child.

Soliloquy

'Bringing the inward outward'*

Griefwork: an example inspired by a terminal hospital in which professionals are required to make home visits, helping the survivor pack away the possessions of the deceased.

Therapist: You are standing silently to one side and letting me do all the packing. What do you really want to say?

Mrs J: I want to tell him what I never said before. How I love him—but how his tight hold on his salary irritated me.

'I'm sorry, Steve, that we fight so much about money. I know it's because you had such a tough time when you were a kid. But I've got to scrimp and save for months before I can get enough together for the kids' Christmas presents. Oh poor Steve—now you are gone I'll be able to do as I please this Christmas [tearful and distressed]. Oh what a wicked thought!

---

* Nicholls, Lindsey & Psychiatric Occupational Therapists, Groote Schuur and Valkenberg Hospitals: Using Role Play in Psychiatric Treatment—A Lecture Demonstration with Video Presented at the Groote Schuur Psychiatric discussion Group, 27 October 1986.

Therapist: It's an absolutely normal thought! Death always leaves bits and
              pieces undone to make us feel illogically guilty.
Mrs J: But why do I always bottle up everything inside me?
Therapist: You don't like to hurt anyone's feelings. That has become your
              natural way of reacting. But it knots you up inside.
                  Why not say to Steve:
                      'You're too secretive and tight with your money.'
Mrs J: That's right. He was secretive and tight-fisted—now he's gone and
              I have to make my own way, I'm going to tell people what *I* want
              for myself.

Application of role play in chronic and long-term psychiatric units

Here the aim is usually to

1. Instil normal emotional reactions in place of that blunt affect characteristic of
    burnt-out psychiatric illness.
2. To teach self-care skills—personal hygiene, table manners, etc, using group
    pressure to achieve conformity.
3. Demonstrate behaviour patterns favourable to the formation and retention of
    relationships. Some must learn to reduce their pressure on others, some to
    become more assertive. Ward situations are acted out, observed, discussed
    and redirected.
4. Restore initiative lost though institutionalization:

    what to do when people stare,
    how to ask prices,
    how to contact the family—to write letters,
    to use the phone.

All these are acted out, discussed, reinforced and introjected.

Music therapy

Clearly, there is aggressive group catharsis in participating in the strident
clamour of a percussion band, and the achievement of considerable group harmony
in playing, listening to or moving with smooth, soothing music.
Music therapy has a role

1. in conjunction with suggestion relaxation therapy:

    (i) in antenatal preparation—it is helpful if the patient takes the tape
         complemented by the instructress' voice with her into labour,
    (ii) in inducing hypnotic states for diagnosis and therapy.
2. In intruding into the isolation and confusion of psychotic or autistic patients.
3. Rhythm and movement, including active music-making 'unfreeze' uplift,
    increase muscle tone, confidence and social awareness in the mentally
    retarded, brain injured and aged.
    (Psychoneurological dysfunction overleaf)

Movement therapy

The contents of this section are contributed by An Fiske, MA Antioch
University, USA, movement therapist.

'My body is the fabric into which all objects are woven, and it is, at least, in relation to the perceived world, the general instrument of my comprehension.' Phenomenology of Perception, Merlau-Ponty.

By the very nature of muscle tension, body action mobilizes the organism to release its tension.

Movement therapy is the psychotherapeutic use of movement as a process which strives towards the physical and psychic integration of the individual.

In common with other forms of psychotherapeutic relationships, movement therapy aims to provide opportunity for:

1. problem identification and catharsis;
2. development of trust in oneself and others;
3. fostering independence;
4. recreating social awareness;
5. developing and maintaining personal integrity and sense of self-worth, while accepting social interactions, controls and skills.

Because *everybody*, irrespective of his diagnosis, *moves*, this therapy is very versatile.

Areas of special usefulness are—

1. **Psychiatry**—*movement dispenses with the necessity for complicated or painful verbalization.*

    'Because dance and emotional expression share the same neuromuscular pathways, it is easy to understand the emotion behind the movement. In reverse, [the therapist's] creation of a dance movement can evoke memories and reveal underlying emotions.
    For example, someone who is angry, and smashes down a ball will find that the expression of anger suddenly releases the pain, and they cry.'*

    Where emotional maladjustments lie deep in destructive developmental experiences, movement therapy offers opportunity for re-experiencing, ventilating and coming to terms with areas of unresolved conflict, pain and stress.

    The abused infant, the academically stressed child, the clumsy, rejected adolescent, the inadequate mother, the frightened old person; all may be guided through movement, to therapeutic regression and hence to more fruitful coping patterns.

2. **Physical diminishment**—because movement is a body-orientated therapy it is particularly appropriate *where emotional problems are focused on body structure and process* as pertaining in:

    (a) sexual maladjustment and abuse
    (b) eating disorders
    (c) destruction of body image by
    amputation
    neck and spinal injuries
    (d) impaired co-ordination and clumsiness resultant upon
    brain injury

* Bernstein, Penny Lewis. ed. *Eight Theoretical Approaches in Dance-movement Therapy.* Iowa: Kendall Hunt, 1979.

cerebro-vascular insult

old age.

In all these areas movement therapy, by helping the client feel graceful, proficient and comfortable, plays an important role in defusing negative body image, building up compensation skills and restoring self-esteem.

Movement therapy techniques derive from the pioneer work of *Marion Chase** who stressed *dance as a vehicle of interpersonal communication* within the unique relationship of subject and therapist *on a movement level.*

Chase extracts four major techniques:

1. body action,   3. the therapeutic movement relationship,
2. symbolism,   4. rhythmic group movements.

1. The goals of **body action** are:

(a) re-creation of a realistic body image,

(b) activation, integration and sensitization of body parts which are normally bound and frozen through tension. Awareness of the power of movement promotes that inner awareness of body parts and sensory-motor organization basic to remediation in psychoneurological dysfunction.

Body action helps reconstruct a postural Gestalt (wholeness).

The resensitization of the body permits *emergence into consciousness of inner sensations and vital body messages* inhibited into the 'unconscious' by negative experiences.

Body action mobilizes energy, develops better control over movements and expands the range and expression of emotion.

'In group situations one aims at daily programmes for hospitalized and day centre populations. At best it gives them a clear understanding of what they are feeling and, at worst, it gives a measure of exercise and relaxation.'*

2. The goals of **symbolism** include:

(a) integration of experience and action,

(b) insight,

(c) resolution of conflict through symbolic action,

(d) recall of the significant past,

(e) perhaps most important of all, the externalizing of inner thoughts and feelings.

'Both the psychotic patient and the dancer make use of symbolic body action to communicate emotions and ideas which defy everyday use of language. However, the intent is different. Whereas the dancer may objectively choose bizarre and exaggerated postures to communicate with an audience, the client is *giving expression to his subjective emotions,* conveying in a single moment the *complexity and depth of feelings that cannot be put into words.*'*

The opportunity afforded by symbolic movement for the *recapitulation of past events* is powerful.

---

* Bernstein, Penny Lewis. ed. *Eight Theoretical Approaches in Dance-movement Therapy.* Iowa: Kendall Hunt, 1979.

'As a movement therapist it is easy to accept the symbolic language offered by the client, because *this message is decoded (introjected) by simply reproducing the movement, posture, expression with your own body.'*

Because movement is slower than verbalization, there is more time to synthesize material.

3. The therapeutic movement relationship

Because dance is communication it fulfils a basic human need.

'*Chase entered a patient's world by re-enacting the essential constellation of movement characterizing his expression.* As she re-created the patient's movements with her own body, she would sense what was possible (in terms of movement) and *further the interaction by doing similar, broader or complementary movements.* . . . By *reproducing* (projecting) the significant gesture at the right time, and for only as long as the patient would accept it (identification) Chase established trust, leading patients to communicate repressed ideas and feelings and to risk new, deeper experiences and relationships.'†

By sharing her own body experience with that of her client, Chase

(a) created an interflow of understanding and empathy
(b) legitimized his deepest emotional upheavals
(c) created the climate for further therapeutic involvement
(d) assessed her own counter-transference (p 67).

Case example

Doris aged 18, clumsy, obese, uncommunicative, withdrawn, isolated and resentful refuses to move from her crouched position on the floor.
Therapist crouches beside her, and tries to hold her hand, but is rebuffed.
Therapist draws her own feet in chalk on the floor, and stands in them.
She draws feet for Doris, enclosing them in a wide circle, to indicate Doris' own 'safe' territory.
With her own body action therapist mirrors Doris' fear, shame, reluctance.
Doris nods her head.
She stands and holds up her hands with those of the therapist.
Therapist moves to a gentle, musical beat. Holding hands Doris identifies with therapist's movements, but only inside her circle where she feel safely contained.
Therapist enters Doris' circle. To a louder beat she takes larger steps, then leaps outside the circle.
It takes several sessions before Doris is able to share therapist's movements outside her chalked circle. Later she is able to communicate, through physical movement, episodes of her history of child abuse.

4. Rhythmic group movement

'Chase recognized rhythm as organizing individual behaviour and creating a feeling of solidarity and contagion among people.'*

---

* Foster, Ruth. *Knowing in My Bones.* London: Adam and Charles Black, 1976.

† Bernstein, Penny Lewis. ed. *Eight Theoretical Approaches in Dance-movement Therapy.* Iowa: Kendall Hunt, 1979.

The goals she saw in using rhythmic activity were:
1. a sense of one's own vitality,
2. participation in group activity,
3. channelling of one's energy into a structure.

People need to be aware of, and responsive to others' disparate feelings and life-styles.

Movement promotes interaction and helps to develop awareness of shared feelings and experiences.

'The more subtle rhythms which underlie expressive, functional and biological movement combine to form a symphony of rhythms. All are vitally important. Among these is breathing pattern. Breath adaptation to a partner, to stresses phrased out in group movement are easily observed.*

Pioneer work at some psychiatric hospitals, has demonstrated many ways in which ward, garden and clinic may utilize movements with sensitivity in order to

observe and evaluate,
encourage and expand.

Staff have shown how, freely expressed, spontaneous group movement and more structured therapeutic situations may ventilate sadness, grief, anger, solitude, conflict, guilt. Tension energy is thus converted into a new stretching out of personal boundaries towards individual and group fulfilment.

These treatment methods, probably administered in varying combinations, have revolutionized the progress and prognosis of mental illness.

Physically restrictive handling of patients in strait-jackets, padded cells, etc, is rendered virtually superfluous in the context of modern drug therapy. In any case it is claimed that less than 5% of mental hospital patients need to be institutionalized for 'public safety'.

TANGIBLE CREATIVITY provides an important *bridge from phantasy back to reality*. It also reintroduces the universal satisfaction to be found in *productivity*. Thus painting, sculpting, weaving, woodwork, pottery, etc are all important aspects of occupational therapy.

Diagnostic and therapeutic value of creativity

The content of creativity:

(a) constitutes a *diagnostic projective technique* (see pp 64, 122), reflecting the subject's deeper-level associations, phantasies, anxieties and conflicts, delusions and hallucinations. Before taking upon herself to interpret to a patient the meaning and import of his actions and creations the nurse should seek guidance. Patients become increasingly sophisticated. Thus the nurse should take pains to avoid what they may consider amateurish or presumptuous intrusions on their privacy;

(b) provides the patient with *tangible representation* of his previously frightening abstract phantasies. Content analysis helps him to come to grips with his

* Foster, Ruth. *Knowing in My Bones*. London: Adam and Charles Black, 1976.

problems at a tangible, concrete level where he can deal with them more effectively;

(c) constitutes an important means of achieving *catharsis*—that emotional release essential to psychotherapy. Creative materials through their flexible, sometimes sensuous, frequently unstructured media—their colours, shapes and dynamic, changing fluidity provide opportunity not only for diagnosis but also for mood expression—aggression, sadness, confusion, hope and mental balance;

(d) *relieves him of the necessity for abstract verbalization*, achieving direct communication with the outside world.

Thus, in reflecting both to the therapist and to the patient, his diagnosis, therapeutic progress and reintegration, creativity constitutes important tangible evidence of the patient's return to mental health.

Activities providing personal and group growth include outdoor sports, walking, shopping expeditions or coach outings; play reading, debating, musical appreciation.

Group identification in singing is a pleasing communal experience, especially when accompanied by the soothing tones of a guitar. (See also Music therapy, Movement therapy, p 629.)

More introverted, and perhaps more highly educated, patients prefer more intellectually oriented occupations such as chess, bridge, political discussions— always geared towards active participation, observation of interactions, the necessity of coming to grips with one's problems, the provision of support, the reassertion of personality, the ability to make decisions, to formulate and to bring to fruition.

Many patients find church services soothing, comforting in their familiarity, and in their childhood associations.

For those seeking relief in physical catharsis, judo is a constructive outlet. Mutually conducted beauty parlours and hairdressing salons are a source of much pleasurable communal activity, and a happy preparation for discharge—above all they provide a 'booster' for that important self-concept which is the basis of mental health. (For Assertiveness Training see p 165.)

Visitors provide an important link between hospital and the patient's long-term familial and communal life. They should certainly be welcomed—even if this involves flexibility of routine.

A pleasant sitting-room, providing a reasonable degree of privacy, is recommended. A sensible, well-guided relative may even help in the social and routine activities of the ward. Parents and spouses may well be included in group activities, thus imparting to the patient a strong feeling of being loved and supported in both the hospital and community situations.

It may be true that family members have contributed, however unconsciously, to the patient's illness. However, they remain part of his ultimate environment, to which he is required to readjust.

Even though he may be disturbed by their visits, these serve to reaffirm that he is still loved and needed. Visits also provide an opportunity for confrontation, problem-solving and growth.

Some relatives, through their involvement in psychiatric situations, have become aware of their own contribution to the patient's illness and feel guilty. In their effort to externalize these *guilt feelings*, unconsciously, they *project* them *on to the staff* or hospital situation, blaming a staff member or the hospital administration for aggravating the patient's illness. It is important that the nurse try to gain insight into this projective mechanism, without taking umbrage.

The student nurse should be careful lest, in her enthusiasm, she inflict upon her patient, or his relatives, her own sometimes inexperienced interpretation of his sayings and doings. Many patients are educated people; many have read a considerable amount of psychologically oriented literature, and will feel affronted and resentful when subjected to somewhat amateurish interpretations of their behaviour. There are seldom 'cut and dried' answers in mental functioning, and the nurse may be wrong!

Many relatives and friends are reasonable, co-operative people, anxious to 'do their bit' for their loved ones. In all probability the patient, in some way or other, *needs* his relatives or friends, who should be treated in a friendly, courteous and kind manner. Human needs should take priority over stringency of visiting hours. Very frequently the visitor can come only in 'out of visiting' hours.

The family need reassurance, and may even appear to 'make a nuisance' of themselves in repeating and manipulating their questions. The nurse, realizing the emotional needs, especially the guilt-feelings, of the family, will, no doubt, do her best to answer such questions or will refer them to the attendant doctor or appropriate specialist member of the psychiatric team. Throughout hospitalization, and in fact on discharge, the psychiatric team co-operates in their many-faceted and complementary participation.

The Psychiatric Nurse's emergency code

In order to create an atmosphere of freedom, while retaining sensible caution, it is important for the Psychiatric Nurse to have available to her a code of *'Psychiatric First Aid'* featuring the following principles:

(a) The nurse should always remain as cool, calm and 'collected' as possible. Should a patient suddenly become agitated, excited, or threaten suicide, *she should not leave him alone*. She should wear a 'bleeper' or some other method of communication by which to summon aid. During the interim she may attempt to soothe him in conversation, and to communicate with him, by physical tactile comfort and emotional level identification—very frequently a soothing hand will prove more helpful than a lengthy intellectualized conversation.

(b) 'No matter how busy she is, time must be made available to cope with an emergency, and the patient should be made to feel that the nurse has all the time in the world for him and that only his problem matters.'

(c) 'Attentive listening is vital and is something which a nurse should develop.'

(d) 'When the problem has been heard out, and not until then, attempts at reassurance should be made.'

(e) 'When the person has settled, some form of activity such as occupational or recreational therapy may be necessary to provide a means of diversion from the problem.'*

Handling physical aggression

Physically restrictive handling of patients in strait-jackets, padded cells, etc is rendered virtually superfluous in the context of modern drug therapy, and may in terms of legislation, render offending hospital staff liable to prosecution.

Episodes of aggressive outbursts occur mostly in the young and physically fit. The patient may break up valuable property or, more seriously, he may attack or injure someone else or himself.

The general rule in dealing with aggressive people is sufficiency of staff.

A nurse should not try to calm a physically aggressive or violent patient on her own, but should summon enough colleagues to ensure efficient handling of the situation without recourse to physical violence. Where possible a patient should be approached from behind, and the staff should stand as close to him as possible so as to limit the strength of his physical movements. If the patient continues to be violent one may seek permission of the medical staff in order to place him in a side-room and close the door. One should try not to lock the doors, and such isolation should be discontinued immediately the patient calms down.[†]

Although it is not always possible to eliminate them, causes of physical outbursts, whether from within the patient himself, or from environmental provocation, should certainly be investigated.

The episode may take place in a period of amnesia—as may occur in the post-epileptic aura. The incident is frequently quite foreign to his general behaviour pattern.

Suicide (see chapter 25)

Family involvement

On admission:

 (i) the patient's involuntarily disruptive behaviour has probably imposed an increasingly unbearable burden upon his family. Resultant 'abandonment' to institutionalization, frequently imposes upon family members feelings of acute guilt, anxiety and distress, which the psychiatric team should seek to relieve by interpretation and reassurance; catharsis and support;

(ii) where the patient is agitated or hallucinated; depressed or otherwise grossly disturbed, the family constitutes an important source of information as to his case-history behaviour patterns, fears and anxieties, etc.

---

* John Sheahan. *Essential Psychiatry*, p 166.
† John Sheahan. *Essential Psychiatry*.

In therapy:

The interplay between the patient and his family is clearly of importance in the achievement of effective living for all concerned.

The patient's problems may well have affected his whole family constellation, imposing stress upon marital relationships with consequent impaired communication; ambivalence, hostility and role-reversal—often to the diminishment of the patient himself.

Marital and other family psychotherapy may well be indicated, eg in alcoholism:
    the wife may be angry
    the 'in-laws' contemptuous
    the children ashamed and fearful
    the son, having usurped the father-role (and now fulfilling certain Oedipal phantasies), may be reluctant to resume his former 'subservient' position.

Clearly family therapy is indicated for both the mental health of family members, and also the establishment of that continuous therapeutic atmosphere which is an essential stepping stone to community rehabilitation.

Preparation for discharge

Especially to the *occupational therapist* falls the task of interpreting the construction and aims of *activity programmes*, that these may extend into family and community situations.

For example, the necessity for including the schizophrenic or geriatric patient in family chores, conversations, decisions and outings; social groups and tangible creative hobbies, should be interpreted and assessed, first by evaluating weekend visits and later by community case-work.

Failure to follow through active participation in programmes initiated during hospitalization may result in the breakdown of constructive behaviour patterns and a return to unmotivated withdrawal and isolation.

The family-orientated duties of the *psychiatric social worker* and *community sister* include

  (i) encouraging and tactful supervision of medication maintenance (stressing its long-term supplementary nature);
 (ii) preparation for possible temporary or permanent amendment of the patient's work-goals, employability and thus financial contribution. Seeing him looking fit, the family may resent his reduced productivity.
(iii) where appropriate bridging day care occupational and social facilities.

Criticism and diminishment should be avoided, lest the patient regress to anxiety, depression, withdrawal and isolation.

The fact that *many families do not wish to reaccept the patient into the family constellation* should be faced. It was, after all, the burden imposed by the patient's disruptive behaviour which originally led them to apply for hospitalization. In their unwillingness to resume their burden, the family may rationalize that mental illness is incurable. It is essential that family members realize that the psychiatric hospital is not a permanent hostel, and that community services are there to support and guide towards rehabilitation.

Should family rejection, or, indeed, unsuitability preclude family placement, small hostels or community homes may be indicated. These may be run or financed by the borough from which the client was admitted.

Specific difficulties of the Nursing Process in the psychiatric setting

1. Because

    (a) emotional problems

        (i) are often more vague and elusive than physiological disruptions,
        (ii) vary widely in symptomatology and behaviour,
        (iii) arise from *multiple* causes,

    (b) many clients are initially unable to describe or identify their problems,
    (c) clients may perceive themselves as powerless victims of their circumstances.

    Therefore assessment and planning stages of the psychiatric nursing process present special, but not insurmountable, difficulties.

2. Although isolation and confusion may be part of her client's maladaptive lifestyle, the nurse should resist the temptation to exclude him from partnership in the problem-solving process.

    Learning and growth are most effective when both partners actively participate in the experience within an agreed 'contract' situation.

    Advantages of client-participation include:

    (a) restoration of the client's sense of control over his life and responsibility for his actions;
    (b) reinforcement of the message that he is capable of continuing to make his own decisions in his battle between adaptive and maladaptive coping mechanisms.

Medication enabling early discharge

The important guiding principle throughout modern psychiatric treatment is to reduce as much as possible stigma, impairment of self-concept, loss of status and job security, and the onset of those various impediments to normal community life which we term 'hospitalism'.

An impediment to early discharge frequently consists in the *patient's failure to maintain his medication*, and the mistaken advice of family and friends that he attempt to 'wean himself from these drugs'.

It is important that the patient and his family realize that *drug treatment is not drug addiction;* just as the faulty metabolism of the diabetic requires that he take insulin for the rest of his life, so the psychotic's faulty biochemistry requires long-term medicinal supplementation. He should not expect significant relief in under three weeks.

When a patient fails to maintain his medication, and thus his revised metabolism, his symptoms usually recur, including a typical paranoid reaction in respect of medication itself, eg: 'You are trying to turn me into a drug addict—you are trying to poison me, because you want to steal my brains out of my head.'

New long-acting phenothiazine drugs, such as Moditen and Modecate, have done much to overcome this problem. Maintenance Moditen injections are required about every two weeks, and Modecate injections every three to four weeks.

The modern prognosis

Today even psychiatric hospitals dealing with advanced cases claim to discharge annually as many patients as are admitted. Figures for readmissions are not as optimistic.

Many psychiatric units have become short-stay hospitals, soon followed by out-patient treatment. Day hospitals, night hospitals, protective 'half-way' hostels and community support all constitute important innovations in out-patient treatment.

Once over the acute stage of his illness, the psychotic patient, like the neurotic, requires the long-term guidance and support of the psychiatric team as described above (see pp 605 et seq).

In general research shows that 80% of *patients show marked improvement:*

in the *severity of psychiatric disease symptoms* and disturbed behaviour, e g deluded and fractional thought processes, etc.

It would appear that these more gross and externalized symptoms are most responsive to medication.

But, in contrast, more subtle and pervasive functional performance in life tasks, such as

decision-making
self-care
maintenance of efficiency
on the open labour market
in household tasks
in the establishment and maintenance of relationships

i e *ability to function efficiently and constructively in real life tasks, remains at a low level* in spite of medication and psychotherapy.

At more subtle, sustained, deeper and pervasive levels patients did not manage in the outside world

either on admission
or after discharge.

Typical responses on the Honey and Stewart rating presented as follows:

Social presentation

Conversation, dress, etc—continued to function at a low level.
Household tasks—not better than 25% of the norm on admission nor on follow-up.
At work—at no time did any group exceed 45% of the norm.
Establishing and maintaining social relationships—performance exceeded only 20% of the norm.

IN SUMMATION, objective assessment showed *personal, work and social life functioning to be 'low' on admission and only 'low to moderate' on follow-up.*

'Many psychiatric patients get used to the path back to hospital.'

Gillis has shown that maintaining *functional efficiency outside the hospital is associated with the number, quality and attendance 'attractiveness' of out-patient clinics.*

Of discharged patients who attended his research clinics, only 20% fell away, but of those who did not attend the incidence of fall-away and gross relapse was 'very high'.*

The emotional support sister—the Psychiatric Nurse in the general wards

Wracked with pain, terrified of the unknown, isolated in the agony of multilation, death and loss patients, family and staff are all, to some extent, in crisis. While staff should not rely upon *them* to provide emotional support for their patients, there is certainly real need for sensitive, warm, empathic nurses, who have a specialized insight into human needs and whose sole job is the emotional support of patients, family and staff.

The role of the Psychiatric Nurse in the general hospital situation includes the following functions:

(1) *Crisis intervention* (see pp 563 et seq)

    (a) within the wide range of emergencies presenting in casualty: attempted suicides, loss by motor accident, etc.

    (b) in out-patient departments: necessity for surgery; cancer or AIDS realization, etc.

    (c) in the wards: emotional trauma associated with hospitalization and surgery, depression, death, etc.

    (d) destructive patient–staff relationships.

(2) *Emotional support and 'on-site' therapy*

    (a) Essential ability to *identify with the feelings* of patients and relatives stimulates appreciation of the acute emotional suffering which accompanies hospitalization. Indeed, fear of mutilation, personal diminishment and depression accompanying surgery often constitutes the patient's major distress area. Failure to provide surgical nursing would be unthinkable, yet *succour for emotional suffering* is frequently uncatered for or left to chance.

        'Mental health is every nurse's responsibility. The coronary thrombosis of today may be the psychiatric patient of tomorrow. Forty per cent of patients in your hospital today could also be classified as suitable for psychiatric hospitalization.'†

    (b) Provision of a 'screening' and psychotherapeutic service, gauging the severity of emotional disturbance, based on assessment of the potency of *inner personal resources* (intelligence; personal philosophy and religious faith; flexibility, optimism, etc.)

        and

        outer resources (familial, hospital and community, financial)

    available to the patient. Assessment includes reference to the patient's *own image of himself*. At this level the Psychiatric Nurse may either

* Gillis, Professor L. Full reference available from the author.
† Bruwer, A M Chief Psychiatric Nursing Officer (for further information refer to author).

(i) request referral to specialist facilities, or

(ii) 'reach out' to patient and family, rendering assistance at an emotional level meaningful to them.

In this capacity the Psychiatric Nurse intervenes directly, acting as a primary therapist, assessing, planning, implementing and evaluating within the *nursing process*.

(3) As a participant in the nursing process the Psychiatric Nurse co-operates with her colleagues by providing a *consultative service* in *assessing* dynamics of underlying problem presentation, and *planning* total patient care.

(4) In *follow-up care* she provides complementary, repetitive reassuring information, thus helping alleviate the anxiety and symptom fixation associated with serious or chronic illness: support, catharsis, comfort and liaison with community facilities.

(5) *Demonstration of emotionally supportive behaviour patterns* which will hopefully be introjected by other staff members ('behaviour spin-off').

(6) *Pertaining to staff members themselves: the provision of immediate, 'hot' on-site catharsis, guidance and emotional support* in times of crisis and stress.

Warm, but not authoritarian, involvement is a basic personality trait in all aspects of the Psychiatric-nurse counsellor role.

The nurse is so often in the front line of crisis presentation. Almost every traumatic or serious illness involves confrontation of patient, family *and nurse* with:

Impact
Turmoil and recoil
Emotional wounding
The necessity of Adjustment and Reconstitution.

(The role of the professional in crisis situation, p 565.)

The nurse experiences *her own crisis within a crisis*, certainly profiting from opportunity for:

Awareness and Sensitivity,
Catharsis and Support,
Involved comfort,
On the spot, 'hot' counteraction of *frightening phantasy, spiralling panic* and *guilt feelings* (pp 565, 580),
Mobilisation of impaired defense mechanisms including professional identification,

offered by a ward-based psychiatric nurse.

This specialized colleague should be independent of routine responsibilities and the disciplinary hierarchy.

Nothing will impede her therapeutic role as surely as temptation to break confidences, nor involvement in staff assessment.

The nurse must feel free to *ventilate* her helplessness or anger at the mercy of senior staff; her fear of having made a mistake; her terror of infection by AIDS or exposure to cancer by radio-activity.

Few other professionals can offer stressed nurses comparable compassion, and insight into *shared vocational perils and satisfactions*. For between nurses there is precious identification to strengthen motivation for personal survival as well as caring service.

CHAPTER 27

MENTAL HEALTH

The World Health Organization Expert Committee on Mental Health (1951) defined mental health as follows:

> 'Mental health as the committee understands it is influenced by both *biological* and *social* factors. It is not a static condition but subject to *variations* and *fluctuations* of degree.'

The committee's conception implied the capacity of an individual

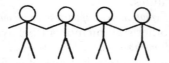

(a) To *form harmonious relations* with others.

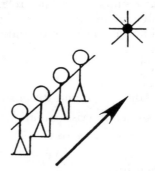

(b) To *participate in*, or contribute *constructively* towards, *changes* in his social and physical environment.

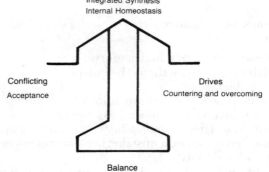

(c) To achieve *internal, personalized homeostasis* (p 103)—a harmonious and balanced satisfaction of his *own potentially conflicting drives* to reach an *integrated synthesis*.

Emphasis is on the *amendment* and *organization* of satisfactions rather than on their frustration and denial.

Clearly mental health implies an internal *balance* between responsibility, the ability to *accept* the burdens, sorrows and disappointments of life, while at the same time possessing the capacity for *counteracting* problems with a certain *optimism, philosophy, hope* and that *sense of proportion* which is bolstered by an active sense of humour.

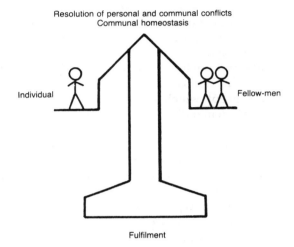

(d) To participate in communal homeostasis.

The World Health Organization has attempted to impart the principle that mental health implies an ability to achieve a balance between the needs of an individual and those of his fellow men, to resolve in a balanced but dynamic manner his own internal motivation satisfactions and those of the environment, with emphasis on fulfilment rather than denial of both personality and community.

Where, one may well ask, may one find this so well-balanced individual? In the stresses, anxieties, the 'rat race' of modern living, I doubt very much whether he exists at all.

Clearly, every one of us is, at some time or other, ready to explode with lack of internal harmony. Who at some time or other, does not lose his 'cool', his sense of proportion, in a state of unhappy tension, anxiety, depression and 'the heartache, and the thousand natural shocks that flesh is heir to'?*

It would appear that, for most of us, a reasonable adjustment—a majority of happy times over sad ones; an ability to realize that depression will lift, and that 'tomorrow will be another day', that our neighbour has needs and rights as important as our own—is as much as we can ask.

---

* Shakespeare. *Hamlet*, III, i.

Some people, as we have seen, appear to *inherit* an easy-going, not too vulnerable personality which makes the achievement of mental health easier. Others must learn to live with whatever internal equipment for homeostasis has been issued to them.

Among *factors contributory* to mental health, are

(a) A personal *philosophy of life, well summarized in the Serenity Prayer of Alcoholics Anonymous:*

'*God grant me the serenity to accept the things I cannot change; the courage to change the things I can, and the wisdom to know the difference.*'

(b) *Religious faith,* a belief in constant and powerful support and compassion, a faith and a hope beyond mortal limitations and failures, helping make the burdens of life more tolerable.

(c) *Intelligence*—the ability to achieve insight, to make purposeful decisions; to generalize, formulate and embark on a constructive behaviour plan; to achieve that healthy self-concept which comes through success and self-respect. Certainly in our high-demanding modern society, intelligence is essential to mental health.

(d) *Education* for life—for the development of intellectual resources, job skills; for the development of interest in music, art, literature, utilization of leisure time; preparation for a serene and fulfilling retirement—all these develop from education in its wider sense.

(e) *A sound, secure, loving and accepting parent–child relationship* probably constitutes the best insurance policy against failure to develop patterns of social conformity, and thus exposure to social rejection; frustration, guilt, anxiety and sorrow. The child who grows up knowing that he is loved, that he can rely on his parents to accept him for what he is; whose parents are able to demonstrate their affection; who is not crushed by early and excessive disciplinary demands; a childhood in which the developing youngster feels safe to experience and express strong emotions, to express his ambivalence without fear of guilt-laden disapproval; parents whose loving relationship motivates the wish to identify strongly and constructively—the girl with her mother in preparation for womanhood, the boy with his father in preparation for manhood; the youngster whose most important lessons in self-discipline are to be found in the constant example of his loved and admired parents—all these contribute to the formation of that important *self-concept* or *self-respect* which is the basis of mental health.

It is essential that a youngster *grow up liking himself,* satisfied in his accomplishments and in his ability to handle life; confident that he is loved and approved of, and thus possessing the generosity, warmth and freedom from inhibition to express his love and caring in long-term human relationships.

BIBLIOGRAPHY
AND SUGGESTED READING

CHAPTER 1

Allport, G.W. *Personality, a Psychological Interpretation.* NY: Holt (1937).
Freud, S. *Outline of Psychoanalysis* (Std Ed, 1964), Vol XXIII. London: Hogarth Press (1940).
Heidegger, M. (1967). *Being and Time.* Oxford: Basil Blackwell. (originally published in 1962).
Hilgard, Ernest R. Atkinson, Richard C. Atkinson, Rita L. *Introduction to Psychology,* Harcourt Brace
    Jovanovich Inc, 8th International Edition (1986).
Howard, W.C. (1948). *Dictionary of Psychology.* Houghton, Mifflin: Riverside Press.
Husserl, E. (1965). *Phenomenology and the Crisis of Philosophy.* New York: Harper and Row.
Layton, L. and Shapiro, B.A. (1988). *Narcissism and the Text: Studies in Literature and Psychology of Self.* New York:
    New York University Press.
Mechanic, D. (1968). *Medical Sociology.* New York: Free Press.
Pavlov, I.P. *Conditional Reflexes,* pp 197, 220. NY: Oxford University Press (1927).
Skinner, B.F. *The Technology of Teaching.* NY: Appleton-Century-Crofts (1968).
Smith, M.B. (1973) 'Is Psychology relevant to new Priorities?' *American Psychologist* **6**, 463–71.
Watson, J.B. *Psychology from the Standpoint of a Behaviourist* (2 ed). Philadelphia: J.B. Lippincott. (1919).

CHAPTER 2

Bowlby, J. *Attachment.* NY: Basic Books (1969).
Dement, W.C. *Some must watch while others sleep.* Stanford Calif. Alumni Association. (1972).
Dunbar, H.F. *Mind and Body.* Random House (1947).
Eysenck, H.J. *The Biological Basis of Personality.* Springfield Ill.: Thomas.
Goldfarb, W. (1945). Effects of psychological deprivation in infancy and subsequent stimulation. *American
    Journal of Psychiatry, 102,* 18–33.
Harlow, H.F. (1971). *Learning to Love.* San Francisco: Albion.
Harlow, H.F. Harlow, M.K. (1966), 'Learning to Love', *American Scientist* **54**: 244–72.
Harlow, H.F. Harlow, M.K. and Meyer, D.R. (1950). Learning motivated by a motivation drive. *Journal of
    Experimental Psychology,* **40**: 228–34.
Hilgard, E.R. Atkinson, R.C. Atkinson, R.L. *Introduction to Psychology.* Harcourt Brace and Jovanovich Inc.
    8th International Edition. (1986).
Holmes, T.H. and Rahe. (1967) 'The Social Readjustment Rating Scale', *Journal of Psychomatic Research,*
    213–18, 437.
Jacobs, Price, Court, Brown, Brittain and Whatmore (1968) 'Chromosome Studies of Men in a maximum
    security hospital', *Annals of Human Genetics* **31**: 339–58.
Kestenberg, J.A. *Psychoanalytic Study of the Adoptive Child.* Tavistock Publications.
Maccoby, E.E. and Feldman, S.S. (1972). Mother attachment and stranger reactions in the third year of life.
    Monograph of the Society for Research in Child Development, No. 1, **37**: 1–86.
Nahir, H.Y. and Yussen, S.R. (1977). Performance of kibbutz- and city-reared Israeli children on two
    role-taking tasks. *Developmental Psychology,* **13**, 450–55.
Price, W.H. 'Sex Determination, Mental Subnormality, Crime and Delinquency in Males'. Medical
    Research Council, Clinical and Population Cytogenics Research Unit and University Dept of Medicine,
    Western General Hospital, Edinburgh 4.
Rabkin, Y. and Rabkin, K. (1969). Children of the kibbutz. *Psychology Today,* **3**, 40–6.
Rheingold, H.L. and Echerman, C.O. (1970). 'The Infant Separates Himself from his Mother', *Science* **168**:
    78–83.
Schaffer, H.R. *The Growth of Sociability.* Harmondsworth: Penguin.
Shaffer, L.F. *The Psychology of Adjustment.* Columbia Teachers' College Bookshop.

CHAPTER 3

Crile, George. *What Every Woman Should Know About the Breast Cancer Controversy.* New York: Macmillan (1973).
Dannenfeldt, G. (1982). The Psychological Aspects of Intensive Care Units. *Curationis,* **5**(3).
Dannenfeldt, G. The Psychological Aspects of Intensive Care Units. *Curationis,* **5**(3) (1982).
Eron, L.D. Huesman, L.R. Lefkowitz, M.M. and Walder, L.O. (1972). How learning conditions in early
    childhood relate to aggression in later childhood. *American Journal of Orthopaedics,* **44**(5), 412–23.
Freud, S. *Introductory Lectures to Psychoanalysis.* Harmondsworth: Penguin.
Gillis, L. *The Emotional Problems of Illness.* Faber and Faber.

Hackett, T. *et al* (1968), The Coronary Care Unit—an appraisal of Psychological Hazards. *New England Journal Med* **279**: 25.
Inman, V.T. 'Conservation of Energy in Ambulation', *Archives of Physical Medicine* **49**: 484.
Kushner, Rose, *Alternative—New Developments in the War on Breast Cancer*. Harcourt Brace and Jovanovich. (1985).
Loon, H. *Below Knee Amputation Surgery*. American Orthotics and Prosthetic Association.
Mital, M.A. Pierce, D.S. *Amputees and their Prostheses*. Boston: Little, Brown and Co.
Nash, E. Stoch, B. Harper, G. *Human Behaviour*. Cape Town. David Philip (1984).
Nobel, (1979). Communication in the ICU—therapeutic or disturbing. *Nursing Outlook*, **27**(3).
Olivier, L. (1982). *Confessions of an Actor*. London: Weidenfeld and Nicholson.
Peters, Vera (1977). 'Wedge Resection with or without Radiation in the Treatment of Early Breast Cancer.' *International Journal of Radiation Oncology*. 1977, **2**: 8.
Schwartz, C.H. *The Psychodynamics of Patient Care*. Prentice-Hall.
Tiffany, F. *Cancer Nursing: Surgical*. Faber (1980).

CHAPTERS 4 and 5

Buss, A.H. (1966). Instrumentality of aggression feedback and frustration as determinants of physical aggression. *Journal of Personality and Social Psychology*, **4**, 153–62.
Coziet and Du Gas, *Fundamentals of Nursing*.
Ekman, P. Friesen, W.W. *Unmasking the Face*. Englewood Cliffs, N.J. Prentice Hall (1975).
Gordon, M. *The Clinical Specialist as a Change Agent*. M. Lewis E.P. Editor.
Groves, J.E. (1978). Taking care of the hateful patient. *New England Journal of Medicine*, **298**, 883–7.
Hilgard, Atkinson and Atkinson, *Op. Cit.*
Holman, Portia, *Psychology and Psychological Medicine for Nurses*. Heinemann (1957).
Jahoda, Marie, 'Nursing as a Profession'. 12th Quadrennial International Congress of Nursing.
Leiffer, A.D. Gordon, N.J. and Graves, S.B. (1974). Children's television: more than mere entertainment. *Harvard Educational Review*, **44**, 213–45.
Loew, C.A. (1967). Acquisition of a hostile attitude and its relationship to aggressive behaviour. *Journal of Personality and Social Psychology*, **5**, 335–41.
Maslow, A. *Motivation and Personality*. Harper and Row. New York. (1970).
Mussen, P.H. Conger, J.J. and Kagan, J. *Child Development and Personality* (5 ed). Harper and Row (1981).
Shaffer, C.F. *The Psychology of Adjustment*. Columbia Teachers' College Bookshop.

CHAPTER 6

Gerbner, G. and L. Gross, 'The Scary World of TV's Heavy Viewer'. (1976) *Psychology Today*. **9**: 41–5, 329–555.
Gray, W. *The Living Brain*. W.W. Norton. New York (1953).
Hilgard, Atkinson and Atkinson. *Introduction to Psychology*. *Op. Cit.*
Hyden, H. *Biochemical Aspects of Learning and Memory* (1969).
Jersild, A. *Child Psychology*. 6th edition . Teachers' College Press, Columbia University, New York (1969).
Kamin, L.J. (1974). *The Science and Politics of I.Q.* Hillsdale, N.J.: Erlbaum.
Miller, J.M. Moody, D.B. and Stebbens, W.C. (1969). A primate restraint and handling system for auditory research. *Behavioral Researethods*, **2**(4), 180.
Pribram, K. (ed), *The Biology of Learning*. New York, Harcourt, Brace and Jovanovich.
Riesen, A.H. (1965). Effects of early deprivation of photic stimulation. In Osler, S. and Cooke, R. (eds) *The Biosocial Basis of Mental Retardation*. Baltimore: Johns Hopkins University Press.
Scarr, S. (1977). Testing minority children: why, how and with what effects? *Proceedings of the National Conference on Testing*. New York Center for Advanced Study in Education.
Skinner, B.F. *Science and Human Behaviour*. Free Press (1953).
Stuart, G.W. and S.J. Sundeen, *Principles and Practice of Psychiatric Nursing*. St Louis, Mosby (1979).
Thurstone, L.L. (1938), *Primary Mental Abilities*. Chicago: Chicago University Press.
Weisman, S. (1966). Enviromental and innate factors and educational attainment. In Meade, J.E. Parkes, A.S. (eds). *Genetic and Environmental Factors in Human Ability*. Edinburgh: Oliver and Boyd.
Wolpe, J. *The Practice of Behaviour Therapy*. New York Paramedical Press, 1969.
Yalom, I. *The Theory and Practice of Group Psychotherapy*. (2 ed) New York. Basic Books Inc (1975).

CHAPTER 7

Bennett, A.E. *Communication between Doctors and Patients* Oxford University Press (Nuffield Provincial Hospitals Trust) (1976).
Berne, E. *Games People Play*. New York. Grove Press Inc. (1964).
Berne, E. *Sex in Human Loving*. Penguin Books (1967).
Berne, E. *Transactional Analysis in Psychotherapy*. New York. Grove Press Inc (1961).

Buber, M. *I and Thou*. New York, Charles Scribner's. (1958).
Coziet and Du Gas, *Fundamentals of Nursing*.
Gillis, L. *Guidelines in Psychiatry*. Juta. (1986).
Gillis, L. *The Emotional Problems of Illness*. Faber and Faber.
Groves, G.E. (1978). Taking Care of the Hateful Patient. *New England Journal of Medicine*, **298**: 883–7.
Lundberg, G.A. Schragg, C.C. and Larsen, O.N. *Sociology*, New York: Harper and Bros (1954).
Schwartz, C.H. O.C. *The Psychodynamics of Patient Care*. Prentice-Hall.
Stuart, G.W. and S.J. Sundeen. *Op Cit*.
Szaz, T.S. and Hollander, M.H. (1956). A Contribution to the Philosphy of Medicine: The basic models of the doctor patient relationship. *Archives of Internal Medicine*; **97**: 585–95.
Watzlawich, P. J.H. Beavin and D.O. Jackson. *Pragmatics of Human Communication*. New York: Norton & Co, Inc. (1967).
Wisser, Susan Hiscoe, (1979) 'When the Walls Listened'. *American Journal of Nursing*, **6**:
Yura, H. and M.B. Walsh, *The Nursing Process* New York: Appleton-Century-Crofts (1978).

CHAPTER 8

Brown, R.J. (1988). *Group Processes*. Oxford: Blackwell.
Clark, K.B. and Clark, M.P. (1947). Racial identification and preference in Negro children. In T.M. Newcomb and E.L. Hartley (Eds). *Readings in Social Psychology*. New York: Holt, Rhinehart and Winston.
Luft, J. *Group Processes: an introduction to Group Dynamics* (2 ed). Palo Alto, Calif.: National Press Books. (1970).
Lundberg, G.A., Schragg, C.C., Larsen, O.N. *Op. Cit*.
Sherif, M. (1966). *Group Conflict and Co-operation*. London: Routledge and Kegan, Paul.
Smith, James P. *Sociology and Nursing*. Livingstone Nursing Texts.
Tajfel, H. (ed) (1982). *Social Identity and Intergroup Relations*. London: Cambridge University Press.
Tuckman, B. (1965) Developmental Sequence in Small Groups. *Psychol. Bull.* **63**: 384.

CHAPTER 9

American Nurses' Association. 1973. *Standards of Nursing Practice*. Kansas City: American Nurses' Association.
Stuart, G.W. and S.J. Sundeen. *Op. Cit*.
Yara, H. and M.B. Walsh. *Op. Cit*.

CHAPTER 10

De Young, C.D. M. Tower *Out of Uniform and Into Trouble.: The nurse's role in Community Health Services*. St. Louis. Mosby.
Horton and Horton, *Introductory Sociology Learning Systems*. Ontario. Irwin-Dorsey Ltd.
Lindberg H. and C.H. Braach (1973). Community Health Nursing in the Changing Mental Health Scene. *J. Nurs Admin* **3**: 41.
Lundberg, G.A. Schragg, C.C. Larsen, O.N. *Op. Cit*.
Nash, E. Stoch, B. Harper, G. *Human Behaviour*. David Philip (1984).
Ruybal, S.: (1978) 'Community Health Planning' *Fam Commun Health* **1**: 9.
Vlok, M. *Manual of Community Health*. Juta. (1984).

CHAPTER 11

Caplan, G.: *Preventive Psychiatry*. Basic Books. (1963).
Erikson, E.H.: *Childhood and Society*. New York: W.W. Norton and Co. (1963).
Erikson, E.H.: *Identity: Youth and Crisis* New York: W.W. Norton and Co. (1968).
Erikson, E.H.: (1956) 'The Problem of Ego-Identity'. *J. Am Psycho-anal Assoc* **4**: 56–121.
Havighurst, R.J.: *Human Development and Education*. New York.: Longman. (1953).
Stuart G.W. and S.J. Sundeen: *Op. Cit*.

CHAPTER 12

Bayley, N. (1970). Development of mental abilities. In Mussen, P. (ed). *Carmichael's manual of Child Psychology*. New York: John Wiley and Sons.
Gesell, A. Ilg, F.C. *The Child from Five to Ten*. Harper.
Gesell, A. *The First Five Years of Life*. London: Methuen. (1950).
Jersild, A.T. *Child Development*. Columbia: University Press.
Mussen, Conger and Kagan. *Op. Cit*.
Piaget, J. *The Origins of Intelligence in Children*. NY: International Universities Press.

CHAPTER 13

Bowlby, J. *Maternal Care and Maternal Health*. Geneva: WHO (1952).
Films: *Grief*: Spitz, R.P. Levy, D.M.
Hawthorn, P.J. (1974). *Nurse — I want my mummy*. London: Royal College of Nursing.
Holman, Portia. *Op. Cit.*
Jolly, H. *Book of Child Care*. Allen and Unwin. London.
Kanner, Leo. *Child Psychiatry*. Blackwell.
Levy, D.M. (1932). Body Interest in Children with Hypochondriasis, *American Journal of Psychiatry* **12**: 295–315.
Lindberg, C. *Helping Children Understand — A Guide for a Parent with Cancer*. Minnesota Division, American Cancer Association.
Robertson, J. *Young Children in Hospital*. Tavistock. London.
Spitz, R.A. *Hospitalism in the Psychoanalytic Study of the Child*. International University Press (1945).
The Two Year Old Goes to Hospital with Mother—The Amersham (UK) Experiment.
Visentainer and Wolfer. (1975) Psychological Preparation for Surgical Pediatric Patients: The Effect on Children and Parents' Stress Responses and Adjustments. *Paediatrics* **56**(2): 187–202.

CHAPTER 14

Bowlby, J. *Maternal Care and Maternal Health*. Geneva WHO, 1951.
Corby, B. (1987). *Working with Child Abuse: Social Work Practice and the Child Abuse System*. Milton Keynes: Open University Press.
Gill, D. (1970). *Violence Against Children: Physical Abuse in the U.S.A.* Harvard, Mass. Harvard University Press.
Gill, D. (1975). Unravelling child abuse. *American Journal of Orthopsychiatry*, **45**(3), 346–65.
Hopkins, J. (1970). The nurse and the abused chid. *Nurs Clin. North Am.* **5**: 589.
Irwin, Claire, The Establishment of a Child Abuse Unit in a Children's Hospital. *SA Medical Journal* **49**: 1142–6.
Kempe, C.H. Droegemuller, W. and Silver, H.K. (1962). The battered child syndrome. *Journal of the American Medical Association*, **181**, 17–24.
Pelton, L.H. (1978). Child abuse and neglect—the myth of classlessness. *American Journal of Orthopsychiatry*, **48**(4), 608–17.

CHAPTER 15

Cole, L. *Psychology of Adolescence*. Rinehart and Co, Inc.
Erikson, E.H. *Childhood and Society* (2 ed). NY: Norton.
Hilgard, E.R. Atkinson, R.C. Atkinson, R.L. *Op. Cit.*
Jersild, A.J. *Psychology of Adolescence*. Teachers' College Bookshop, Columbia University Press. (1963).
Kinsey, A.C. Pomeroy, W.B. Martin, C.E. and Gebhard, P.H. *Sexual Behaviour in the Human Male* (1948).
Mead, M. *Culture and commitment: a study of the generation gap*. NY: Basic Books Inc. (1970).
Mussen, Conger and Kagan. *Op. Cit.*
Survison, K.C. *Psychology of Adolescence*. Prentice-Hall. (1977).
Thornburg, H.: *Development in adolescence*. Monterey. Calif.: Brooks/Cole. (1975).

CHAPTER 16

American Psychiatric Association. Quick reference to the Diagnostic Criteria from Diagnostic and Statistical Manual of Mental Disorders. (3rd ed). (DSM III) Washington, D.C. APA 1980.
Burgess A.W. and Holmstrom L.L. (1973). The Rape Victim in the Emergency Ward. *Am J. Nursing* **73**: 1744.
Burgess A.W. and Holmstrom L.L. (1974). Crisis and Counselling Requests of Rape Victims. *Nurs Res* **23**: 196.
Burgess A.W. Groth A.N. Holmstrom L.L. and Sgroi S.M.: *Sexual assault of children and adolescents*. Lexington Mass: D.C. Heath and Co. (1978).
Burgess A.W. Groth A.N. Rape Crisis Center of Syracuse, Inc. *Training Manual*. Sept. 1976 601 Allen Street, Syracuse NY 13210.
Cole, L. *Psychology of Adolescence*. Rinehart and Co. Inc.: New York.
Gillis, L.S. *Guidelines in Psychiatry*. Juta: (1986).
King, N. and Rodin. *Venereal Diseases: 1964–1980*. Bailliere. London.
Kinsey, A.C. Pomeroy, W.B. Martin, C.E. and Gebbard, P.H. *Sexual Behaviour in the Human Female*. Philadelphia: Saunders (1953).
Miller, D. Weber, J. and Green, J. (1986). *The Management of AIDS Patients*. London: MacMillan Press.
Ounsted, C. and Taylor, D.C. *Gender Differences: Their Ontogeny and Significance*. Churchill-Livingstone (1972).
Scheinfeld, A. *You and Heredity*. Garden City Publishing.
Schlesinger B. From A to Z with adolescent sexuality. *Can. Nurse*. Oct. 1977.

Simonton, O.C. Mathews-Simonton, S. and Creighton, J.C. (1978). Getting Well Again. Toronto: Bantam Books.
Sorenson, R. *Adolescent Sexuality in Contemporary America* NY: World Publishing. (1973).

CHAPTER 17

AA World Services Inc: *A Message to Teenagers* PO Box 459, Grand Central Station New York NY 10163.
Estes, N.J. and Heinemann, M.E. (eds): *Alcoholism: development, consequences and interventions*. St. Louis: Mosby. (1977).
Fraser, R.W. *Hurdles in Continuing Sobriety*. Alcoholism Foundation of Alberta.
Gamage, J.R. (ed), *Management of Adolescent drug misuse: Clinical, Psychological and Legal Perspectives*. Beloit, Wis: Reach Press. (1973).
Gareri, E. (1979). Assertiveness Training for Alcoholics *J Psychiatr Nursing* **17**: 31.
Morgan, A.J. and Moreno J.W. (1973). Attitudes Towards Addiction, *Am J Nurs* **73**: 497.
Ray, O.S.: *Drugs, Society and Human Behaviour* 2 ed. St. Louis: Mosby. (1970).

CHAPTER 18

Boberg, P.Q.R. *Law of Persons and the Family*. Juta: (1981).
Dalton, K. *Depression after Childbirth*. Oxford: Oxford University Press. (1980).
Fine, S.H. Krell, R. and Tsung-yi Lin (eds), *Today's Priorites in Mental Health—Children and families—Needs, Rights and Action*. Reidel, Dordrecht: Boston.
Lieberman, S. *Transgenerational Family Therapy*. London. Croom Helm (1979).
Morton, A.J. and Glick, P.S. *Marital Instability in America. Past and Present in Divorce and Separation. Context, Causes and Consequences*. New York: Basic Books. (1979).
Spiro, E. *The Law of Parent and Child*. Juta. (1981).
Wallerstein, J.S. & Kelly, J.B. (1977). "Divorce Counselling. A community service for families in the midst of divorce". *American Journal of Orthopsychiatry* **47**(4).
Wallerstein, J.S. & Kelly, J.E. (1976). The Effects of Parental Divorce. Experience of the Child in Later Latency. *American Journal of Orthopsychiatry* **36**(2) 256–69.
Wallerstein, J.S. & Kelly, J.E. (1975). The Effects of Parental Divorce: Experiences of the Pre-school Child. *Journal of American Academy of Child Psychiatry* **14**: 600–16.
Wallerstein, J.S. & Kelly, J.E. 'The Effects of Parental Divorce. The Adolescent Experience'. In: *The Child in his Family* Anthony, E.J. & Kouterlik, A. (eds) vol 3. John Wiley & Son New York (1974).

CHAPTER 19

Family Doctor Publications: *Hysterectomy*. British Medical Association.
Goddard, J. *Middle Age Crisis—a self-fulfilling prophesy*. Plato Health Care Promotions.
Hilgard, Atkinson and Atkinson. *Op. Cit.*
Kaplan, H.S.: *The New Sex Therapy*. New York: Brunner/Mazel Inc. (1974).
Kinsey, Pomeroy, Martin and Gebhard, *Sexual Behaviour in the Human Female* (1953).
Llewellyn-Jones, Derek. *Hysterectomy—A Book to Help You Deal with the Physical and Emotional Aspects* (Oxford Medical Publishers).
Masters, W.H. and Johnson V.E. *Human Sexual Response* Boston: Little, Brown and Co. (1966).
Schwartz, C.H. J.C. *The Psychodynamics of Patient Care*. Prentice-Hall.

CHAPTER 20

Abramowitz, L.J. Sexuality in the Ageing. *Continuing Medical Education*. **1**(5).
Adams, G. *Essentials of Geriatric Medicine*. Oxford Medical Publications.
Conti, M.L. (1970) The Loneliness of Old Age. *Nurs Outlook* **18**: 28.
Davis, L. 'As in Life'. *Senior News*. **16**(1).
Dunham, A. Sengupta, S.B. Nusberg, C. Planning for the Elderly in Local Communities, An International Perspective, International Federation on Ageing, 1909 K Street, NW Washington DC, 20049, USA.
Gillis, Lynn. *Guidelines in Psychiatry*. David Philip (1986).
Gray, W. *The Living Brain*. W. W. Norton: New York. (1953).
Jack, R. (1983). Out from the Geriatric Ghetto. *Social Work Today*, **14**(20).
Lynch, J.J. *The Broken Heart, the Medical Consequences of Loneliness*. New York: Basic Books Inc.
Manchester Area Health Authority. *The Arts in Hospital: Edgar Wood Centre Conference Report*. December 1981.
Parkes, C.M. Benjamin, B. and Fitzgerald, R.C. (1969). Broken heart—a statistical study of increased mortality among widowers. *British Medical Journal*, **1**(5646), 740.
Stuart, G.W. and S.J. Sundeen. *Op Cit.*
— Gillis, L. *The Emotional Problems of Illness*. Faber & Faber.

The International Federation on Ageing, International Survey of Periodicals in Gerontology, IFA yearly, 1909 K Street, NW Washington DC, 20049, USA.

CHAPTER 21

Hilgard, E.R. Atkinson R.C. Atkinson R.L. *Op. Cit.*
Lewis, E.P. (1975). The Stuff of which Nursing is Made. *Nursing Outlook* **23**(2).
McLaughlin, A.M. *Coping in Context—Adaptation Group for Chronic Pain Patients.* Bryn Mawr Rehabilitation Hospital, Malvern, Penn. USA.
Saunders, Cicly. *Care of the Dying.* Macmillan.
Wechsler, I.S. *Textbook of Clinical Neurology.* Saunders.
Wisser, S.H. When the walls listened. *American Journal of Nursing* **78**(6).

CHAPTER 22

Cohen, S. (1977). Helping Depressed patients in general Nursing Practice *Am J Nurs* **77**: 1007.
DeCato, C.M. and Wicks, R.J. (1976). Psychological Testing referrals: a guide for psychiatrists, psychiatric nurses, physicians in general practice and allied health personnel. *J Psychiatr Nurs* **14**:
Fisher, B. (et al) (1985). Five year results of a randomized clinical trial comparing total mastectomy and segmental mastectomy with or without radiation in the treatment of breast cancer. *New England Journal of Medicine*, **312**(111).
Frostig, M. Lefever, W. and Whittlesey, J.R.B. *Marianne Frostig Developmental Test of Visual Perception* Consulting Psychologists' Press. Palo Alto. California.
Gray, W. *The Living Brain.* New York: W.W. Norton (1953).
Griffith, E.R. and Trieschmann, R.R. *Sexual Training of the Spinal Cord-injured Male and his Partner: Human Sexuality Rehabilitation Medicine.* Baltimore: Williams & Williams. (1983).
Gruendemann, B. (1975). The Impact of Surgery on Body Image. *Nurs Clin North Am* **10**: 635.
Hamilton, A. (1978). The Sexual Problems of the Disabled. *British Journal Family Planning* **4**: 12–13.
Immelman, E.J. Surgery and Sexual Dysfunction, *Continuing Medical Education,* Vol 1, May 1983.
Kephart, N.C. *The slow Learner in the Classroom.* Columbus, Ohio: Charles E. Merril Books (1960).
Mital and Pierce, *Amputees and their Prostheses.* Boston: Little, Brown and Co.
Mooney, T.O. Cole, T. and Chileren, R.A. *Sexual Options for Paraplegics and Quadraplegics.* Boston: Little Brown. (1975).
Sadok, B.A. *Organic Brain Syndromes: introduction.* In Freedman A.M. Kaplan, H.I. and Sadock, B.J. *Comprehensive Textbook of Psychiatry* Baltimore. Williams and Wilkins (1975).
Sapire, K.E. Disease, Disability and Sexuality, *Continuing Medical Education,* Vol 1, May 1983.
Siegel, E. *Helping the Brain-Injured Child,* Association for the Brain-Injured, New York. (1962).
Tansley A.E. *Reading and Remedial Reading.* Unwin.

CHAPTER 23

Black, D. (1983). Bereaved Children—Family Intervention. *Bereavement Care.* **2**(2).
Cope Magazine for Cancer Patients, their families and Physicians, September 1986. 12600 W. Colfax. Suite B-400. Denver Colo. 80215.
Freihofer, P. and Fetton G. (1976) Nursing Behaviours in Bereavement: an exploratory Study. *Nurs Res* **25**: 332.
Hinton, J. *Dying.* Penguin Books (1967).
Hodge, J. (1972) They that Mourn, *J Religious Health* **11**: 229.
Kaufman, F. and Ellzur, E. Children's Bereavement Reactions Following Death of the Father. *International Journal Family Therapy.* **3**: 203–29.
Kauffman, M. and Ellzur, E. (1984). Children's Bereavement Reactions Following Death of the Father. *International Journal Family Therapy,* **6**(4), 259–83.
Kübler, Ross, E. *On Death and Dying.* London: Tavistock Publications (1970).
Saunders, Cicely. *Care of the Dying.* Macmillan. (1962).
Schiff, Harriet Sarnoff. *The Bereaved Parent.*
Schoenberg, B. Irwin, G. Wiener, A. Kutscher, H. Perets, D. Carr, A. *Bereavement—Its Psycho-Social Aspects.* Columbia: University Press.
Stanislave, G. Halifax, J. *The Human Encounter with Death.* Souvenir Press.

CHAPTER 24

Gillis, L.S. *Guidelines in Psychiatry.* David Philip. 1986.
Hall, J. and Weaver, B. (1974). *Nursing of familes in Crisis. Philadelphia: Lippincott. (1974).*
Savage, P.E.A. *Disasters: Hospital Planning.* Pergamon Press. (1979).
Shields, L. (1975). Crisis Intervention: implications for the Nurse. *J Psychiatr Nurs* **13**: 37.

Values, Sherrill. *Mission, Operation Peace*. Therapy for Vietnam Combat Veterans. Veteran Administration Outpatient Clinic, 5599 North Dixie Highway, Oakland Park, Florida USA 33334.

CHAPTER 25

Babra, R.J. (1975). The Potential for Suicide. *Am J Nurs* **75**: 1782.
Jourard, S. (1970). Suicide: An invitation to Die. *Am J Nurs* **70**: 269.
Perlin, *A Handbook for the Study of Suicide*. Oxford University Press.

CHAPTER 26

Publications of the Joseph P. Kennedy Foundation, 719 Thirteenth Street,Suite 510, Washington, DC 20005, N.W.
American Nurses' Association. 1973. *Standards of Nursing Practice*. Kansas City: American Nurses' Association.
American Psychiatric Association. *Quick Reference to the Diagnostic Criteria from Diagnostic and Statistical Manual of Mental Disorders. 3rd Ed. Division of Publications and Marketing (DSM III)*. American Psychiatric Association, 1700, 18th Street, N.W. Washington, D.C. USA. 20009.
Arnhons, F.N. (1975). Social Consequences of Policy towards Mental Illness. *Science* **188**: 1277.
Ayllon, T. and Michael, J. The Psychiatric Nurse as a Behavioural Engineer. *Journal of Experimental Analls Behav* **2**: 323. 1959.
Bellak, L. Hurvich, M. and Gediman H.K. (1973). *Ego Functions in Schizophrenics, Neurotics and Normals*. New York: John Wiley.
Bentovim, A. and Kinston, W. (1978) Brief focal family therapy when the child is the referred patient. *Journal of Child Psychology and Psychiatry* **19**.
Bernstein, P.L. ed. *Eight Theoretical Approaches to Dance Movement Therapy*. Iowa. Kendall Hunt (1979).
Cantela, J. Behaviour Therapy. In L. Herschel (ed). *Your Psychotherapist*. New York: Appleton Century Crofts. (1970).
Caplan, G. *Preventive Psychiatry*. Basic Books. (1963).
Carkhoff, R and Truax, C. *Toward Effective Counseling and Psychotherapy*. Chicago; Aldine. (1967).
Carmichael's *Manual of Child Psychology*, Ed Museen, P.H. Wiley (1970).
Cheetham, R.W.S. Sibisi, H. and Cheetham, R.J. (1974) psychiatric problems encountered in urban zulu adolescents. *Australia and New Zealand Journal of Psychiatry* **8**: 41.
Clayton, Barbara. *The Use of Diagnostic Biochemical Tests in Severe Mental Retardation*.
Collis, Eirene. *A Way of Life for the Handicapped Child*. Faber.
Dalton, K. *Depression after Childbirth*. Oxford University Press. (1980).
Donovan, Bonny, *The Caesarian Birth Experience*. Beacon Press. Boston. (1978).
Elliot, P. *Childbirth*. Fontana Collins.
Emery, A.E.H. *Risks for Some Common Congenital Disorders*. Livingstone.
Foster, Ruth, *Knowing in my Bones*. London. Adam and Charles Black.
Friedman, A.M. Kaplan, H.I. Sadock, B.J. *Comprehensive Textbook of Psychiatry*. Baltimore. Williams and Wilkins (1981).
Gillis, L.S. *Guidelines to Psychiatry*. David Philip. (1986).
Hackett, T. et. al. (1964). The Coronary Care Unit—an appraisal of psychological hazards. *New Eng. J. Med.* 279 (25).
Hanson, J.W. *Alcohol and the Fetus*. University of Iowa.
Hanson, J.W. Jones, K.C. and Smith, D.W. (1976). Fetal alcohol syndrome: experience with 41 patients. *Journal of American Medical Association 235*.
Higgins, J. and Peterson, J.C. (1966) Concept of Process—reactive schizophrenia—a critique. *Psychological Bulletin*, 66: 201–06.
Hilgard, Atkinson and Atkinson. *Op. Cit.*
Hutchinson, E. and Lanctot, Elizabeth. *Handbook on Physical Therapy for Cerebral Palsy*.
Jolly, H. *Book of Child Care*. Allen and Unwin, London.
Kanner, L. *Child Psychiatry*. Oxford: Blackwell Scientific Publications.
Klaus, M. and J. Kendall. *Maternal Infant Bonding*. St. Louis: Mosby. (1976).
Kneisl, C.L. & Wilson, H.S. *Current Perspectives in Psychiatric Nursing*. vol 2. St. Louis: Mosby and Co (1978).
Kritzinger, S. *The Experience of Childbirth*. Penguin.
Launer, J. (1978). Taking medical histories through interpreters: practice in a Nigerian out-patients' department. *British Medical Journal*, **2**, 934–5.
Leavitt, M. (1975). The Discharge Crisis—the experience of families of psychiatric patients. *Nurs Res* **24**: 33.
Leboyer, Frederick, *Birth Without Violence*. Collins.
Lee, D. (1969) An adjunct to training psychiatric aides in behavioural modification techniques. *Journal of Psychiatric Nursing* **7**: 169.
Lieberman, S. *Transgenerational Family Therapy*. London: Croom Helm. (1979).
Lieberman, S. Yalom, I. and Miles. *Encounter Group—First Facts*. New York: Basic books. (1973).

652 BIBLIOGRAPHY AND SUGGESTED READING

—*Loving Hands*. Collins

MacFarlane, A. *The Psychology of Childbirth*. London: Open Books.

Maher, B.A. *Principles of Psycho-therapy; an experimental approach*. NY: McGraw-Hill (1966).

Newman, H.H. Freeman, F.N. Holzinger, K.J. *Twins—a Study of Heredity and Environment*. Chicago: University Press (1937).

Ounsted and Taylor. *Gender Differences—their Ontogeny and Significance*. Churchill-Livingstone (1972).

Peplau, H. (1962). Interpersonal techniques: the crux of psychiatric nursing. *American Journal of Nursing*.

Read, Grantly-Dick, *Childbirth without Fear*.

Rogers, C.R.: *Client-Centred Therapy*, Boston, 1951. Houghton-Mifflin.

Sheahan, John, *Essential Psychiatry*. Thanet Press, Margate: Eyre and Spotti Swoorde (1973).

Skinner, B.F.: *Science and Human Behavior*. Free Press. (1953).

Spock, B. *Baby and Child Care*.

Stephens, J. Astrup, C. and Mangrum, J.C. (1967). Prognosis in Schizophrenia. *Archives of General Psychiatry* **16**: 693–8.

Stuart, G.W. and S.J. Sundeen. *Op. Cit.*

Stuart, G.W. and Sundeen, S.J. (1979) *Principles and Practice of Psychiatric Nursing*. St. Louis: Mosby.

Wechsler, D. *The Measurement of Adult Intelligence*.

Welburne, J., Purgold, J. *The Eating Stickness: Anorexia, Bulimia and the Myth of Suicide by Slimming*. Harvester Press (1984).

Wolpe, J. *The Practice of Behavior Therapy* (2 ed) New York: Pergamon Press. (1973).

Yalom, I. *Inpatient Group Psychotherapy*. New York: Basic Books.

Yalom, I. *The Theory and Practice of Group Psychiatry Op. Cit.*

Yura, H. and M.B. Walsh. *Op. Cit.*

CHAPTER 27

Fann, W.E. Goshen, C.E. *The Language of Mental Health*. St. Louis: Mosby.